HEAD TRAUMA

HEAD TRAUMA
BASIC, PRECLINICAL, AND CLINICAL DIRECTIONS

Edited by

LEONARD P. MILLER
San Diego, California

RONALD L. HAYES
University of Florida Brain Institute
  Gainesville, Florida

Co-edited by

JENNIFER K. NEWCOMB
University of Texas Health Science Center
  Houston, Texas

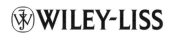

A JOHN WILEY & SONS, INC., PUBLICATION

New York / Chichester / Weinheim / Brisbane / Singapore / Toronto

For ordering and customer service, call 1-800-CALL-WILEY.

Library of Congress Cataloging-in-Publication Data:

Head trauma : basic, preclinical, and clinical directions / edited by
Leonard P. Miller, Ronald L. Hayes; co-edited by Jennifer K. Newcomb.
    p. ; cm.
Includes index.
    ISBN 0-471-36015-5 (cloth : alk. paper)
  1. Brain damage. 2. Brain damage–Molecular aspects.
    [DNLM: 1. Brain Injuries–therapy. 2. Craniocerebral
Trauma–therapy. 3. Brain Injuries–etiology. 4. Cranocerebral
Trauma–complications. WL 354 H4327 2000] I. Miller, Leonard P., 1946-
II. Hayes, Ronald L. (Ronald Lawrence) III. Newcomb, Jennifer K.
  RC387.5 .H446 2000
  617.4'81044–dc21   00-068632

Printed in the United States of America.

10 9 8 7 6 5 4 3 2 1

We would like to dedicate this book to our families:
Mary, Emily, and Brian (Dr. Miller)
and Linda, Austin, and Adrienne (Dr. Hayes)

CONTENTS

II. PRECLINICAL STUDIES

FOREWORD

Drs. Miller and Hayes have produced an important book that provides the reader a unique opportunity to quickly review advances in three major areas in head injury research. The chapter by Lenzlinger provides a very useful overview of the basic pathophysiologic mechanisms underlying the sequelae of brain injury. This is followed by a review of both in vitro and in vivo models of brain injury, a particularly important focus given our need to more thoroughly test treatments in well controlled experimental paradigms.

The second section of the book is devoted to a detailed exploration of a number of potential mechanisms of secondary brain damage. These chapters, written by leaders in their fields provide a very comprehensive review of the basic biological mechanisms felt to be important in the progression of brain damage following injury. Particularly impressive are the chapters on ionic alterations and their relationship to metabolic dysfunction following brain injury, and the review of the role of calpains and caspases in producing cell death, as well as the detailed review by Povlishock and Stone on traumatic axonal injury. Axonal injury has been somewhat neglected in head injury research because of the mistaken belief that such damage is irreversible. The demonstration from this laboratory that axonal injury is potentially reversible is very important and is particularly timely given those observations.

The third and final section of the book deals with clinical issues in traumatic head injury. Particularly noteworthy are two chapters on clinical trials in head injury in the United States and in Europe. The third section also contains a detailed description of guidelines for medical surgical management in head injured patients. Such guidelines have recently been promulgated in both Europe and the United States and serve as useful series of buoys in the water to guide neurosurgeons and intensivists in the care of these patients. As advances from the basic research described in section two of this book become available these guidelines are likely to change, but they are extremely useful in providing a template upon which clinical care can go forward.

Lawrence F. Marshall, M.D.
Professor of Surgery and Chief,
Division of Neurosurgery,
U.C.S.D. School of Medicine,
La Jolla, CA

PREFACE

The conceptual framework for this book is derived from an attempt on the part of the editors to present the readers with a collection of important works covering head trauma therapeutics along the bench-to-bedside continuum. To accomplish this goal we selected topics ranging from basic research studies to the identification of compounds presently under investigation in clinical trials. Readers of this book will already be familiar to varying extents with some topics addressed in the various chapters. However, we felt it necessary to provide readers with a book that covered as much information as possible over three major areas of head trauma research. In this regard, authors were solicited who possessed expertise in specific areas of research such as preclinical models, investigations of specific drugs with defined mechanisms of action, and application of drugs in clinical trials.

In addition to providing readers with a broad presentation of the head trauma landscape, we also felt that the contents of this book will allow readers to gain an appreciation of the difficulties associated with efforts at all levels of research related to head trauma therapeutics. These various levels include identification of basic mechanisms underlying the neuropathological consequences of head trauma and extension of these results to man as a means of justifying therapeutic application of new investigatory drugs.

We have attempted to present a book containing numerous topics designed to spark the interest of readers ranging in disciplines from basic researchers to clinicians. This task was greatly facilitated by the contributions of numerous world-renowned authors who have pioneered investigations into their respective areas of expertise. Thus, we act merely as facilitators in this process and ascribe credit for any success of this book to all the contributing authors. Unfortunately, however, as in most endeavors of this kind, some topics and works by other investigators are not presented in the breadth and depth they merit. This shortcoming on our part is merely a practical consequence of page limitation. To assist the reader, at the end of each chapter there is a list of abbreviations used throughout the text.

This book is divided into three major areas of head trauma research. These areas are Basic, Preclinical and Clinical Directions of head trauma. In the basic section, the first chapter is devoted to an integrated overview of basic mechanisms identified to date that underlie the pathological consequences of head trauma. Subsequent chapters in this section cover both in vitro and in vivo preclinical models that are utilized to assess mechanisms of damage along with the potential of drugs to ameliorate brain damage associated with head trauma.

The second main section of this book, Preclinical Directions, is devoted to an in depth presentation of various processes associated with the neuropathological consequences of head trauma and specific pharmacological approaches testing potential for efficacy. In these chapters the authors review evidence supporting the involvement of various processes at the cellular level in head trauma-related damage. In addition, some chapters outline specific drug development efforts targeted at identifying pharmacophores for intervention at specific steps in the neuropathological cascade. Within this section we have attempted to progress the topics of the individual chapters from actions at cell surface receptors (and channels) such as acetylcholine, glutamate, adenosine, etc. to intracellular events such as proteases, DNA changes, etc. Other topics of related importance, such as vascular events and traumatic axonal injury, which are outside of this general theme, are also presented.

The third section of the book, Clinical Directions, is devoted to presenting not only aspects of clinical trials in head trauma, but also past and present clinical efforts to identify the effectiveness of compounds in humans that had shown efficacy in preclinical animal models. Furthermore, we have attempted to overview clinical trials conducted around the world by having three separate chapters covering the U.S., Europe, and Asia. Also included are chapters that focus on the epidemiology and neuropsychological consequences of head trauma. In addition, of great importance to all clinicians involved in the field, is a chapter that presents a detailed description of guidelines for medical surgical management in head injured patients.

As a new addition, we have included an appendix section that contains a list of WEB sites, hopefully of interest to most investigators involved in neurotrauma research. These sites were compiled with the grateful assistance of numerous authors within this book. In this appendix section we have also included the e-mail addresses of most of the contributors to this book to facilitate ease of contact with them should readers so desire.

Leonard P. Miller
Ronald L. Hayes

CONTRIBUTORS

SHARON A. BROWN, Ph.D., Department of Physical Medicine and Rehabilitation, Scurlock Tower, Room 1144, Baylor College of Medicine, Houston, TX 77030-3405

TIMOTHY M. CARLOS, M.D., Department of Medicine, University of Pittsburgh, 3434 Fifth Avenue, Pittsburgh, PA 15260

ROBERT S. B. CLARK, M.D., Department of Anasthesiology and Critical Care Medicine, University of Pittsburgh, 3434 Fifth Avenue, Pittsburgh, PA 15260

DOMINICO D'AVELLA, M.D., Department of Neurosciences, Neurosurgical Clinic, University of Mersina Medical School, Italy

S. M. DEFORD, M.D., Department of Neuroscience, University of Florida Brain Institute, Center for Traumatic Brain Injury Studies, 100 Newell Road, Box 100244, Gainesville, FL 32610-0244

STEVEN T. DEKOSKY, M.D., Department of Psychiatry and Neurology, University of Pitttsburgh, 3434 Fifth Avenue, Pittsburgh, PA 15260

EDWARD DIXON, Ph.D., Department of Neurological Surgery, University of Pittsburgh, 3434 Fith Avenue, Pittsburgh, PA 15260

ALAN I. FADEN, M.D., Departments of Neuroscience and Neurology, Institute of Cognitive and Computational Science, Georgetown University Medical Center, Washington, D.C. 20007

SETH P. FINKLESTEIN, M.D., C.S.N. Growth Factor Laboratory, Department of Neurology, Massachusetts General Hospital, Warren 408, Boston, Massachusetts

CHRISTOPHER C. GIZA, M.D., Neurotrauma Laboratory, Division of Neurosurgery, UCLA School of Medicine, Los Angeles, CA 90095

RONALD L. HAYES, Ph.D., Department of Neuroscience, University of Florida Brain Institute, Center for Traumatic Brain Injury Studies, 100 Newell Road, Box 100244 Gainesville, FL 32610-0244

DAVID A. HOVDA, Ph.D., Neurotrauma Laboratory, Division of Neurosurgery, UCLA School of Medicine, Los Angeles, CA 90095

YOICHI KATAYAMA, M.D., Ph.D., Department of Neurological Surgery, Nihon University School of Medicine, Ohyaguchi Kami-Machi 30-1, Itabashi-Ku, Tokyo, Japan

ANTHONY E. KLINE, Ph.D., Brain Trauma Research Center, Department of Neurosurgery, University of Pittsburgh, 3434 Fifth Avenue, Pittsburgh, PA 15260

PATRICK KOCHANEK, M.D., Departments of Anesthesiology and Critical Care Medicine, University of Pittsburgh, 3434 Fifth Avenue, Pittsburgh, PA 15260

C. P. LEE, Ph.D., Department of Biochemistry and Molecular Biology, School of Medicine, Wayne State University, Detroit, MI 48201

PHILIPP M. LENZLINGER, M.D., Head Injury Center, Department of Neurosurgery, University of Pennsylvania and Veterans Administration Medical Center, 105 Hayden Hall, 3320 Smith Walk, Philadelphia, PA 19104-6316

HARVEY S. LEVIN, Ph.D., Department of Physical Medicine and Rehabilitation, Baylor College of Medicine, Houston, Texas

BRUCE LYETH, Ph.D., Department of Neurological Surgery, University of California at Davis, 1515 Newton Court, One Shields Avenue, Davis, CA 95616

A. I. R. MAAS, M.D., Department of Neurosurgery, Academic Hospital of Rotterdam, Molewaterplein 40, 3015 GD Rotterdam, The Netherlands

SADAHIRO MAEJIMA, M.D., Ph.D., Department of Neurological Surgery, Nihon University School of Medicine, Ohyaguchi Kami-Machi 30-1, Itabashi-Ku, Tokyo, Japan

DONALD W. MARION, M.D., Department of Neurological Surgery, University of Pittsburgh, 3434 Fifth Avenue, Pittsburgh, PA 15260

ANTHONY MARMAROU, Ph.D., Division of Neurosurgery, Medical College of Virginia, Virginia Commonwealth University, P.P. Box 980 508, Richmond, VA 23298-0508

TRACY K. MCINTOSH, Ph.D., Head Injury Center, Department of Neurosurgery, University of Pennsylvania and Veterans Administration Medical Center, 105 Hayden Hall, 3320 Smith Walk, Philadelphia, PA 19104-6316

LEONARD P. MILLER, Ph.D., San Diego, California

AMY H. MOORE, Ph.D., Neurotrauma Laboratory, Division of Neurosurgery, UCLA School of Medicine, Los Angeles, CA 90095

J. PAUL MUIZELAAR, Ph.D., Department of Neurological Surgery, University of California, Davis, 4860 Y Street, Suite #3740, Sacramento, CA 95817

JENNIFER K. NEWCOMB, Ph.D., Deparment of Neurosurgery, Vivian L. Smith Center for Neurological Research, University of Texas, Houston Health Science Center, Houston, TX 77030

DEIRDRE M. O'LEARY, Ph.D., Departments of Neuroscience and Neurosurgery, Institute of Cognitive and Computational Science, Georgetown University Medical Center, Washington D.C. 20007

P. L. PETERSON, M.D., Department of Neurology, School of Medicine, Wayne State University, Detroit, MI 48201

BRIAN R. PIKE, Ph.D., E. F. and W. L. McKnight Brain Institute of the University of Florida, Center for Traumatic Brain Injury Studies, Department of Neuroscience, Gainesville, Florida

ANDRAIKI PLOMARITOGLOU, M.D., Department of Neurology, Massachusetts General Hospital, Warren 408, Boston, MA 02114

JOHN T. POVLISHOCK, Ph.D., Department of Anatomy, Medical College of Virginia, Campus of Virginia Commonwealth University, Richmond, VA 232 98-0709

RAMESH RAGHUPATHI, Ph.D., Department of Neurosurgery, University of Pennsylvania, School of Medicine, Hayden Hall, 3320 Smith Walk, Philadelphia, PA 19104-6316

KATHRYN E. SAATMAN, Ph.D., Head Injury Center, Department of Neurosurgery, University of Pennsylvania and Veterans Administration Medical Center, 105 Hayden Hall, 3320 Smith Walk, Philadelphia, PA 19104-6316

AMIR SAMII, M.D., Department of Neurosurgery, Norstaelt Medical Center, Haltezhoffstraße 41, 30167 Hannover, Germany

JAMES R. STONE, Ph.D., Department of Anatomy, Medical College of Virginia, Campus of Virginia Commonwealth University, Richmond, VA 23298-0709

MEREDITH D. TEMPLE, Ph.D., Departments of Neuroscience and Neurosurgery, Institute of Cognitive and Computational Science, Georgetown University Medical Center, Washington D.C. 20007

DAVID J. THURMAN, M.D., M.P.H., Rehabilitation Research and Disability Prevention, National Center for Injury Prevention and Control, 4770 Buford Highway NE, Atlanta, GA 30341-3742

GIASTINO TOMEI, M.D., Institute of Neurosurgery, Ospedale Maggiore Polichinico, IRCCS, Milano, Italy

Y. XIONG, M.D., Ph.D., Department of Biochemistry and Molecular Biology, School of Medicine, Wayne State University, Detroit, MI 48201

MARIKE ZWIENENBERG, M.D., Department of Neurological Surgery, University of California, Davis, Sacramento, CA 95817

PART I

BASIC SCIENCE: OVERVIEW

CHAPTER 1

OVERVIEW OF BASIC MECHANISMS UNDERLYING NEUROPATHOLOGICAL CONSEQUENCES OF HEAD TRAUMA

PHILIPP M. LENZLINGER M.D., KATHRYN E. SAATMAN Ph.D., RAMESH RAGHUPATHI Ph.D., and TRACY K. MCINTOSH Ph.D.
Department of Neurosurgery, University of Pennsylvania School of Medicine and Veterans Administration Medical Center, Philadelphia, Pennsylvania

INTRODUCTION AND EPIDEMIOLOGY

Traumatic brain injury (TBI) remains one of the leading causes of injury-related deaths in the Western hemisphere, accounting for 26 percent of all trauma-associated deaths in the United States (between 17 and 25 per 100,000 residents) (Sosin et al., 1989, 1995). Of the 1.5 to 2 million people who sustain TBI in the United States each year, approximately 70,000 to 90,000 will suffer from long-term disability with dramatic impacts on the lives of the individuals and their families and enormous socioeconomic costs. Young men between the ages of 15 and 24 years are affected most commonly, and children below the age of 5 and the elderly above 65 years of age are also at increased risk (Kraus, 1993). According to the most recent statistics from the National Institutes of Health (NIH), the major causes of TBI are vehicular accidents, falls, acts of violence, and sports injuries (NIH Consensus Development Panel on Rehabilitation of Persons with Traumatic Brain Injury, 1999). While motor vehicle-related brain injuries have apparently been on a steady decline since the beginning of the 1980s, firearm-induced brain injuries have increased sharply, somewhat masking the benefit of increased preventive efforts in traffic-related brain injury in the overall statistics (Sosin et al., 1995).

Traumatic brain damage is a result of direct (immediate mechanical disruption of brain tissue, or primary injury) and indirect (delayed or secondary) mechanisms. The primary injury can be influenced largely through preventive measures, such as

Head Trauma: Basic, Preclinical, and Clinical Directions, Edited by Leonard P. Miller and Ronald L. Hayes, Co-edited by Jennifer K. Newcomb
ISBN 0-471-36015-5 © 2001 John Wiley & Sons, Inc.

education of potential victims, use of safety equipment (airbags, helmets), and enforcement of laws enhancing individual and public safety. For example, increased use of helmets has significantly reduced the frequency and severity of bicycle-related head injuries (Benz et al., 1993; Rivara et al., 1994; Thompson et al., 1997). In contrast, secondary injuries, because of their delayed onset and progression over minutes to months after the initial trauma, are potentially amenable to postinjury therapeutic intervention. Despite an ever-expanding knowledge of the pathophysiological mechanisms involved in secondary brain injury, an effective treatment strategy has yet to be developed. Moreover, given the complex nature of the neurochemical cascade initiated after head injury, it appears unlikely that a single type of intervention at one time point within this multifactorial pathway will efficiently attenuate secondary injuries. In this introductory chapter, we give an overview of the current understanding of these mechanisms and highlight similarities with other neuropathological conditions. All of the topics will be further addressed in greater detail and length in the subsequent chapters of this textbook.

CURRENT UNDERSTANDING OF MOLECULAR MECHANISMS OF TBI PATHOPHYSIOLOGY

Excitatory Amino Acid Receptors

Excitatory amino acids (EAAs) and their receptors have been the focus of TBI research for over a decade. The release of EAA neurotransmitters glutamate and aspartate leads to the activation of specific receptors coupled to a sodium/calcium ionophore, causing an influx of these cations to the cytosol. Elevated extracellular levels of glutamate have been observed after experimental TBI (Faden et al., 1989; Globus et al., 1995; Katayama et al., 1990; Nilsson et al., 1990; Palmer et al., 1993) as well as in the cerebrospinal fluid (CSF) (Stover et al., 1999) or the extracellular compartment of the cortical brain tissue of head-injured patients (Brown et al., 1998; Bullock et al., 1998; Vespa et al., 1998). Cell death associated with the release of EAA has been suggested to be a staged process with acute and delayed components. The acute influx of sodium and chloride leads to neuronal swelling, the early hallmark of excitotoxicity. The second component, marked by gradual neuronal damage and delayed cell death, is dependent on calcium influx (Choi, 1987). The N-methyl-D-aspartate (NMDA) receptor contains multiple sites, which are accessible to potential antagonistic compounds. Besides competitive blockade of the glutamate-binding site, this receptor complex may be modulated either by blocking the channel itself, or by interaction of compounds at different secondary binding sites such as those for magnesium, glycine, or polyamines.

Both competitive and noncompetitive NMDA antagonists as well as non-NMDA antagonists have been shown to be efficacious in the treatment of experimental TBI (Bullock and Fujisawa, 1992; Okiyama et al., 1998). In an in vitro model of mechanical shearing injury, blockage of the NMDA receptor with the noncompetitive NMDA receptor blocker dizocilipine maleate (MK-801) reduced the intracellular calcium increase associated with cell death in this model by almost half

(LaPlaca and Thibault, 1998). In rats, preinjury administration of MK-801 improved postinjury neurologic function significantly (McIntosh et al., 1989a), while postinjury administration has been shown to attenuate neurochemical sequelae and edema formation (McIntosh et al., 1990; Shapira et al., 1990). Several presynaptic glutamate release inhibitors, which also block sodium channels, have been investigated in experimental TBI. The compound BW1003C87 significantly reduced focal brain edema in the injured cortex and hippocampus, when given after lateral fluid percussion (FP) injury in rats (Okiyama et al., 1995), while BW619C89 administered 15 min before FP injury significantly attenuated behavioral deficits at 24 h and 1 week and protected neurons in the CA1 and CA3 regions of the hippocampus at 2 weeks postinjury (Sun and Faden, 1995). Another drug in this class, riluzole, has been shown to reduce brain lesion size and attenuate neurologic impairment after experimental TBI in rats when given in repetitive doses after brain injury (McIntosh et al., 1996; Wahl et al., 1997; Zhang et al., 1998). The magnesium ion functions as an essential endogenous modulator of the NMDA receptor, but its role in bioenergetic and cellular metabolic and genomic activity must be considered when evaluating the importance of this ion in brain trauma. Besides influencing NMDA-mediated neurotransmission, the loss of intracellular magnesium following experimental brain injury (Vink et al., 1987, 1988, 1997) may have profound effects on posttraumatic repair mechanisms, including protein, RNA, and DNA synthesis. Both pre- and postinjury treatments with magnesium salts ($MgCl_2$ or $MgSO_4$) have been shown to improve neurologic motor and cognitive function and decrease regional cerebral edema formation (Bareyre et al., 1999a; Heath and Vink, 1998; McIntosh et al., 1988, 1989b; Okiyama et al., 1995; Smith et al., 1993). The efficacy of magnesium in experimental trauma models, coupled with its existing clinical use in obstetrics and cardiology, makes this ion an attractive compound for the treatment of clinical brain injury, and single-center clinical trials have been initiated. The clinical use of EAA receptor blockers in TBI, however, has shown rather discouraging results (Morris et al., 1999), and unfavorable side effect profiles, namely, psychotropic actions, of many of these substances further complicate their clinical application (Choi, 1995).

Cholinergic Receptors

The hippocampus receives cholinergic innervation from cell bodies located in the basal forebrain. Lateral FP injury has been shown to cause structural damage to the basal forebrain septohippocampal pathway, which terminates in specific hippocampal regions (Leonard et al., 1997). Schmidt and Grady (1995) have related the loss of forebrain cholinergic neurons following lateral FP brain injury to cognitive dysfunction associated with closed head injury.

Recent research supports a theory of an injury-induced change from cholinergic hyperfunction in the acute posttraumatic period to a hypofunctional cholinergic state that develops much later after injury (Dixon et al., 1995a, b; Hamm et al., 1993; Pike and Hamm, 1995; Saija et al., 1998a, b). Immunohistochemical staining for basal forebrain choline acetyltransferase (ChAT)-positive neurons has been shown to be significantly reduced following central (Schmidt and Grady, 1995) and lateral FP injury in the rat (Gorman et al., 1996; Leonard et al., 1994; Sinson et al., 1996). Dixon et al. (1994) have shown that hippocampal high-affinity choline uptake is reduced following cortical impact brain injury, suggestive of a decreased ability of cholinergic neurons to take up choline. Studies employing postmortem human tissue have validated and extended these observations by reporting a depletion of ChAT activity but preservation of M1 and M2 muscarine receptor binding sites in the temporal cortex following severe clinical head injury (Dewar and Graham, 1996).

Earlier studies employed anticholinergics, based on the hypothesis that some components of neurologic disturbances following TBI were attributable to increased functional activity of cholinergic systems within specific brain regions (Hayes et al., 1986; Katayama et al., 1984). Administration of the anticholinergic scopolamine was observed to effectively attenuate both the transient (Lyeth et al., 1988a) and long-term motor deficits observed following experimental brain injury in the rat (Lyeth et al., 1988b). Scopolamine administration has also recently been shown to attenuate beam balance (motor) deficits in rats subjected to a combined injury of midline FP injury with entorhinal cortical lesion (Phillips et al., 1997). Furthermore, scopolamine administration has been shown to block both the spontaneous recovery of decreased cerebral blood flow (CBF) in the ipsilateral (injured) hemisphere and the hyperemic increase in CBF in the contralateral hemisphere observed following weight drop brain injury in the rat (Scremin et al., 1997).

In contrast to anticholinergic therapy, which appears to improve neurologic motor deficits and alter posttraumatic cerebrovascular response, cholinergic agonists have recently been evaluated for their effects in experimental brain injury, based upon observations that cognitive deficits commonly observed in the posttraumatic recovery period may be temporally related to neuronal cholinergic hypofunction. To this end, daily postinjury administration of BIBN 99, a selective presynaptic antagonist of the M2 muscarinic cholinergic autoreceptor, or LU 25-109-T, a partial M1 muscarinic cholinergic receptor (mAChR) agonist with associated M2 antagonist effects, has been demonstrated to improve cognitive function following midline FP brain injury in the rat (Hamm et al., 1993; Pike and Hamm, 1995). Another recent strategy has focused on the use of compounds that are hydrolyzed or metabolized to form choline, the precursor of ACh. Dixon et al. (1997a) have shown that administration of CDP-choline can reduce cognitive deficits following TBI. Taken together, the above data suggests that, following brain trauma, treatment with anticholinergic agents may restore reflexive and motor function in the acute posttraumatic period while cholinomimetic therapy may improve cognitive dysfunction. Since these strategies are diametrically opposed with respect to their pharmacological effects, the timing of therapy with these agents will be critical.

Free Radicals

Free radicals are highly reactive molecules that cause an almost instantaneous peroxidation of neuronal, glial, and vascular membrane phospholipids as well as the oxidation of cellular proteins and nucleic acids, thereby contributing to widespread cellular and vascular damage. Potential sources of oxygen radicals within the traumatically injured brain include the arachidonic acid cascade, the xanthine oxidase pathway, activated white blood cells, catecholamine oxidation, and mitochondrial leakage (Hall et al., 1992; Traystman et al., 1991). Their formation has been reported in various models of experimental brain injury (Ellis et al., 1991; Hall et al., 1993; Inci et al., 1998; Kontos and Povlishock, 1986; Lewen and Hillered, 1998; Petty et al., 1996). Althaus and colleagues (1993) demonstrated that the formation of hydroxyl radicals within minutes of moderately severe concussive head injury in mice could be attenuated by the administration of the 21-aminosteroid tirilazad mesylate. The same group showed that the observed breakdown of the blood–brain barrier (BBB) after controlled cortical impact (CCI) injury in the rat is related to the formation of hydroxyl radicals and can be attenuated by antioxidant therapy (Smith et al., 1994). Alpha-tocopherol and its analog MDL 74,180 have been shown to be protective against radical-mediated lipid peroxidation and edema formation after experimental TBI (Inci et al., 1998; Petty et al., 1996). Among the drugs that have been evaluated for their ability to protect the brain against the onslaught of free oxygen radicals are superoxide dismutase (SOD) and its polyethylene glycol-conjugate (PEG-SOD, or pegorgotein), which has a longer biological half-life. PEG-SOD has been shown to improve cortical blood flow and to reduce posttraumatic motor dysfunction after lateral FP injury in rats (Hamm et al., 1996; Muir et al., 1995). However, a large multicenter study with more than 450 patients did not show a significantly improved outcome in patients who received PEG-SOD compared to those who received placebo (Young et al., 1996).

Adenosine

Adenosine, which in its phosphorylated forms is ubiquitous as a nucleoside in DNA and as an intracellular second messenger, is now widely accepted as a major inhibitory neuromodulator in the central nervous system (CNS) and an endogenous neuroprotective metabolite. In situations of metabolic stress, for example, ischemia, adenosine decreases energy demand and increases energy supply. Of particular relevance in the context of TBI is the ability of adenosine to modulate glutamate release (Deckert and Gleiter, 1994). Adenosine is released from neurons into the extracellular fluid, where it markedly inhibits the release of excitatory neurotransmitters and has direct inhibitory effects on postsynaptic excitability. Adenosine also modulates neuronal sensitivity to acetylcholine and catecholamines (Higgins et al., 1994). Within the CNS the A2A and A3 receptor subtypes are most prevalent (Fredholm and Altiok, 1994; Miller, 1999). Adenosine is believed to originate from ATP breakdown in ischemic tissue and to exert its neuroprotective role through a concurrent reduction in cerebral metabolic rate and an increase in cerebral blood flow, in addition to its antiexcitotoxic effects (Bell et al., 1998; Deckert and Gleiter, 1994; Kochanek et al., 1997). In experimental TBI, extracellular adenosine was found to be elevated within 10 minutes after trauma, and reverted to preinjury levels by 1 h, while metabolic disturbances as measured by mitochondrial capacity for oxidative phosphorylation were prolonged and maximal at 2 to 3 h postinjury

(Headrick et al., 1994). Intracerebroventricular (ICV) injections of 2-chloroadenosine prior to TBI dose-dependently attenuated metabolic disturbances and significantly improved posttraumatic neurologic outcome in that study.

Growth Factors

The peptide neurotrophic or growth factors, including nerve growth factor (NGF), basic fibroblast growth factor (bFGF), ciliary neurotrophic factor (CNTF), brain-derived neurotrophic factor (BDNF), insulin-like growth factor 1 (IGF-1), and neurotrophin-3 (NT-3) all function in the developing and normal adult brain to support neuronal survival, induce sprouting of neurites (neuronal plasticity), and facilitate the guidance of neurons to their proper target sites. Alterations in neurotrophic factors following brain injury may occur in a response designed to facilitate neuronal repair and reestablish functional connections in the healing brain (Varon et al., 1991). Recent studies have reported a marked increase in NGF mRNA and NGF protein in the acute posttraumatic period following experimental brain injury in rats (DeKosky et al., 1994; Goss et al., 1998), although a significant reduction in p75 NGFR (NGF receptor) has been observed in the chronic postinjury period (Leonard et al., 1994). Basic FGF concentrations in brain tissue have also been observed to be elevated following brain trauma (Eckenstein et al., 1991; Gomez-Pinilla et al., 1992; Logan and Berry, 1993; Logan et al., 1992), and CSF concentrations of both NGF and bFGF have been reported to increase following human head injury as well (Longo et al., 1984; Patterson et al., 1993). More recently, hippocampal expression of mRNA for BDNF was reported to increase with a concomitant decrease in mRNA for NT-3 (Hicks et al., 1997a). Walter et al. (1997) demonstrated that penetrating brain injury induces regionally distinct upregulation in gene and protein expression for IGF-1, IGF-binding proteins, and IGF receptors, suggesting that IGF-1 acts in an autocrine/paracrine manner to regulate cell responses.

As a pharmacotherapeutic strategy, posttraumatic administration of neurotrophic factors has been shown to be efficacious in models of TBI. Several laboratories report that intraparenchymal administration of NGF can attenuate cognitive but not neurobehavioral motor deficits or hippocampal cell loss following FP brain injury (Sinson et al., 1995, 1996) and CCI brain injury in rats (Dixon et al., 1997b). Other studies demonstrate that central NGF administration can reduce the extent of apoptotic cell death in septal cholinergic neurons following experimental brain trauma (Sinson et al., 1997) and can reverse the trauma-induced reductions in scopolamine-evoked ACh release (Dixon et al., 1997b).

Dietrich et al. (1996) reported that acute administration of bFGF could attenuate cortical cell loss following lateral FP brain injury in rats, while McDermott and co-workers (1997), using the same model, demonstrated that delayed intraparenchymal administration of bFGF, beginning 24 h after injury, can significantly improve posttraumatic cognitive deficits in the rat. Intracerebroventricular administration of IGF-1 has been reported to reduce neuronal loss in vulnerable areas following hypoxic-ischemic injury, via mechanisms found to be independent of systemic glucose concentrations or brain temperature (Gluckman et al., 1992; Guan et al.,

1993, 1996), and to attenuate hippocampal cell loss following transient forebrain ischemia in rats (Zhu and Auer, 1994). Saatman et al. (1997) have reported that continuous subcutaneous administration of IGF-1 for 7 days accelerated neurologic motor recovery and attenuated cognitive deficits following lateral FP brain injury in rats.

Inflammatory Events

Increased evidence points to the potentially deleterious—and paradoxically bene-ficial—role of posttraumatic inflammation in CNS injury. Infiltration and accumula-tion of polymorphonuclear leukocytes (PMNs) into brain parenchyma have been documented to occur in the acute posttraumatic period, reaching maximal accumula-tion by 24 h post injury (Soares et al., 1995). Zhuang et al. (1993) have suggested a relationship between cortical PMN accumulation and secondary brain injury, including lowered CBF, increased edema, and elevated intracranial pressure (ICP). The entry of macrophages into brain parenchyma following brain injury has been shown to be maximal by 24 to 48 h following lateral FP brain injury in rats and after human TBI (Holmin et al., 1995, 1998; Soares et al., 1995).

The specific cytokines that have been implicated in posttraumatic neuropatholo-gical damage include tumor necrosis factor (TNF) and the interleukin (IL) family of peptides (see below) (Hans et al., 1999a; Morganti-Kossmann et al., 1997; Ott et al., 1994; Rothwell and Hopkins, 1995). Alterations in circulating and CSF concentra-tions of cytokines such as IL-1, IL-6, IL-8, IL-10, IL-12, and TNF-α have been reported to occur in human patients following severe head injury (Cohen et al., 1991; Csuka et al., 1999; Goodman et al., 1990; Kossmann et al., 1995, 1997a; McClain et al., 1987; Morganti-Kossmann et al., 1997; Ott et al., 1994; Young et al., 1988), and regional mRNA and protein concentrations of these cytokines have been shown to increase markedly in the acute posttraumatic period following experimental brain trauma in the rat (Fan et al., 1995, 1996; Hans et al., 1999b; Knoblach et al., 1999; Shohami et al., 1994; Taupin et al., 1993; Woodroofe et al., 1991). The increase in IL-1α, IL-1β, and TNF-α following stab wound injury to the rat brain has been related to trauma-induced astrogliosis (Rostworowski et al., 1997). Upregulation of gene (mRNA) expression for both IL-1β and TNF has been reported as early as 1 to 2 h following lateral FP brain injury in the rat (Fan et al., 1995, 1996), suggesting that these cytokines may play a role in the pathophysiological sequelae of brain trauma. IL-6 mRNA has been shown to be upregulated in a weight drop model of TBI in rats in infiltrating macrophages as well as in cortical and thalamic neurons as early as 1 h post injury, while IL-6 immunoreactivity and protein levels in rat CSF peaked within the first 24 h after the trauma (Hans et al., 1999b). Even though the presence of these mediators is generally believed to be deleterious for the injured brain, recent studies point toward a beneficial role of certain cytokines following TBI. For example, work with transgenic brain-injured mice deficient in TNF (TNF$-/-$) shows that while the neurologic motor scores of these animals were initially better than those of brain-injured wild-type (WT) controls in the acute posttraumatic period, the trend was reversed from 7 to 28 days post injury (Scherbel et al., 1999), suggesting a differential action depending on the time point of its release. Mice deficient in both subtypes of TNF receptors were shown to be more vulnerable to TBI than wild-type animals, further indicating a neuroprotective role for TNF-α in the pathological sequelae of head injury (Sullivan et al., 1999).

There is increasing evidence that the complement system plays an important role in tissue damage associated with brain trauma (Mollnes and Fosse, 1994; Stahel et al., 1998), and upregulation of complement factor C5a mRNA has been shown in infiltrating blood leukocytes as well as in cerebellar and cortical neurons after weight drop experimental TBI in rats (Stahel et al., 1997). Complement factors C3 and B, two central components of the alternative activation pathway, have been found to be significantly elevated after severe TBI in humans as compared to control subjects (Kossmann et al., 1997b).

The migration of leukocytes into damaged tissue typically requires the adhesion of these cells to the endothelium and therefore the expression of the intercellular adhesion molecule ICAM-1, a member of the immunoglobulin supergene family. An upregulation of ICAM-1 has been described in a variety of experimental TBI models (Carlos et al., 1997; Isaksson et al., 1997; Shibayama et al., 1996), and in humans soluble ICAM-1 (sICAM-1) in CSF has been associated with the breakdown of the BBB after severe isolated TBI (Pleines et al., 1998).

Only recently has research concerning the possible beneficial effects of cytokine blockade or anti-inflammatory compounds been initiated. The soluble human recombinant complement (sCR-1) receptor BRL-55730 has been used with success to inhibit PMN accumulation and improve neurobehavioral recovery following controlled cortical impact (CCI) injury in the rat (Kaczorowski et al., 1995). Posttraumatic ICV administration of IL-1 receptor antagonist (IL-1ra), which competitively binds to the IL-1 receptor and inhibits its physiological function, has been shown to reduce the extent of neuronal death in cortex and hippocampus and to improve cognitive function following lateral FP brain injury in the rat (Sanderson et al., 1999; Toulmond and Rothwell, 1995). DeKosky et al. (1996) have shown that implantation of fibroblasts transfected with a retroviral vector containing the human IL-1ra gene can significantly reduce microglial proliferation and NGF upregulation induced by weight drop injury. Inhibition of TNF-α activity in rat brain has been shown to significantly reduce edema and to improve motor function following weight drop brain injury (Shohami et al., 1996), while antibodies against MAC-1, the leukocyte counterreceptor of ICAM-1, have shown promising effects in reducing the accumulation of PMNs after cortical impact injury in rats (Clark et al., 1996).

Ion Channels

Among the agents involved in the neurochemical "maelstrom" that occurs following TBI, the calcium ion (Ca^{2+}) has probably drawn the most attention. This ion has been implicated in regional cerebral edema, vasospasm, and acute as well as delayed cell death following injury to the CNS (Goldberg and Choi, 1993; McIntosh et al., 1997; Shapira et al., 1989; Siesjo and Bengtsson, 1989). Sustained intracellular elevations of Ca^{2+} are toxic, which is not surprising in the face of the many biological processes regulated by Ca^{2+} availability. The specific events triggered by an excess of intracellular Ca^{2+} include activation of proteases and lipases, the generation of free radicals, depletion of energy reserves through the activation of Ca^{2+}-ATPase, and impairment of mitochondrial oxidative phosphorylation (Cheung et al., 1986). Anoxic injury of gray matter appears to be associated with potassium-induced release of EAA, such as glutamate (see above), leading to the opening of glutamate-associated ion channels (NMDA receptors), resulting in a pathological influx of Ca^{2+} (Choi, 1988; Rothman and Olney, 1987). Depolarization of cell membranes leads to entry of Ca^{2+} through voltage-gated Ca^{2+} channels (Tsien et al., 1988), and in white matter, in conjunction with a reduction of the transmembrane sodium (Na^+) gradient, results in the reversal of the Na^+/Ca^{2+} exchanger (Nachshen et al., 1986; Stys et al., 1992). Other mechanisms suggested to further elevate cytosolic $[Ca^{2+}]$ are direct transmembrane entry through leaks caused by cell swelling and intracellular mobilization of Ca^{2+} from intracellular organelles, including the endoplasmic reticulum (Choi, 1988). Significantly increased calcium concentrations have been observed in injured tissue (Fineman et al., 1993; Shapira et al., 1989), and in areas with marked morphological damage this Ca^{2+} overload can persist for a prolonged period of time (Nilsson et al., 1993, 1996).

Despite the pivotal role of Ca^{2+} in the pathophysiology of brain injury (see above and below), the use of calcium channel blockers in clinical head injury has not lived up to expectation. Only a subgroup of severely brain-injured patients with traumatic subarachnoid hemorrhage and concomitant vasospasm has been observed to benefit from the administration of these drugs, conceivably due to their hypotensive side effects, which may mask their potential neuroprotective action (Bailey et al., 1991; Langham et al., 1999; Teasdale et al., 1992). Furthermore, an uncontrolled reduction of intracellular Ca^{2+} may also have deleterious effects (Choi, 1995), since $[Ca^{2+}]_i$ has been shown to significantly influence the positive effect of NGF on sympathetic neurons (Koike et al., 1989).

Proteolytic Mechanisms of Cell Death

Calcium also plays an important role in activation of intracellular proteases. The nonlysosomal cysteine proteases calpains are irreversibly activated by elevated intracellular $[Ca^{2+}]$. Calpains proteolyze a wide range of cytoskeletal proteins such as spectrin, tubulin, microtubule-associated proteins (MAPs), and neurofilamental proteins (McIntosh et al., 1998) and are involved in the degradation of other enzymes (kinases, phosphatases) and membrane associated proteins, including ion channels, EAA receptors, and adhesion molecules (Takahashi, 1990). The major isoenzymes found in the CNS are μ-calpain and m-calpain. While the former has a sensitivity to intracellular calcium in the micromolar range and is located primarily in the neuronal cell body and dendrites and only to a lesser degree in axons and glia, the latter is activated by a thousandfold higher calcium levels and is found in glia and in low concentrations in axons (Kampfl et al., 1997). The prolonged and unregulated activation of calpains produces irreversible structural damage and functional alterations that have been implicated in neuronal toxicity (Bartus, 1997). Activated μ-calpain has been demonstrated as early as 15 minutes after CCI injury in the ipsilateral hemisphere (Kampfl et al., 1996). Calpain-mediated spectrin breakdown has been observed in several models of experimental TBI (Buki et al., 1999a; Kampfl et al., 1996; Newcomb et al., 1997; Saatman et al., 1996a). Saatman and colleagues (1996a) have observed calpain proteolytic activity following TBI in the lateral FP model in the rat, specifically in regions that sustain neuronal loss and axonal injury. Given the ubiquitous distribution of calpain in the brain and its association with posttraumatic cytotoxicity related to increased $[Ca^{2+}]_i$, strategies to block calpain or antagonize its proteolytic actions on the cytoarchitecture would seem to hold some promise for the protection of neural tissue following TBI. Administration of the calpain inhibitor AK295 significantly attenuates both motor and cognitive deficits at 1 week after lateral FP injury in rats (Saatman et al., 1996b). Somewhat surprisingly, these behavioral effects do not seem to be associated with a reduction in spectrin proteolysis or regional cell death 48 h or 1 week post injury (Saatman et al., 2000). In the CCI model of TBI in rats, Posmantur and colleagues (1997) were able to show that administration of calpain inhibitor-2 over 24 h post injury attenuates loss of neurofilament protein and calpain-mediated spectrin breakdown.

Another family of cysteine proteases, the caspases, have recently received much attention for their potential role in cell death following TBI. Caspases are involved in central pathways of neuronal apoptosis (Schwartz and Milligan, 1996). Activated caspase-3 and elevated levels of caspase-3 mRNA have been observed after experimental TBI in rats (Yakovlev et al., 1997). Differentiating the roles of calpains and caspases in cell death is facilitated by the fact that these protease families, while sharing many common substrates, tend to cleave proteins into unique proteolytic fragments (Wang, 2000). For example, spectrin fragments generated by calpain are different from those resulting from caspase-mediated spectrin breakdown. Pike and colleagues (Pike et al., 1998) reported distinct regional and temporal patterns of calpain and caspase-3 processing of α-spectrin following CCI injury in rats. While calpain-mediated spectrin breakdown products were found acutely in the injured cortex and later (for up to 2 weeks) in hippocampus and thalamus, caspase-3-mediated spectrin breakdown products were absent in cortex and limited to hippocampus and striatum early after injury.

Apoptosis and DNA Damage

Although necrotic cell death has been extensively documented in TBI (Adams et al., 1989; Cortez et al., 1989; Sutton et al., 1993), the underlying mechanisms of posttraumatic neuronal death are not well understood. It has been hypothesized recently that the chronic cell death observed after brain trauma (Bramlett et al., 1997; Colicos and Dash, 1996; Smith et al., 1997) may be related to programmed cell death (PCD), which, in contrast to necrosis, requires the active initiation of transcription- and translation-dependent pathways (Arends and Wyllie, 1991). Apoptosis is generally regarded as the morphological hallmark of PCD. In experimental brain injury, apoptotic cell death in cortex and hippocampus was first described in the acute posttraumatic period by Rink and colleagues (Rink et al., 1995), and confirmed in a number of subsequent studies (Colicos and Dash, 1996; Colicos et al., 1996; Fox et al., 1998; Kaya et al., 1999; Newcomb et al., 1999;

Pravdenkova et al., 1996). Distinct regional and temporal patterns of apoptotic cell death have been observed in the cortex, hippocampus, white matter, and thalamus of brain-injured rats (Conti et al., 1998). Recently, Clark and co-workers (1999) were the first to show apoptotic cell death in the acute phase of severe human TBI.

The Bcl-2 family of genes comprise those that inhibit (e.g. *bcl-2*, *bcl-xL*, *bcl-w*) or promote (e.g. *bax*, *bad*, *bcl-xS*, *bak*) apoptosis. Differential expression of the genes in this family appears to be an important factor in mediating trauma-induced cell death in the CNS. Strauss et al. (1997) have shown that loss of neuronal immunohistochemical staining for Bcl-2 in cortical and hippocampal neurons by 2 h after TBI was unique to those cells that appear to be destined to die within 24 h. The proapoptotic bax mRNA has been shown to be upregulated at 3 days following FP injury in the rat (Strauss et al., 1997). Clark and colleagues (1997) have shown that *bcl-2* mRNA and protein are expressed in surviving cells in the injured cortex, hippocampus, and dentate gyrus after experimental TBI. A recent study of human brain tissue after TBI found an increase in Bcl-2 but not Bcl-x_L or Bax (Clark et al., 1999). These data suggest that a dysbalance in pro- and antiapoptotic gene expression may play an important role in cellular damage following TBI.

The caspase gene family appears to play an essential role in neuronal apoptosis (Schwartz and Milligan, 1996). Yakovlev et al. (1997) observed a fivefold increase in caspase-3 mRNA in injured cortex and hippocampus at 24 h after lateral FP injury in rats. Caspase-1 mRNA was also found elevated, but at lower levels than caspase-3. Administration of z-DEVD-fmk, a specific inhibitor of caspase-3, has been shown to significantly reduce posttraumatic apoptosis and neurologic deficits after lateral FP injury in rats, implicating an important role for caspase-3-like proteases in apoptotic pathways following TBI (Yakovlev et al., 1997). DNA fragmentation occurs in apoptotic and necrotic cell death following TBI (Newcomb et al. 1999; Rink et al., 1995). Early DNA fragmentation may be initiated by caspase-3, which is believed to activate and release DNA fragmentation factor 40 (DFF40) through the cleavage of DFF45. Zhang and co-workers (1999) observed a translocation of DFF40 from the cytosol to the nucleus together with changes in the breakdown products of DFF45 after lateral FP injury in the rat, suggesting that this pathway plays a role in the DNA fragmentation observed after experimental TBI. Caspase-3 will mediate cleavage of poly(ADP-ribose) polymerase (PARP), thereby preventing the DNA repair enzyme from identifying DNA strand breaks (Ashkenas and Werb, 1996; Schwartz and Milligan, 1996). PARP activity has been shown to be enhanced early (30 min) after lateral FP injury, and cleavage of this enzyme was shown to gradually increase up to 7 days post injury (LaPlaca et al., 1999). A recent study on human brain tissue obtained from decompressive brain surgery after TBI showed cleavage of caspase-1 and caspase-3, and an upregulation of caspase-3 together with DNA fragmentation, supporting the importance of this gene family in the pathophysiology of human brain trauma (Clark et al., 1999).

Mitochondrial Damage

Mitochondria play a central role in the survival as well as the death of neurons. They are key players in several pathways implicated in the pathophysiology of TBI, such as glutamate toxicity, reactive oxygen species and Ca^{2+} homeostasis (Nicholls and Budd, 2000). Mitochondria have the ability to buffer posttraumatic cytosolic Ca^{2+} overload. However, once the sequestration capacity of the mitochondria is exhausted or oxidative damage to the mitochondrial membrane has occurred, Ca^{2+} is released back into the cytosol (Kontos, 1989; Nicholls and Budd, 2000). Cytosolic Ca^{2+} overload, in turn, has been shown to be linked to mitochondrial dysfunction induced by CCI brain injury in the rat (Xiong et al., 1997a), which may be reversed by administration of N-type calcium channel blockers and/or antioxidant agents (Verweij et al., 1997; Xiong et al., 1997b, 1998). In rats subjected to lateral FP brain injury, mitochondrial dysfunction is correlated with the severity of injury and progresses over the first 72 h, indicating a secondary bioenergetic deterioration (Jiang et al., 1999). Pathological mitochondrial swelling has been identified as one of the earliest hallmarks of axonal damage following experimental TBI in cats (Pettus and Povlishock, 1996). Furthermore, the calcium-induced release of mitochondrial cytochrome c is believed to be a critical step in the process of apoptosis. A recent study on cytochrome c distribution and DNA laddering after cerebral cold injury indicates that cytochrome c released from mitochondria is involved in trauma-induced apoptosis (Morita-Fujimura et al., 1999).

Most recently, cyclosporin A (CsA), an immunosuppressant drug used widely in organ transplantation patients, has become a focus of attention in the field of TBI research, due to its ability to block the mitochondrial permeability transition (MPT) pore, a multimeric transmembrane protein that assembles on the inner mitochondrial membrane as a result of oxidative stress and Ca^{2+} accumulation (Halestrap et al., 1997; Zoratti and Szabo, 1995). Cyclosporin A given as an intrathecal bolus to rats before impact acceleration brain injury was shown to preserve the integrity of mitochondria and to protect axons from degeneration (Okonkwo and Povlishock, 1999). In the same model, when given as posttreatment, CsA was able to limit axonal damage and disconnection at 24 h post injury (Buki et al., 1999b). Furthermore, both immediate pre- as well as posttreatment with CsA resulted in a significant reduction of lesion volume after CCI injury in rats and mice (Scheff and Sullivan, 1999). Observations from our laboratory suggest that CsA may attenuate neurologic deficits after lateral FP injury in rats when given for a prolonged period after trauma (Riess et al., 1999). The above investigations emphasize the pivotal role of mitochondria in the events following TBI.

Diffuse Axonal Injury

Axons are exquisitely vulnerable to damage following closed head injury. Localized axonal swellings and axonal disconnection can be visualized in human postmortem brain tissue, and are common to mild, moderate, and severe TBI (Adams et al., 1989; Blumbergs et al., 1995; Gentleman et al., 1995). While a subset of injured axons may undergo primary axotomy during a traumatic insult (Graham et al., 2000; Maxwell et al., 1993), the majority exhibit progressive morphological and ultra-structural damage leading to secondary axotomy (Grady et al., 1993; Maxwell et al., 1997; Povlishock and Christman, 1995). A number of techniques for visualization of traumatic axonal injury (Adams et al., 1989; Buki et al., 1999a; Pettus et al., 1994; Povlishock et al., 1983; Schweitzer et al., 1993; Sherriff et al., 1994; Yaghmai and Povlishock, 1992) have yielded insight into potential mechanisms underlying axonal dysfunction and disconnection after trauma, such as alterations in axolemmal integrity, activation of calpain, disruption of microtubules and axonal transport, alterations in neurofilament structure and phosphorylation status, and mitochondrial damage (Buki et al., 1999a; Maxwell et al., 1997; Okonkwo et al., 1998; Povlishock and Christman, 1995; Saatman et al., 1996a). Quantitative evaluation of axonal pathology has recently become an important outcome parameter with which to assess potential therapeutic strategies (Buki et al., 1999c; Koizumi and Povlishock, 1998; Marion and White, 1996; Okonkwo and Povlishock, 1999).

Vascular Aspects of Head Injury

The cerebral vascular bed plays an important role in the pathogenesis of elevated ICP, a clinical hallmark of severe TBI, and posttraumatic ischemia. ICP elevations occur as a result of a disturbance of CBF and brain swelling (Bouma and Muizelaar, 1992). Studies in brain-injured humans have shown a profound disturbance of CBF due to a dysfunction of vascular autoregulation and CO_2 responsiveness (Bouma et al., 1991, 1992; Bouma and Muizelaar, 1995; Nawashiro et al., 1994). There is increasing evidence that compromise of the microvasculature may be even more important than vasospasms of the larger vessels in the distortion of CBF patterns (Cobbs et al., 1997; Schroder et al., 1998). Calcium entry blockers increase vascular diameter and cerebral blood flow by their direct action on the smooth muscle cells of the cerebroarterial wall (Alborch et al., 1995). The effects of calcium channel blockers on regional cerebral blood flow (rCBF) have been extensively investigated in humans and in animal models of ischemia (Infeld et al., 1999; Mohamed et al., 1984; Tanaka et al., 1996; Zumkeller et al., 1997). In low doses, nimodipine, a dihydropyridine L-channel antagonist, has been shown to increase rCBF in cerebral cortex, hippocampus, hypothalamus, and thalamic nuclei, but not in brain stem, pons, and cerebellum. With higher doses this potentially beneficial effect disappeared, possibly due to increased systemic hypotension (Mohamed et al., 1984). Little experimental work has been performed to evaluate the influence of calcium channel blockers on CBF after TBI. However, the administration of the Ca^{2+} antagonist (S)-emopamil has been shown to reduce regional cerebral edema, attenuate neurologic motor and cognitive impairment, and improve rCBF after experimental lateral FP injury in the rat (Okiyama et al., 1992, 1994). The swelling of brain tissue after TBI is believed to be the result of cellular edema formation, due to complex cytotoxic events (see above), and, to a lesser extent, vascular edema following the breakdown of the BBB (Baskaya et al., 1997; Unterberg et al., 1997).

A profound disruption of the BBB has been observed in a variety of experimental TBI models (Barzo et al., 1996; Baskaya et al., 1997; Fukuda et al., 1995; Hicks et al., 1997b; McIntosh et al., 1987), as well as in humans (Csuka et al., 1999; Morganti-Kossmann et al., 1999; Pleines et al., 1998). Initial breakdown of the BBB due to trauma occurs within minutes and lasts approximately 6 h, while secondary hypoxia may lead to a prolonged BBB impairment, which may persist for several days (Barzo et al., 1996; Baskaya et al., 1997; Fukuda et al., 1995; Hicks et al., 1997b; Tanno et al., 1992). While activation of white blood cells (WBC) may influence cerebral microcirculation and therefore CBF (Hartl et al., 1997a), WBCs do not appear to be involved in mediating early BBB breakdown (Hartl et al., 1997a,b; Whalen et al., 1999).

Other than mediating WBC extravasation through expression of adhesion molecules (see above), the vascular endothelium may also participate in the posttraumatic inflammatory process through the production of cytokines. Using cultured human cerebral microvascular endothelium, Gourin and Shackford (1997) have shown that percussive injury to these cells in vitro induces a significant release of TFN and IL-1β.

NOVEL CONCEPTS IN TRAUMATIC BRAIN INJURY RESEARCH

As the underlying cellular mechanisms that lead to neuronal and glial dysfunction and death are beginning to be elucidated, it is becoming increasingly clear that the pathophysiology of TBI is complex. The data that are reviewed in this chapter and addressed in detail in subsequent chapters of this book suggest that there may be multiple pathways that are affected following a mechanical insult to the brain. Thus more than likely, therapies targeted at two or more of these pathways may ultimately be most effective in alleviating the pathological consequences of the trauma. In the following sections we propose a more integrative conceptual approach to TBI pathology as opposed to the single-pathway approach.

Is TBI an Inflammatory Disease?

There remains little doubt that a role exists for postinjury inflammation in mediating delayed neuronal damage following TBI. Alterations in blood-borne immunocompetent cells have been described in head-injured patients (Hoyt et al., 1990; Piek et al., 1992; Quattrocchi et al., 1990, 1992a,b), and since the BBB is pathologically opened during the acute posttraumatic period, entry into the brain may directly affect neuronal death and/or survival. Infiltration and accumulation of PMNs into brain parenchyma has been documented early after experimental and human TBI. Immunocytochemical studies have demonstrated the presence of macrophages, natural killer (NK) cells, helper T cells, and T-cytotoxic suppressor cells by 2 days postinjury, and both macrophages and microglia have been proposed as key cellular elements in the progressive tissue necrosis following both spinal cord and brain trauma. The presence of activated immunocompetent cells within the injured brain causes the release of inflammatory mediators, and alterations in systemic and CSF concentrations as well as local expression of cytokines have indeed been reported after experimental and human TBI. Other aspects of the inflammatory response to trauma include expression of adhesion molecules and the activation of the complement system (Fig. 1.1). Both have recently been implicated in events

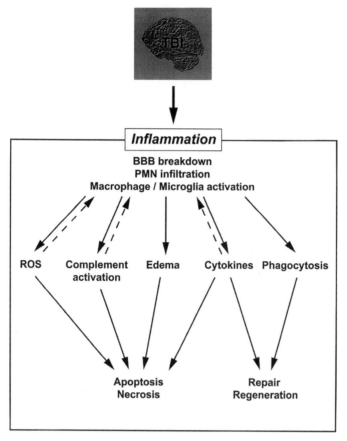

Figure 1.1   Inflammation after traumatic brain injury (TBI). The complex inflammatory response to TBI may have detrimental as well as beneficial effects for the damaged brain (BBB, blood–brain barrier; PMN, polymorphonuclear leukocyte; ROS, reactive oxygen species).

following human and experimental TBI. Common features of inflammation such as edema formation and generation of oxygen free radicals are also observed after brain trauma. These inflammatory events may lead to further cell death and tissue destruction, but may also lay the foundation for repair and regeneration. In fact, some of the inflammatory mediators may have both beneficial and deleterious effects, depending on their concentration and on the time point in the neurochemical cascade at which they are released. Some studies suggest that cytokines released intrathecally may also affect systemic responses to trauma, such as the acute phase response. In conclusion, there is increased evidence of a major inflammatory response to head trauma. However, little is known about its effects in the acute and in the chronic stages of TBI pathology, and further research in this area may lead to novel approaches in the therapy of TBI.

Is TBI a Neurodegenerative Disorder?

Beta-Amyloidosis and Alzheimer-like Pathology. Epidemiological studies have suggested that head injury may be a risk factor for Alzheimer's disease (Mayeux et al., 1993; Mortimer et al., 1991). Alzheimer's disease is characterized by declining cognitive (memory) ability and the accumulation of extracellular β-amyloid ($A\beta$) deposits. Cognitive dysfunction, evident as deficits in both memory and learning, is a well-established consequence of TBI. Histopathological examination of brains from patients who died as a consequence of head trauma has revealed $A\beta$ deposition (Roberts et al., 1994). It is interesting to note that dementia pugilistica (punch-drunk syndrome) is also associated with memory loss and diffuse $A\beta$ deposits (Tokuda et al., 1991).

Upregulation or accumulation of β-amyloid precursor protein (β-APP) similar to that noted after human TBI (Graham et al., 1996) has been observed in a variety of experimental TBI models (Lewen et al., 1995; Pierce et al., 1996; Van den Heuvel et al., 1999). Accumulation of both $A\beta$ and β-APP has been observed in damaged axons and in neuronal perikarya in pigs subjected to nonimpact acceleration brain injury, underlining the similarities between the neuropathology of trauma and of neurodegenerative disease (Smith et al., 1999). Brain-injured transgenic mice that overexpressed *mutant* human β-APP exhibited exacerbated neuronal cell loss in vulnerable hippocampal regions, impaired cognition, and increased regional concentrations of $A\beta$ 1-42 (an amyloid beta-peptide species terminating at amino acid residue 42) (Smith et al., 1998). $A\beta$ 1-42 has been found to be elevated in the CSF of severely head-injured patients (Raby et al., 1998). It is interesting to note that the expression and synthesis of β-APP is induced by cytokines, such as IL-1, which are known to be upregulated directly within the injured CNS or by peripheral immune cells after trauma (Goldgaber et al., 1989). Increased numbers of neurons expressing β-APP have been correlated with increases in activated microglia immunopositive for IL-1 in the acute period following human head injury (Griffin et al., 1994).

Apolipoprotein E Genotyping. Carriers of the apolipoprotein E4 (apo E4) allele, which may play a direct role in $A\beta$ deposition in vivo, have been shown to be at an increased risk for developing Alzheimer's disease (Poirier et al., 1993; Strittmatter et al., 1993). The frequency of apo E4 in individuals with $A\beta$ deposits following head injury is higher than in most studies of Alzheimer's disease, suggesting a genetic susceptibility to the effects of head injury (Mayeux et al., 1995; Nicoll et al., 1995). Head-injured patients with apo E ε4 are more than twice as likely as those without apo E ε4 to have an unfavorable outcome at 6 months (Teasdale et al., 1997).

Cytoskeleton-related Neurodegenerative Pathology. In addition to amyloid plaques, Alzheimer's disease is characterized by neurofibrillary tangles, which are comprised of abnormally phosphorylated tau protein (Grundke-Iqbal et al., 1986). Neurofibrillary tangles in brains from ex-boxers also immunolabel for tau, suggesting that tau pathology may be a feature of dementia pugilistica-associated neurodegeneration as well (Tokuda et al., 1991). In brain-injured humans, cleaved forms of tau proteins are elevated in the CSF (Zemlan et al., 1999). Although relatively little is known about alterations in tau in the traumatically injured brain, there is some indication in animals that phosphorylated tau may accumulate in injured axons and cell bodies (Hoshino et al., 1998; Smith et al., 1999). In addition, increased tau immunoreactivity has been observed in oligodendrocytes in the acute posttraumatic period in humans (Irving et al., 1996). Several neurodegenerative diseases are associated with disorganization of the neurofilamentous cytoskeleton. For example, abnormal accumulations of neurofilament proteins and/or changes in NF phosphorylation occur in diffuse Lewy body disease, Parkinson's disease, certain variants of Alzheimer's disease, and amyotrophic lateral sclerosis (Julien and Mushynski, 1998). In addition, neurofilament proteins have been localized to axonal swellings in motoneuron disease (Schmidt et al., 1987). Many aspects of the NF alterations which accompany neurodegenerative diseases are also present in the pathology of TBI (Fig. 1.2). Increased NF immunoreactivity in axonal swellings, indicative of NF protein accumulation, is a well-established consequence of traumatic axonal injury (Maxwell et al., 1997). A transient increase in neurofilament immunoreactivity precedes loss of NF proteins in regions of gray and white matter following TBI (Posmantur et al., 1994; Saatman et al., 1998). Abnormal phosphorylation of NF proteins in neuronal cell bodies and dephosphorylation of NF proteins in axons has been noted after experimental TBI (Chen et al., 1999; Dunn-Meynell and Levin, 1997; Ross et al., 1994; Yaghmai and Povlishock, 1992). Recently, in a model of diffuse axonal injury, NF-rich inclusions were reported in brain-injured pigs that also exhibited $A\beta$-immunopositive plaquelike profiles (Smith et al., 1999). While it is not well understood how and to what extent disturbances in the neurofilament cytoskeleton contribute to the morbidity or mortality of TBI, abnormal NF organization may be related to significantly worsened outcome after experimental brain injury. Transgenic mice expressing a NF fusion protein and exhibiting perikaryal NF accumulation had greater initial neuromotor dysfunction, slower recovery of function, and larger cortical lesions than their wild-type littermates after TBI (Nakamura et al., 1999a). Together these data suggest that the study of neurodegenerative disease may provide great insight into the mechanisms and treatment of cytoskeletal pathology associated with TBI.

Does TBI Recapitulate Neurodevelopmental Changes?

Although necrotic cell death has been extensively documented following both clinical and experimental TBI, it has been suggested that one component of the diffuse and progressive cell death observed following TBI is related to the induction of neurodevelopmental cascades including PCD (Fig. 1.3). Unlike necrosis, PCD involves the initiation and active expression of transcription- and translation-dependent pathways where apoptosis is regarded as the primary pathological hallmark (see Chapter 11). Apoptosis has been classically associated with the formation of the normal CNS during development. Although necrosis and apoptosis have been more traditionally considered as distinct mechanisms, it may be possible

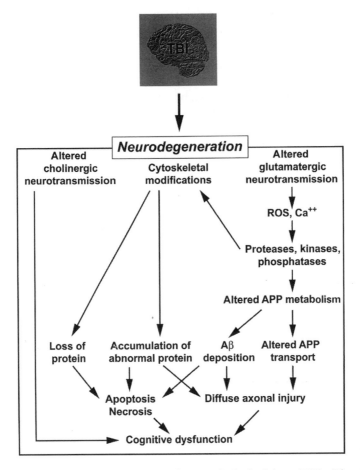

Figure 1.2 Neurodegenerative aspects of traumatic brain injury (TBI). Disturbances in neurotransmission and derangement of the cytoskeleton after TBI lead to morphological hallmarks and cognitive dysfunction similar to the ones observed in neurodegenerative diseases (ROS, reactive oxygen species; Aβ, beta-amyloid; APP, amyloid precursor protein).

to consider them part of the same continuum of cell death, particularly within the context of traumatic CNS injury. A number of studies have now convincingly identified the presence of apoptotic cells following experimental brain injury in rodents (Colicos and Dash, 1996; Rink et al., 1995; Yakovlev et al., 1997), and apoptotic, TUNEL-positive neurons and oligodendrocytes in human head-injured tissue (Smith et al., 2000).

The pattern of alterations in apoptosis-related cell death/survival genes recently documented following TBI supports the importance of these cascades in the pathobiology of head injury (see Chapter 11). Increased expression of the anti-apoptotic protein Bcl-2 has been observed in surviving neurons following both

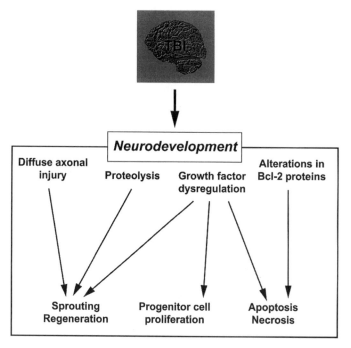

Figure 1.3   Neurodevelopment and traumatic brain injury (TBI). Many alterations observed after TBI share similarities with processes initiated during neurodevelopment.

experimental and clinical TBI (Clark et al., 1997, 1999), while Strauss et al. (1997) have reported an acute downregulation of bcl-2 in hippocampal and cortical neurons destined to die following experimental TBI. Transgenic mice overexpressing human Bcl-2 protein exhibit significantly less neuronal loss in the injured cortex and hippocampus following experimental TBI (Nakamura et al., 1999b; Raghupathi et al., 1998). Bcl-2 proteins may also participate in control of cell death and survival by regulating release of cytochrome c from the mitochondria, which itself participates in the activation of members of the caspase family of death-related proteases.

The caspase family contains up to 12 known members, which, during CNS development, are associated with the final steps in the apoptotic cascade. Specific caspases, including caspase-3, may cleave substrates associated with DNA damage and repair, including DNA-fragmentation factor (DFF45/40), poly(ADP-ribose) polymerase (PARP), and cytoskeletal proteins actin and laminin. Both activated caspase and caspase-associated cleavage products of these substrates have been observed following experimental (Bareyre et al., 1999b; LaPlaca et al., 1999; Pike et al., 1998; Yakovlev et al., 1997; Zhang et al., 1999) and human (Clark et al., 1999) brain injury.

In the CNS, it has been established that neurotrophic molecules have a profound influence on the development and maintenance of neuronal innervation, differentiation and process outgrowth. Nerve growth factor plays a major role during normal neuronal development in supporting neurons which have made appropriate connections, while bFGF has trophic effects during CNS development and promotes neurite outgrowth and astrocyte/oligodendroglial proliferation. Several recent studies suggest that these growth factors including NGF (DeKosky et al., 1994; Goss et al., 1997; Morrison et al., 2000; Oyesiku et al., 1999), bFGF (Gomez-Pinilla et al., 1992), and BDNF (Hicks et al., 1997a) are altered following TBI, perhaps in a response designed to facilitate neuronal repair and reestablish functional connections in the injured brain (see Chapter 7). In addition to the injury-induced response of trophic factors, convergent evidence from several laboratories suggests that an upregulation of several growth-related proteins such as growth-associated protein 43 (GAP-43), microtubule-associated protein 1B (MAP1B), and polysialylated neural-cell adhesion molecule (PSA-NCAM) occurs following brain injury (Emery et al., 2000; Hulse-bosch et al., 1998), providing further support for a "recapitulation" of early CNS developmental events. It is possible that this developmentally appropriate injury response represents a regenerative response by the adult CNS to traumatic injury.

Does Brain Injury Replicate Oncogenesis?

Oncogenesis is typically characterized by sustained alterations in intracellular signaling pathways that control growth and/or death of cells. Importantly, cells with oncogenic potential are unable to stringently regulate these intracellular events, and therefore communication between the environment and the cell is disrupted. Dysregulation of signaling mechanisms may be the result of either functional mutations in, and/or overexpression of, certain critical genes. Examples include transcription factors (c-Fos, c-Jun, p53, c-Myc), cellular proteins (Bcl-2), and receptor kinases (c-erB). The current theory states that rather than being caused by aberrant regulation of a single gene, oncogenesis occurs as a result of changes in at least two genes (i.e., a null mutation in an antioncogene, which is accompanied by the overexpression or functional mutation in a protooncogene). Interestingly, a number of studies have reported that both in the acute and in the chronic posttraumatic period, neural cells respond to a traumatic insult by upregulating genes that have putative oncogenic potential (i.e., protooncogenes). Moreover, TBI results in coordinated changes in expression of multiple protooncogenes. These observations do lead to the speculation that there is much we can learn from the field of oncogenesis and cancer research and apply to the study of the traumatically injured brain. While alterations in gene expression have been evaluated to a significant extent, more recent investigations have attempted to address the issue whether cellular DNA damage may be associated with the pathobiology of TBI. Neural cell DNA may be subjected to oxidative DNA damage and DNA strand breaks, which if unrepaired may lead to either cell death or the expression of mutated proteins. It has been proposed that, as observed during oncogenesis and tumor formation, these repair mechanisms are compromised in CNS injury. While oncogenic mechanisms may mediate the cellular response of existing pools of neurons and glia to a traumatic insult, the increased proliferation of neural precursor cells in response to an injury or stress has only recently become the focus of interest. It is conceivable that in an attempt to repair itself, and replace the dead cells, the

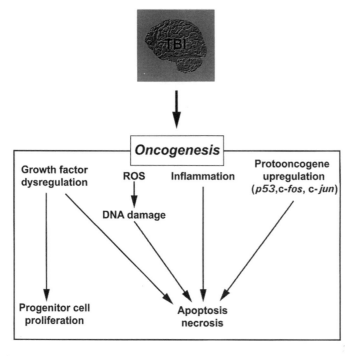

Figure 1.4 Oncogenesis and traumatic brain injury (TBI). TBI may lead to similar changes in gene expression and damage of the DNA as observed in oncogenesis (ROS, reactive oxygen species).

traumatically injured brain may increase the numbers of proliferating progenitor cells. In addition, the brain may also attempt to support the survival of these newly formed cells by increasing extracellular levels of trophic factors (Fig. 1.4).

It may even be possible that the mechanisms controlling the population of precursor cells go awry, leading in fact to an increase in cell numbers within injured regions of the brain. While these preliminary and retrospective comparisons between oncogenesis and TBI provide for an interesting discussion, we suggest that a more careful prospective analysis of the cellular mechanisms underlying cancer should provide novel avenues to better understand the pathophysiology of TBI.

Concluding Remarks

Despite almost three decades of basic preclinical research, by no means have we fully understood the pathological manifestations of TBI. It appears to bear hallmarks of many different disorders of the CNS—of the inflammatory system, of cancer, of neurodegeneration, of senescence, or of aberrant development. "Horizontal thinking" about TBI pathology in the context of these well-characterized disease states raises a number of interesting and important issues. Does the traumatically injured brain attempt to save itself and is the ultimate pathology a manifestation of putative protective processes gone awry? This may certainly be true in light of observations that developmental processes such as neurite outgrowth (axonal regrowth versus aberrant sprouting) and programmed cell death (apoptosis) are observed in the traumatically injured brain. By activating inflammatory mechanisms, is the brain attempting to remove potentially lethal substances that are released from dying neurons and glia? Recent reports describing the reduction of the extent of ischemia-induced neuronal damage by compounds that promote apoptosis, or the exacerbation of trauma-induced tissue damage in mice that are deficient in certain cytokines such as TNF, would suggest that not all putative destructive mechanisms are "bad." Such "out-of-the-box" approaches to evaluating brain trauma may lead to the identification of novel therapeutic targets, particularly to attenuate the chronic consequences of TBI in patients that survive the traumatic insult.

ACKNOWLEDGMENT

This work was supported, in part, by NIH grants NINDS P50-NS08803, NIGMS RO1-GM34690 and a Merit Review grant from the United States Veterans Administration. P.M. Lenzlinger was supported by a research fellowship from the Swiss National Science Foundation (SNF).

ABBREVIATIONS

$A\beta$	Beta-amyloid
apo E	Apolipoprotein E
β-APP	Beta-amyloid precursor protein
ATP	Adenosine triphosphate
BBB	Blood–brain barrier
BER	Base excision repair
BDNF	Brain-derived neurotrophic factor
bFGF	Basic fibroblast growth factor
(r)CBF	(regional) Cerebral blood flow
CCI	Controlled cortical impact
CDP-choline	Cytidine-5′-diphosphate-choline
ChAT	Choline acetyltransferase
CNS	Central nervous system
CNTF	Ciliary neurotrophic factor
CsA	Cyclosporin A
CSF	Cerebrospinal fluid
DFF	DNA fragmentation factor
DNA	Deoxyribonucleic acid

EAA	Excitatory amino acid
FP	Fluid percussion
GAP-43	Growth-associated protein 43
(s)ICAM-1	(soluble) Intercellular adhesion molecule-1
ICP	Intracranial pressure
ICV	Intracerebroventricular
IGF-1	Insulin-like growth factor 1
IL-(1 to 14)	Interleukins-1 to 14
mAChR	Muscarinic acetylcholine receptor
MAP	Microtubule associated protein
MTP	Mitochondrial permeability transition
NER	Nucleotide excision repair
NF	Neurofilament
NGF	Nerve growth factor
NGFR	Nerve growth factor receptor
NK	Natural killer (cells)
NMDA	N-methyl-D-aspartate
NT-3	Neurotrophin-3
PARP	Poly(ADP-ribose) polymerase
PCD	Programmed cell death
PEG	Polyethylene glycol
PMN	Polymorphonuclear leukocytes
PSA-NCAM	Polysialylated neural-cell adhesion molecule
(m)RNA	(messenger) Ribonucleic acid
sCR-1	Soluble complement receptor 1
SOD	Superoxide dismutase
TBI	Traumatic brain injury
TGF	Transforming growth factor
TNF	Tumor necrosis factor
TUNEL	Terminal deoxynucleotidyl transferase-mediated nick end-labeling
WBC	White blood cells
WT	Wild-type

REFERENCES

J. H. Adams, D. Doyle, I. Ford, T. A. Gennarelli, D. I. Graham, and D. R. McLellan, *Histopathology*, 15, 49–59 (1989).

E. Alborch, J. B. Salom, and G. Torregrosa, *Pharmacol. Ther.*, 68, 1–34 (1995).

J. S. Althaus, P. K. Andrus, C. M. Williams, P. F. VonVoigtlander, A. R. Cazers, and E. D. Hall, *Mol. Chem. Neuropathol.*, 20, 147–162 (1993).

M. J. Arends and A. H. Wyllie, *Int. Rev. Exp. Pathol.*, 32, 223–254 (1991).

J. Ashkenas and Z. Werb, *J. Exp. Med.*, 183, 1947–1951 (1996).

I. Bailey, A. Bell, J. Gray, R. Gullan, O. Heiskanan, P. V. Marks, H. Marsh, D. A. Mendelow, G. Murray, and J. Ohman, *Acta Neurochir.*, 110, 97–105 (1991).

F. M. Bareyre, R. Raghupathi, K. E. Saatman, and T. K. McIntosh, *J. Neurotrauma*, 16, 1004 (1999b).

F. M. Bareyre, K. E. Saatman, M. A. Helfaer, G. Sinson, J. D. Weisser, A. L. Brown, and T. K. McIntosh, *J. Neurochem.*, 73, 271–280 (1999a).

R. T. Bartus, *Neuroscientist*, 3, 314–327 (1997).

P. Barzo, A. Marmarou, P. Fatouros, F. Corwin, and J. Dunbar, *J. Neurosurg.*, 85, 1113–1121 (1996).

M. K. Baskaya, A. M. Rao, A. Dogan, D. Donaldson, and R. J. Dempsey, *Neurosci. Lett.*, 226, 33–36 (1997).

M. J. Bell, P. M. Kochanek, J. A. Carcillo, Z. Mi, J. K. Schiding, S. R. Wisniewski, R. S. Clark, C. E. Dixon, D. W. Marion, and E. Jackson, *J. Neurotrauma*, 15, 163–170 (1998).

G. Benz, A. McIntosh, D. Kallieris, and R. Daum, *Eur. J. Pediatr. Surg.*, 3, 259–263 (1993).

P. C. Blumbergs, G. Scott, J. Manavis, H. Wainwright, D. A. Simpson, and A. J. McLean, *J. Neurotrauma*, 12, 565–572 (1995).

G. J. Bouma and J. P. Muizelaar, *J. Neurotrauma*, 9 (Suppl. 1), S333–S348 (1992).

G. J. Bouma and J. P. Muizelaar, *New Horizons*, 3, 384–394 (1995).

G. J. Bouma, J. P. Muizelaar, S. C. Choi, P. G. Newlon, and H. F. Young, *J. Neurosurg.*, 75, 685–693 (1991).

G. J. Bouma, J. P. Muizelaar, K. Bandoh, and A. Marmarou, *J. Neurosurg.*, 77, 15–19 (1992).

H. M. Bramlett, W. D. Dietrich, E. J. Green, and R. Busto, *Acta Neuropathol.*, 93, 190–199 (1997).

J. I. Brown, A. J. Baker, S. J. Konasiewicz, and R. J. Moulton, *J. Neurotrauma*, 15, 253–263 (1998).

A. Buki, R. Siman, J. Q. Trojanowski, and J. T. Povlishock, *J. Neuropathol. Exp. Neurol.*, 58, 365–375 (1999a).

A. Buki, D. O. Okonkwo, and J. T. Povlishock, *J. Neurotrauma*, 16, 511–521 (1999b).

A. Buki, H. Koizumi, and J. T. Povlishock, *Exp. Neurol.*, 159, 319–328 (1999c).

R. Bullock and H. Fujisawa, *J. Neurotrauma*, 9 (Suppl. 2), S443–S462 (1992).

R. Bullock, A. Zauner, J. J. Woodward, J. Myseros, S. C. Choi, J. D. Ward, A. Marmarou, and H. F. Young, *J. Neurosurg.*, 89, 507–518 (1998).

T. M. Carlos, R. S. Clark, D. Franicola-Higgins, J. K. Schiding, and P. M. Kochanek. *J. Leukoc. Biol.*, 61, 279–285 (1997).

X. H. Chen, D. F. Meaney, B. N. Xu, M. Nonaka, T. K. McIntosh, J. A. Wolf, K. E. Saatman, and D. H. Smith, *J. Neuropathol. Exp. Neurol.*, 58, 588–596 (1999).

J. Y. Cheung, J. V. Bonventre, C. D. Malis, and A. Leaf, *N. Engl. J. Med.*, 314, 1670–1676 (1986).

D. W. Choi, *J. Neurosci.*, 7, 369–379 (1987).

D. W. Choi, *Trends Neurosci.*, 11, 465–469 (1988).

D. W. Choi, *Trends Neurosci.*, 18, 58–60 (1995).

R. S. Clark, T. M. Carlos, J. K. Schiding, M. Bree, L. A. Fireman, S. T. DeKosky, and P. M. Kochanek, *J. Neurotrauma*, 13, 333–341 (1996).

R. S. Clark, J. Chen, S. C. Watkins, P. M. Kochanek, M. Chen, R. A. Stetler, J. E. Loeffert, and S. H. Graham, *J. Neurosci.*, 17, 9172–9182 (1997).

R. S. Clark, P. M. Kochanek, M. Chen, S. C. Watkins, D. W. Marion, J. Chen, R. L. Hamilton, J. E. Loeffert, and S. H. Graham, *FASEB J.*, 13, 813–821 (1999).

C. S. Cobbs, A. Fenoy, D. S. Bredt, and L. J. Noble, *Brain Res.*, 751, 336–338 (1997).

D. Cohen, R. Phillips, L. Ott, and B. Young, *J. Lab. Clin. Med.*, 118, 225–231 (1991).

M. A. Colicos and P. K. Dash, *Brain Res.*, 739, 120–131 (1996).

M. A. Colicos, C. E. Dixon, and P. K. Dash, *Brain Res.*, 739, 111–119 (1996).

A. C. Conti, R. Raghupathi, J. Q. Trojanowski, and T. K. McIntosh, *J. Neurosci.*, 18, 5663–5672 (1998).

S. C. Cortez, T. K. McIntosh, and L. J. Noble, *Brain Res.*, 482, 271–282 (1989).

E. Csuka, M. C. Morganti-Kossmann, P. M. Lenzlinger, H. Joller, O. Trentz, and T. Kossmann, *J. Neuroimmunol.*, 101, 211–221 (1999).

J. Deckert and C. H. Gleiter, *J. Neural Trans., Suppl.*, 43, 23–31 (1994).

S. T. DeKosky, J. R. Goss, P. D. Miller, S. D. Styren, P. M. Kochanek, and D. Marion, *Exp. Neurol.*, 130, 173–177 (1994).

S. T. DeKosky, S. D. Styren, M. E. O'Malley, J. R. Goss, P. Kochanek, D. Marion, C. H. Evans, and P. D. Robbins, *Ann. Neurol.*, 39, 123–127 (1996).

D. Dewar and D. I. Graham, *J. Neurotrauma*, 13, 181–187 (1996).

W. D. Dietrich, O. Alonso, R. Busto, and S. P. Finklestein, *J. Neurotrauma*, 13, 309–316 (1996).

C. E. Dixon, J. Bao, J. S. Bergmann, and K. M. Johnson, *Neurosci. Lett.*, 180, 127–130 (1994).

C. E. Dixon, S. J. Liu, L. W. Jenkins, M. Bhattachargee, J. S. Whitson, K. Yang, and R. L. Hayes, *Behav. Brain Res.*, 70, 125–131 (1995a).

C. E. Dixon, J. Bao, K. M. Johnson, K. Yang, J. Whitson, G. L. Clifton, and R. L. Hayes, *Neurosci. Lett.*, 198, 111–114 (1995b).

C. E. Dixon, X. Ma, and D. W. Marion, *J. Neurotrauma*, 14, 161–169 (1997a).

C. E. Dixon, P. Flinn, J. Bao, R. Venya, and R. L. Hayes, *Exp. Neurol.*, 146, 479–490 (1997b).

A. A. Dunn-Meynell and B. E. Levin, *Brain Res.*, 761, 25–41 (1997).

F. P. Eckenstein, G. D. Shipley, and R. Nishi, *J. Neurosci.*, 11, 412–419 (1991).

E. F. Ellis, L. Y. Dodson, and R. J. Police, *J. Neurosurg.*, 75, 774–779 (1991).

D. L. Emery, R. Raghupathi, K. E. Saatman, I. Fischer, M. S. Grady, and T. K. McIntosh, *J. Comp. Neurol.*, 424, 521–531 (2000).

A. I. Faden, P. Demediuk, S. S. Panter, and R. Vink. *Science*, 244, 798–800 (1989).

L. Fan, P. R. Young, F. C. Barone, G. Z. Feuerstein, D. H. Smith, and T. K. McIntosh, *Mol. Brain Res.*, 30, 125–130 (1995).

L. Fan, P. R. Young, F. C. Barone, G. Z. Feuerstein, D. H. Smith, and T. K. McIntosh, *Mol. Brain Res.*, 36, 287–291 (1996).

I. Fineman, D. A. Hovda, M. Smith, A. Yoshino, and D. P. Becker, *Brain Res.*, 624, 94–102 (1993).

G. B. Fox, L. Fan, R. A. Levasseur, and A. I. Faden, *J. Neurotrauma*, 15, 599–614 (1998).

B. B. Fredholm and N. Altiok, *Neurochem. Int.*, 25, 99–102 (1994).

K. Fukuda, H. Tanno, Y. Okimura, M. Nakamura, and A. Yamaura, *J. Neurotrauma*, 12, 315–324 (1995).

S. M. Gentleman, G. W. Roberts, T. A. Gennarelli, W. L. Maxwell, J. H. Adams, S. Kerr, and D. I. Graham, *Acta. Neuropathol.*, 89, 537–543 (1995).

M. Y. Globus, O. Alonso, W. D. Dietrich, R. Busto, and M. D. Ginsberg, *J. Neurochem.*, 65, 1704–1711 (1995).

P. Gluckman, N. Klempt, J. Guan, C. Mallard, E. Sirimanne, M. Dragunow, M. Klempt, K. Singh, C. Williams, and K. Nikolics, *Biochem. Biophys. Res. Commun.*, 182, 593–599 (1992).

M. P. Goldberg and D. W. Choi, *J. Neurosci.*, 13, 3510–3524 (1993).

D. Goldgaber, H. W. Harris, T. Hla, T. Maciag, R. J. Donnelly, J. S. Jacobsen, M. P. Vitek, and D. C. Gajdusek, *Proc. Natl. Acad. Sci. USA*, 86, 7606–7610 (1989).

F. Gomez-Pinilla, J. W. Lee, and C. W. Cotman, *J. Neurosci.*, 12, 345–355 (1992).

J. C. Goodman, C. S. Robertson, R. G. Grossman, and R. K. Narayan, *J. Neuroimmunol.*, 30, 213–217 (1990).

L. K. Gorman, K. Fu, D. A. Hovda, M. Murray, and R. J. Traystman, *J. Neurotrauma*, 13, 457–463 (1996).

J. R. Goss, M. E. O'Malley, L. Zou, S. D. Styren, P. M. Kochanek, and S. T. DeKosky, *Exp. Neurol.*, 149, 301–309 (1998).

J. R. Goss, K. M. Taffe, P. M. Kochanek, and S. T. DeKosky, *Exp. Neurol.*, 146, 291–294 (1997).

C. G. Gourin and S. R. Shackford, *J. Trauma*, 42, 1101–1107 (1997).

M. S. Grady, M. R. McLaughlin, C. W. Christman, A. B. Valadka, C. L. Fligner, and J. T. Povlishock, *J. Neuropathol. Exp. Neurol.*, 52, 143–152 (1993).

D. I. Graham, S. M. Gentleman, J. A. Nicoll, M. C. Royston, J. E. McKenzie, G. W. Roberts, and W. S. Griffin, *Acta Neurochir. (Suppl.)*, 66, 96–102 (1996).

D. I. Graham, R. Raghupathi, K. E. Saatman, D. Meaney, and T. K. McIntosh, *Acta Neuropathol.*, 99, 117–124 (2000).

W. S. Griffin, J. G. Sheng, S. M. Gentleman, D. I. Graham, R. E. Mrak, and G. W. Roberts, *Neurosci. Lett.*, 176, 133–136 (1994).

I. Grundke-Iqbal, K. Iqbal, Y. C. Tung, M. Quinlan, H. M. Wisniewski, and L. I. Binder, *Proc. Natl. Acad. Sci. USA*, 83, 4913–4917 (1986).

J. Guan, C. Williams, M. Gunning, C. Mallard, and P. Gluckman. *J. Cereb. Blood Flow Metab.*, 13, 609–616 (1993).

J. Guan, C. E. Williams, S. J. Skinner, E. C. Mallard, and P. D. Gluckman, *Endocrinology*, 137, 893–898 (1996).

A. P. Halestrap, C. P. Connern, E. J. Griffiths, and P. M. Kerr, *Mol. Cell. Biochem.*, 174, 167–172 (1997).

E. D. Hall, P. A. Yonkers, P. K. Andrus, J. W. Cox, and D. K. Anderson, *J. Neurotrauma*, 9 (Suppl. 2), S425–S442 (1992).

E. D. Hall, P. K. Andrus, and P. A. Yonkers, *J. Neurochem.*, 60, 588–594 (1993).

R. J. Hamm, B. G. Lyeth, L. W. Jenkins, D. M. O'Dell, and B. R. Pike. *Behav. Brain Res.*, 59, 169–173 (1993).

R. J. Hamm, M. D. Temple, B. R. Pike, and E. F. Ellis, *J. Neurotrauma*, 13, 325–332 (1996).

V. H. Hans, T. Kossmann, H. Joller, V. Otto, and M. C. Morganti-Kossmann, *Neuroreport*, 10, 409–412 (1999a).

V. H. Hans, T. Kossmann, P. M. Lenzlinger, R. Probstmeier, H. G. Imhof, O. Trentz, and M. C. Morganti-Kossmann, *J. Cereb. Blood Flow Metab.*, 19, 184–194 (1999b).

R. Hartl, M. B. Medary, M. Ruge, K. E. Arfors, and J. Ghajar, *J. Cereb. Blood Flow Metab.*, 17, 1210–1220 (1997a).

R. Hartl, M. Medary, M. Ruge, K. E. Arfors, and J. Ghajar, *Acta Neurochir. (Suppl.)*, 70, 240–242 (1997b).

R. L. Hayes, H. H. Stonnington, B. G. Lyeth, C. E. Dixon, and T. Yamamoto, *CNS Trauma*, 3, 163–173 (1986).

J. P. Headrick, M. R. Bendall, A. I. Faden, and R. Vink, *J. Cereb. Blood Flow Metab.*, 14, 853–861 (1994).

D. L. Heath and R. Vink, *J. Neurotrauma*, 15, 183–189 (1998).

R. R. Hicks, S. Numan, H. S. Dhillon, M. R. Prasad, and K. B. Seroogy, *Mol. Brain Res.*, 48, 401–406 (1997a).

R. R. Hicks, S. A. Baldwin, and S. W. Scheff, *Mol. Chem. Neuropathol.*, 32, 1–16 (1997b).

M. J. Higgins, H. Hosseinzadeh, D. G. MacGregor, H. Ogilvy, and T. W. Stone, *Pharm. World Sci.*, 16, 62–68 (1994).

S. Holmin, T. Mathiesen, J. Shetye, and P. Biberfeld, *Acta. Neurochir.*, 132, 110–119 (1995).

S. Holmin, J. Soderlund, P. Biberfeld, and T. Mathiesen, *Neurosurgery*, 42, 291–298 (1998).

S. Hoshino, A. Tamaoka, M. Takahashi, S. Kobayashi, T. Furukawa, Y. Oaki, O. Mori, S. Matsuno, S. Shoji, M. Inomata, and A. Teramoto, *Neuroreport*, 9, 1879–1883 (1998).

D. B. Hoyt, A. N. Ozkan, J. F. Hansbrough, L. Marshall, and M. vanBerkum-Clark, *J. Trauma*, 30, 759–766 (1990).

C. E. Hulsebosch, D. S. DeWitt, L. W. Jenkins, and D. S. Prough, *Neurosci. Lett.*, 255, 83–86 (1998).

S. Inci, O. E. Ozcan, and K. Kilinc, *Neurosurgery*, 43, 330–335 (1998).

B. Infeld, S. M. Davis, G. A. Donnan, M. Yasaka, M. Lichtenstein, P. J. Mitchell, and G. J. Fitt, *Stroke*, 30, 1417–1423 (1999).

E. A. Irving, J. Nicoll, D. I. Graham, and D. Dewar, *Neurosci. Lett.*, 213, 189–192 (1996).

J. Isaksson, A. Lewen, L. Hillered, and Y. Olsson, *Acta Neuropathol.*, 94, 16–20 (1997).

X. B. Jiang, T. Kuroiwa, K. Ohno, L. Duan, M. Aoyagi, and K. Hirakawa, *Neurol. Med. Chir.*, 39, 649–656 (1999).

J. P. Julien and W. E. Mushynski, *Prog. Nucleic Acids Res. Mol. Biol.*, 61, 1–23 (1998).

S. L. Kaczorowski, J. K. Schiding, C. A. Toth, and P. M. Kochanek, *J. Cereb. Blood Flow Metab.*, 15, 860–864 (1995).

A. Kampfl, R. Posmantur, R. Nixon, F. Grynspan, X. Zhao, S. J. Liu, J. K. Newcomb, G. L. Clifton, and R. L. Hayes, *J. Neurochem.*, 67, 1575–1583 (1996).

A. Kampfl, R. M. Posmantur, X. Zhao, E. Schmutzhard, G. L. Clifton, and R. L. Hayes, *J. Neurotrauma*, 14, 121–134 (1997).

Y. Katayama, D. S. DeWitt, D. P. Becker, and R. L. Hayes, *Brain Res.*, 296, 241–262 (1984).

Y. Katayama, D. P. Becker, T. Tamura, and D. A. Hovda, *J. Neurosurg.*, 73, 889–900 (1990).

S. S. Kaya, A. Mahmood, Y. Li, E. Yavuz, M. Goksel, and M. Chopp, *Brain Res.*, 818, 23–33 (1999).

S. M. Knoblach, L. Fan, and A. I. Faden, *J. Neuroimmunol.*, 95, 115–125 (1999).

P. M. Kochanek, R. S. Clark, W. D. Obrist, J. A. Carcillo, E. K. Jackson, Z. Mi, S. R. Wisniewski, M. J. Bell, and D. W. Marion, *Acta Neurochir. (Suppl.)*, 70, 109–111 (1997).

T. Koike, D. P. Martin, and E. M. Johnson, Jr, *Proc. Natl. Acad. Sci. USA*, 86, 6421–6425 (1989).

H. Koizumi and J. T. Povlishock, *J. Neurosurg.*, 89, 303–309 (1998).

H. A. Kontos, *Chem. Biol. Interac.*, 72, 229–255 (1989).

H. A. Kontos and J. T. Povlishock, *CNS Trauma*, 3, 257–263 (1986).

T. Kossmann, V. H. Hans, H. G. Imhof, R. Stocker, P. Grob, O. Trentz, and C. Morganti-Kossmann, *Shock*, 4, 311–317 (1995).

T. Kossmann, P. F. Stahel, P. M. Lenzlinger, H. Redl, R. W. Dubs, O. Trentz, G. Schlag, and M. C. Morganti-Kossmann, *J. Cereb. Blood Flow Metab.*, 17, 280–289 (1997a).

T. Kossmann, P. F. Stahel, M. C. Morganti-Kossmann, J. L. Jones, and S. R. Barnum, *J. Neuroimmunol.*, 73, 63–69 (1997b).

J. F. Kraus and D. L. McArthur "Epidemiology of Head Injury", in P. R. Cooper, Ed., *Head Injury*, Williams & Wilkins, Baltimore, 1993, pp. 1–26.

J. Langham, C. Goldfrad, G. Teasdale, D. Shaw, and K. Rowan, The Cochrane Database of Systematic Reviews, Issue 4 (2000).

M. C. LaPlaca and L. E. Thibault, *J. Neurosci. Res.*, 52, 220–229 (1998).

M. C. LaPlaca, R. Raghupathi, A. Verma, A. A. Pieper, K. E. Saatman, S. H. Snyder, and T. K. McIntosh, *J. Neurochem.*, 73, 205–213 (1999).

J. R. Leonard, D. O. Maris, and M. S. Grady, *J. Neurotrauma*, 11, 379–392 (1994).

J. R. Leonard, M. S. Grady, M. E. Lee, J. C. Paz, and L. E. Westrum, *Exp. Neurol.*, 143, 177–187 (1997).

A. Lewen and L. Hillered, *J. Neurotrauma*, 15, 521–530 (1998).

A. Lewen, G. L. Li, P. Nilsson, Y. Olsson, and L. Hillered, *Neuroreport*, 6, 357–360 (1995).

A. Logan and M. Berry, *Trends Pharmacol. Sci.*, 14, 337–342 (1993).

A. Logan, S. A. Frautschy, A. M. Gonzalez, and A. Baird, *J. Neurosci.*, 12, 3828–3837 (1992).

F. M. Longo, I. Selak, J. Zovickian, M. Manthorpe, S. Varon, and H. S. U, *Exp. Neurol.*, 84, 207–218 (1984).

B. G. Lyeth, C. E. Dixon, R. J. Hamm, L. W. Jenkins, H. F. Young, H. H. Stonnington, and R. L. Hayes, *Brain Res.*, 448, 88–97 (1988a).

B. G. Lyeth, C. E. Dixon, L. W. Jenkins, R. J. Hamm, A. Alberico, H. F. Young, H. H. Stonnington, and R. L. Hayes, *Brain Res.*, 452, 39–48 (1988b).

D. W. Marion and M. J. White, *J. Neurotrauma*, 13, 139–147 (1996).

W. L. Maxwell, C. Watt, D. I. Graham, and T. A. Gennarelli, *Acta Neuropathol.*, 86, 136–144 (1993).

W. L. Maxwell, J. T. Povlishock, and D. L. Graham, *J. Neurotrauma*, 14, 419–440 (1997).

R. Mayeux, R. Ottman, M. X. Tang, L. Noboa-Bauza, K. Marder, B. Gurland, and Y. Stern, *Ann. Neurol.*, 33, 494–501 (1993).

R. Mayeux, R. Ottman, G. Maestre, C. Ngai, M. X. Tang, H. Ginsberg, M. Chun, B. Tycko, and M. Shelanski, *Neurology*, 45, 555–557 (1995).

C. J. McClain, D. Cohen, L. Ott, C. A. Dinarello, and B. Young, *J. Lab. Clin. Med.*, 110, 48–54 (1987).

K. L. McDermott, R. Raghupathi, S. C. Fernandez, K. E. Saatman, A. A. Protter, S. P. Finklestein, G. Sinson, D. H. Smith, and T. K. McIntosh, *J. Neurotrauma*, 14, 191–200 (1997).

T. K. McIntosh, L. Noble, B. Andrews, and A. I. Faden, *CNS Trauma*, 4, 119–134 (1987).

T. K. McIntosh, A. I. Faden, I. Yamakami, and R. Vink, *J. Neurotrauma*, 5, 17–31 (1988).

T. K. McIntosh, R. Vink, H. Soares, R. Hayes, and R. Simon, *J. Neurotrauma*, 6, 247–259 (1989a).

T. K. McIntosh, R. Vink, I. Yamakami, and A. I. Faden, *Brain Res.*, 482, 252–260 (1989b).

T. K. McIntosh, R. Vink, H. Soares, R. Hayes, and R. Simon, *J. Neurochem.*, 55, 1170–1179 (1990).

T. K. McIntosh, D. H. Smith, M. Voddi, B. R. Perri, and J. M. Stutzmann, *J. Neurotrauma*, 13, 767–780 (1996).

T. K. McIntosh, K. E. Saatman, and R. Raghupathi, *Neuroscientist*, 3, 169–175 (1997).

T. K. McIntosh, K. E. Saatman, R. Raghupathi, D. I. Graham, D. H. Smith, V. M. Lee, and J. Q. Trojanowski, *Neuropathol. Appl. Neurobiol.*, 24, 251–267 (1998).

L. P. Miller, Ed., *Stroke Therapy: Basic, Preclinical and Clinical Directions*, Wiley-Liss, New York, 1999, pp. 131–156.

A. A. Mohamed, J. McCulloch, A. D. Mendelow, G. M. Teasdale, and A. M. Harper, *J. Cereb. Blood Flow Metab.*, 4, 206–211 (1984).

T. E. Mollnes and E. Fosse, *Shock*, 2, 301–310 (1994).

M. C. Morganti-Kossmann, P. M. Lenzlinger, V. Hans, P. Stahel, E. Csuka, E. Ammann, R. Stocker, O. Trentz, and T. Kossmann, *Mol. Psychiatry*, 2, 133–136 (1997).

M. C. Morganti-Kossmann, V. H. Hans, P. M. Lenzlinger, R. Dubs, E. Ludwig, O. Trentz, and T. Kossmann, *J. Neurotrauma*, 16, 617–628 (1999).

Y. Morita-Fujimura, M. Fujimura, M. Kawase, S. F. Chen, and P. H. Chan, *Neurosci. Lett.*, 267, 201–205 (1999).

G. F. Morris, R. Bullock, S. B. Marshall, A. Marmarou, A. Maas, and L. F. Marshall, *J. Neurosurg.*, 91, 737–743 (1999).

B. Morrison, J. H. Eberwine, D. F. Meaney, and T. K. McIntosh, *Neuroscience*, 96, 131–139 (2000).

J. A. Mortimer, C. M. Van Duijn, V. Chandra, L. Fratiglioni, A. B. Graves, A. Heyman, A. F. Jorm, E. Kokmen, K. Kondo, and W. A. Rocca, *Int. J. Epidemiol.*, 20 (Suppl. 2), S28–S35 (1991).

J. K. Muir, M. Tynan, R. Caldwell, and E. F. Ellis, *J. Neurotrauma*, 12, 179–188 (1995).

D. A. Nachshen, S. Sanchez-Armass, and A. M. Weinstein, *J. Physiol.*, 381, 17–28 (1986).

M. Nakamura, K. E. Saatman, J. E. Galvin, U. Scherbel, R. Raghupathi, J. Q. Trojanowski, and T. K. McIntosh, *J. Cereb. Blood Flow Metab.*, 19, 762–770 (1999a).

M. Nakamura, R. Raghupathi, D. E. Merry, U. Scherbel, K. E. Saatman, and T. K. McIntosh, *J. Comp. Neurol.*, 412, 681–692 (1999b).

H. Nawashiro, K. Shima, and H. Chigasaki, *Acta Neurochir. (Suppl.)*, 60, 440–442 (1994).

J. K. Newcomb, A. Kampfl, R. M. Posmantur, X. Zhao, B. R. Pike, S. J. Liu, G. L. Clifton, and R. L. Hayes, *J. Neurotrauma*, 14, 369–383 (1997).

J. K. Newcomb, X. Zhao, B. R. Pike, and R. L. Hayes, *Exp. Neurol.*, 158, 76–88 (1999).

D. G. Nicholls and S. L. Budd, *Physiol. Rev.*, 80, 315–360 (2000).

J. A. Nicholl, G. W. Roberts, and D. I. Graham, *Nat. Med.*, 1, 135–137 (1995).

NIH Consensus Development Panel on Rehabilitation of Persons With Traumatic Brain Injury, *J. Am. Med. Assoc.*, 282, 974–983 (1999).

P. Nilsson, L. Hillered, U. Ponten, and U. Ungerstedt, *J. Cereb. Blood Flow Metab.*, 10, 631–637 (1990).

P. Nilsson, L. Hillered, Y. Olsson, M. J. Sheardown, and A. J. Hansen, *J. Cereb. Blood Flow Metab.*, 13, 183–192 (1993).

P. Nilsson, H. Laursen, L. Hillered, and A. J. Hansen, *J. Cereb. Blood Flow Metab.*, 16, 262–270 (1996).

K. Okiyama, D. H. Smith, M. J. Thomas, and T. K. McIntosh, *J. Neurosurg.*, 77, 607–615 (1992).

K. Okiyama, T. S. Rosenkrantz, D. H. Smith, T. A. Gennarelli, and T. K. McIntosh, *J. Neurotrauma*, 11, 83–95 (1994).

K. Okiyama, D. H. Smith, T. A. Gennarelli, R. P. Simon, M. Leach, and T. K. McIntosh, *J. Neurochem.*, 64, 802–809 (1995).

K. Okiyama, D. H. Smith, W. F. White, and T. K. McIntosh, *Brain Res.*, 792, 291–298 (1998).

D. O. Okonkwo and J. T. Povlishock, *J. Cereb. Blood Flow Metab.*, 19, 443–451 (1999).

D. O. Okonkwo, E. H. Pettus, J. Moroi, and J. T. Povlishock, *Brain Res.*, 784, 1–6 (1998).

L. Ott, C. J. McClain, M. Gillespie, and B. Young, *J. Neurotrauma*, 11, 447–472 (1994).

N. M. Oyesiku, C. O. Evans, S. Houston, R. S. Darrell, J. S. Smith, Z. L. Fulop, C. E. Dixon, and D. G. Stein, *Brain Res.*, 833, 161–172 (1999).

A. M. Palmer, D. W. Marion, M. L. Botscheller, P. E. Swedlow, S. D. Styren, and S. T. DeKosky, *J. Neurochem.*, 61, 2015–2024 (1993).

S. L. Patterson, M. S. Grady, and M. Bothwell, *Brain Res.*, 605, 43–49 (1993).

E. H. Pettus and J. T. Povlishock, *Brain Res.*, 722, 1–11 (1996).

E. H. Pettus, C. W. Christman, M. L. Giebel, and J. T. Povlishock, *J. Neurotrauma*, 11, 507–522 (1994).

M. A. Petty, P. Poulet, A. Haas, I. J. Namer, and J. Wagner, *Eur. J. Pharmacol.*, 307, 149–155 (1996).

L. L. Phillips, B. G. Lyeth, R. J. Hamm, J. Y. Jiang, J. T. Povlishock, and T. M. Reeves, *J. Neurosci. Res.*, 49, 197–206 (1997).

J. Piek, R. M. Chesnut, L. F. Marshall, M. Berkum-Clark, M. R. Klauber, B. A. Blunt, H. M. Eisenberg, J. A. Jane, A. Marmarou, and M. A. Foulkes, *J. Neurosurg.*, 77, 901–907 (1992).

J. E. Pierce, J. Q. Trojanowski, D. I. Graham, D. H. Smith, and T. K. McIntosh, *J. Neurosci.*, 16, 1083–1090 (1996).

B. R. Pike and R. J. Hamm, *Brain Res.*, 686, 37–43 (1995).

B. R. Pike, X. Zhao, J. K. Newcomb, R. M. Posmantur, K. K. Wang, and R. L. Hayes, *Neuroreport*, 9, 2437–2442 (1998).

U. E. Pleines, J. F. Stover, T. Kossmann, O. Trentz, and M. C. Morganti-Kossmann, *J. Neurotrauma*, 15, 399–409 (1998).

J. Poirier, J. Davignon, D. Bouthillier, S. Kogan, P. Bertrand, and S. Gauthier, *Lancet*, 342, 697–699 (1993).

R. Posmantur, R. L. Hayes, C. E. Dixon, and W. C. Taft, *J. Neurotrauma*, 11, 533–545 (1994).

R. Posmantur, A. Kampfl, R. Siman, J. Liu, X. Zhao, G. L. Clifton, and R. L. Hayes, *Neuroscience*, 77, 875–888 (1997).

J. T. Povlishock and C. W. Christman, *J. Neurotrauma*, 12, 555–564 (1995).

J. T. Povlishock, D. P. Becker, C. L. Cheng, and G. W. Vaughan, *J. Neuropathol. Exp. Neurol.*, 42, 225–242 (1983).

S. V. Pravdenkova, A. G. Basnakian, S. J. James, and B. J. Andersen, *Brain Res.*, 729, 151–155 (1996).

K. B. Quattrocchi, E. H. Frank, C. H. Miller, J. P. MacDermott, L. Hein, L. Frey, and F. C. Wagner, Jr, *J. Neurotrauma*, 7, 77–87 (1990).

K. B. Quattrocchi, C. H. Miller, F. C. Wagner, Jr., S. J. DeNardo, G. L. DeNardo, K. Ovodov, and E. H. Frank, *J. Neurosurg.*, 77, 694–699 (1992a).

K. B. Quattrocchi, B. W. Issel, C. H. Miller, E. H. Frank, and F. C. Wagner, Jr, *J. Neurotrauma*, 9, 1–9 (1992b).

C. A. Raby, M. C. Morganti-Kossmann, T. Kossmann, P. F. Stahel, M. D. Watson, L. M. Evans, P. D. Mehta, K. Spiegel, Y. M. Kuo, A. E. Roher, and M. R. Emmerling, *J. Neurochem.*, 71, 2505–2509 (1998).

R. Raghupathi, S. C. Fernandez, H. Murai, S. P. Trusko, R. W. Scott, W. K. Nishioka, and T. K. McIntosh, *J. Cereb. Blood Flow Metab.*, 18, 1259–1269 (1998).

P. Riess, F. M. Bareyre, J. A. Cheney, J. C. Gensel, R. Raghupathi, K. E. Saatman, and T. K. McIntosh, *J. Neurotrauma*, 16, 1016 (1999).

A. Rink, K. M. Fung, J. Q. Trojanowski, V. M. Lee, E. Neugebauer, and T. K. McIntosh, *Am. J. Pathol.*, 147, 1575–1583 (1995).

F. P. Rivara, D. C. Thompson, R. S. Thompson, L. W. Rogers, B. Alexander, D. Felix, and A. B. Bergman, *Pediatrics*, 93, 567–569 (1994).

G. W. Roberts, S. M. Gentleman, A. Lynch, L. Murray, M. Landon, and D. I. Graham, *J. Neurol. Neurosurg. Psychiatry*, 57, 419–425 (1994).

D. T. Ross, D. F. Meaney, M. K. Sabol, D. H. Smith, and T. A. Gennarelli, *Exp. Neurol.*, 126, 291–299 (1994).

M. Rostworowski, V. Balasingam, S. Chabot, T. Owens, and V. W. Yong, *J. Neurosci.*, 17, 3664–3674 (1997).

S. M. Rothman and J. W. Olney, *Trends Neurosci.*, 10, 299–302 (1987).

N. J. Rothwell and S. J. Hopkins, *Trends Neurosci.*, 18, 130–136 (1995).

K. E. Saatman, D. Bozyczko-Coyne, V. Marcy, R. Siman, and T. K. McIntosh, *J. Neuropathol. Exp. Neurol.*, 55, 850–860 (1996a).

K. E. Saatman, H. Murai, R. T. Bartus, D. H. Smith, N. J. Hayward, B. R. Perri, and T. K. McIntosh, *Proc. Natl. Acad. Sci. USA*, 93, 3428–3433 (1996b).

K. E. Saatman, P. C. Contreras, D. H. Smith, R. Raghupathi, K. L. McDermott, S. C. Fernandez, K. L. Sanderson, M. Voddi, and T. K. McIntosh, *Exp. Neurol.*, 147, 418–427 (1997).

K. E. Saatman, D. I. Graham, and T. K. McIntosh, *J. Neurotrauma*, 15, 1047–1058 (1998).

K. E. Saatman, C. Zhang, R. T. Bartus, and T. K. McIntosh, *J. Cereb. Blood Flow Metab.*, 20, 66–73 (2000).

A. Saija, R. L. Hayes, B. G. Lyeth, C. E. Dixon, T. Yamamoto, and S. E. Robinson, *Brain Res.*, 452, 303–311 (1988a).

A. Saija, S. E. Robinson, B. G. Lyeth, C. E. Dixon, T. Yamamoto, G. L. Clifton, and R. L. Hayes, *J. Neurotrauma*, 5, 161–170 (1988b).

K. L. Sanderson, R. Raghupathi, K. E. Saatman, D. Martin, G. Miller, and T. K. McIntosh, *J. Cereb. Blood Flow Metab.*, 19, 1118–1125 (1999).

S. W. Scheff and P. G. Sullivan, *J. Neurotrauma*, 16, 783–792 (1999).

U. Scherbel, R. Raghupathi, M. Nakamura, K. E. Saatman, J. Q. Trojanowski, E. Neugebauer, M. W. Marino, and T. K. McIntosh, *Proc. Natl. Acad. Sci. USA*, 96, 8721–8726 (1999).

D. T. Schmidt, M. J. Carden, V. M. Y. Lee, and J. Q. Trojanowski, *Lab. Invest.*, 56, 282–294 (1987).

R. H. Schmidt and M. S. Grady, *J. Neurosurg.*, 83, 496–502 (1995).

M. L. Schroder, J. P. Muizelaar, P. Fatouros, A. J. Kuta, and S. C. Choi, *Acta Neurochir. (Suppl.)*, 71, 127–130 (1998).

L. M. Schwartz and C. E. Milligan, *Trends Neurosci.*, 19, 555–562 (1996).

J. B. Schweitzer, M. R. Park, S. L. Einhaus, and J. T. Robertson, *Acta Neuropathol.*, 85, 503–507 (1993).

O. U. Scremin, M. G. Li, A. M. Scremin, and D. J. Jenden, *Brain Res. Bull.*, 42, 59–70 (1997).

Y. Shapira, G. Yadid, S. Cotev, and E. Shohami, *Neurol. Res.*, 11, 169–172 (1989).

Y. Shapira, G. Yadid, S. Cotev, A. Niska, and E. Shohami, *J. Neurotrauma*, 7, 131–139 (1990).

F. E. Sherriff, L. R. Bridges, S. M. Gentleman, S. Sivaloganathan, and S. Wilson, *Acta Neuropathol.*, 88, 433–439 (1994).

M. Shibayama, H. Kuchiwaki, S. Inao, K. Yoshida, and M. Ito, *J. Neurotrauma*, 13, 801–808 (1996).

E. Shohami, M. Novikov, R. Bass, A. Yamin, and R. Gallily, *J. Cereb. Blood Flow Metab.*, 14, 615–619 (1994).

E. Shohami, R. Bass, D. Wallach, A. Yamin, and R. Gallily, *J. Cereb. Blood Flow Metab.*, 16, 378–384 (1996).

B. K. Siesjo and F. Bengtsson, *J. Cereb. Blood Flow Metab.*, 9, 127–140 (1989).

G. Sinson, M. Voddi, and T. K. McIntosh, *J. Neurochem.*, 65, 2209–2216 (1995).

G. Sinson, M. Voddi, E. S. Flamm, and T. K. McIntosh, *Clin. Neurosurg.*, 43, 219–227 (1996).

G. Sinson, B. R. Perri, J. Q. Trojanowski, E. S. Flamm, and T. K. McIntosh, *J. Neurosurg.*, 86, 511–518 (1997).

D. H. Smith, K. Okiyama, T. A. Gennarelli, and T. K. McIntosh, *Neurosci. Lett.*, 157, 211–214 (1993).

D. H. Smith, X. H. Chen, J. E. Pierce, J. A. Wolf, J. Q. Trojanowski, D. I. Graham, and T. K. McIntosh, *J. Neurotrauma*, 14, 715–727 (1997).

D. H. Smith, M. Nakamura, T. K. McIntosh, J. Wang, A. Rodriguez, X. H. Chen, R. Raghupathi, K. E. Saatman, J. Clemens, M. L. Schmidt, V. M. Lee, and J. Q. Trojanowski, *Am. J. Pathol.*, 153, 1005–1010 (1998).

D. H. Smith, X. H. Chen, M. Nonaka, J. Q. Trojanowski, V. M. Lee, K. E. Saatman, M. J. Leoni, B. N. Xu, J. A. Wolf, and D. F. Meaney, *J. Neuropathol. Exp. Neurol.*, 58, 982–992 (1999).

F. M. Smith, R. Raghupathi, M.-A. MacKinnon, T. K. McIntosh, K. E. Saatman, D. F. Meaney, and D. I. Graham, *Acta Neuropathol.*, 100, 537–545 (2000).

S. L. Smith, P. K. Andrus, J. R. Zhang, and E. D. Hall, *J. Neurotrauma*, 11, 393–404 (1994).

H. D. Soares, R. R. Hicks, D. Smith, and T. K. McIntosh, *J. Neurosci.*, 15, 8223–8233 (1995).

D. M. Sosin, J. J. Sacks, and S. M. Smith, *J. Am. Med. Assoc.*, 262, 2251–2255 (1989).

D. M. Sosin, J. E. Sniezek, and R. J. Waxweiler, *J. Am. Med. Assoc.*, 273, 1778–1780 (1995).

P. F. Stahel, T. Kossmann, M. C. Morganti-Kossmann, V. H. Hans, and S. R. Barnum, *Brain Res. Mol. Brain Res.*, 50, 205–212 (1997).

P. F. Stahel, M. C. Morganti-Kossmann, and T. Kossmann, *Brain Res. Rev.*, 27, 243–256 (1998).

J. F. Stover, M. C. Morganti-Kossmann, P. M. Lenzlinger, R. Stocker, O. S. Kempski, and T. Kossmann, *J. Neurotrauma*, 16, 135–142 (1999).

K. I. Strauss, R. Raghupathi, S. Karjewski, J. C. Reed, and T. K. McIntosh, *J. Neurotrauma*, 13, 620 (1997).

W. J. Strittmatter, A. M. Saunders, D. Schmechel, M. Pericak-Vance, J. Enghild, G. S. Salvesen, and A. D. Roses, *Proc. Natl. Acad. Sci. USA*, 90, 1977–1981 (1993).

P. K. Stys, S. G. Waxman, and B. R. Ransom, *J. Neurosci.*, 12, 430–439 (1992).

P. G. Sullivan, A. J. Bruce-Keller, A. G. Rabchevsky, S. Christakos, D. K. Clair, M. P. Mattson, and S. W. Scheff, *J. Neurosci.*, 19, 6248–6256 (1999).

F. Y. Sun and A. I. Faden, *Brain Res.*, 673, 133–140 (1995).

R. L. Sutton, L. Lescaudron, and D. G. Stein, *J. Neurotrauma*, 10, 135–149 (1993).

K. Takahashi, in R. L. Mellgren and T. Murachi, eds., *Intracellular Calcium-dependent Proteolysis*, CRC Press, Boca Raton, 1990, pp. 55–74.

R. Tanaka, Y. Miyasaka, S. Maruyama, S. Nagai, and K. Fujii, *Neurol. Res.*, 18, 325–328 (1996).

H. Tanno, R. P. Nockels, L. H. Pitts, and L. J. Noble, *J. Neurotrauma*, 9, 335–347 (1992).

V. Taupin, S. Toulmond, A. Serrano, J. Benavides, and F. Zavala, *J. Neuroimmunol.*, 42, 177–185 (1993).

G. Teasdale, I. Bailey, A. Bell, J. Gray, R. Gullan, O. Heiskanan, P. V. Marks, H. Marsh, D. A. Mendelow, and G. Murray, *J. Neurotrauma*, 9 (Suppl. 2), S545–S550 (1992).

G. M. Teasdale, J. A. Nicoll, G. Murray, and M. Fiddes, *Lancet*, 350, 1069–1071 (1997).

D. C. Thompson, F. P. Rivara, and R. S. Thompson, *J. Am. Med. Assoc.*, 277, 883–884 (1997).

T. Tokuda, S. Ikeda, N. Yanagisawa, Y. Ihara, and G. G. Glenner, *Acta Neuropathol.*, 82, 280–285 (1991).

S. Toulmond and N. J. Rothwell, *Brain Res.*, 671, 261–266 (1995).

R. J. Traystman, J. R. Kirsch, and R. C. Koehler, *J. Appl. Physiol.*, 71, 1185–1195 (1991).

R. W. Tsien, D. Lipscombe, D. V. Madison, K. R. Bley, and A. P. Fox, *Trends Neurosci.*, 11, 431–438 (1988).

A. W. Unterberg, R. Stroop, U. W. Thomale, K. L. Kiening, S. Pauser, and W. Vollman, *Acta Neurochir. (Suppl.)*, 70, 106–108 (1997).

C. Van den Heuvel, P. C. Blumbers, J. W. Finnie, J. Manavis, N. R. Jones, P. L. Reilly, and R. A. Pereira, *Exp. Neurol.*, 159, 441–450 (1999).

S. Varon, T. Hagg, and M. Manthorpe, *Adv. Exp. Med. Biol.*, 296, 267–276 (1991).

B. H. Verweij, J. P. Muizelaar, F. C. Vinas, P. L. Peterson, Y. Xiong, and C. P. Lee, *Neurol. Res.*, 19, 334–339 (1997).

P. Vespa, M. Prins, E. Ronne-Engstrom, M. Caron, E. Shalmon, D. A. Hovda, N. A. Martin, and D. P. Becker, *J. Neurosurg.*, 89, 971–982 (1998).

R. Vink, T. K. McIntosh, P. Demediuk, and A. I. Faden, *Biochem. Biophys. Res. Commun*, 149, 594–599 (1987).

R. Vink, A. I. Faden, and T. K. McIntosh, *J. Neurotrauma*, 5, 315–330 (1988).

R. Vink, E. M. Golding, J. P. Williams, and T. K. McIntosh, *J. Cereb. Blood Flow Metab.*, 17, 50–53 (1997).

F. Wahl, E. Renou, V. Mary, and J. M. Stutzmann, *Brain Res.*, 756, 247–255 (1997).

H. J. Walter, M. Berry, D. J. Hill, and A. Logan, *Endocrinology*, 138, 3024–3034 (1997).

K. K. W. Wang, *Trends Neurosci.*, 23, 20–26 (2000).

M. J. Whalen, T. M. Carlos, P. M. Kochanek, R. S. Clark, S. Heineman, J. K. Schiding, D. Franicola, F. Memarzadeh, W. Lo, D. W. Marion, and S. T. DeKosky, *J. Neurotrauma*, 16, 583–594 (1999).

M. N. Woodroofe, G. S. Sarna, M. Wadhwa, G. M. Hayes, A. J. Loughlin, A. Tinker, and M. L. Cuzner, *J. Neuroimmunol.*, 33, 227–236 (1991).

Y. Xiong, Q. Gu, P. L. Peterson, J. P. Muizelaar, and C. P. Lee, *J. Neurotrauma*, 14, 23–34 (1997a).

Y. Xiong, P. L. Peterson, J. P. Muizelaar, and C. P. Lee, *J. Neurotrauma*, 14, 907–917 (1997b).

Y. Xiong, P. L. Peterson, B. H. Verweij, F. C. Vinas, J. P. Muizelaar, and C. P. Lee, *J. Neurotrauma*, 15, 531–544 (1998).

A. Yaghmai and J. Povlishock, *J. Neuropathol. Exp. Neurol.*, 51, 158–176 (1992).

A. G. Yakovlev, S. M. Knoblach, L. Fan, G. B. Fox, R. Goodnight, and A. I. Faden, *J. Neurosci.*, 17, 7415–7424 (1997).

A. B. Young, L. G. Ott, D. Beard, R. J. Dempsey, P. A. Tibbs, and C. J. McClain, *J. Neurosurg.*, 69, 375–380 (1988).

B. Young, J. W. Runge, K. S. Waxman, T. Harrington, J. Wilberger, J. P. Muizelaar, A. Boddy, and J. W. Kupiec, *J. Am. Med. Assoc.*, 276, 538–543 (1996).

F. P. Zemlan, W. S. Rosenberg, P. A. Luebbe, T. A. Campbell, G. E. Dean, N. E. Weiner, J. A. Cohen, R. A. Rudick, and D. Woo, *J. Neurochem.*, 72, 741–750 (1999).

C. Zhang, R. Raghupathi, K. E. Saatman, D. H. Smith, J. M. Stutzmann, F. Wahl, and T. K. McIntosh, *J. Neurosci. Res.*, 52, 342–349 (1998).

C. Zhang, R. Raghupathi, K. E. Saatman, M. C. LaPlaca, and T. K. McIntosh, *J. Neurochem.*, 73, 1650–1659 (1999).

C. Z. Zhu and R. N. Auer, *J. Cereb. Blood Flow Metab.*, 14, 237–242 (1994).

J. Zhuang, S. R. Shackford, J. D. Schmoker, and M. L. Anderson, *J. Trauma*, 35, 415–422 (1993).

M. Zoratti and I. Szabo, *Biochim. Biophys. Acta*, 1241, 139–176 (1995).

M. Zumkeller, H. E. Heissler, and H. Dietz, *Neurosurg. Rev.*, 20, 259–268 (1997).

CHAPTER 2

IN VITRO MODELS OF TRAUMATIC BRAIN INJURY

BRIAN R. PIKE

E.F. & N.L. McKight Brain Institute of the University of Florida, Center for Traumatic Brain Injury Studies, Department of Neuroscience, Gainesville, Florida

INTRODUCTION

The goal of in vivo models of traumatic brain injury (TBI) is to reproduce, with as much fidelity as possible, the behavioral and pathological sequelae associated with TBI in humans. Importantly, these animal models have generated much knowledge about the pathological responses to brain injury and have led to better emergency management of the human brain-injured patient. However, the study of cellular pathological responses to mechanical brain trauma is difficult in vivo due to various secondary central and systemic responses to the initial injury. For example, primary mechanical head injury elicits a host of relatively delayed secondary injuries such as anoxia, ischemia, increased cerebral perfusion pressure, edema, and so on, that complicate interpretation of the effects of mechanical brain injury per se. In addition, the presence of the circulatory system can further complicate results due to its close interaction with the brain parenchyma (metabolite removal/delivery, hemorrhage, host for neutrophil infiltration, etc.). Similarly, the blood–brain barrier hampers investigation of potential therapeutic agents that do not readily enter the brain due to poor lipid solubility or absence of specific transporters. Finally, mechanical impact itself is a dynamic variable that generates complex forces on brain tissues such as brain volume compression, tissue shearing (torque), and linear tensile strain (stretch), each of which can have different effects on cellular function (Gennarelli and Thibault, 1985). Thus, because of the complex responses observed after TBI in vivo, it is extremely difficult to study with rigor the effects of any individual pathological component of TBI. For this reason, in vitro approaches of neuronal injury have been developed that model different mechanical or neurochemical insults commonly associated with TBI, allowing more precise control over intracellular and

Head Trauma: Basic, Preclinical, and Clinical Directions, Edited by Leonard P. Miller and Ronald L. Hayes, Co-edited by Jennifer K. Newcomb
ISBN 0-471-36015-5 © 2001 John Wiley & Sons, Inc.

extracellular environments than is possible in vivo. These in vitro models typically employ cultured central nervous system (CNS) cells or ex vivo preparations of CNS tissues and include, but are not limited to, (1) mechanical cell injury, (2) ischemia (hypoglycemia + hypoxia), and (3) glutamate toxicity. The purpose of this chapter is to provide an overview of the most commonly used in vitro models of mechanical cell injury currently employed by neurotraumatologists and to provide a review of the rapidly evolving pharmacological strategies for preserving cell viability and function after mechanical cell injury in these models. See Table 2.1 for a summary of the various in vitro models of traumatic brain injury reviewed in this chapter.

MODELS OF MECHANICAL CELL INJURY

Several in vitro models have been developed for mechanically deforming cultured cells or tissue slices and these can be classified according to the method used to induce mechanical injury. For example, tensile strain may be induced by stretching the substrate to which adherent CNS cells are attached (Cargill and Thibault, 1996; Ellis et al., 1995; Morrison et al., 1998a). Rapid acceleration injury can be used to examine the effects of inertia on cultured cells (Lucas and Wolf, 1991). Shear strain injury has been investigated by using angular velocity (torque) to force fluid over stationary cells (LaPlaca and Thibault, 1997; LaPlaca et al., 1997; Triyoso and Good, 1999). Cultured cells or tissue slice preparations have been mechanically deformed by subjecting them to a pressurized environment produced by a fluid percussion barotrauma chamber used by Shepard and colleagues (1991), which uses a fluid percussion device similar to that used in in vivo TBI studies. Other systems of mechanical insult model transection-type injuries and involve scratching cultured cell layers with a stylet (Regan and Choi, 1994; Mitchell et al., 1995) or punching cells with small stainless steel blades (Mukhin et al., 1997a; Mukhin et al., 1996). Because the transection type models cause primary injury only to a subpopulation of cultured cells, these models can be used to examine the effects of injury to neighboring cells not exposed to the primary mechanical injury. A brief description of the most common models used in in vitro CNS injury is provided below.

Tensile Strain (Stretch) Models

A major biomechanical stress encountered by CNS tissues in vivo during compressive injury is that of rapid deformation and tensile strain, or stretch. Models designed to mimic this type of cellular injury involve culturing of primary fetal or neonatal CNS cells or human immortalized neuronal cell lines onto deformable substrates. The adherent cells are then exposed to an applied load, such as compressed nitrogen gas, which deforms the substrate, thus stretching the cells. Examples of this type of model include those of Cargill and Thibault (1996), Ellis et al. (1995), and Morrison et al. (1998a). For example, in the model developed by Ellis et al. (1995), CNS cells are plated onto collagen-coated silastic membranes (25 mm diameter, 2 mm thick) that form the bottom surface of six-well plates. A Cell Injury Controller (model 94A)

TABLE 2.1 In Vitro Models of Traumatic Brain Injury

Model	Injury	Features	Biomechanical Force Modeled
Tensile strain (stretch)	Adherent cells cultured on flexible membranes are stretched by controlled application of a pressurized gas (e.g., nitrogen) that produces a rapid biaxial deformation of the cells	Each well of six-well plates can be injured independently or serve as uninjured control (e.g., Ellis et al., 1995)	Models tensile component of inertial loading
Shear strain (torque)	Culture medium is rapidly accelerated over adherent cultured cells that are injured by the resulting tangential frictional force	Allows real-time monitoring of strain and strain rates on cells during controlled hydrodynamic stress (e.g., LaPlaca and Thibault, 1997; LaPlaca et al., 1997)	Models shear component of inertial loading
Rapid acceleration	Trauma to adherent cultured cells is induced by a ballistic pendulum device that rapidly accelerates culture flasks containing adherent CNS cell monolayers	Injury is more severe when flasks are accelerated tangentially to the plane of cell growth. Removal of culture medium just prior to injury eliminates injury due to fluid shear stress or pressure wave effects	Models acceleration component of inertial loading. Axotomy is minimal, allowing investigation of effects of acceleration on soma and dendrites
Fluid percussion barotrauma	Adherent cell cultures or tissue slice preparations are injured by compression from a modified fluid percussion device	With cell cultures, a sealed system prevents cross contamination of saline from fluid percussion device with culture medium	Models compression injury
Transection	Various injury techniques have been utilized and include scratching cell monolayers with a 20-gauge needle or transection of individual dendrites with a UV microbeam	Technique permits investigation of secondary injury effects to cells distal from site of primary transection injury	Models simple mechanical disruption of cells
Organotypic tissue slice	In most models discussed above, dissection and maintenance of adult tissue slices or culturing of fetal tissue slices can be used in lieu of cell culture	Preserves functional and anatomical relationships between cells. Greater variety of cell types, e.g., granule and pyramidal neuronal cells	Complexity of in vivo biomechanical insults may be better represented in slices; however, uniform injury across cells is compromised in thick sections

that is connected to a tank of compressed gas produces the cell injury. The delivered gas is immediately vented, which allows for a rapid deformation and rebound of the silastic membrane (Ellis et al., 1995).

Shear Strain (Torque) Models

Another biomechanical stress encountered by CNS tissues is shear strain due to inertial loading of the head during blunt trauma or rapid acceleration of the head. The model of cell shear injury developed and characterized by LaPlaca and Thibault (1997) offers the advantage of allowing measurement of actual cell strain during the injury as well as immediate response of the cell to injury (LaPlaca and Thibault, 1997; LaPlaca et al., 1997). The Cell Shearing Injury Device (CSID) employed by LaPlaca et al. (1997) is a parallel disk viscometer. Cells are grown on glass coverslips (25 mm diameter) and then kept stationary by vacuum in a buffer filled chamber. A top cylindrical disk is made to come in complete contact with the buffer in the lower chamber. Shear injury is caused by the rapid rotation of the top disk resulting in fluid shear stress on the adherent cells. With this model, actual strain rates can be determined by coating cells with 0.5 μm diameter carboxyl-coated FluoSpheres (Molecular Probes, Eugene, OR). Triyoso and Good (1999) developed another in vitro fluid shear injury device that was used to injure neuronally derived SH-SY5Y cells.

Rapid Acceleration Models

Rapid acceleration and/or deceleration of the head and neck is a major cause of CNS injury (Frankowski, 1986) and is associated with diffuse axonal injury (Adams et al., 1982; Povlishock, 1985). An in vitro model of rapid acceleration injury (RAI) was developed and characterized by Lucas and Wolf (1991). In this model, adherent CNS cell cultures were grown in 25 cm^2 plastic culture flasks. Injury was induced by means of a ballistic pendulum apparatus by which one pendulum was made to strike a second pendulum that housed an attached culture flask. The culture medium was removed immediately prior to injury or control injury (approximately 1 min deprivation).

Fluid Percussion Barotrauma Models

The fluid percussion barotrauma chamber (Shepard et al., 1991) uses the same fluid percussion device commonly employed for production of in vivo traumatic brain injury (see Dixon et al., 1987). Shepard and colleagues modified a fluid percussion device to deliver a fluid pulse to cell cultures grown in 60-mm-diameter petri dishes. Briefly, a petri dish is fitted snugly in a stainless steel lower chamber. A second upper chamber containing rubber gaskets with a waterproof latex membrane connects the injury device to the lower chamber. This provides a sealed system and prevents saline from the saline-filled fluid percussion device from mixing with cell culture medium. However, the force of the fluid pulse is transmitted between the two chambers. As in in vivo fluid percussion injury, injury is produced when a pendulum strikes a Plexiglas piston mounted at the end of the device. The fluid percussion device has also been modified for use with tissue slice preparations (e.g., Girard et al., 1996; Wallis and Panizzon, 1995).

Transection Models

Perhaps the simplest in vitro model of mechanical cell injury involves the use of a stylet to scratch cultured CNS cells. Although the technique may vary between investigators, in its simplest form, transection injury is caused by the generation of one or more tears in culture monolayers using a stylet, such as a 20-gauge needle (e.g., Mitchell et al., 1995; Regan and Choi, 1994; Regan and Panter, 1995; Shah et al., 1997) or a plastic pipette tip (e.g., Tecoma et al., 1989). A model employed by Lucas et al. (1990) employed a UV microbeam to transect primary dendrites from individual neurons, while Mukhin et al. (1996, 1998) have used a band of 28 stainless steel blades controlled with an electromagnetic device to transect cultured cells. Another model developed by Mukhin et al. (1997b) used a cylinder fitted with needles and attached to an electric screwdriver to produce concentric circular cuts in cultured CNS cells.

Organotypic Tissue Slice Preparations

An alternative to cell culture is the use of organotypic tissue slices. With this approach, intact brain or spinal cord regions can be sectioned and functionally maintained for relatively short periods in physiological buffers. The advantage to this method is that the in vivo anatomic relationship between astrocytes, neurons, and their projections is maintained while in vitro control of the environment is possible. For example, Wallis and Panizzon (1995) employed hippocampal slice preparations in a model of fluid percussion barotrauma to study electrophysiological function of CA1 neuronal responses. Leybaert and Hempti nne (1996) used lumbar spinal cord slices in a mechanical lesion model, while Agrawal and Fehlings (1996) examined spinal cord compression in dissected dorsal column strips.

CELL VIABILITY IN MODELS OF MECHANICAL CELL INJURY

The extent of cell death or damage after in vitro mechanical injury can be assayed by a variety of relatively simple assays. The most commonly used techniques include the use of vital dyes such as trypan blue, propidium iodide (PI) or ethidium homodimer, or enzymatic assays of lactate dehydrogenase (LDH) release into the culture medium. Trypan blue, PI, and ethidium homodimer are normally excluded from normal healthy cells but readily permeate cell membranes when cells die or when plasma membrane integrity is compromised (Jones and Senft, 1985). The fluorescent dyes like PI and ethidium homodimer are more commonly used as these dyes are not sensitive to serum proteins in culture medium and have a greater interobserver reliability (Singh and Stephens, 1986). In contrast to dye exclusion detection of cell injury/death, fluorescein diacetate (FDA) is a vital dye that is taken up by healthy cells. Thus, FDA (green fluorescence) can be used concurrently with PI (red fluorescence) to monitor the ratio of living to dead cells. LDH is a stable large molecular weight cytoplasmic enzyme present in all cells and is rapidly released into culture medium upon disruption of plasma membranes due to injury (Murphy and Horrocks, 1994). The LDH assay is very sensitive and relatively small quantities (50 μL) of culture medium may be used, allowing for repeated sampling of the same cell culture medium over time. A disadvantage of the LDH assay is that different cell types express different levels of intracellular LDH; thus, the amount of released LDH does not always correlate with the number of dead cells, especially when mixed culture systems (e.g., glial + neuronal) are used.

As would be expected, the percentage of nonviable cells after in vitro traumatic injury increases correspondingly with severity of injury regardless of the injury model employed (Ellis et al., 1995; LaPlaca et al., 1997; Lucas and Wolf, 1991; Mukhin et al., 1997a; Pike et al., 1999; 2000; Shepard et al., 1991). In models of stretch injury, PI staining and/or LDH release typically reach maximal levels immediately or soon after injury (Ellis et al., 1995; Pike et al., 1999; 2000). For example, in astrocyte cultures, Ellis et al. (1995) found that the majority of LDH release occurred between 10 and 30 min after injury and that no further release of LDH was detectable from 2 to 24 h after stretch injury. In agreement with Ellis' results, our laboratory also observed peak LDH release and PI uptake at the earliest postinjury time points assayed after stretch injury to neuronal + glial cocultures (Pike et al., 1999; 2000). However, we also detected smaller but significant levels of LDH still being released into culture medium up to 5 days after the injury. We attributed these lower levels of LDH release to delayed apoptotic cell death that was evident to at least 5 days post injury. This hypothesis is supported by Ellis and colleagues who reported that PI uptake after stretch injury is primarily localized to astrocytes immediately after injury and that neurons do not stain predominately for PI until 24 to 48 h after the injury (Willoughby et al., 1998). Similarly, Triyoso and Good (1999) observed apoptotic-like DNA fragmentation in neurons prior to detection of significant LDH release that was not detected until 24 h after pulsatile fluid shear stress injury. Thus, cell type-specific vulnerability to mechanical injury may be an important pathological feature of trauma and this phenomenon warrants further research regarding mechanisms of cell death including delayed apoptotic cell death.

Similarly to the differences in astrocyte versus neuronal cell viability reported by Willoughby et al. (1998) after stretch injury, Mukhin et al. (1998) found that mechanical punch injury caused a significantly larger increase in LDH release from neuronal + glial cocultures than in enriched astrocyte cultures 16 to 18 h after injury. Interestingly, Mukhin and colleagues replenished their culture medium 30 min after injury in order to examine the effects of delayed secondary injury. Using ethidium homodimer to label injured or dead cells, these investigators found that both injured neuronal + glial and glial cultures had significantly higher numbers of stained nuclei than did uninjured controls 30 min after injury. However, by 16 to 24 h after injury, little or no staining was evident in glial cultures whereas neuronal + glial cultures displayed significantly elevated staining. Using NT2 neuronal cell lines, LaPlaca and Thibault (1997) also found that LDH concentrations continued to accumulate from 1 min to 24 h after fluid shear injury and that nuclear binding of ethidium homodimer was greatest at 24 h post injury, indicating continued cellular degeneration occurring after the traumatic insult. In summary, in vitro mechanical injury models provide investigators the flexibility to examine traumatic injury in a wide variety of cell types and tissues from various brain and spinal cord regions. In vitro models allow rapid and continuous monitoring of cell viability in living, nonfixed cultures with a simple LDH assay or staining with vital dyes. These important features of in vitro injury models will further the understanding of pathological responses in individual cell subtypes as well as complex interaction effects that may exist in mixed culture systems.

PHARMACOLOGICAL PROTECTION IN MODELS OF MECHANICAL CELL INJURY

A major advantage to the employment of in vitro cell injury models is the ability for high-throughput screening of potential neuroprotective compounds. This approach can provide investigators with an enormous amount of important information regarding a drug's effects prior to administration in animals, for example, mechanism of action, cell type affected, dose response, therapeutic window, and so on. Thus, use of in vitro models may offer a strategic advantage in the identification of efficacious pharmacotherapies for clinical traumatic brain injury. To date, the number of compounds tested in in vitro mechanical cell injury models are not as numerous as those tested in vivo. However, the growing popularity of in vitro systems ensures an expansion of therapeutic screening in the near future. A review of some of the compounds that have been tested in mechanical cell injury are discussed below and outlined in Table 2.2.

Glutamate Receptor Antagonists

It is well established that excessive activation of ionotropic glutamate receptors after brain injury can lead to pathological influx of calcium through N-methyl-D-aspartate (NMDA) and voltage-sensitive calcium channels (see Chapter 4). Numerous in vivo models of traumatic brain injury have reported neuroprotective effects with the administration NMDA antagonists (for reviews see Hayes et al., 1992; McIntosh, 1993; McIntosh et al., 1998a). Similarly to the neuroprotective effect in in vivo traumatic brain and spinal cord injury, NMDA receptor antagonists have been shown to be protective against CNS injury and cell loss in various in vitro mechanical cell injury models. For example, using a model of rapid acceleration injury, Lucas and Wolf (1991) observed a near 30 percent reduction in cell death when spinal cord CNS cultures were treated with the noncompetitive NMDA antagonist ketamine (100 μM). Tecoma and co-workers (1989) observed a concentration-dependent neuroprotective effect with both noncompetitive (dextrorphan; $EC_{50} \cong 10\,\mu M$) and

TABLE 2.2 Pharmacological Strategies for Treatment of In Vitro CNS Trauma

Agent	Site or Mechanism of Action	Model	Protective?	Source
NMDA Glutamate Receptor Antagonists				
Ketamine	Noncompetitive	Rapid acceleration	Yes	Lucas and Wolf (1991)
Dextrorphan	Noncompetitive	Stylet transection	Yes	Tecoma et al. (1989)
MK-801	Noncompetitive	Stylet transection	Yes	Regan and Choi (1994)
MK-801	Noncompetitive	Stylet transection	No	Shah et al. (1997)
MK-801	Noncompetitive	Stylet transection	Yes	Mitchell et al. (1995)
MK-801	Noncompetitive	Punch transection	Yes	Faden et al. (1997)
MK-801	Noncompetitive	Punch transection	Yes	Mukhin et al. (1998)
MK-801	Noncompetitive	Stretch	Yes	Zhao et al. (1998)
D-APV	Competitive	Stylet transection	Yes	Tecoma et al. (1989)
Felbamate	Glycine site	Barotrauma	Yes	Wallis and Panizzon (1995)
AMPA/kainate Glutamate Receptor Antagonists				
CNQX	Competitive	Stylet transection	Yes	Regan and Choi (1994)
CNQX	Competitive	Stylet transection	No	Shah et al. (1997)
NBQX	Competitive	Stylet transection	No	Regan and Choi (1994)
Metabotropic Glutamate Receptor (mGluR) Agonists				
DHPG	mGluR1	Punch transection	No	Mukhin et al. (1996)
L-AP4	Group III mGluR	Punch transection	Yes	Mukhin et al. (1996)
L-SOP	Group III mGluR	Punch transection	Yes	Mukhin et al. (1996)
Metabotropic Glutamate Receptor (mGluR) Antagonists				
MCPG	Nonselective mGluR	Punch transection	Yes	Mukhin et al. (1996)
4CPG	Selective group I mGluR	Punch transection	Yes	Mukhin et al. (1996)
AIDA	Selective group I mGluR	Punch transection	Yes	Mukhin et al. (1997a)
MSOP	Selective group III mGluR	Punch transection	No	Faden et al. (1997)
MAP4	Selective group III mGluR	Punch transection	No	Faden et al. (1997)
A_1 Adenosine Receptor Agonists/Antagonists				
Cyclopentyl adenosine	Specific A_1 adenosine agonist	Stylet transection	Yes	Mitchell et al. (1995)

Agent	Function	Injury model	Protective	Reference
CPT	Specific A_1 adenosine antagonist	Stylet transection	No	Mitchell et al. (1995)
Calcium Channel Blockers, Inhibitors, and Chelators				
Nimodipine	Voltage-sensitive channels	Stylet transection	Yes	Regan and Choi (1994)
Nifedipine	Voltage-sensitive channels	Stylet transection	Yes	Regan and Choi (1994)
Nifedipine	Voltage-sensitive channels	Tissue slice lesion	Yes	Leybaert and Hemptinne (1996)
Cadmium	Voltage-sensitive channels	Tissue slice lesion	No	Leybaert and Hemptinne (1996)
Flunarizine	Voltage-sensitive channels	Tissue slice lesion	No	Leybaert and Hemptinne (1996)
Cobalt	Voltage-sensitive channels	Stylet transection	Yes	Regan and Choi (1994)
Diltiazem	Voltage-sensitive channels	Stylet transection	No	Regan and Choi (1994)
Thapsigargin	Inhibitor of Ca^{2+} storage	Tissue slice lesion	No	Leybaert and Hemptinne (1996)
Dantrolene	Inhibitor of Ca^{2+} release	Tissue slice lesion	Yes	Leybaert and Hemptinne (1996)
EGTA	Chelating agent	Fluid shear stress	Yes	Triyoso and Good (1999)
Sodium Channel/Pump Blockers				
Tetrodotoxin	Channel blockers	Compression	Yes	Agrawal and Fehlings (1996)
Procaine	Channel blockers	Compression	Yes	Agrawal and Fehlings (1996)
Oubain	Na^+-K^+-ATPase inhibitor	Compression	No	Agrawal and Fehlings (1996)
Amiloride	Na^+-H^+ exchange blocker	Compression	Yes	Agrawal and Fehlings (1996)
Harmaline	Na^+-H^+ exchange blocker	Compression	Yes	Agrawal and Fehlings (1996)
Benzamil	Na^+-Ca^{2+} exchange blocker	Compression	No	Agrawal and Fehlings (1996)
Bepridil	Na^+-Ca^{2+} exchange blocker	Compression	No	Agrawal and Fehlings (1996)
Protease Inhibitors				
Calpain inhibitor II	Inhibits calpain proteases	Stretch	Yes	Zhao et al. (1998)
Z-D-DCB	Pan caspase-inhibitor	Stretch	No	Zhao et al. (1998)
Bcl-2[20–34] peptide	unknown	Barotrauma	Yes	Panizzon et al. (1998)
BAF	Pan caspase-inhibitor	Punch transection	Yes	Allen et al. (1999)
z-DEVD-fmk	Caspase-3 inhibitor	Punch transection	Yes	Allen et al. (1999)
z-YVAD-fmk	Caspase-1 inhibitor	Punch transection	No	Allen et al. (1999)
Inhibitors of G Protein Activation				
Pertussis toxin	Specific inhibitor of GTP hydrolysis	Fluid shear stress	Yes	Triyoso and Good (1999)

(continued)

TABLE 2.2 (continued)

Agent	Site or Mechanism of Action	Model	Protective?	Source
Antisense Oligonucleotides				
Against: NMDAR1	Downregulate target protein	Punch transection	Yes	Mukhin et al. (1998)
Against: mGluR1	Downregulate target protein	Punch transection	Yes	Mukhin et al. (1996)
Against: mGluR5	Downregulate target protein	Punch transection	No	Mukhin et al. (1996)
Against: GFAP	Downregulate target protein	Stylet transection	Yes	Lefrancois et al. (1997)
Antioxidants and Inhibitors of Lipid Peroxidation				
Methylprednisolone	Inhibits lipid peroxidation	Dendritic transection	Yes	Rosenberg-Schaffer and Lucas (1993)
U74389F	Inhibits lipid peroxidation	Stylet transection	Yes	Regan and Panter (1995)
U74500A	Inhibits lipid peroxidation	Stylet transection	Yes	Regan and Panter (1995)
PEG-superoxide dismutase	Antioxidant	Stretch (neurons)	No	McKinney et al. (1996)
PEG-superoxide dismutase	Antioxidant	Stretch (endothelial cells)	Yes	McKinney et al. (1996)
Superoxide dismutase	Antioxidant	Stylet transection	Yes	Shah et al. (1997)
N-acetylcysteine	Antioxidant	Stretch	Yes	Lamb et al. (1997)
Vitamin E phosphate	Antioxidant	Stretch	Yes	Lamb et al. (1997)
Vitamin E succinate	Antioxidant	Stretch	Yes	Lamb et al. (1997)
Vitamin E	Antioxidant	Stretch	Yes	Lamb et al. (1997)
Melatonin	Antioxidant	Stretch	Yes	Lamb et al. (1997)
Tin-protoporphyrin	Antioxidant (metalloporphyrin)	Barotrauma	Yes	Panizzon et al. (1996)
Tin-mesoporphyrin	Antioxidant (metalloporphyrin)	Barotrauma	Yes	Panizzon et al. (1996)
Zinc-protoporphyrin	Antioxidant (metalloporphyrin)	Barotrauma	Yes	Panizzon et al. (1996)
Dimethyl sulfoxide (DMSO)	Solvent, antioxidant	Stylet transection	Yes	Shah et al. (1997)
Methyl-L-arginine	Inhibits nitric oxide synthase	Barotrauma	Yes	Wallis et al. (1996)
Hemoglobin	Inhibits nitric oxide synthase	Barotrauma	Yes	Wallis et al. (1996)
L-NAME	Inhibits nitric oxide synthase	Fluid shear stress	Yes	Triyoso and Good (1999)
Inhibitors of mono- and poly-ADP-ribosylation				
Nicotinamide	Multiple: may prevent cell	Barotrauma	Yes	Wallis et al. (1996)
3-amino-benzamide	Energy failure and provide	Barotrauma	Yes	Wallis et al. (1996)

3-methoxybenzamide	Microtubule stabilization	Barotrauma	Yes	Wallis et al. (1996)
m-Indobenzylguanidine		Barotrauma	Yes	Wallis et al. (1996)
Novobiocin		Barotrauma	Yes	Wallis et al. (1996)
Lipoxygenase and Leukotriene Inhibitors				
Azelastine	Leukotriene LTC4 inhibitor	Barotrauma	Yes	Girard et al. (1996)
MK-571	Leukotriene LTD4 inhibitor	Barotrauma	Yes	Girard et al. (1996)
MK-886	5-lipoxygenase inhibitor	Barotrauma	Yes	Girard et al. (1996)
Inhibitors of DNA/RNA Transcription or Protein Translation				
Cyclohexamide	Protein synthesis inhibitor	Fluid shear stress	Yes	Triyoso and Good (1999)
Cyclohexamide	Protein synthesis inhibitor	Stylet transection	Yes	Shah et al. (1997)
Cyclohexamide	Protein synthesis inhibitor	Punch transection	Yes	Allen et al. (1999)
Actinomycin D	RNA synthesis inhibitor	Stylet transection	Yes	Shah et al. (1997)
Modulators of Intercellular Communication				
Halothane	Gap junction blocker	Tissue slice lesion	Yes	Leybaert and Hemptinne (1996)
Octanol	Gap junction blocker	Tissue slice lesion	Yes	Leybaert and Hemptinne (1996)
Paraffin oil	Increases concentration of released substances in extracellular space	Tissue slice lesion	No	Leybaert and Hemptinne (1996)
Nonpharmacological: Hypothermia				
17°C (2 h)	Multiple: may reduce levels of excitatory neurotransmitters and inhibit protease activation	Microbeam dendrotomy	Yes	Lucas et al. (1990)
17°C (2 h +rewarming)		Microbeam dendrotomy	Yes	Lucas et al. (1994)

competitive (D-APV, D-2-amino-5-phosphonovalerate, $EC_{50} \cong 10 \, \mu M$) NMDA antagonists following stylet transection injury in neuronal + glial cell cultures. The anticonvulsant felbamate (2-phenyl-1,3-propanediol dicarbamate), an antagonist of the NMDA-associated glycine site, provided significant CA1 neuronal protection ($EC_{50} = 136 \, mg/L$) to organotypic hippocampal slice preparations following fluid percussion barotrauma injury (Wallis and Panizzon, 1995). In models of stylet transection injury, Regan and Choi (1994) and Mitchell et al. (1995) reported that the noncompetitive NMDA antagonist MK-801 (dizocilpine) (3 to $10 \, \mu M$) attenuated neuronal death. Similarly, Faden and colleagues found that MK-801 provided protection against LDH release across a range of concentrations ($EC_{50} = 55 \, nM$) in neuronal + glial cultures in their mechanical punch transection model (Faden et al., 1997; Mukhin et al., 1998). In addition, these investigators also found that significant protection was afforded when functional NMDA receptors were downregulated with an antisense oligonucleotide directed against the NMDAR1 subunit (Mukhin et al., 1998). Our laboratory has also reported that MK-801 ($50 \, \mu M$) significantly attenuated LDH release by 26% after stretch injury in neuronal + glial cocultures (Zhao et al., 1998). However, in a model of stylet transection injury to hippocampal cultures, Shah and colleagues (1997) found that pretreatment with the combination of MK-801 ($10 \, \mu M$) and CNQX ($30 \, \mu M$) provided no protection against cell death when naive cultures were exposed to the extracellular fluid from the traumatized cultures. Interestingly, when the same concentrations of MK-801 and CNQX were prepared in the solvent dimethyl sulfoxide (DMSO; 0.1%), a significant protective effect was observed that was almost identical to the protective effect of DMSO alone. Thus, the authors concluded that this protective effect was attributed solely to DMSO, perhaps due to its antioxidant properties (Shah et al., 1997). Pharmacological modulation of glutamate release also provides neuroprotection. For example, the ribonucleoside adenosine causes presynaptic inhibition of glutamate release (Thompson et al., 1992; Yoon and Rothman, 1991), and treatment with the specific A_1 adenosine receptor agonist CPA (cyclopentyl adenosine; $10 \, \mu M$) significantly attenuated neuronal loss after stylet transection injury while the specific A_1 adenosine receptor antagonist CPT (cyclopentyl-1,3-dimethylxanthine; $1 \, \mu M$) exacerbated cell death (Mitchell et al., 1995).

In addition to excessive glutamate stimulation of NMDA ionotropic glutamate receptors, prolonged activation of non-NMDA ionotropic glutamate receptors, that is, AMPA/kainate receptors, may also contribute to neuronal pathology after traumatic CNS injury (see Chapter 4 for an extensive review of the various glutamate receptor subtypes). The AMPA/kainate ionophore permits Na^+ influx and K^+ efflux from cells (Foster and Fagg, 1987) and is also thought to be associated with Ca^{2+} influx (Iino et al., 1990). However, to date few investigations have examined the role of AMPA/kainate receptors in the pathobiology of traumatic CNS injury. In vitro, Regan and Choi (1994) employed transection injury to neuronal cell cultures and reported that the competitive AMPA/kainate receptor antagonist 6-cyano-7-nitro-quinoxaline-2,3-dione (CNQX, 10 to $100 \, \mu M$) provided about 50% protection against neuronal damage. However, much of the neuroprotective effect may have been due to nonselective antagonism of NMDA receptors as no additional protective effects were observed when MK-801 was added with CNQX. Moreover, the related quinoxalinedione NBQX [2,3-dihydroxy-6-nitro-7-sulfamoylbenzol(F)quinoxaline], which does not share an affinity with NMDA receptors, failed to provide neuroprotection after transection injury (Regan and Choi, 1994).

In addition to the important role of ionotropic glutamate receptors in brain injury, increasing evidence indicates that G protein-coupled metabotropic glutamate receptors (mGluR) may also be important modulators of cell pathology in CNS injury. For example, antagonists of group I mGluR (mGluR1 and mGluR5) have been shown to provide neuroprotection after traumatic brain injury in vivo (Gong et al., 1995), whereas group I mGluR agonists exacerbate damage after traumatic brain injury (Mukhin et al., 1996). In vitro, LDH release after mechanical punch injury to neuronal + glial cultures was exacerbated by the mGluR1 agonist DHPG [(R,S)-3,5-dihydroxyphenylglycine], whereas the nonselective mGluR antagonist MCPG ((+)-α-methyl-4-carboxyphenylglycine) attenuated this effect (Mukhin et al., 1996). LDH release in this trauma model was also attenuated with the more selective group I antagonists 4CPG [(S)-4-carboxyphenylglycine] (Mukhin et al., 1996) and AIDA [(±)-1-aminoindan-1,5-dicarboxylic acid] (Mukhin et al., 1997b). To further examine the role of mGluR1 and mGluR5 group I receptors, cell cultures were treated with antisense oligonucleotides directed at either the mGluR1 or mGluR5 receptor. Mukhin et al. (1996) found that downregulation of mGluR1, but not mGluR5, provided significant protection against injury-induced LDH release.

Activation of group II mGluR (mGluR2 and mGluR3) and group III mGluR (mGluR4, mGluR6, mGluR7, and mGluR8) appears to provide a neuroprotective effect by presynaptic inhibition of glutamate release (Pin and Duvoisin, 1995). Using their in vitro model of mechanical punch injury (Mukhin et al., 1996), Faden and colleagues (1997) examined the effects of a variety of group III mGluR agonists and antagonists on cell viability after injury in neuronal + glial cell cultures. The relatively specific group III mGluR agonists L-AP4 [L-(+)-2-amino-4-phosphono-butyric acid] or L-SOP (L-serine-O-phosphate) provided significant neuroprotection (EC_{50} = 0.34 μM and 6 μM, respectively) as measured by LDH assay and with the vital dye ethidium homodimer. In contrast, treatment with the group III mGluR antagonists MSOP (α-methylserine-O-phosphate) or MAP4 (α-methyl-AP4) caused a significant and dose-dependent exacerbation of LDH release after injury that was attenuated by the addition of L-AP4 or L-SOP. Importantly, MSOP and MAP4 were not neurotoxic to uninjured control cultures (Faden et al., 1997).

Calcium Channel Blockers

Numerous investigations have provided compelling evidence that alterations in calcium homeostasis is an important pathological sequela in a variety of CNS injuries and neurodegenerative diseases (for reviews see McIntosh et al., 1997; Nicotera et al., 1992; Siesjo and Bengtsson, 1989; Tymianski and Tator, 1996). In addition, calcium channel blockers have been used to attenuate various pathologies associated with traumatic brain injury in vivo (Bodie et al., 1993; McBurney et al., 1992; Okiyama et al., 1992; Verweij et al., 1997). The role of calcium channel blockade on neuronal function and viability after mechanical trauma in vitro has also been investigated recently. For example, in a model of stylet transection injury to neuronal cell cultures, Regan and Choi (1994) found that the dihydropyridine voltage-sensitive calcium channel antagonists nimodipine (10 or 30 μM) or nifedipine (100 μM) afforded neuroprotection and that the combination of nimodipine or nifedipine with MK-801 resulted in an additive neuroprotection. Cobalt (100 μM), an inorganic calcium channel antagonist was weakly, but significantly, protective, whereas diltiazem, a benzothiazepine calcium channel antagonist, provided no protection up to its highest nontoxic concentration (30 μM) (Regan and Choi, 1994). Leybaert and Hemptinne (1996) examined the effects of a variety of voltage- and receptor-mediated calcium channel blockers on injury-induced changes in intracellular free calcium using a blunt lesion model of mechanical trauma to spinal cord organotypic tissue slice preparations. These investigators found that nifedipine (10 μM) reduced injury-induced increases in free calcium concentrations (detected by fura-2) by almost 25%. However, cadmium (50 μM), an L-, N-, and P-type calcium channel blocker, and flunarizine (10 μM), a nonspecific calcium channel blocker, were ineffective in reducing injury-induced increases in intracellular free calcium. Interestingly, MK-801 (100 μM) had no effect on injury-induced intracellular free calcium concentrations in this model. Thus, the authors suggest the possibility that the NMDA receptor may not be a major source of excessive calcium flux after primary mechanical injury and that the neuroprotective benefits of MK-801 observed in vivo may not involve inhibition of calcium entry. Leybaert and Hemptinne (1996) also reported that thapsigargin (1 μM), an inhibitor of intracellular calcium storage, was ineffective in this model, whereas dantrolene (10 μM), an inhibitor of intracellular calcium release, reduced intracellular calcium levels by nearly 25%. Using a model of fluid shear stress, Triyoso and Good (1999) reported that the chelating agent EGTA (1 mM), provided significant protection against injury-induced LDH release and attenuated apoptotic-like DNA fragmentation.

Although increased calcium concentrations are generally regarded as being detrimental to cell viability and function, Rzigalinski et al. (1997) reported that increased levels of total cell-associated calcium were protective to astrocytes after stretch injury. Thus, knowledge of calcium's role in normal and pathological cell function is far from complete, and the work of Rzigalinski et al. (1997) underscores the importance of examining the effects of mechanical trauma in different cell types (e.g., astrocytes, neurons, endothelial cells).

There is also evidence that increased cellular calcium concentrations after injury may be due in part to increases in intracellular sodium that are mediated by "reverse mode" Na^+–Ca^{2+} exchange (Stys et al., 1992; Ziegelstein et al., 1992). Agrawal and Fehlings (1996) used aneurysm clips to injure (compression injury) dorsal spinal cord columns dissected from rodents to examine the role of Na^+ on compound action potential (CAP) waveforms. CAPs are used to determine nerve conduction velocities and are the summation of all electrically stimulated action potentials of nerve fibers that are recorded from two or more equally spaced electrodes placed along the length of the nerve. These authors found that removal of extracellular Na^+ provided significant protection against the loss of CAP waveform amplitude compared to injured cords bathed in Ringer's solution. Significant protection of the CAP waveform was also afforded by the Na^+ channel blockers tetrodotoxin (TTX; 10 nM) and procaine (1 mM). The Na^+K^+-ATPase pump is important to the maintenance of intracellular Na^+. Oubain (25 μM), a potent Na^+K^+-ATPase pump inhibitor, significantly worsened recovery of the CAP waveform, whereas blockade of the Na^+–H^+ exchanger by amiloride (100 μM) or harmaline (100 μM) was neuroprotective (Agrawal and Fehlings, 1996). Benzamil (100 to 500 μM) and bepridil (50 μM), potent blockers of the Na^+–Ca^{2+} exchanger, were ineffective in this model.

Protease Inhibitors

Recently, two major families of cysteine proteases, the calpains and caspase-3-like proteases, have been the focus of intensive investigation of their roles in mediating cellular dysfunction and/or cell death in numerous pathological conditions. The calcium-activated family of cysteine proteases, the calpains, are found ubiquitously in mammalian cells, are activated after traumatic brain injury (Newcomb et al., 1997; Pike et al., 1998a; Posmantur et al., 1997; Saatman et al., 1996) and are thought to be an important effector of cell death following injury-induced calcium overload. Caspase-3-like proteases, and especially caspase-3, are important effectors of apoptotic cell death in numerous cell types and have recently been found to be activated after traumatic brain injury in vivo (Pike et al., 1998a; Yakovlev et al., 1997). In addition, our laboratory has recently found that both calpains and caspase-3 are activated after in vitro stretch injury in neuronal + glial cocultures (Pike et al., 1999; 2000). We also found that administration of the calpain inhibitor, calpain inhibitor II (37.5 μM), significantly attenuated LDH release by 38% after injury (Zhao et al., 1998). However, while the pan-caspase inhibitor also attenuated LDH release by 19%, this did not reach statistical significance, most likely due to the relatively lower level of caspase-3 activity compared to calpain activity in this model (Zhao et al., 1998).

Products of the *bcl-2* protooncogene family are important regulators of apoptotic cell death and the Bcl-2 protein is a potent suppressor of cell death in many cell types (Reed, 1994). Although the molecular mechanisms of Bcl-2 cellular interaction are complex, several mechanisms of protection afforded by the Bcl-2 protein have been postulated. These include potential regulatory effects on cellular proteases such as calpains and caspases. For example, evidence suggests that Bcl-2 regulates calcium homeostasis (Lam et al., 1994), which could effect calpain activation, and Bcl-2 overexpression in neuronal cells blocks activation of caspase-3-like proteases (Srinivasan et al., 1996). Panizzon and co-workers (1998) examined the effects of the Bcl-2[20–34] peptide sequence in hippocampal slices after fluid percussion barotrauma injury. This peptide sequence is contained within the N-terminal region and deletion of the N-terminus of Bcl-2 exacerbates cell death in fibroblasts (Hunter et al., 1996). When the Bcl-2[20–34] peptide was added to the extracellular perfusion fluid 1 min after trauma, significant neuroprotection of hippocampal CA1 orthodromic and antidromic evoked responses were observed (Panizzon et al., 1998). In addition, Bcl-2^{20-34} also preserved CA1 pyramidal LTP (long-term potentiation) responses after trauma. Importantly, this peptide sequence also provided protection against hypoxic injury as well as exposure to NMDA, nitric oxide, and AMPA (Panizzon et al., 1998), indicating that the protective effects of Bcl-2^{20-34} may extend well beyond those associated with apoptosis (see Chapter 11). Indeed, Bcl-2 overexpression has been shown to attenuate necrotic cell death induced by glutathione depletion (Kane et al., 1995).

Antioxidants and Inhibitors of Lipid Peroxidation

Destructive oxygen free radical formation occurs after numerous CNS injuries and has thus been the focus of numerous in vivo and in vitro investigations (Braughler and Hall, 1992; Clark et al., 1995). Oxygen free radicals can be generated via the arachidonic acid cascade, by mitochondrial disruption, or by neutrophil infiltration into the brain parenchyma. Free radicals cause the formation of lipid peroxides within cell membranes, which alters membrane phospholipids and affects phospholipid-dependent systems and ion gradients. The lipid peroxide inhibitors methylprednisolone and the 21-aminosteroids (lazaroids) have been used effectively in the treatment of experimental and clinical spinal cord injury (Clark et al., 1995; Hall, 1992; Villa and Gorini, 1997). In in vitro mechanical injury models, inhibition of lipid peroxidation has also been shown to be neuroprotective. For example, 30 μg/mL methylprednisolone increased survival of cultured spinal neurons after dendritic transection (Rosenberg-Schaffer and Lucas, 1993). Interestingly, lower (10 or 20 μg/mL) or higher (60 μg/mL) concentrations were ineffective, suggesting a narrow dose range for methylprednisolone treatment. These biphasic drug effects in vitro parallel observations made in vivo where treatment with a single intravenous bolus of 30 mg/kg methylprednisolone, but not lower or higher concentrations, prevented a rise in lactate content in injured cat spinal cord (Braughler and Hall, 1983). For this reason, an intravenous bolus of 30 mg/kg was used for both the second and third National Acute Spinal Cord Injury Study (NASCIS) (Bracken et al., 1990, 1997). Also noteworthy in the in vitro study by Rosenberg-Schaffer and Lucas (1993) was that methylprednisolone was neuroprotective in an environment absent of many factors that would favor lipid peroxidation in vivo, such as hypoxia, acidosis, and vascular changes. This fact led the authors to speculate that the cholesterol-derived methylprednisolone may act as a membrane stabilizer by inserting itself into damaged plasma membranes. In other studies of mechanical trauma, the 21-aminosteroids U74389F (10 μM) and U74500A (1 to 10 μM) were found to provide significant protection against LDH release from murine cortical cultures subjected to stylet transection injury (Regan and Panter, 1995). An additive protection was afforded when MK-801 (10 μM) was coadministered, suggesting that the 21-aminosteroids do not act via NMDA receptor blockade.

Shah et al. (1997) reported that the extracellular fluid collected from traumatized hippocampal cultures injured by stylet transection was toxic to naive cultures and that this toxicity could be attenuated by the antioxidant superoxide dismutase (5 U/mL). Following a moderate level of mechanical stretch injury (6.3 mm deformation) to astrocyte or neuronal + glial cells, polyethylene glycol-conjugated superoxide dismutase (PEG-SOD, 300 U/mL) provided no significant protection against cell injury assayed by propidium iodide (PI) uptake (McKinney et al., 1996). However, this same study found that PEG-SOD did reduce PI uptake by 51% in stretched aortic endothelial cells. In addition, a subsequent study by this group found a number of antioxidants, including N-acetylcysteine, vitamin E phosphate, melatonin, vitamin E succinate, and vitamin E, reduced the level of postinjury phosphatidylcholine (PC) biosynthesis (Lamb et al., 1997). PC biosynthesis is a cellular indicator of membrane repair that occurs after free radical-induced lipid peroxidation. Thus, inhibition of PC biosynthesis may be a more sensitive indicator of the effect of free radical scavengers than PI uptake.

The excitotoxic response that occurs as a result of excessive NMDA receptor activation after trauma is mediated in part by generation of the free radical nitric oxide (NO). Neuronal production of NO can pose a number of challenges to cell survival through generation of peroxynitrite, one of the more potent cellular radicals, and as a mediator of poly-ADP-ribosylation via poly(ADP-ribose) polymerase (PARP) activation and mono-ADP-ribosylation via mono(ADP-ribosyl) transferase (Kawaichi et al., 1981; Moss et al., 1981). Mono- and poly-ADP-ribosylation can affect cell function by enzymatic inhibition, microtubule destabilization, and/or depletion of cellular energy reserves (Brune et al., 1994; Dimmeler et al., 1993; Zhang et al., 1994). For example, activation of PARP causes depletion of NAD and ATP that can lead to cell death due to energy failure (Berger, 1985). Subjecting organotypic hippocampal slices to fluid percussion barotrauma, Wallis and co-workers (1996) found that the NO synthase (NOS) inhibitor methyl-L-arginine (170 μM) and hemoglobin (50 μM) (which directly binds NO) provided significant protection against CA1 neuronal injury. In addition, inhibitors of poly-ADP-ribosylation, nicotinamide (10 mM), 3-aminobenzamide (1 mM), 3-methoxybenzamide (0.5 mM), and of mono-ADP-ribosylation, m-indobenzylguanidine (20 μM) and nivobiocin (95 μM) also provided marked protection against CA1 neuronal cell injury after fluid percussion barotrauma injury (Wallis et al., 1996). The NOS inhibitor L-NAME provided significant protection against LDH release and attenuated apoptotic-like DNA fragmentation in a model of fluid shear stress (Triyoso and Good, 1999).

The metalloporphyrins are a novel class of catalytic antioxidants that are known to have scavenging effects across a variety of reactive oxygen species such as lipid peroxyl, peroxide, peroxynitrite, and superoxide radicals (Patel and Day, 1999). Thus, the development of metalloporphyrins that have specific activities greater than superoxide dismutases have emerged as potential candidates for treatment of numerous diseases and traumas involving free radical production. Panizzon and colleagues (1996) used a model of fluid percussion barotrauma to injure hippocampal tissue slices and examined the neuroprotective effects of several classes of metalloporphyrins. In this model, tin-protoporphyrin (EC_{50} 10 μM), tin-mesoporphyrin (EC_{50} 4 μM), and zinc-protoporphyrin (EC_{50} 32 μM) were each found to provide significant recovery of hippocampal CA1 antidromic population spikes compared to untreated control slices.

Lipoxygenase and Leukotriene Inhibitors

The liberation of arachidonic acid from membrane phospholipids after cellular injury can initiate activation of lipoxygenases which form leukotrienes (e.g., LTA_4, LTB_4, LTC_4, LTD_4, and LTE_4) (Samuelsson et al., 1987). Increased levels of LTC_4 have been observed after cerebral ischemia in animals and humans (Aktan et al., 1991a,b; Moskowitz et al., 1984), and cortical and hippocampal tissue levels of LTC_4 were found to be elevated after lateral fluid percussion brain injury in rats (Dhillon et al., 1996). The deleterious effects of leukotriene production after cerebral ischemia in vivo have been shown to be mediated, at least in part, by increased vasoconstriction and vascular permeability (Aktan et al., 1991a,b). However, these vascular altera-tions are not encountered in in vitro systems. Thus, leukotriene formation is also thought to be associated with the NMDA-mediated excitotoxic response as inhibitors of LTC_4 protect against NMDA-induced injury (Wallis and Panizzon, 1993). In vitro, cultured human astroglial cells had increased levels of LTC_4 (40 to 200 pg/mL) 15 min after fluid percussion barotrauma injury (Shepard et al., 1990). Employing in vitro fluid percussion barotrauma injury to organotypic hippocampal slice preparations, Girard and co-workers (1996) found that the LTC_4 inhibitor azelastine (15 μM) was protective against CA1 neuronal injury. In addition, other leukotriene inhibitors such as the specific LTD_4 receptor antagonist MK-571 (15 μM) and the 5-lipoxygenase inhibitor MK-886 (30 μM) were also neuroprotective in this model (Girard et al., 1996).

Hypothermia

Although the mechanism of protection afforded by hypothermic cooling of the CNS is unknown, several possibilities have been postulated in the literature. For example, in several models of concussive brain injury in vivo, hypothermia has been reported to reduce opening of the blood–brain barrier (Jiang et al., 1992; Smith and Hall, 1996), inflammation (Goss et al., 1995), cerebral ICP (Pomeranz et al., 1993), and motor and cognitive deficits (Dixon et al., 1998). Moderate hypothermia has also been reported to reduce levels of excitatory neurotransmitters such as glutamate and aspartate (Globus et al., 1995; Palmer et al., 1993) and acetylcholine (Lyeth et al., 1993). Hypothermia may also provide protection by inhibition of proteases such as the calpains, which have a high affinity for numerous cytoskeletal proteins such as the neurofilament proteins, microtubule associated protein-2 (MAP-2), and α-spectrin. Indeed, hypothermia has been shown to provide protection against MAP-2 loss after traumatic brain injury in vivo (Taft et al., 1993). In vitro, Lucas and co-workers (1990, 1994) found that hypothermic cooling of cultured spinal neurons to 17°C for 2 h provided significant protection against laser microbeam dendrotomy. Hypothermic protection was maintained even after rewarming to 37°C following 2 h of hypothermia; however, protection was lost when cooling was extended to 6 h (Lucas et al., 1994).

APOPTOTIC CELL DEATH IN MODELS OF MECHANICAL CELL INJURY

Mechanisms of cell death have recently drawn the attention of basic and clinical scientists alike. Although Flemming's (1885) camera lucida drawings were the first to clearly illustrate pathological cells that would today be termed apoptosis (see Majno and Joris, 1995, for a historical review), it was not until recently that an eruption of research into apoptotic cell death occurred. Apoptotic cell death has now been reported after traumatic brain injury (Clark et al., 1997a,b, 1999; Colicos and Dash, 1996; Conti et al., 1996; Eldadah et al., 1996; Fox et al., 1998; Joashi et al., 1999; Kaya et al., 1999; McIntosh et al., 1998b; Newcomb et al., 1999; Pohl et al., 1999; Pravdenkova et al., 1996; Rink et al., 1995; Sinson et al., 1997; Yakovlev et al., 1997), traumatic spinal cord injury (Crowe et al., 1997; Kato et al., 1997), cerebral ischemia (Charriaut-Marlangue et al., 1998), and in a variety of neuro-degenerative diseases including Alzheimer's disease (Anderson et al., 1996) and Huntington's disease (Portera-Cailliau et al., 1995). However, the relative importance of apoptosis (versus necrosis) to overall pathology and morbidity is unknown. Thus, furthering our understanding of apoptotic cascades could result in promising therapeutic opportunities for a diversity of neurobiological disorders including traumatic CNS injuries and neurodegenerative diseases. Importantly, the development of in vitro models of CNS trauma, by allowing more precise control and access to intracellular and extracellular environments, will provide an ideal arena for the study of regulatory mechanisms mediating apoptotic and necrotic cell death after traumatic cell injury.

Although apoptotic cell death has been reported after neurotrauma in vivo, investigation of apoptosis after mechanical injury in vitro has not been extensively characterized. In addition, it should be emphasized that traumatic brain injury in vivo is characterized by *both* necrotic and apoptotic cell death. Therefore, our laboratories have begun to examine cell death by utilizing an assortment of in vitro models to systematically examine apoptosis and necrosis in isolation or in more complex systems where both apoptotic and necrotic cell death occur. These injury paradigms have been developed to examine the effects of different pathological signaling events in relation to necrotic and apoptotic cell death. For example, maitotoxin is a highly potent marine toxin that activates both voltage-sensitive and receptor-mediated calcium channels, resulting in calcium overload and rapid necrotic cell death (Gusovsky and Daly, 1990; Wang et al., 1996; Zhao et al., 1999). In contrast, staurosporine is a broad-range protein kinase inhibitor that induces apoptosis in a variety of in vitro cell systems (Bertrand et al., 1994; Nath et al., 1996; Pike et al., 1998b). Use of these model systems (or other similar necrotic or apoptotic inducers) to reliably induce necrosis or apoptosis provides important systems for comparing biochemical and morphological alterations that occur only during necrosis or apoptosis and after excitotoxic, hypoxic, or mechanical injury whereby both necrotic and apoptotic cell death may occur.

To this end, our laboratory employed the Ellis model of mechanical stretch injury (Ellis et al., 1995) to determine whether stretch injury applied to septo-hippocampal cultures (neuronal + glial) was associated with apoptotic or necrotic nuclear morphological phenotypes (Pike et al., 1999; 2000). Using the vital dye Hoechst 33258, we observed that during the acute postinjury period (1 to 6 h), numerous cell nuclei stained intensely but were necrotic in appearance, that is, hyperchromatic nuclei that maintained normal size and shape as compared to unstretched control cells. In contrast, between 24 h and 5 days after stretch injury, populations of nuclei could be discerned in various stages of apoptotic nuclear disassembly. Nuclei of apoptotic cells appeared shrunken or had fragmented nuclei and formation of discrete apoptotic bodies was clearly evident (Pike et al., 1999; 2000). In addition, other indicators of apoptosis such as caspase-3 activation and DNA ladder formation were also associated with apoptotic nuclear phenotypes but not with necrotic nuclear phenotypes.

Apoptotic cell death was also observed following mechanical punch injury to neuronal + glial cocultures (Allen et al., 1999). Interestingly, mechanical trauma alone resulted in a significant twofold increase in the number of Hoechst 33258-stained nuclei with apoptotic-like characteristics. However, mechanical punch injury to cells with metabolic impairment, induced by 3-nitropropionic acid (3NP) and glucose deprivation (GD), resulted in a fourfold increase in the number of apoptotic cells. Release of LDH into culture medium after trauma + 3NP/GD was attenuated by the administration of the broad-range protein synthesis inhibitor cycloheximide (10 μg/mL), which further suggests a role for apoptosis in this model system (Allen et al., 1999). In addition, the pan-caspase inhibitor BAF (100 μM) and the relatively selective caspase-3 inhibitor z-DEVD-fmk (160 μM) also attenuated trauma + 3NP/GD-induced LDH release. Administration of z-DEVD-fmk decreased the number of apoptotic cells, while the relatively specific caspase-1 inhibitor z-YVAD-fmk was ineffective in this model (Allen et al., 1999).

It has recently been demonstrated that, following traumatic cell injury, apoptotic cell death signals can be propagated through the extracellular milieu. For example, Shah and co-workers (1997) reported that the extracellular fluid collected 5 min after stylet transection to neuronal + glial cocultures induced neuronal apoptotic cell death when naive cultures were bathed in the same medium. Stereotypical apoptotic nuclear phenotypes, including chromatin aggregation and nucleosome formation, were detected with in situ nick translation or Hoechst 33342 (similar to Hoechst 33258 above). Apoptotic cell death in this model was attenuated with DMSO, and by inhibitors of protein synthesis (cycloheximide) and RNA synthesis (actinomycin D). The authors conclude that a yet unknown substance mediated the apoptotic response induced by the extracellular fluid (Shah et al., 1997).

Triyoso and Good (1999) examined the effects of pulsatile shear stress injury using various markers of apoptotic cell death in a differentiated human SH-SY5Y neuroblastoma cell line. These investigators reported that short durations (10 min) of high shear stress (100 dyn/cm^2) produced greater DNA fragmentation than did long durations (90 min) at more moderate levels of shear stress (10 dyn/cm^2). Furthermore, the highest increases in TUNEL-positive cells were observed immediately after shear injury and remained elevated to at least 24 h after the injury. In contrast, increased LDH levels were not detected immediately after injury but increased only at 24 h after shear injury, indicating that plasma membrane integrity was not compromised during the early apoptotic phase but was disturbed during later stages of apoptotic cell death. This also indicates that this model of shear stress does not induce necrotic cell death immediately after injury (Triyoso and Good, 1999). Cycloheximide, pertussis toxin, L-NAME, and EGTA in Ca^{2+}-free medium (inhibitors of protein synthesis, G_o/G_i protein activation, nitric oxide production, and Ca^{2+} influx, respectively) were each effective in attenuating apoptotic-like DNA fragmentation in this model.

The results of the investigations described above indicate that mechanical injury to CNS cultures causes apoptotic cell death in at least three different injury models. Thus, for neurotrauma researchers, in vitro models of traumatic cell injury are an attractive alternative to currently employed pharmacological models of apoptosis. In addition, mechanical cell injury models may facilitate elucidation of cell death mechanisms that may contribute to in vivo necrotic and apoptotic cell death. However, although in vitro pharmacological and mechanical cell injury models provide a simple and more controlled method for studying cell death mechanisms related to in vivo traumatic brain injury, the relative importance of apoptotic cell death to traumatic brain injury will ultimately be determined in the whole animal and in human brain-injured patients.

SUMMARY

The major goal of whole-animal models of traumatic brain or spinal cord injury is to provide valid and reliable models that replicate the gross anatomical, physiological, and neurobehavioral responses observed in the clinical setting. A major drawback of these models is that injury mechanisms caused by the primary injury (blunt mechanical trauma) are difficult to study as they are complicated by a host of secondary events (anoxia, hypoxia, hemorrhage, edema, etc.) that exacerbate the initial injury response. Thus, to address this problem, several in vitro model systems have been developed that allow researchers to examine the effects of mechanical trauma in a wide variety of cell types (e.g., neurons, glia, cocultures, and human cell lines) and tissues (e.g., hippocampal and spinal cord slices). In addition, these models allow precise control over extracellular environmental conditions and provide an ideal system for high-throughput pharmacological screening that is unaffected by systemic complications such as systemic metabolism and blood–brain barrier permeability.

While there are numerous advantages to in vitro traumatic injury models, these models are not meant to replace current in vivo systems. In vitro models of traumatic CNS injury will never mimic the clinical pathology that is an important feature of in vivo models. Instead, in vitro models serve to complement in vivo models and increase knowledge of traumatic CNS pathology by facilitating understanding of the pathophysiological mechanisms that ultimately contribute to cellular dysfunction and death. It is hoped that use of in vitro mechanical injury models will facilitate more rapid screening of a greater number of candidate pharmacotherapeutics designed for selective application in animal traumatic brain injury models that will ultimately lead to judicious administration in the human head-injured patient.

ACKNOWLEDGMENTS

A portion of the work reviewed in this chapter was supported by NIH grants NINDS RO1-NS21458 and F32-NS10857 and by the State of Florida Brain and Spinal Cord Injury Rehabilitation Trust Fund (BSCIRTF).

ABBREVIATIONS

AIDA	$(\pm)$-1-Aminoindand-1,5-dicarboxylic acid
AMPA	α-Amino-3-hydroxy-5-methyl-4-isoxazole-4-propionic acid
ATP	Adenosine triphosphate
CAP	Compound action potential
CNS	Central nervous system
CPA	Cyclopentyl adenosine
CSID	Cell shearing injury device
4CPG	(S)-4-carboxyphenylglycine
CPT	Clopentyl-1,3-dimethylxanthine
CNQX	6-Cyano-7-nitroquinoxaline-2,3-dione
DHPG	(R,S)-3,5-Dihydroxyphenylglycine
DMSO	Dimethylsulfoxide
DNA	Deoxyribonucleic acid
EGTA	Ethylene-bis(oxyethyleneitrilo)tetraacetic acid
FDA	Fluorescein diacetate
GD	Glucose deprivation
ICP	Intracranial pressure
L-AP4	L-($+$)-2-Amino-4-phosphonobutyric acid
LDH	Lactate dehydrogenase
L-NAME	N^{ω}-nitro-L-arginine methyl ester
L-SOP	L-Serine-O-phosphate
LTP	Long-term potentiation
MAP-2	Microtubule-associated protein-2
MAP4	α-Methyl-AP4

MCPG	(+)-α-Methyl-4-carboxyphenylglycine
mGluR	Metabotropic glutamate receptors
MSOP	α-Methylserine-O-phosphate
NAD	Nicotinamide adenine dinucleotide
NBQX	2,3-Hydroxy-6-nitro-7-sulfamoylbenzol(F)quinoxaline
NMDA	N-methyl-D-aspartate
3NP	3-Nitropropionic acid
NO	Nitric oxide
NOS	Nitric oxide synthase
PARP	poly(ADP-ribose) polymerase
PC	Phosphatidylcholine
PEG-SOD	Polyethylene glycol-conjugated superoxide dismutase
PI	Propidium iodide
RAI	Rapid acceleration injury
RNA	Ribonucleic acid
TBI	Traumatic brain injury
TTX	Tetrodotoxin
TUNEL	Terminal deoxynucleotidyl transferase-mediated dUTP-biotin nick end labeling
UV	Ultraviolet

REFERENCES

J. H. Adams, D. I. Graham, L. S. Murray, and G. Scott, *Ann. Neurol.*, 12, 557–563 (1982).

S. K. Agrawal and M. G. Fehlings, *J. Neurosci.*, 16(2), 545–552 (1996).

S. Aktan, C. Aykut, and S. Ercan, *Prostaglandins Leukot. Essent. Fatty Acids*, 43(4), 247–249 (1991a).

S. Aktan, C. Aykut, S. Oktay, B. Yegen, E. Keles, I. Aykac, and S. Ercan, *Prostaglandins Leukot. Essent. Fatty Acids*, 42(1), 67–71 (1991b).

J. W. Allen, S. M. Knoblach, and A. I. Faden, *FASEB J.*, 13, 1875–1882 (1999).

A. J. Anderson, J. H. Su, and C. W. Cotman, *J. Neurosci.*, 16, 1710–1719 (1996).

N. A. Berger, *Radiat. Res.*, 101, 4–15 (1985).

R. Bertrand, E. Solary, P. O'Connor, K. W. Kohn, and Y. Pommier, *Exp. Cell Res.*, 211, 314–321 (1994).

H. Bodie, K. Fu, A. Sanit, and D. Hovda, *J. Neurotrauma*, 10, S161 (1993).

M. B. Bracken, M. J. Shepard, W. F. Collins, T. R. Holford, W. Young, D. S. Baskin, H. M. Eisenberg, E. Flamm, L. Leo-Summers, J. Maroon, L. F. Marshall, P. L. Perot, J. Piepmeier, V. K. H. Sonntag, F. C. Wagner, J. E. Wilberger, and H. R. Winn, *N. Engl. J. Med.*, 322, 1405–1411 (1990).

M. B. Bracken, M. J. Shepard, T. R. Holford, L. Leo-Summers, E. F. Aldrich, M. Fazi, M. Fehlings, D. L. Herr, P. W. Hitchon, L. F. Marshall, R. P. Nockels, V. Pascale, P. L. Perot, J. Piepmeier, V. K. H. Sonntag, F. Wagner, J. E. Wilberger, H. R. Winn, and W. Young, *J. Am. Med. Assoc.*, 277(20), 1597–1604 (1997).

J. M. Braughler and E. D. Hall, *J. Neurosurg.*, 59, 256–261 (1983).

J. M. Braughler and E. D. Hall, *J. Neurotrauma*, 9, S1–S7 (1992).

B. Brune, S. Dimmeler, Y. Molina, L. Vedia, and E. G. Lapetina, *Life Sci.*, 54, 61–70 (1994).

R. S. Cargill and L. E. Thibault, *J. Neurotrauma*, 13, 396–407 (1996).

C. Charriaut-Marlangue, S. Remolleau, D. Aggoun-Zouaoui, and Y. Ben-Ari, *Biomed. Pharmacother.*, 52(6), 264–269 (1998).

R. S. Clark, J. Chen, S. C. Watkins, P. M. Kochanek, M. Chen, R. A. Stetler, J. E. Loeffert, and S. H. Graham, *J. Neurosci.*, 17(23), 9172–9182 (1997a).

R. S. Clark, P. M. Kochanek, C. E. Dixon, M. Chen, D. W. Marion, S. Heineman, S. T. DeKosky, and S. H. Graham, *J. Neurotrauma*, 14(4), 179–189 (1997b).

R. S. Clark, P. M. Kochanek, M. Chen, S. C. Watkins, D. W. Marion, J. Chen, R. L. Hamilton, J. E. Loeffert, and S. H. Graham, *FASEB J.*, 13(8), 813–821 (1999).

W. M. Clark, S. Hazel, and B. M. Coull, *Drugs*, 50, 971–983 (1995).

M. A. Colicos and P. K. Dash, *Brain Res.*, 739(1–2), 120–131 (1996).

A. C. Conti, R. Raghupathi, J. Q. Trojanowski, and T. K. McIntosh, *J. Neurosci.*, 18(15), 5663–5672 (1998).

M. J. Crowe, J. C. Bresnahan, S. L. Shuman, J. N. Masters, and M. S. Beattie, *Nat. Med.*, 3, 73–76 (1997).

H. S. Dhillon, J. M. Dose, and M. R. Prasad, *J. Neurotrauma*, 13(12), 781–789 (1996).

S. Dimmeler, M. Ankarcrona, P. Nicotera, and B. Brune, *J. Immunol.*, 150, 2964–2971 (1993).

C. E. Dixon, B. G. Lyeth, J. T. Povlishock, R. L. Findling, R. J. Hamm, A. Marmarou, H. F. Young, and R. L. Hayes, *J. Neurosurg.*, 67, 110–119 (1987).

C. E. Dixon, C. G. Markgraf, F. Angileri, B. R. Pike, B. Wolfson, J. K. Newcomb, M. M. Bismar, A. J. Blanco, G. L. Clifton, and R. L. Hayes, *J. Neurotrauma*, 15(2), 95–103 (1998).

E. F. Ellis, J. S. McKinney, K. A. Willoughby, S. Liang, and J. T. Povlishock, *J. Neurotrauma*, 12, 325–339 (1995).

B. A. Eldadah, A. G. Yakovlev, and A. I. Faden, *Nucleic Acids Res.*, 24(20), 4092–4093 (1996).

A. I. Faden, S. A. Ivanova, A. G. Yakovlev, and A. G. Mukhin, *J. Neurotrauma*, 14(12), 885–895 (1997).

W. Flemming, *Arch. Anat. EntwGesch.*, 221–224 (1885).

A. Foster and G. Fagg, *Nature*, 329, 395–396 (1987).

G. B. Fox, L. Fan, R. A. Levasseur, and A. I. Faden, *J. Neurotrauma*, 15(8), 599–614 (1998).

R. F. Frankowski, *Adv. Psychosom. Med.*, 16, 153–172 (1986).

T. A. Gennarelli and L. E. Thibault, "Biological Models of Head Injury," in J. Povlishock and D. Becker, Eds., *Central Nervous System Trauma Status Report*, National Institute of Neurological and Communicative Disorders and Strokes, National Institutes of Health, Bethesda, MD, 1985, pp. 392–405.

J. Girard, K. Panizzon, and R. A. Wallis, *Eur. J. Pharmacol.*, 300, 43–49 (1996).

M. Y. Globus, O. Alonso, W. D. Dietrich, R. Busto, and M. D. Ginsberg, *J. Neurochem.*, 65(4), 1704–1711 (1995).

Q. Z. Gong, T. M. Delahunty, R. J. Hamm, and B. G. Lyeth, *Neurosci. Lett.*, 203, 211–213 (1995).

J. R. Goss, S. D. Styren, P. D. Miller, P. M. Kochanek, A. M. Palmer, D. W. Marion, and S. T. DeKosky, *J. Neurotrauma*, 12(2), 159–167 (1995).

F. Gusovsky and J. W. Daly, *Biochem. Pharmacol.*, 39, 1633–1639 (1990).

E. D. Hall, *J. Neurosurg.*, 76, 13–22 (1992).

R. L. Hayes, L. W. Jenkins, and B. G. Lyeth, *J. Neurotrauma*, 9(Suppl. 1), S173–187 (1992).

J. J. Hunter, B. L. Bond, and T. G. Parslow, *Mol. Cell Biol.*, 16(3), 877–883 (1996).

M. Iino, S. Ozawa, and K. Tsuki, *J. Physiol.*, 424, 151–165 (1990).

J. Y. Jiang, B. G. Lyeth, M. Z. Kapasi, L. W. Jenkins, and J. T. Povlishock, *Acta Neuropathol.*, 84(5), 495–500 (1992).

U. C. Joashi, K. Greenwood, D. L. Taylor, M. Kozma, N. D. Mazarakis, A. D. Edwards, and H. Mehmet, *Eur. J. Neurosci.*, 11(1), 91–100 (1999).

K. H. Jones and A. J. Senft, *J. Histochem. Cytochem.*, 33, 77–79 (1985).

D. J. Kane, T. Ord, R. Anton, and D. E. Bredesen, *J. Neurosci.*, 40, 269–275 (1995).

H. Kato, G. K. Kanellopoulos, S. Matsuo, Y. J. Wu, M. F. Jacquin, C. Y. Hsu, D. W. Choi, and N. T. Kouchoukos, *J. Thorac. Cardiovasc. Surg.*, 114, 609–618 (1997).

M. Kawaichi, K. Ueda, and O. Hayaishi, *J. Biol. Chem.*, 256, 9483–9489 (1981).

S. S. Kaya, A. Mahmood, Y. Li, E. Yavuz, M. Goksel, and M. Chopp, *Brain Res.*, 818(1), 23–33 (1999).

M. Lam, G. Dubyak, L. Chen, G. Nunez, R. L. Miesfeld, and C. W. Distelhorst, *Proc. Natl. Acad. Sci. USA*, 91, 6569–6573 (1994).

R. G. Lamb, C. C. Harper, J. S. McKinney, B. A. Rzigalinski, and E. F. Ellis, *J. Neurochem.*, 68, 1904–1910 (1997).

M. C. LaPlaca and L. E. Thibault, *Ann. Biomed. Eng.*, 25, 665–677 (1997).

M. C. LaPlaca, V. M. Lee, and L. E. Thibault, *J. Neurotrauma*, 14, 355–368 (1997).

T. Lefrancois, C. Fages, M. Peschanski, and M. Tardy, *J. Neurosci.*, 17(11), 4121–4128 (1997).

L. Leybaert and A. Hemptinne, *Exp. Brain Res.*, 112, 392–402 (1996).

J. H. Lucas and A. Wolf, *Brain Res.*, 543, 181–193 (1991).

J. H. Lucas, D. G. Emery, G. Wang, L. J. Rosenberg-Schaffer, R. S. Jordan, and G. W. Gross, *J. Neurotrauma*, 11(1), 35–61 (1994).

J. H. Lucas, G. F. Wang, and G. W. Gross, *Brain Res.*, 517(1–2), 354–357 (1990).

B. G. Lyeth, J. Y. Jiang, S. E. Robinson, H. Guo, and L. W. Jenkins, *Mol. Chem. Neuropathol.*, 18(3), 247–256 (1993).

G. Majno and I. Joris, *Am. J. Pathol.*, 146(1), 3–15 (1995).

R. N. McBurney, D. Daly, J. B. Fischer, L. Y. Hu, K. Subbarao, A. G. Knapp, K. Kobayashi, L. Margolin, N. L. Reddy, S. M. Goldin, *J. Neurotrauma*, 9, S531–S543 (1992).

T. K. McIntosh, *J. Neurotrauma*, 10(3), 215–261 (1993).

T. K. McIntosh, K. E. Saatman, and R. Raghupathi, *Neuroscientist*, 3, 169–175 (1997).

T. K. McIntosh, M. Juhler, and T. Wieloch, *J. Neurotrauma*, 15(10), 731–769 (1998a).

T. K. McIntosh, K. E. Saatman, R. Raghupathi, D. I. Graham, D. W. Smith, V. M. Lee, and J. Q. Trojanowski, *Neuropathol. Appl. Neurobiol.*, 24(4), 251–267 (1998b).

J. S. McKinney, K. A. Willoughby, S. Liang, and E. F. Ellis, *Stroke*, 27, 934–940 (1996).

H. L. Mitchell, W. A. Frisella, R. W. Brooker, and K.-W. Yoon, *Neurosurgery*, 36(5), 1003–1008 (1995).

B. Morrison III, D. F. Meaney, and T. K. McIntosh, *Ann. Biomed. Eng.*, 26, 381–390 (1998a).

B. Morrison III, K. E. Saatman, D. F. Meaney, and T. K. McIntosh, *J. Neurotrauma*, 15(11), 911–928 (1998b).

M. A. Moskowitz, K. J. Kiwak, K. Hekimian, and L. Levine, *Science*, 224(4651), 886–889 (1984).

J. Moss and S. J. Stanley, *J. Biol. Chem.*, 256, 7830–7883 (1981).

A. Mukhin, L. Fan, and A. I. Faden, *J. Neurosci.*, 16, 6012–6020 (1996).

A. G. Mukhin, S. A. Ivanova, and A. I. Faden, *Neuroreport*, 8, 2561–2566 (1997a).

A. G. Mukhin, S. A. Ivanova, S. M. Knoblach, and A. I. Faden, *J. Neurotrauma*, 14(9), 651–663 (1997b).

A. G. Mukhin, S. A. Ivanova, J. W. Allen, and A. I. Faden, *J. Neurosci. Res.*, 51, 748–758 (1998).

E. J. Murphy and L. A. Horrocks, "Models of Neurotrauma Ex Vivo," in S. K. Salzman and A. I. Faden, Eds., *The Neurobiology of Central Nervous System Trauma*, Oxford University Press, New York, 1994, pp. 28–40.

R. Nath, K. J. Raser, D. Stafford, I. Hajimohammadreza, A. Posner, H. Allen, R. V. Talanian, P. Yuen, R. B. Glibertsen, and K. K. W. Wang, *Biochem. J.*, 319, 683–690 (1996).

J. K. Newcomb, A. Kampfl, R. M. Posmantur, X. Zhao, B. R. Pike, S. J. Liu, G. L. Clifton, and R. L. Hayes, *J. Neurotrauma*, 14(6), 369–383 (1997).

J. K. Newcomb, X. Zhao, B. R. Pike, and R. L. Hayes, *Exp. Neurol.*, 158, 76–88 (1999).

P. Nicotera, G. Bellomo, and S. Orrenius, *Annu. Rev. Pharmacol. Toxicol.*, 32, 449–470 (1992).

K. Okiyama, D. H. Smith, M. J. Thomas, and T. K. McIntosh, *J. Neurosurg.*, 77, 607–615 (1992).

A. M. Palmer, D. W. Marion, M. L. Botscheller, and E. E. Redd, *J. Neurotrauma*, 10(4), 363–372 (1993).

K. L. Panizzon, B. E. Dwyer, R. N. Nishimura, and R. A. Wallis, *Neuroreport*, 7(2), 662–666 (1996).

K. L. Panizzon, D. Shin, S. Frautschy, and R. A. Wallis, *Neuroreport*, 9, 4131–4136 (1998).

M. Patel and B. J. Day, *Trends Pharmacol. Sci.*, 20(9), 359–364 (1999).

B. R. Pike, X. Zhao, J. K. Newcomb, R. M. Posmantur, K. K. W. Wang, and R. L. Hayes, *Neuroreport*, 9, 2437–2442 (1998a).

B. R. Pike, X. Zhao, J. K. Newcomb, K. K. W. Wang, R. M. Posmantur, and R. L. Hayes, *J. Neurosci. Res.*, 52, 505–520 (1998b).

B. R. Pike, X. Zhao, J. K. Newcomb, and R. L. Hayes, *J. Neurochemistry*, 72(Suppl.), S53 (1999).

B. R. Pike, X. Zhao, J. K. Newcomb, C. C. Glenn, D. K. Andrson, and R. L. Hayes, *J. Neurotrauma*, 17(4), 283–298 (2000).

J.-P. Pin and R. Duvoisin, *Neuropharmacology*, 34, 1–26 (1995).

D. Pohl, P. Bittigau, M. J. Ishimaru, D. Stadthaus, C. Hubner, J. W. Olney, L. Turski, and C. Ikonomidou, *Proc. Natl. Acad. Sci. USA*, 96(5), 2508–2513 (1999).

S. Pomeranz, P. Safar, A. Radovsky, S. A. Tisherman, H. Alexander, and W. Stezoski, *J. Neurosurg.*, 79(2), 241–251 (1993).

C. Portera-Cailliau, J. C. Hedreen, D. L. Price, and V. E. Koliatsos, *J. Neurosci.*, 15, 3775–3787 (1995).

R. M. Posmantur, A. Kampfl, R. Siman, S. J. Liu, X. Zhao, G. L. Clifton, and R. L. Hayes, *Neuroscience*, 77(3), 875–888 (1997).

J. T. Povlishock, "The Morphopathologic Response to Head Injuries of Varying Severity," in D. P. Becker and J. T. Povlishock, Eds., *Central Nervous System Trauma Status Report*, Bethesda MD, National Institute of Neurological and Communicative Disorders and Stroke, National Institutes of Health, 1985, pp. 443–452.

S. V. Pravdenkova, A. G. Basnakian, S. J. James, and B. J. Andersen, *Brain Res.*, 729(2), 151–155 (1996).

J. C. Reed, *J. Cell Biol.*, 124, 1–6 (1994).

R. F. Regan and D. W. Choi, *Brain Res.*, 633, 236–242 (1994).

R. F. Regan and S. S. Panter, *Brain Res.*, 682, 144–150 (1995).

A. Rink, K. M. Fung, J. Q. Trojanowski, V. M. Lee, E. Neugebauer, and T. K. McIntosh, *Am. J. Pathol.*, 147(6), 1575–1583 (1995).

L. J. Rosenberg-Schaffer and J. H. Lucas, *Brain Res.*, 605, 327–331 (1993).

B. A. Rzigalinski, S. Liang, J. S. McKinney, K. A. Willoughby, and E. F. Ellis, *J. Neurochem.*, 68, 289–296 (1997).

K. E. Saatman, D. Bozyczko-Coyne, V. Marcy, R. Siman, and T. K. McIntosh, *J. Neuropathol. Exp. Neurol.*, 55, 850–860 (1996).

B. Samuelsson, S. E. Dahlen, J. A. Lindgren, C. A. Rouzer, and C. N. Serhan, *Science*, 237(4819), 1171–1176 (1987).

P. T. Shah, K. W. Yoon, X. M. Xu, and L. D. Broder, *Neuroscience*, 79(4), 999–1004 (1997).

S. R. Shepard, R. J. Hariri, R. Giannuzzi, K. Pomerantz, D. Hajjar, and J. B. Ghajar, *Acta Neurochir. Suppl. (Wien)*, 51, 58–60 (1990).

S. R. Shepard, J. B. G. Ghajar, R. Giannuzzi, S. Kupferman, and R. J. Hariri, *J. Surg. Res.*, 51, 417–424 (1991).

B. K. Siesjo and F. Bengtsson, *J. Cereb. Blood Flow Metab.*, 9, 127–140 (1989).

N. P. Singh and R. E. Stephens, *Stain Technol.*, 61, 315–318 (1986).

G. Sinson, B. R. Perri, J. Q. Trojanowski, E. S. Flamm, and T. K. McIntosh, *Neurosurgery.* 86(3), 511–518 (1997).

S. L. Smith and E. D. Hall, *J. Neurotrauma*, 13(1), 1–9 (1996).

A. Srinivasan, L. M. Foster, M. P. Testa, T. Ord, R. W. Keane, D. E. Bredesen, and C. Kayalar, *J. Neurosci.*, 16, 5654–5660 (1996).

P. K. Stys, S. G. Waxman, and B. R. Ransom, *J. Neurosci.*, 12, 430–439 (1992).

W. C. Taft, K. Yang, C. E. Dixon, G. L. Clifton, and R. L. Hayes, *J. Cereb. Blood Flow Metab.*, 13(5), 796–802 (1993).

E. S. Tecoma, H. Monyer, M. P. Goldberg, and D. W. Choi, *Neuron*, 2, 1541–1545 (1989).

S. M. Thompson, H. L. Haas, and B. H. Gahwiler, *J. Physiol.*, 451, 347–363 (1992).

D. H. Triyoso and T. A. Good, *J. Physiol.*, 515(2), 355–365 (1999).

M. Tymianski and C. H. Tator, *Neurosurgery*, 38, 1176–1195 (1996).

B. H. Verweij, J. P. Muizelaar, F. C. Vinas, P. L. Peterson, Y. Xiong, and C. P. Lee, *Neurol. Res.*, 19, 334–339 (1997).

R. F. Villa and A. Gorini, *Pharmacol. Rev.*, 49, 99–136 (1997).

R. A. Wallis and K. L. Panizzon, *Eur. J. Pharmacol.*, 238, 165–171 (1993).

R. A. Wallis and K. L. Panizzon, *Eur. J. Pharmacol.*, 294, 475–482 (1995).

R. A. Wallis, K. L. Panizzon, and J. M. Girard, *Brain Res.*, 710, 169–177 (1996).

K. K. W. Wang, R. Nath, K. J. Raser, and I. Hajimohammadreza, *Arch. Biochem. Biophys.*, 331, 208–214 (1996).

K. A. Willoughby, B. A. Rzigalinksi, and E. F. Ellis, *J. Neurotrauma*, 15(10), 902 (1998).

A. G. Yakovlev, S. M. Knoblach, L. Fan, G. B. Fox, R. Goodnight, and A. I. Faden, *J. Neurosci.*, 17(19), 7415–7424 (1997).

K.-W. Yoon and S. M. Rothman, *J. Neurosci.*, 11, 1375–1380 (1991).

J. Zhang, V. L. Dawson, T. M. Dawson, and S. H. Snyder, *Science*, 263, 687–689 (1994).

X. Zhao, B. R. Pike, J. K. Newcomb, K. K. W. Wang, and R. L. Hayes, *J. Neurotrauma*, 15(10), 904 (1998).

X. Zhao, B. R. Pike, J. K. Newcomb, K. K. Wang, R. M. Posmantur, and R. L. Hayes, *Neurochem. Res.*, 24(3), 371–382 (1999).

R. C. Ziegelstein, J. L. Zweier, E. D. Mellits, A. Younes, E. G. Lakatta, M. D. Stern, and H. S. Silverman, *Circ. Res.*, 70, 804–811 (1992).

CHAPTER 3

CONTEMPORARY IN VIVO MODELS OF BRAIN TRAUMA AND A COMPARISON OF INJURY RESPONSES

ANTHONY E. KLINE and C. EDWARD DIXON
Brain Trauma Research Center, Department of Neurosurgery,
University of Pittsburgh, Pittsburgh, Pennsylvania

INTRODUCTION

For over a century, various in vivo animal models of traumatic brain injury (TBI) have been employed to systematically produce and study TBI pathology (Kramer, 1896; Cannon, 1901; Denny-Brown and Russell, 1941; Rinder and Olsson, 1968; Ommaya et al., 1971; Govons et al., 1972; Ommaya and Gennarelli, 1974; Sullivan et al., 1976; Nilsson et al., 1977; Parkinson, 1982; Gennarelli et al., 1982; Dixon et al., 1987; Lighthall, 1988; Dixon et al., 1991; Marmarou et al., 1994). There has never been such a wide array, as at present, of relevant TBI devices for researchers to characterize, modify, and implement in their laboratories. With the advent of such models, the aim of elucidating brain injury mechanisms and the development and testing of relevant clinical therapies is facilitated. Although several injury devices currently exist, this chapter will focus on the most commonly used as evidenced by peer-reviewed publications. The three main contemporary in vivo TBI models that will be described, compared, and contrasted are the fluid-percussion, controlled cortical impact, and weight drop (closed skull—acceleration/deceleration and open skull). We will describe the injury devices and how TBI is produced, as well as functional responses and histopathological consequences of the injury. We will also briefly discuss the application of the devices to immature rats and mice. Lastly, we will focus briefly on large animal models of TBI and conclude with a discussion of anesthetic agents routinely used with these contemporary in vivo models of TBI. As a caveat, it should be noted that although the terms "model" and "device" will be

Head Trauma: Basic, Preclinical, and Clinical Directions, Edited by Leonard P. Miller and Ronald L. Hayes, Co-edited by Jennifer K. Newcomb
ISBN 0-471-36015-5 © 2001 John Wiley & Sons, Inc.

used interchangeably throughout the chapter, it is not the intention of the authors to imply that a model of TBI is only a means of producing an insult. Rather, we believe that a model of TBI is, at a minimum, a combination of device, species of animals used, location and severity of injury, and choice of anesthesia.

DESCRIPTION OF THE MODELS

Fluid Percussion

First described by Lindgren and Rinder (1965) using a rabbit model of TBI, the fluid percussion (FP) device has since been utilized in several other animal species, including cats (Sullivan et al., 1976; Thibault et al., 1992), rats (Dixon et al., 1987, 1998; McIntosh et al., 1987), pigs (Pfenninger et al., 1989; Zink et al., 1993; Armstead and Kurth, 1994), and more recently mice (Carbonell et al., 1998). The FP device (Fig. 3.1) consists of a Plexiglas cylinder (however, see Yamaki et al., 1994) filled with physiological saline and enclosed at one end by a male Luer-Loc fitting that is subsequently paired with a female Luer-Loc, which is typically affixed approximately 24 h prior to the induction of brain trauma to the skull in either the region of the sagittal sinus for midline injury or the parietal cortex for lateral percussive injury. On the day of surgery, the animal is reanesthetized and the Luer-Loc fittings are coupled. Injury is produced when a metal pendulum strikes the piston of the injury device from a predetermined height and causes a rapid injection of saline into the closed cranium. The resulting pressure pulse induces a brief increase in intracranial pressure with associated displacement and deformation of neural tissue. Severity of injury is regulated by varying the height of the pendulum, which corresponds to variations of extracranial pressure pulses expressed in atmospheres (atm). Increased magnitudes of tissue deformation are associated with increased brain injury.

The original FP model has undergone several modifications since first described. These include altering the length and material of the tubing that connects the device to the animal and moving the injury site (midline versus lateral). Perhaps the main reason for moving from midline to lateral percussive injury is that the lateral FP, as well as the controlled cortical impact model, benefit from not mechanically injuring the central sagittal sinus. Concerns regarding pressure pulse variability stemming from a reservoir that is prone to temperature-dependent elasticity prompted one group to replace the Plexiglas cylindrical reservoir with one fabricated from stainless steel (Yamaki et al., 1994).

The FP device reproduces a number of clinically relevant injury responses. Specifically, midline FP has been used to induce concussive injuries (Dixon et al., 1987; Hayes et al., 1987), while lateral FP is advantageous for producing hippocampal cell death and cortical contusions (McIntosh et al., 1987). Furthermore, FP injury in the rat has been shown to produce vascular and blood–brain barrier (BBB) disruption (Cortez et al., 1989), alterations in cerebral blood flow (CBF) (Yamakami and McIntosh, 1991), cerebral edema, tissue shearing (Graham et al., 2000), and

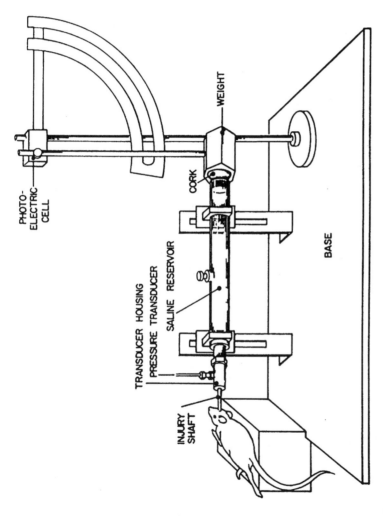

Figure 3.1 Diagram of the fluid percussion model of brain injury in the rat consisting of a Plexiglas cylindrical reservoir, 60 cm long and 4.5 cm in diameter (filled with 37°C isotonic saline), with a transducer mounted at one end. At the other end of the cylinder is a Plexiglas cork mounted on O-rings. Injury is produced by striking the cork with a 4.8 kg pendulum dropped from a predetermined height. The resulting pressure causes a rapid injection of saline into the closed cranium and induces a brief increase in intracranial pressure with associated displacement and deformation of neural tissue. Severity of injury is regulated by varying the height of the pendulum, which results in corresponding variations of extracranial pressure pulses, expressed in atmospheres (atm).

TABLE 3.1 **Summary of Morphological and Cerebrovascular Responses Observed with Contemporary Rodent TBI Models**

	LFP	LCCI	WDO	WDC
Cortical contusion	+	+	+	−
Subarachnoid hemorrhage	+	+	+	+
Subdural hematoma	+	+	+	+
Intraparenchymal hematoma	+	+	+	+
Hippocampal cell loss	+	+	+	−
Axonal injury	+	+	+	+
Edema	+	+	+	+
Altered CBF	+	+	+	+
Ischemia	−	+	+	−
Altered metabolism	+	+	+	+
BBB dysfunction	+	+	+	+
Inflammation	+	+	+	−

+, observed; −, not observed. LFP, lateral fluid percussion; LCCI, lateral controlled cortical impact; WDO, weight drop–open skull; WDC, weight drop–closed skull.

intraparenchymal hemorrhage (Table 3.1), all of which contribute to the formation of a focal lesion in the injured cortex (Tanno et al., 1992a,b; Schmidt and Grady, 1993; Hicks et al., 1996; Qian et al., 1996; Iwamoto et al., 1997; Dietrich et al., 1998). Furthermore, the FP device is able to produce neurobehavioral and cognitive deficits that are commonly seen after brain injury in human patients (see subsequent section).

Controlled Cortical Impact

Experimental TBI employing a pneumatic impactor was first introduced for use in laboratory ferrets by Lighthall and colleagues (Lighthall, 1988; Lighthall et al., 1990) and subsequently adapted for rat by Dixon et al. (1991) in an attempt to better control the biomechanical parameters of brain injury. Unlike the FP injury device, which disperses a stream of solution intracranially that cannot be readily quantified, the controlled cortical impact (CCI) model of experimental brain injury takes advantage of biomechanical events contributing to injury. These biomechanical events can be analyzed by establishing a quantifiable relationship between measurable engineering parameters, such as force, velocity, and tissue deformation, and the magnitude of tissue damage and/or functional impairment. These controlled mechanical variables enable accurate, reliable, and independent control of the deformation parameters over a wide range of contact velocities.

The CCI injury device (Fig. 3.2) consists of a small-bore (1.975 cm), double-acting stroke-constrained pneumatic cylinder with a 5.0 cm stroke. The cylinder is rigidly mounted on a crossbar in either an angled or vertical position. The lower rod end has an impact tip attached that varies in shape (rounded or flat edge) and diameter (5 to 6 mm) and the upper rod end is attached to the transducer core of a linear velocity displacement transducer (LVDT). The impactor tip is pneumatically driven at a predetermined velocity, depth, and duration of tissue deformation. A penetration depth of 2.5–2.7 mm with a velocity of 4.0 m/s, and a deformation of 50 ms consistently produces an injury of moderate severity. However, exact injury parameters are laboratory-dependent. The velocity of the impacting shaft is controlled by gas pressure and measured directly by the LVDT, which produces an analog signal that is recorded by a PC-based data acquisition system for analysis of time/displacement parameters of the impact. Unlike the FP model, animals undergoing a CCI injury do not have to endure two surgery episodes.

Like the FP model of experimental brain injury, the CCI model also produces morphological and cerebrovascular injury responses that resemble certain aspects of human TBI (Table 3.1). Commonly observed are graded histological and axonal derangements (Lighthall, 1988; Lighthall et al., 1990; Dixon et al., 1991; Goodman et al., 1994; Meaney et al., 1994), as well as disruption of the BBB (Dhillon et al., 1994), subdural and intraparenchymal hematoma, edema, inflammation, and alterations in CBF (Kochanek et al., 1995). Similarly, the CCI model also produces neurobehavioral and cognitive impairments like those observed in human patients (see subsequent section). In contrast to FP injury, the CCI device produces a significantly more pronounced cortical contusion.

Weight Drop

Weight drop models can be used with either an open or closed skull, with the choice resting primarily on the type of injury one is interested in obtaining (focal versus diffuse). For example, injury with the open skull weight drop device (Feeney et al., 1981; Fig. 3.3) produces a focal lesion that progresses from hemorrhages in the white matter directly under the contusion site during the first few hours after injury to the evolution of a necrotic cavity by 24 h. Additionally, the lesion continues to expand over the subsequent 2 weeks with maximal size attained by 15 days. On the other hand, the closed skull injury model (Fig. 3.4) developed by Marmarou and colleagues (1994) produces a diffuse injury without noticeable contusions or hippocampal cell loss. In both models a weight is attached to a string and, when the predetermined distance is obtained, the weight is released through a guide tube and subsequently strikes a footplate resting directly on the exposed brain (open skull) or directly on a cemented disk on the skull (closed skull). For the closed head injury model the weight is dropped from a Plexiglas guide tube that is significantly longer (2 m) than the 40 cm stainless steel tube of the model of Feeney et al. The height and mass of the falling weight are adjusted according to the desired severity of injury, with further distances and increased weights producing more injury than less distant and lighter weights.

Like the FP and CCI models, the weight drop techniques have also been shown to produce characteristics of human brain injury. Disturbances in regional CBF have been observed following either open skull weight drop (Nilsson et al., 1996; Scremin et al., 1997) or diffuse injury (Prat et al., 1998). Diffuse axonal injury (Okonkwo and

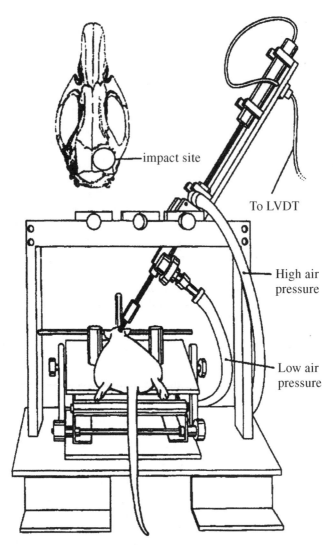

Figure 3.2 Diagram of a rat undergoing a right-hemisphere injury via the lateral controlled cortical impact injury device (CCI). The CCI injury device consists of a small (1.975 cm) bore with a double-acting stroke-constrained pneumatic cylinder and a 5.0 cm stroke. The cylinder is rigidly mounted in either an angled (depicted) or vertical position on a crossbar. The lower rod end that comes into contact with the dura has an impact tip attached that varies in size and shape and that can be precisely adjusted for varying tissue deformation levels. The upper rod end is attached to the transducer core of a linear velocity displacement transducer (LVDT). The velocity of the impacting shaft is controlled by gas pressure and measured directly by the LVDT that produces an analog signal that is recorded by a PC-based data acquisition system. The skull image depicts the impact site following a craniotomy. (Reprinted from Cherian et al., 1994, with publishers permission, Mary Ann Liebert, Inc.)

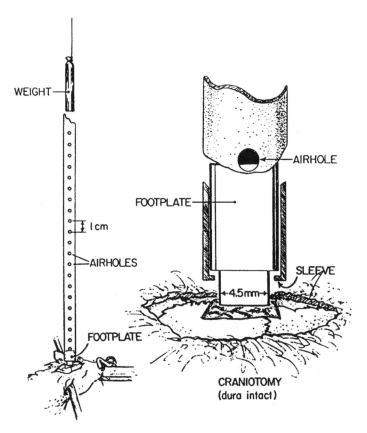

WEIGHT

1 cm

AIRHOLES

FOOTPLATE

AIRHOLE

FOOTPLATE

SLEEVE

←4.5mm→

CRANIOTOMY
(dura intact)

Figure 3.3   Diagram of the open skull weight drop device by Feeney et al. (1981), designed to produce a focal cortical contusion. A 40 cm stainless steel tube positioned at a 90° angle and perforated at 1 cm intervals to prevent air compression guides a falling weight onto a footplate resting on the dura. A string is used to lower the weight to the proper height in the tube, using the perforations to visually position the weight. A sleeve at the base of the tube is set to a height permitting a maximum of 2.5 mm depression of cortex. Force of the impact is expressed as weight × distance dropped (e.g., a 20 g weight dropped from 10 cm equals a force of 200 g-cm, which produces a moderate injury). (Reprinted with permission from *Brain Research*).

Povlishock, 1999) and elevations in intracranial pressure (Engelborghs et al., 1998) have also been observed following closed head injury (Table 3.1). The weight drop models are similar to the CCI injury device in that they too do not require two days of surgery. Additionally, the open skull weight drop model is quite similar to the CCI in terms of morphological, cerebrovascular, and neurobehavioral and cognitive alterations following impact.

Unlike in the CCI and lateral FP models, the potential for producing repeatable injury is lessened by factors inherent to the weight drop technique. Specifically, variations in weight drop velocity are possible because the impact is not pneumatically controlled, but rather is dependent on physical properties of the weight, the

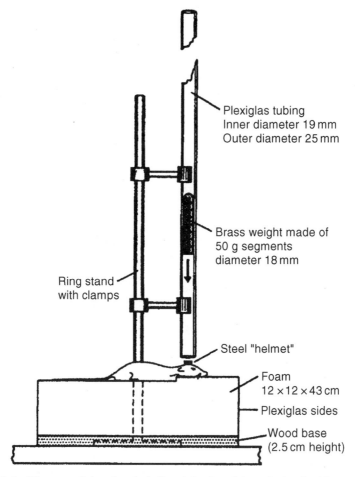

Figure 3.4   Diagram of the closed skull weight drop injury device by Marmarou et al. (1994), designed to produce a diffuse injury. The bottom opening of the 2 m, vertically aligned Plexiglas tube is positioned in close proximity to the head of the rat and centered so that the weight falls directly on the stainless steel disk (10 mm in diameter and 3 mm thick) cemented to the skull. The brass weight is attached to a guide string that is released from various heights to produce injuries of various severity. Immediately after the weight makes contact with the disk, the Plexiglas box (foam bed) containing the rat is quickly removed to prevent a rebound impact. (Reprinted with permission from *J. Neurosurgery*).

guide tube, and, in the case of the closed skull model, the rigidity of the foam bedding. For example, even a slight misalignment of the string holding the weight could cause drag, which would slow the velocity of the falling weight and ultimately affect the impact. Additionally, continued use of the foam bedding can decrease its stiffness and alter impact parameters (Piper et al., 1996). However, it should be noted that these potential problems can be remedied easily by ensuring that the supporting weight line does not drag against the side of the tube and by regularly changing the foam bedding. Lastly, the potential for a second, albeit slight, impact is possible due to rebounding of the weight. This phenomenon is more likely to occur with the open skull weight drop device because the guide tube is mounted on a stereotaxic frame that does not facilitate removing the rat immediately after impact, as can be done with the closed skull model by simply moving the Plexiglas box holding the rat.

FUNCTIONAL OUTCOME MEASURES

Table 3.2 is intended as a brief, nonexhaustive, summary of tasks that are used following TBI to assess neurobehavioral and cognitive outcome in rodents. The tasks assess functions that are known to be impaired in human TBI patients, such as memory and locomotion. The single plus sign next to the task indicates that it has been utilized before, but is not meant to be an indication of frequency. Additionally, a score of minus indicates that to our knowledge the particular task has not been incorporated after a certain TBI, but does not necessarily suggest that it would not be a viable measure.

Acute Neurological Responses

Studies employing short-acting anesthetics have the advantage over those using anesthesia's of long duration that animals can undergo acute neurological assessments using tests that have been shown to be sensitive to varying magnitudes of FP (Dixon et al., 1987; Lyeth, 1988) and CCI injury. These tests are analogous to motor components of the Glasgow Coma Scale (Teasdale and Jennett, 1974) and allow quantification of various features of the suppression of the animal's responsiveness to external stimuli and relationships between durations of behavioral suppression

TABLE 3.2 Summary of Neurobehavioral and Cognitive Assessment Tools Utilized with Contemporary Rodent TBI Models

	LFP	LCCI	WDO	WDC
Neuroreflexes	+	+	?	?
Beam balance	+	+	+	+
Beam walk	+	+	+	+
MWM acquisition	+	+	?	+
MWM retention	+	+	?	?
MWM working memory	+	+	?	?
Barnes maze	−	+	−	−

and magnitudes of injury. Assessments of simple nonpostural somatomotor functions include measurements of corneal and pinna reflex suppression. Simple postural somatomotor functions include measuring the duration of suppression to flexion responses, such as the latency of hind paw flexion following the gradual application of pressure, and the time to recover the righting reflex (Dixon et al., 1987).

Motor Deficits

Vestibulomotor. Both the beam-balance (BB) and the beam-walking (BW) tasks have been utilized to assess gross and fine motor function, respectively. The BB task consists of measuring the animal's latency to balance on a beam for up to 60 s. The scoring criteria vary from laboratory to laboratory, with some scoring only the latency of an animal on the beam regardless of how it balances itself, while other laboratories assign a rating score depending on the nature of the balancing act (i.e., an animal balancing with both limbs on the beam is given a better neurological score than one that is draped over the beam). The BW task, originally devised by Feeney et al. (1982), allows for the assessment of refined locomotor activity. Briefly, the task consists of training animals using a negative-reinforcement paradigm to escape a bright light and loud white noise by traversing a narrow wooden beam to enter a darkened goal box at the opposite end. The termination of the adverse stimuli (noise and light) serves as reinforcement (reward). Like the BB task, the rating scales for the BW task vary from simply recording the time to traverse the beam regardless of the nature of the traversal to counting the actual number of foot slips, with the latter being more sensitive to motor ability and the former more sensitive to overall behavior following brain trauma (i.e., ability and motivation).

Composite Scores. Composite neurological scores have frequently been used to assess the extent of global neurological deficits following lateral FP brain injury (McIntosh et al., 1989). Briefly, animals are given a score from 0 (complete loss of function) to 4 (normal function) in the following neuromotor tasks (neuroreflexes): (i) ability to stand on an inclined angled board, (ii and iii) forelimb contraflexion and hindlimb flexion response during suspension by the tail, and (iv) resistance to right and left lateral pulsion. Composite scores are derived by summing the totals from all tests to a single numerical value.

Rotarod Performance. Assessment of rotarod performance has also been shown to be an indicator of injury-induced motor disability in rats subjected to central FP (Hamm et al., 1994) and mice following CCI (Raghupathi et al., 1998). Briefly, the animal is placed on a rotating rod or rotating bars that increase in both speed and the number of revolutions over time. The duration for which the animal remains on the rotarod is considered to be indicative of the severity of damage, with shorter durations indicating greater impairment. Hamm et al. (1994) report that, compared to BB and BW, the rotarod task is a more sensitive and efficient index for assessing motor impairment produced by central FP in rats. However, the sensitivity of the rotarod task to experimental therapies is not yet known.

Cognitive Deficits

Morris Water Maze. Memory deficits are one of the most persistent sequelae of nonmissile head injury in humans (Levin et al., 1979). These memory disturbances include a period of transient posttraumatic amnesia characterized by gross confusion and inability to commit new information to memory. After the resolution of posttraumatic amnesia, many patients exhibit persistent memory disturbances. The animal models of TBI presented in this chapter have been used extensively to examine cognitive deficits following injury. In 1992, Hamm and colleagues employed what was then a recently adapted CCI injury model (Dixon et al., 1991) to assess cognitive function in rats following CCI brain injury using the Morris water maze (MWM) procedure (Morris, 1981). Following isoflurane anesthesia, and endotracheal intubation, mechanically ventilated rats were subjected to a mild CCI injury (1.5 to 2.0 mm deformation at 6 m/s). Beginning on postoperative day 11, rats were provided with a daily block of four trials for five consecutive days. Briefly, the rats began a trial from one of four possible start locations (east, west, north, south) and were given a maximum of 120 s to find a submerged platform (positioned in either the northeast, southeast, southwest, or northwest quadrant of the pool) using spatial cues as a guide. On postoperative days 30 to 34, the rats were once again tested in the maze, but this time the platform was situated in a location that differed from previous testing. The authors report that following CCI injury, rats showed spatial memory performance deficits on days 11 to 15 and 30 to 34. Additionally, the deficits were observed despite the lack of structural damage as assessed by qualitative light-microscope examination (Hamm et al., 1992). Recent studies investigating spatial learning following the CCI injury model have since been reported (Dixon et al., 1999a; Kline et al., 2000). Spatial memory performance deficits in the MWM are also observed following FP injury (Bramlett et al., 1995; Pierce et al., 1998; Sanders et al., 1999). In a study examining the long-term effects of TBI, Pierce et al. (1998) showed that one year after the initial trauma fluid-percussed rats were still significantly impaired compared to sham controls.

To determine whether working memory is affected following TBI, Hamm et al. (1996) subjected rats to FP injury and assessed them in a working memory paradigm in the MWM. Briefly, the task consisted of providing eight pairs of trials per day. Start points (E, W, N, S) and platform placements were quasi-randomly assigned each day such that an animal began from each location twice and also had to locate the platform at one of four locations two times. The animal is given a maximum of 2 min to find the platform (trial 1); if it does not do so in the allotted time, it is set on the platform by the experimenter for 10 s, then promptly placed back in the water from the same location as the previous trial (same platform location; trial 2). Following a 4 min intertrial interval the rat is placed back in the pool to search for another location. The authors report that FP injured rats performed significantly worse than sham controls. Using the same procedure as Hamm et al. (1996), Kline et al. (1999) assessed working memory in animals subjected to a CCI injury of moderate severity (2.7 mm deformation, 4 m/s) and found that the CCI injured animals exhibited significantly longer latencies, compared to sham controls, to find the hidden platform over several days. That the finding was similar to that of Hamm et al. indicates, that at least for this type of cognitive behavior, the FP and CCI injury models produce similar injury responses. Morris water maze performance is also impaired following bilateral frontal cortical impact injury (Hoffman et al., 1994). Thus, several independent laboratories have shown that TBI can produce memory deficits in rats as assessed in the MWM. Importantly, spatial memory may represent a rodent analogue for declarative memory studied in humans and is thought to be mediated by temporal lobe function (Zola-Morgan and Squire, 1985). However, the neural substrates subserving spatial memory in rats are not entirely clear. While hippocampal function seems to be important for spatial memory, other data in rats suggest that the cortex may also be critical for spatial memory performance (Berger-Sweeney et al., 1994).

Barnes Circular Maze. The Barnes maze was first described by Carol Barnes as a new method for examining memory impairments associated with senescence (Barnes, 1979), and has recently been adapted by Fox et al. (1998b) for assessment of cognitive function following CCI injury in mice. The device consists of a hidden escape tunnel located beneath one of the 40 holes at the perimeter of a large circular platform. As in the MWM training, numerous extramaze visual cues are provided. The advantages of the Barnes maze is that rodents can be tested for spatial learning without the repetitive swimming that may not only be stressful but may also be compromised by sensorimotor impairment.

MORPHOLOGICAL RESPONSES

With the possible exception of the weight drop (closed skull) model, the other TBI models (FP, CCI, weight drop–open skull) all have been shown to consistently produce a cortical contusion. However, the degree of contusion size differs between models. The CCI and weight drop (open skull) injury models, for example, generally produce greater contusion volumes than seen with the FP device. Aside from subdural and intraparenchymal hematomas and axonal injury, the models described also produce hippocampal cell loss. In a recent study, Bramlett et al. (1997) looked at chronic histopathology in rats 8 weeks after parasagittal percussion injury and found significant hippocampal cell loss in the ipsilateral dentate hilar region. Additionally, quantitative volume measurements showed significant decreases in cortical, thalamic, and hippocampal volume ipsilateral to the lesion. Cortical atrophy and ventricular enlargement were observed in the traumatized hemisphere. In rats undergoing mild (1.1 to 1.3 atm), moderate (2.0 to 2.3 atm), or severe (2.4–2.6 atm) lateral FP injury, Perri et al. (1997) showed a significant correlation between cerebral cortical lesion volume and severity of brain injury 48 h after insult. Mean lesion volumes were 12.1 mm^3 following mild injury, 33.8 mm^3 following moderate injury and 45.1 mm^3 after severe percussive injury.

In a long-term assessment study, Smith et al. (1997) demonstrated a temporal profile of histopathological changes following parasagittal FP injury in rats over a one-year period. Specifically, rats were subjected to a percussion injury of high severity (2.5 to 2.9 atm) and sacrificed for histopathological assessment at 1, 2, or 48 h, 1 and 2 weeks, and 1, 2, 6, or 12 months. Brain sections were analyzed to determine the extent of cortical tissue loss and shrinkage of the hippocampal pyramidal cell layer. The authors also conducted cell counts of the dentate hilus and immunostained for glial fibrillary acidic protein to reveal reactive astrocytes. A significant progressive loss of cortical tissue as well as shrinkage of the hippocampal pyramidal cell layer was observed over one year following injury in the ipsilateral hemisphere. The data suggest that following FP brain injury there is a progressive degenerative process. Dixon et al. (1999b) also showed that a long-term degenerative process exists utilizing the CCI injury model. Animals were subjected to a moderate CCI injury and contusion volume was measured at either 3 weeks or 1 year after injury. A hemispheric loss of 30.4 mm^3 was seen at 3 weeks, with a more pronounced hemispheric loss of 51.5 mm^3 observed at 12 months. Progressive tissue loss was also reflected by a threefold to fourfold increase in ipsilateral ventricular volume between 3 weeks and 1 year after injury.

APPLICATION OF THE MODELS TO IMMATURE RATS

Head trauma is a leading cause of disability in children, producing long-lasting functional deficits following moderate or severe trauma (Levin et al., 1979, 1982). It has generally been thought that recovery from brain injury is facilitated in children because of neuroplasticity-mediated events. However, younger children have been shown to exhibit poorer functional outcomes than older children suffering the same degree of brain damage (Koskiniemi et al., 1995). Clearly there is a need for further research into the mechanisms of the immature brain such that potential pharmacotherapies can be implemented. Adelson et al. (1997) have utilized a model of diffuse brain injury in immature rats that produces acute motor and cognitive deficits. Briefly, the model consists of dropping a weight onto the closed skull of 17-day-old rat pups. In a subsequent study, Adelson and colleagues (2000) investigated long-term functional ability after diffuse injury in the immature 17-day-old rat. Reduced latencies on the BB and inclined plane were observed in injured animals (compared to shams) at 24 h and persisted for 10 days post injury. Diffuse injury also produced a marked and sustained impairment in MWM performance that lasted 90 days after injury. In another study evaluating functional outcome in the immature subject, Prins and Hovda (1998) reported that postnatal day-17 injured rats showed no significant difference from age-matched controls in terms of escape latency or time to criterion performance following closed head injury. This finding suggests that if the animals survive the brain injury they are apt to show remarkable sparing. The outcome from these studies suggests that the immature model could be useful for testing novel therapies and their effect on chronic outcome and development in the immature rat.

APPLICATION OF THE MODELS TO MICE

Historically, animal models of TBI have tended to focus more on the laboratory rat, but as described in the subsequent section, large animals have also been utilized. However, genetically altered mice are becoming increasingly useful in the study of normal and pathological consequences of brain function and the adaptation of injury devices for these smaller animals has resulted in several mouse models of brain injury. The well established rat CCI injury model (Dixon et al., 1991) was first adapted for mice by Smith and colleagues (1995) and more recently by Fox et al. (1998a) and Hannay et al. (1999). Utilizing the Morris water maze and the Barnes circular maze, Fox et al. (1998a,b) have shown that mice subjected to CCI injury exhibit marked impairment in cognitive performance. Deficits in motor function have also been described utilizing a BW task in which the number of foot faults is counted. Mice have also been used following CCI injury to assess pathological consequences of brain injury such as apoptotic cell death (Fox et al., 1998a). Clearly, in such a short period the CCI/mouse model of TBI has made significant contributions to experimental brain injury research. The closed head injury model, like the CCI device, causes cognitive and histopathological sequelae. The FP model of TBI has recently been adapted for mice by Carbonell et al. (1998). The authors indicate that, despite the usefulness of the CCI and closed head injury models, they chose to adapt the FP injury device for mice for several reasons. Some of the reasons provided range from the fact that there is no need to modify the FP model, the decreased variability of damage due to skull fractures (closed head injury), plus the strong support for the FP injury device in rat as a viable model of TBI. They have reported that following a parasagittal FP injury mice showed significant impairments in spatial learning and memory as assessed in the MWM at 5 and 6 days post injury that was associated with cortical cell death, axonal degeneration, and gliosis. Hence it appears that either the FP, CCI or weight-drop injury devices may be particularly useful models to study the behavioral, histopathological, and molecular mechanisms of TBI in wild-type and genetically altered mice (Fox and Faden, 1998; Raghupathi et al., 1998; Fox et al., 1999; Sinz et al., 1999; Sullivan et al., 1999; Whalen et al., 1999).

LARGE-ANIMAL MODELS

A number of large-animal TBI models have recently been implemented. The disadvantages of large-animal models include their lack of normative biochemical and molecular data and high expense relative to rodent models of TBI. However, the primary advantages of large-animal models of TBI are in their greater brain mass, having a biomechanical fidelity that more closely matches that of humans. Brain injury tolerances to mechanical stresses may be more easily calculated in large animals than in rodents. Also, the larger brain size is easier to image using magnetic resonance imaging (MRI) or positron emission tomography (PET). However, new technological advances have recently allowed researchers to generate scientifically useful MRI and PET images in rodents (Hendrich et al., 1999; Myers et al., 1999) and the selective vulnerability of neuronal populations to injury (cell death) across species is amazingly consistent.

Cat and pig models constitute the primary contemporary large-animal models of TBI. The cat fluid percussion model, originally described by Sullivan and colleagues (1976) remains an important tool for studying cerebrovascular responses (DeWitt et al., 1996) and axonal injury (Povlishock et al., 1999). The immature pig FP model is useful for studying CBF, pial artery diameter, and cerebral oxygenation (Armstead, 1999). The diffuse inertial model of TBI, originally characterized in sub-human primates (Ommaya and Gennarelli, 1974), has recently been reproduced in the miniature swine by applying a nonimpact, coronal plane, rotational acceleration to the head (Kimura et al., 1996). This pig model of diffuse brain injury produces diffuse axonal injury, neurofilament damage, and increases in beta-amyloid and tau immunoreactivity (Smith et al., 1999). Using proton and phosphorus magnetic resonance spectroscopy (MRS) following inertial TBI to the immature pig, Smith et al. (1998) observed an acute 60% loss of intracellular Mg^{2+} levels, which gradually resolved by 7 days post injury while levels of the neuron marker N-acetylaspartate (NAA), dropped acutely by 20% and remained persistently decreased for at least 7 days post injury.

ANESTHETICS

When designing experimental studies, the effect of anesthetic agents should be given much thought beyond whether the subject will achieve and maintain a surgical level of anesthesia. Specifically, the physiological responses to different anesthetics should be of concern to TBI investigators. As seen in Table 3.3, the anesthetics routinely utilized with rodent TBI models are pentobarbital, halothane, and isoflurane. The long-acting anesthesias such as pentobarbital produce extended depressed consciousness levels compared to the volatile gases such as halothane and isoflurane. This factor certainly influences acute neurological assessments. Discontinuing isoflurane anesthesia after injury has allowed investigators to accurately assess acute neurologic outcomes (e.g., hindpaw flexion and righting reflex; Dixon et al., 1991) within seconds in sham-injured animals and minutes in CCI injured animals.

TABLE 3.3   Brief Summary of Anesthetics Utilized with Contemporary Rodent TBI Models

	LFP	LCCI	WDO	WDC
Pentobarbital	+	+	+	−
Halothane	+	+	+	+
Isoflurane	+	+	+	+
Fentanyl	−	+	−	+
Ketamine	+	+	+	?

+, utilized; −, not utilized; ? unknown. LFP, lateral fluid percussion; LCCI, lateral controlled cortical impact; WDO, weight drop–open skull; WDC, weight drop–closed skull.

Anesthesia may also be neuroprotective by lowering intracranial pressure, by reducing cerebral metabolic rate, and by inducing hypothermia. In an excellent review, McPherson et al. (1994) suggest that halothane neuroprotection appears to be preferentially expressed in instances of neural trauma due to contusion, where its vasodilatory effects can prevent the slow onset of ischemia. Ketamine-induced anesthesia may also be neuroprotective via its actions as an N-methyl-D-aspartate (NMDA) antagonist by inhibiting the action of the excitatory amino acids glutamate and aspartate. In a comparative study of CCI injury in rats, Statler et al. (2000) have demonstrated significant differences in motor, cognitive, and histopathological outcome between isoflurane and fentanyl anesthesia. Specifically, the authors have shown that isoflurane-anesthetized animals performed better on the neurobehavioral tasks and exhibited attenuated damage to CA1 hippocampal neurons. The data suggest that the improvements observed may be attributable to beneficial actions of isoflurane or/and detrimental effects of fentanyl. The beneficial effects of isoflurane may be attributed to a decrease in excitotoxicity or an augmentation of cerebral blood flow. On the other hand, the deleterious effect of fentanyl may be due to its neural suppressive effect. This finding clearly has significant implications, particularly for TBI researchers interested in assessing behavioral outcome following pharmacotherapies, because it suggests that a routinely employed anesthetic may be neuroprotective and as such may be masking the potential efficacy of clinical drugs.

SUMMARY

We have described the three most commonly used injury devices (fluid percussion, controlled cortical impact, and weight drop) currently available for experimentally induced brain injury. Several differences and similarities between the in vivo models have been presented. Based on these comparisons of the models, we contend that the observed differences between them are associated with differences in the primary injury. This is most apparent in the morphological response to experimental TBI. We further contend that the similarities between the models are associated with a relatively universal cascade of secondary injury processes that occur regardless of the physical initiator of TBI. Despite not mimicking all the characteristics of human TBI, all the in vivo models described in this chapter have been instrumental in enhancing our knowledge about the mechanisms of TBI and have been useful for screening potential pharmacotherapies.

ABBREVIATIONS

atm	Atmospheres
BB	Beam-balance
BBB	Blood–brain barrier

BW	Beam-walk
CBF	Cerebral blood flow
CCI	Controlled cortical impact
FP	Fluid percussion
LVDT	Linear velocity displacement transducer
MRS	Magnetic resonance spectroscopy
MRI	Magnetic resonance imaging
MWM	Morris water maze
NAA	N-Acetylaspartate
NMDA	N-Methyl-D-aspartate
PET	Positron emission tomography
TBI	Traumatic brain injury

REFERENCES

P. D. Adelson, C. E. Dixon, P. Robichaud, and P. M. Kochanek, *J. Neurotrauma*, 14, 99–108 (1997).

P. D. Adelson, C. E. Dixon, and P. M. Kochanek, *J. Neurotrauma*, 17, 273–282 (2000).

W. M. Armstead, *Exp. Toxicol. Pathol.*, 51, 137–142 (1999).

W. M. Armstead and C. D. Kurth, *J. Neurotrauma*, 11, 487–497 (1994).

C. A. Barnes, *J. Comp. Physiol. Psychol.*, 93, 74–104 (1979).

T. Berger-Sweeney, S. Heckers, M. M. Mesulam, R. G. Wiley, D. A. Lappi, and M. Sharma, *J. Neurosci.*, 14, 4507–4519 (1994).

H. M. Bramlett, W. D. Dietrich, E. J. Green, and R. Busto, *Acta Neuropathol.*, 93, 190–199 (1997).

H. M. Bramlett, E. J. Green, W. D. Dietrich, R. Busto, M. Y.-T. Globus and M. D. Ginsberg, *J. Neurotrauma*, 12, 289–298 (1995).

W. B. Cannon, *Am. J. Physiol.*, 6, 91–121 (1901).

W. S. Carbonell, D. O. Maris, T. McCall, and M. S. Grady, *J. Neurotrauma*, 15, 217–229 (1998).

S. Cortez, T. K. McIntosh, and L. Noble, *Brain Res.*, 482, 271–282 (1989).

D. Denny-Brown and W. R. Russell, *Brain*, 64, 93–164 (1941).

D. S. DeWitt, D. S. Prough, D. D. Deal, S. M. Vines, and H. Hoen, *Crit. Care Med.*, 24, 109–117 (1996).

H. S. Dhillon, D. Donaldson, R. J. Dempsey, and M.R. Prasad, *J. Neurotrauma*, 11, 405–415 (1994).

W. D. Dietrich, O. Alonso, R. Busto, R. Prado, W. Zhao, M. K. Dewanjee, and M. D. Ginsberg, *Neurosurgery*, 43, 585–594 (1998).

C. E. Dixon, B. G. Lyeth, J. T. Povlishock, R. L. Findling, R. J. Hamm, A. Marmarou, H. F. Young, and R. L. Hayes, *J. Neurosurg.*, 67, 110–119 (1987).

C. E. Dixon, J. W. Lighthall, and T. E. Anderson, *J. Neurotrauma*, 5, 91–104 (1988).

C. E. Dixon, G. L. Clifton, J. W. Lighthall, A. A. Yaghmai, and R. L. Hayes, *J. Neurosci. Methods*, 39, 253–262 (1991).

C. E. Dixon, M. F. Kraus, A. E. Kline, X. Ma, H. Q. Yan, R. G. Griffith, B. M. Wolfson, and D. W. Marion, *Res. Neurol. Neurosci.*, 14, 285–294 (1999a).

C. E. Dixon, P. M. Kochanek, H. Q. Yan, J. K. Schiding, R. G. Griffith, E. Baum, D. W. Marion, and S. T. DeKosky, *J. Neurotrauma*, 16, 109–122 (1999b).

K. Engelborghs, J. Verlooy, J. Van Reempts, B. Van Deuren, M. Van De Ven, and M. Borgers, *J. Neurosurg.*, 89, 796–806 (1998).

D. M. Feeney, M. G. Boyeson, R. T. Linn, H. M. Murray, and W. G. Dail, *Brain Res.*, 211, 67–77 (1981).

D. M. Feeney, A. Gonzalez, and W. A. Law, *Science*, 217, 855–857 (1982).

G. B. Fox and A. I. Faden, *J. Neurosci. Res.*, 53, 718–727 (1998).

G. B. Fox, L. Fan, R. A. LeVasseur, and A. I. Faden, *J. Neurotrauma*, 15, 599–614 (1998a).

G. B. Fox, L. Fan, R. A. LeVasseur, and A. I. Faden, *J. Neurotrauma*, 15, 1037–1046 (1998b).

G. B. Fox, R. A. LeVasseur, and A. I. Faden, *J. Neurotrauma*, 16, 377–389 (1999).

T. A. Gennarelli, L. E. Thibault, J. H. Adams, D. I. Graham, C. J. Thompson, and R. P. Marcincin, *Ann. Neurol.*, 12, 564–574 (1982).

J. C. Goodman, L. Cherian, R. M. Bryan, Jr., and C. S. Robertson, *J. Neurotrauma*, 11, 587–597 (1994).

S. R. Govons, R. B. Govons, W. D. Van Huss, and W. W. Heusner, *Exp. Neurol.*, 34, 121–128 (1972).

D. I. Graham, R. Raghupathi, K. E. Saatman, D. F. Meaney, and T. K. McIntosh, *Acta Neuropathol.*, 99, 117–124 (2000).

R. J. Hamm, C. E. Dixon, D. M. Gbadebo, A. K. Singha, L. W. Jenkins, B. G. Lyeth, and R. L. Hayes, *J. Neurotrauma*, 9, 11–20 (1992).

R. J. Hamm, B. R. Pike, D. M. O'Dell, B. G. Lyeth, and L. W. Jenkins, *J. Neurotrauma*, 11, 187–196 (1994).

R. J. Hamm, M. D. Temple, B. R. Pike, D. M. O'Dell, D. L. Buck, and B. G. Lyeth, *J. Neurotrauma*, 13, 317–323 (1996).

H. J. Hannay, Z. Feldman, P. Phan, A. Keyani, N. Panwar, J. C. Goodman, and C. S. Robertson, *J. Neurotrauma*, 16, 1103–1114 (1999).

R. L. Hayes, D. Stalhammer, J. T. Povlishock, A. M. Allen, B. J. Galinat, D. P. Becker, and H. H. Stonnington, *Brain Inj.*, 1, 93–112 (1987).

K. S. Hendrich, P. M. Kochanek, D. S. Williams, J. K. Schiding, D. W. Marion, and C. Ho, *Magn. Reson. Med.*, 42, 673–681 (1999).

R. Hicks, H. Soares, D. Smith, and T. McIntosh, *Acta Neuropathol.*, 91, 236–246 (1996).

S. W. Hoffman, Z. Fulop, and D. G. Stein, *J. Neurotrauma*, 11, 417–431 (1994).

Y. Iwamoto, T. Yamaki, N. Murakami, M. Umeda, C. Tanaka, T. Higuchi, I. Aoki, S. Naruse, and S. Ueda, *Neurosurgery*, 40, 163–167 (1997).

H. Kimura, D. F. Meaney, J. C. McGowan, R. I. Grossman, R. E. Lenkinski, D. T. Ross, T. K. McIntosh, T. A. Gennarelli, and D. H. Smith, *J. Comput. Assist. Tomogr.*, 20, 540–546 (1996).

A. E. Kline, H. Q. Yan, J. Yu, X. Ma, D. W. Marion, and C. E. Dixon, *Soc. Neurosci. Abstr.*, 25, 312 (1999).

A. E. Kline, H. Q. Yan, J. Bao, D. W. Marion, and C. E. Dixon, *Neurosci. Lett.*, 280, 163–166 (2000).

P. M. Kochanek, D. W. Marion, W. Zhang, J. K. Schiding, M. White, A. M. Palmer, R. S. Clark, M. E. O'Malley, S. D. Styren, C. Ho, and S. T. DeKosky, *J. Neurotrauma*, 12, 1015–1025 (1995).

M. Koskiniemi, T. Kyykka, T. Nybo, and L. Jarho, *Arch. Pediatr. Adolesc. Med.*, 149, 249–254 (1995).

S. P. Kramer, *Ann. Surg.*, 23, 163–173 (1896).

H. S. Levin, R. G. Grossman, J. E. Rose, and G. Teasdale, *J. Neurosurg.*, 50, 412–422 (1979).

H. S. Levin, H. M. Eisenberg, N. R. Wigg, and K. Kobayashi, *Neurosurgery*, 11, 668–673 (1982).

J. W. Lighthall, *J. Neurotrauma*, 5, 1–15 (1988).

J. W. Lighthall, H. G. Goshgarian, and C. R. Pindeerski, *J. Neurotrauma*, 7, 65–76 (1990).

S. Lindgren and L. Rinder, *Biophysik*, 2, 320–329 (1965).

B. G. Lyeth, C. E. Dixon, R. J. Hamm, L. W. Jenkins, H. F. Young, H. H. Stonnington, and R. L. Hayes, *Brain Res.*, 452, 39–48 (1988).

A. Marmarou, M. A. Abd-Alfattah Fod, W. van den Brink, J. Campbell, H. Kita, and K. Demetriadou, *J. Neurosurg.*, 80, 291–300 (1994).

R. W. McPherson, J. R. Kirsch, S. K. Salzman, and R. J. Traystman, *The Neurobiology of Central Nervous System Trauma*, Oxford University Press, New York, 1994, pp. 12–27.

T. K. McIntosh, L. Noble, B. Andrews, and A. I. Faden, *Cent. Nerv. Syst. Trauma*, 4, 119–134 (1987).

T. K. McIntosh, R. Vink, L. Noble, I. Yamakami, S. Fernyak, H. Soares, and A. I. Faden, *Neuroscience*, 28, 233–244 (1989).

D. F. Meaney, D. T. Ross, B. A. Winklestein, J. Brasko, D. Goldstein, L. B. Bilston, L. E. Thibault, and T. A. Gennarelli, *J. Neurotrauma*, 11, 599–612 (1994).

R. G. M. Morris, *Learning Motiv.*, 12, 239–260 (1981).

R. Myers, S. Hume, P. Bloomfield, and T. Jones, *J. Psychopharmacol.*, 13, 352–357 (1999).

B. Nilsson, U. Ponten, and G. Voight, *J. Neurosurg.*, 47, 241–251 (1977).

P. Nilsson, B. Gazelius, H. Carlson, and L. Hillered, *J. Neurotrauma*, 13, 201–207 (1996).

D. O. Okonkwo and J. T. Povlishock, *J. Cereb. Blood Flow Metab.*, 19, 443–451 (1999).

A. K. Ommaya, A. Geller, and L. C. Parsons, *Int. J. Neurosci.*, 1, 371–378 (1971).

A. K. Ommaya and T. A. Gennarelli, *Brain*, 97, 633–654 (1974).

D. Parkinson, *Clin. Neurosurgery*, 29, 131–145 (1982).

B. R. Perri, D. H. Smith, H. Murai, G. Sinson, K. E. Saatman, R. Raghupathi, R. T. Bartus, and T. K. McIntosh, *J. Neurotrauma*, 14, 15–22 (1997).

E. G. Pfenninger, A. Reith, D. Breitig, A. Grunert, and F. W. Ahnefeld, *J. Neurosurg.*, 70, 774–779 (1989).

J. E. S. Pierce, D. H. Smith, J. Q. Trojanowski, and T. K. McIntosh, *Neuroscience*, 87, 359–369 (1998).

I. R. Piper, D. Thomson, and J. D. Miller, *J. Neurosci. Methods*, 69, 171–174 (1996).

J. T. Povlishock, A. Buki, H. Koiziumi, J. Stone, and D. O. Okonkwo, *Acta Neurochir. Suppl. (Wien)*, 73, 15–20 (1999).

R. Prat, V. Markiv, M. Dujovny, and M. Misra, *Acta Neurochir. Suppl. (Wien)*, 71, 123–126 (1998).

M. L. Prins and D. A. Hovda, *J. Neurotrauma*, 15, 799–811 (1998).

L. Qian, K. Ohno, T. Maehara, B. Tominaga, K. Hirakawa, T. Kuroiwa, K. Takakuda, and H. Miyairi, *Acta Neurochir. (Wien)*, 138, 90–98 (1996).

R. Raghupathi, S. C. Fernandez, H. Murai, S. P. Trusko, R. W. Scott, W. K. Nishioka, and T. K. McIntosh, *J. Cereb. Blood Flow Metab.*, 18, 1259–1269 (1998).

L. Rinder and Y. Olsson, *Acta Neuropathol. (Berl.)*, 11, 183–200 (1968).

M. J. Sanders, W. D. Dietrich, and E. J. Green, *J. Neurotrauma*, 16, 915–925 (1999).

R. H. Schmidt and M. S. Grady, *J. Neurotrauma*, 10, 415–430 (1993).

O. U. Scremin, M. G. Li, and D. J. Jenden, *J. Neurotrauma*, 14, 573–586 (1997).

G. Sinson, M. Voddi, and T. K. McIntosh, *J. Neurochem.*, 65, 2209–2216 (1995).

E. H. Sinz, P. M. Kochanek, C. E. Dixon, R. S. B. Clark, J. A. Carcillo, J. K. Schiding, M. Chen, S. R. Wisniewski, T. M. Carlos, D. Williams, S. T. DeKosky, S. C. Watkins, D. W. Marion, and T. R. Billiar, *J. Clin. Invest.*, 104, 647–656 (1999).

D. H. Smith, H. D. Soares, J. S. Pierce, K. G. Perlman, K. E. Saatman, D. F. Meaney, C. E. Dixon, and T. K. McIntosh, *J. Neurotrauma*, 12, 169–178 (1995).

D. H. Smith, X.-H. Chen, J. E. S. Pierce, J. A. Wolf, J. Q. Trojanowski, D. I. Graham, and T. K. McIntosh, *J. Neurotrauma*, 14, 715–727 (1997).

D. H. Smith, K. M. Cecil, D. F. Meaney, X.-H. Chen, T. K. McIntosh, T. A. Gennarelli, and R. E. Lenkinski, *J. Neurotrauma*, 15, 665–74 (1998).

D. H. Smith, X.-H. Chen, M. Nonaka, J. Q. Trojanowski, V. M. Lee, K. E. Saatman, M. J. Leoni, B. N. Xu, J. A. Wolf, and D. F. Meaney, *J. Neuropathol. Exp. Neurol.*, 58, 982–992 (1999).

K. D. Statler, P. M. Kochanek, C. E. Dixon, H. L. Alexander, D. S. Warner, R. S. B. Clarke, S. R. Wisniewski, S. H. Graham, L. W. Jenkins, D. W. Marion, and P. J. Safar, *J. Neurotrauma*, 17, 1179–1189 (2000).

H. G. Sullivan, J. Martinez, D. P. Becker, J. D. Miller, R. Griffith, and A. O. Wist, *J. Neurosurg.*, 45, 520–534 (1976).

P. G. Sullivan, A. J. Bruce-Keller, A. G. Rabchevsky, S. Christakos, D. K. St. Clair, M. P. Mattson, and S. W. Scheff, *J. Neurosci.*, 19, 6248–6256 (1999).

H. Tanno, R. P. Nockels, L. H. Pitts, and L. J. Noble, *J. Neurotrauma*, 9, 21–321 (1992a).

H. Tanno, R. P. Nockels, L. H. Pitts, and L. J. Noble, *J. Neurotrauma*, 9, 335–347 (1992b).

G. Teasdale and B. Jennett, *Lancet*, 2, 81–84 (1974).

L. E. Thibault, D. F. Meaney, B. J. Anderson, and A. Marmarou, *J. Neurotrauma*, 9, 311–322 (1992).

M. J. Whalen, R. S. B. Clark, C. E. Dixon, P. Robichaud, D. W. Marion, V. Vagni, S. H. Graham, L. Virag, G. Hasko, R. Stachlewitz, C. Szabo, and P. M. Kochanek, *J. Cereb. Blood Flow Metab.*, 19, 835–842 (1999).

T. Yamaki, N. Murakami, Y. Iwamoto, E. Yoshino, Y. Nakagawa, S. Ueda, J. Horikawa, and T. Tsujii, *J. Neurotrauma*, 11, 613–622 (1994).

I. Yamakami and T. K. McIntosh, *J. Cereb. Blood Flow Metab.*, 11, 655–660 (1991).

B. J. Zink, R. F. Walsh, and P. J. Feustel, *J. Neurotrauma*, 10, 275–286 (1993).

S. Zola-Morgan and L. R. Squire, *Behav. Neurosci.*, 99, 22–34 (1985).

PART II

PRECLINICAL STUDIES

CHAPTER 4

THE ROLE OF GLUTAMATE RECEPTORS IN THE PATHOPHYSIOLOGY OF TRAUMATIC CENTRAL NERVOUS SYSTEM INJURY

MEREDITH D. TEMPLE, DEIRDRE M. O'LEARY, and
ALAN I. FADEN
Departments of Neuroscience and Neurology and The Institute for Cognitive and
Computational Science, Georgetown University Medical Center, Washington, DC

INTRODUCTION

Traumatic injuries to the central nervous system (CNS) cause reactive, biochemical changes, which include the release or activation of both neurotoxic and neuroprotective factors. The balance between endogenous autodestructive and protective secondary events determines the degree of posttraumatic tissue damage and associated functional deficits. Release of excitatory amino acids (EAA), particularly L-glutamate (Glu), and the subsequent activation of Glu receptors appear to play a critical modulatory role in delayed posttraumatic cell death and subsequent behavioral dysfunction. While activation of certain classes of Glu receptors contributes to so-called excitotoxic cell damage, activation of other groups of Glu receptors may reduce cell death. These topics will be reviewed in detail in the present chapter.

GLUTAMATE RECEPTORS

Glu, the most abundant excitatory neurotransmitter in the central nervous system (CNS), exerts its complex neurotransmitter function through two major classes of receptors—ionotropic glutamate receptors (iGluRs) and metabotropic glutamate

Head Trauma: Basic, Preclinical, and Clinical Directions, Edited by Leonard P. Miller and
Ronald L. Hayes, Co-edited by Jennifer K. Newcomb
ISBN 0-471-36015-5 © 2001 John Wiley & Sons, Inc.

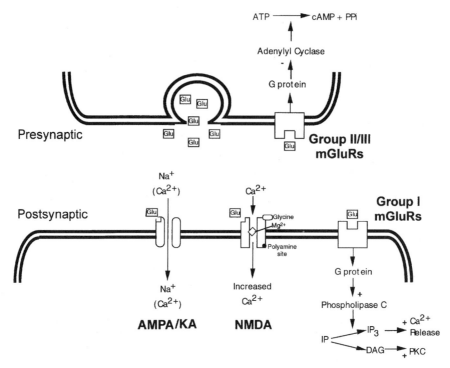

Figure 4.1   Characterization of the signaling process of the iGluRs and the mGluRs. NMDA receptors have multiple binding sites, located on both sides of the membrane as well as within the ion channel. NMDA receptor activation results in Ca^{2+} influx into the cell. AMPA/KA receptors are important for the transmembrane flux of ions, in particular Na^+, with some subtypes allowing Ca^{2+} into the cell. Group I mGluRs, which are primarily located postsynaptically, are coupled to the IP_3/Ca^{2+} pathway. Group II/III mGluRs, which are predominantly located presynaptically, are negatively coupled to the adenylyl cyclase pathway. ATP, adenosine triphosphate; cAMP, cyclic adenosine monophosphate; PP_i, biphosphate; IP, phosphatidylinositol; DAG, diacylglycerol; PKC, protein kinase C.

receptors (mGluRs). The iGluRs form membrane-bound receptors with ligand-gated ion channels that allow direct flux of ions such as potassium (K^+), sodium (Na^+), and calcium (Ca^{2+}) across the membrane, whereas the mGluRs are coupled to second messenger systems via G proteins and regulate complex signal transduction cascades (Monaghan et al., 1989) (see Fig. 4.1).

Ionotropic Receptors

The iGluRs are defined by their pharmacological and electrophysiological properties and are named for the primary ligand that binds to them: (1) N-methyl-D-aspartate (NMDA), (2) α-amino-3-hydroxy–5-methyl-4-isoxazole propionate (AMPA) and (3) kainate (KA) receptors (Monaghan et al., 1989). NMDA receptors are voltage and ligand-gated ion channels. They have multiple binding sites, located on both sides of the membrane as well as within the ion channel (D'Souza et al., 1993), and are ubiquitously distributed throughout the CNS primarily on postsynaptic sites (Wyszynski et al., 1999). These receptors are composed of two primary subunit families. NMDAR1 is found in most, if not all, NMDA receptor complexes and must be present for a functional receptor complex. In contrast, the various NMDAR2 subunits (A, B, C, or D) are more discretely localized within the CNS; they function to modify certain characteristics of the receptor complexes, such as potentiation of evoked currents, sensitivity to Mg^{2+} blockade of Ca^{2+} influx, or sensitivity to different antagonists (Morrison et al., 1996). A variety of types of NMDA receptor antagonists have been developed: competitive antagonists that bind at the Glu/NMDA agonist site; glycine site antagonists; noncompetitive antagonists that bind within the ion channel; and other antagonists that function to block the polyamine site or ion sites (Mg^{2+}, Zn^{2+}) (Watkins, 1991; Wong and Kemp, 1991) (see Table 4.1).

AMPA/KA receptors are also membrane-bound ion channels, but unlike NMDA receptors are not voltage-dependent (Cooper et al., 1996). These receptors are also important for the transmembrane flux of ions, in particular Na^+ and K^+, with some subtypes also allowing Ca^{2+} into the cell (Bettler and Mulle, 1995; Cooper et al.,

TABLE 4.1   Classification of iGluRs[a]

	NMDA	AMPA/KA
Subtype	NMDAR1 NMDAR2A, B, C, D	GluR1, 2, 3, 4 (AMPA) KA1, 2 (KA) GluR5, 6, 7, 8 (KA)
Transmembrane signaling process	Allows Ca^{2+} into cell	Allows Na^+ into cell (some subtypes may allow Ca^{2+} into cell)
Agonist	Glutamate NMDA Glycine Spermidine	Glutamate AMPA Kainate
Antagonist	MK801 Mg^{2+} compounds APV CPP Dextrorphan PCP CGS-19755 Ketamine KYN	NBQX CNQX GYKI-52466

[a] iGluRs may be divided into two groups, NMDA receptors and AMPA/KA receptors. A limited number of agonists and antagonists discussed in the present chapter have been included in this summary table. It should be noted that there are many more iGluR modulators not mentioned in this table; mentioning all of these modulators is beyond the scope of this chapter.

1996). Several subtypes of AMPA/KA receptors have been identified (GluR1–7, KA1–2). GluR1–4 represent the primary AMPA subunits, whereas GluR5–7 and KA1–2 are the major KA subunits (Martin et al., 1993; Bettler and Mulle, 1995). These subtypes form either homomeric or heteromeric receptor configurations, producing receptor complexes with varied characteristics (Bettler and Mulle, 1995). All AMPA/KA subtypes are expressed in the hippocampus, cortex and cerebellum, but show varying degrees of concentration (Martin et al., 1993; Cooper et al., 1996). These receptors are frequently colocalized with NMDA receptors on the postsynaptic membrane (Cooper et al., 1996; Wyszynski et al., 1999).

Antagonists for AMPA/KA receptors are few but include CNQX (6-cyano-7-nitroquinoxaline-2,3-dione), NBQX (2,3-dihydroxy-6-nitro-7-sulfamoylbenzol), as well as GYKI-52466 (see Table 4.1). CNQX is somewhat nonselective, also binding at the glycine site on NMDA receptors. NBQX and GYKI-52466 appear to be more selective for AMPA/KA receptors. Other more recently developed selective AMPA/KA antagonists have not been reported in CNS trauma.

Metabotropic Receptors

The existence of mGluRs was first suggested in 1985 when it was demonstrated that Glu stimulated phospholipase C (PLC) in cultured striatal neurons via a receptor that did not belong to the NMDA, AMPA, or KA families (Sladeczek et al., 1985). The suggestion that Glu activated not only iGluRs but a new family of receptors coupled to G proteins was confirmed in 1987 (Sugiyama et al., 1987), and the cloning of the first mGluR (now thought to be mGluR1a) was achieved in 1991 (Masu et al., 1991). The second messengers that mGluRs are coupled to are capable of producing long-lasting effects on cell excitability.

To date, at least eight different subtypes of mGluRs have been described, mGluR1–8 (Knöpfel et al., 1995; Pin and Duvoisin, 1995; Riedel et al., 1996; Saugstad et al., 1997). These eight subtypes can be divided into three groups (group I, group II and group III) based on sequence homology, signal transduction pathways, and agonist sensitivity. Group I mGluRs, which include subtypes mGluR1 and mGluR5, are coupled via PLC to the inositol trisphosphate $(IP_3)/Ca^{2+}$ pathway. They are selectively activated by (R,S)-3,5-dihydroxy phenyl-glycine [(R,S)-DHPG; Schoepp et al., 1994]. Activation of these receptors, particularly mGluR1, may also serve to increase adenylyl cyclase and phospholipase A_2 (PL A_2) activity. Group II receptors, comprising mGluR2 and mGluR3, are negatively coupled to the adenylyl cyclase second messenger system and are sensitive to agonists such as $(2S,1'R,2'R,3'R)$-2-$(2',3'$-dicarboxy)cyclopropylglycine (DCG-IV). Group III mGluRs, which include mGluR4, mGluR6, mGluR7, and mGluR8, are also negatively coupled to adenylyl cyclase but are differentiated by their sensitivity to L-AP4 (L-2-amino-4-phosphanobutanoic acid). Group I mGluRs are predominantly located postsynaptically, whereas group II and III mGluRs are largely located presynaptically (Knöpfel et al., 1995; Pin and Duvoisin, 1995; Riedel et al., 1996; Saugstad et al., 1997; Shigemoto et al., 1997) (see Table 4.2).

TABLE 4.2   Classification of mGluRs[a]

	Group I	Group II	Group III
Subtype	1, 5	2, 3	4, 6, 7, 8
Second messenger system	Activates IP_3/Ca^{2+}	Inhibits adenylyl cyclase	Inhibits adenylyl cyclase
Agonist	(1S,3R)-ACPD	(1S,3R)-ACPD	L-AP4
	t-ACPD	t-ACPD	L-SOP
	(S)-DHPG	L-CCG-1	
	CHPG	DCG-IV	
	t-ADA	4C3HPG	
		(2R,4R)-APDC	
		LY354740	
Antagonist	MCPG	MCPG	MAP-4
	4C3HPG	MCCG-1	MSOP
	AIDA	MSOPPE	
	CPCCOEt	L-AP3	
	MPEP		
	LY367366		
	LY367385		

[a] mGluRs may be divided into three groups, based on sequence similarities, transduction mechanisms and pharmacological profile. Agonists and antagonists discussed in the present chapter have been included in the table. The pharmacological profile has been somewhat simplified for the purpose of the table.

EVIDENCE OF INVOLVEMENT OF Glu RECEPTORS IN THE PATHOPHYSIOLOGY OF HEAD TRAUMA

There is compelling evidence implicating Glu release and activation of Glu receptors in the pathophysiological mechanisms of CNS injury. Trauma to the brain or spinal cord causes marked elevations in the extracellular levels of EAAs, including Glu and aspartate, in both animal models and humans (Faden et al., 1988, 1989; Katayama et al., 1990; Panter and Faden, 1992; Bullock et al., 1998). Subsequent activation of both iGluRs and mGluRs serves to modulate posttraumatic cell death and its associated functional deficits.

NMDA Receptors and CNS/Neuronal Injury

In Vitro Studies. Considerable experimental evidence implicates Glu release and Glu receptor activation as contributors to cell death in several models of in vitro injury, including hypoxia, oxygen–glucose deprivation, Glu exposure/toxicity, and traumatic injury (Choi et al., 1988, 1990; Monyer et al., 1989; Choi, 1992; Regan and Choi, 1994; Ellis et al., 1995; Gwag et al., 1995; Mukhin et al., 1997a,b, 1998). Many laboratories have shown that NMDA receptor antagonists attenuate Glu-induced neuronal cell death (Choi et al., 1990; Choi, 1992). Similarly, treatment with

NMDA antagonists reduces neuronal cell death caused by transient oxygen–glucose deprivation (Monyer et al., 1989; Gwag et al., 1995).

Recently, several in vitro models have been developed to study mechanisms related to traumatic neuronal injury (Regan and Choi, 1994; Ellis et al., 1995; Mukhin et al., 1997a,b; 1998; see Chapter 2). Regan and Choi (1994) found that multiple tears of rat neuronal/glial cocultures produced extensive cell death. Approximately 50 to 75 percent of cell death was blocked by the NMDA antagonist MK801. Mukhin et al. (1997b) characterized the effects of a moderately severe circular scratch injury on mixed neuronal/glial cultures of rat cortex. In this model, administration of MK801 significantly attenuated neuronal cell death. Mukhin et al. (1998) also used another injury device that produces a series of parallel cuts uniformly distributed throughout the cell layer in 96-well plates. This model is characterized by progressive neuronal cell death around each cut, which is markedly reduced by treatment with MK801 in a pH-dependent manner.

Ellis and colleagues (1995) developed a model in which cultured astrocytes or neurons are injured by stretching them on a silastic membrane. Such injury decreases Mg^{2+} blockade of NMDA receptors, resulting in significantly larger ionic currents as well as increased intracellular Ca^{2+} (Zhang et al., 1996). A follow-up study showed that 24 h post insult, NMDA-stimulated Ca^{2+} is increased, indicating an enhanced sensitivity of the NMDA receptors following injury (Rzigalinski et al., 1998).

Together, these studies demonstrate that Glu and NMDA receptor activation may cause neuronal cell death in vitro. Although it has long been assumed that Glu toxicity causes primarily necrotic cell death, in vitro work from a number of laboratories has shown that NMDA receptors may contribute to either necrotic or apoptotic cell death, depending upon the experimental conditions (Gwag et al., 1995; Nicotera and Lipton, 1999). For example, blockade of iGluRs may unmask Glu-induced apoptosis (Gwag et al., 1995), and alterations in underlying cellular bioenergetic state may shift cell death into primarily necrotic or apoptotic types (Nicotera and Lipton, 1999; Allen et al., 1999). Relating to posttraumatic injury, Allen et al. (1999) found that on combining a mild metabolic insult (brief exposure to 3-nitropropionic acid and glucose deprivation) with trauma, cell death shifted from primarily necrotic to substantially apoptotic.

In Vivo Studies. Numerous studies have shown that treatment with NMDA receptor antagonists reduces posttraumatic tissue damage and associated behavioral changes. Protective effects have been demonstrated with structurally different antagonists that act at different sites on the NMDA receptor complex (see Table 4.3; McIntosh et al., 1998 for review). For example, several competitive antagonists of the Glu/NMDA site, such as APV (2-amino-5-phosphovaleric acid), CPP [3-(2-carboxypiperizin-4-yl)-propyl-1-phosphonic acid], and CGS-19755 can attenuate metabolic dysfunction, decrease concentrations of extracellular Glu, reduce cerebral edema, and improve behavioral outcome following lateral fluid percussion injury (FPI) (Faden et al., 1989; Panter and Faden, 1992; Kawamata et al., 1992; Okiyama et al., 1997). However, because many of these drugs do not easily cross the blood–

brain barrier (BBB), they may not be as potentially useful from a clinical perspective.

Numerous noncompetitive ion channel blockers have been effective in reducing pathological changes or improving behavioral outcome after traumatic CNS injury. These drugs, which include dextrorphan, phenylcyclidine, MK801, ketamine and dextromethorphan, as well as others, reduce brain edema, restore ionic homeostasis and metabolic function, and improve functional recovery after experimental TBI (Hayes et al., 1988; Faden et al., 1989; Panter and Faden, 1992; McIntosh et al., 1989a, 1990; Shapira et al., 1990; Hamm et al., 1993; Smith et al., 1993a,b; Golding and Vink, 1995) (see Table 4.3). MK801 and other NMDA antagonists also produce beneficial effects in models of spinal cord trauma, suggesting that Glu and modulation of Glu receptors is important in spinal cord injury as well as TBI (Faden et al., 1988; Haghighi et al., 1996). Unfortunately, noncompetitive antagonists have potentially undesirable side effects, including increased vacuole size in the cell and psychotomimetic effects (Olney et al., 1989; Kornhuber and Weller, 1997). Some more recently developed noncompetitive antagonists have lower binding affinities within the ion channel, which may result in fewer unwanted side effects (Beal, 1995; McIntosh et al., 1998). One example is remacemide HCl [2-amino-*N*-(1-methyl-1,2-diphenylethyl)acetamide hydrochloride], which reduced lesion volume in rats subjected to lateral FPI (Smith et al., 1997).

Another approach is to use antagonists that modulate other binding sites on the NMDA receptor, such as glycine, Mg^{2+}, or polyamine (see Table 4.3). For example, the glycine site antagonists kynurenate (KYN) and indole-2-carboxylic acid (I2CA) reduce neurobehavioral deficits as well as decrease edema (I2CA) and protect against hippocampal cell loss (KYN) following lateral FPI in rats (Smith et al., 1993a; Hicks et al., 1994). However, it should be noted that although KYN is frequently characterized as a glycine site antagonist, it binds nonselectively at other Glu receptors. Polyamine site antagonists, such as Eliprodil and Ifenprodil derivatives (e.g., CP-101,606; CP-101,581; CP-98,113), reduce lesion volume, edema, and motor/cognitive function following lateral FPI (Toulmond et al., 1993; Hogg et al., 1998; Okiyama et al., 1998). Inhibition of ODC (ornithine decarboxylase), an enzyme necessary for polyamine synthesis, also decreases injury-induced edema (Baskaya et al., 1996). In addition, treatment with different Mg^{2+} compounds (i.e., $MgCl_2$ and $MgSO_4$) is effective in improving motor and cognitive recovery, decreasing edema, and normalizing brain bioenergetics following lateral FPI (Mcintosh et al., 1988, 1989b; Smith et al., 1993b; Okiyama et al., 1995; Heath and Vink, 1998, 1999). Both Eliprodil and $MgSO_4$ have extended therapeutic windows (up to 24 h post injury), which may enhance their clinical utility (Toulmond et al., 1993; Hogg et al., 1998; Heath and Vink, 1999).

Antisense oligodeoxynucleotides (as-ODN) directed against NMDAR1 subunits have also been used to address the role of NMDA receptors in the pathophysiology of posttraumatic brain injury (Sun and Faden, 1995b). When given prior to lateral FPI, as-ODN NMDAR1 decreased mortality, motor dysfunction, and reactive gliosis.

TABLE 4.3 Animal Studies Examining NMDA Antagonists in Traumatic Brain Injury

Site of Action	Compound	Injury Model	Outcome	References
Competitive NMDA antagonist	APV	CFP	↓ Glucose utilization	Kawamata et al. (1992)
	CPP	LFP	↑ Motor function	Faden et al. (1989)
	CGS-19755	LFP	↓ Glutamate release	Panter and Faden, (1992)
Non competitive channel blocker	Dextrorphan	LFP	↓ Glu release; ↑ Bioenergetic status; ↑ Motor function; ↑ Mg^{2+} homeostasis	Faden et al. (1989); Panter and Faden (1992)
	Dextromethorphan	LFP	↑ Mg^{2+} homeostasis; ↑ Bioenergetic status	Golding and Vink (1995)
	PCP	CFP	↑ Motor function	Hayes et al. (1998)
	MK801	CFP, LFP, WD	↑ Bioenergetic status; ↑ Motor/cognitive function; ↓ Edema; ↑ Ionic homeostasis	McIntosh et al. (1989a, 1990); Shapira et al. (1990); Hamm et al. (1993)
	Ketamine	LFP	↑ Motor/cognitive function; ↓ Edema	Shohami et al. (1993); Smith et al. (1993b, 1997)
	Remacemide HCl	LFP	↓ Lesion volume	Kroppenstedt et al. (1998)
	CNS-1102 (Cerestat)	CCI	↓ Contusion volume; ↓ Edema; ↓ H_2O content	
Glycine site	Kynurenate[a]	LFP, CFP	↑ Motor/cognitive function; ↑ Ionic homeostasis	Hicks et al. (1994); Smith et al. (1993a);

Site	Drug	Model	Effects	References
Mg²⁺ site	Indole-2-carboxylic acid	LFP	↓ Edema	Kawamata et al. (1992)
	MgCl₂	LFP	↓ Cell loss ↓ Glucose utilization ↑ Motor/cognitive function ↓ Edema ↑ Ionic homeostasis	Smith et al. (1993a) McIntosh et al. (1989b); Smith et al. (1993b); Okiyama et al. (1995); Heath and Vink (1998)
	MgSO₄	LFP, WD	↑ Motor/cognitive function ↓ Edema ↑ Mg²⁺ homeostasis ↑ Motor/cognitive function ↓ Edema ↑ Bioenergetic status ↑ Mg²⁺ homeostasis	McIntosh et al. (1988); Okiyama et al. (1995); Heath and Vink (1998, 1999)
Polyamine site	Eliprodil	LFP	↓ Lesion volume ↑ Cognitive function	Toulmond et al. (1993); Hogg et al. (1998)
	CP-101,606	LFP	↑ Cognitive function	Okiyama et al. (1997)
	CP-101,581	LFP	↑ Cognitive function	
	CP98,113	LFP	↑ Motor/cognitive function ↓ Edema	Okiyama et al. (1997, 1998)
	ODC synthesis inhibitor (DFMO)	CCI	↓ Edema	Baskaya et al. (1996)

All studies were carried out in the rat model.

ᵃ Kynurenate also has activity at other non-NMDA receptor sites.

LFP, lateral fluid percussion; CFP, central fluid percussion; WD, weight drop.

Several other drugs with purported actions on the Glu receptor system can reduce injury-associated cellular and behavioral damage (see Table 4.4). For example, HU-211 (7-hydroxy-tetrahydrocannabinol 1,1-dimethylheptyl), a cannabinoid, can enhance motor and cognitive function, reduce edema, and decrease BBB breakdown following weight drop injury in rats (Shohami et al., 1993, 1995). HU-211 has a therapeutic window of up to 4 h. However, this compound has multiple potential neuroprotective actions, including inhibition of TNF-α (Shohami et al., 1997). Use-dependent sodium channel blockers also function to block Glu release (Graham et al., 1994). Recent studies indicate that several of these compounds, such as 619C89, BW1003C87, and Riluzole, restore neurobehavioral function, reduce hippocampal cell loss and reactive gliosis, as well as decreasing edema and lesion volume (Sun and Faden, 1995a; Okiyama et al., 1995; Voddi et al., 1995; McIntosh et al., 1996; Bareyre et al., 1997; Wahl et al., 1997). Although these drugs function to inhibit Glu release or block NMDA receptor activation, it is important to stress that the aforementioned drugs have additional mechanisms of action that may be a significant component of their observed neuroprotective effects.

In the last decade, the primary emphasis has been the development and testing of NMDA targeted therapies. However, little is known about *how* the NMDA receptor system is altered following traumatic injury. Miller et al. (1990) found a significant decrease in [^{3}H]NMDA binding to the NMDA receptor in the hippocampus 3 h after central FPI in rats. Reductions were also observed in the neocortex at 5 min, 3 h, and 24 h post TBI. These reductions in NMDA receptor binding may reflect a compensatory downregulation of receptor binding affinity following the postinjury excitotoxic surge of Glu. In addition, decreased [^{3}H]MK801 receptor binding has been observed following trauma to the spinal cord (Sun and Faden, 1994). Temple et al. (1997) also found that there were decreases in immunoreactivity for hippocampal NMDAR1 subunits and NMDAR2A/B subunits at 24 h, 8 days, and 16 days following lateral FPI. The most profound decreases were observed in the NMDAR1 subunit at 24 h post injury, suggesting that NMDAR1 subunits may be more sensitive to TBI than one NMDAR2 subunits. These decreases in protein levels may also reflect an endogenous response to the acute surge of Glu. Together, these studies suggest that NMDA receptors undergo changes after injury that continue for prolonged periods of time, affecting the actions of therapies targeting this receptor.

An Alternative Therapeutic Strategy? There are several concerns with using NMDA antagonists following CNS injury. First, studies using NMDA antagonists have focused on very early (postinjury) treatment or even preinjury treatment models. While this is useful for elucidating early mechanisms of injury, there may be limited clinical relevance. Second, many of these drugs have substantial side effects. Because trauma may serve to downregulate NMDA receptors, which may affect cognitive performance late after injury, a recent study examined whether chronic *enhancement* of NMDA receptors could provide an alternative therapeutic approach. Temple and Hamm (1996) found that chronic administration (30 mg/kg, i.p.; starting 24 h post injury through 15 days post injury) of D-cycloserine (DCS), a *positive* modulator of the NMDA-associated glycine site, significantly improved

TABLE 4.4 Animal Head Trauma Studies Examining Glutamate/NMDA Inhibitors That Also Have Other Potential Neuroprotective Actions

Mechanism of Action	Compound	Injury Model	Outcome	References
Noncompetitive NMDA Antagonist	HU211	WD	↑ Motor/cognitive function ↓ Edema ↓ Blood–brain barrier breakdown	Shohami et al. (1993, 1995)
Inhibition of Glu release	619C89	LFP	↑ Motor/cognitive function ↓ Cell death ↓ Gliosis	Sun and Faden (1995a); Voddi et al. (1995)
	BW1003C87	LFP	↓ Edema	Okiyama et al. (1995) McIntosh et al. (1996); Zhang et al. (1998);
	Riluzole	LFP	↑ Motor/cognitive function ↓ Edema ↓ Lesion volume	Barerye et al. (1997) Wahl et al. (1997)

All studies were carried out in the rat model.
LFP, lateral fluid percussion; WD, weight drop.

cognitive performance of injured rats (lateral FPI) to the level of sham-injured rats. These results suggest that later, chronic positive modulation at the NMDA receptor may provide an additional therapeutic option.

AMPA/KA Receptors and CNS/Neuronal Injury

Whereas the role of the NMDA receptor system in TBI has been well studied, much less is understood about the contribution of AMPA/KA receptors to posttraumatic pathophysiology. Limited studies are available to determine postinjury changes in AMPA/KA receptors or the therapeutic efficacy of modulating these receptors (see Table 4.5). Recent in vivo studies corroborate positive findings of treatment with AMPA/KA antagonists in ischemia (Bullock et al., 1994; Gill, 1994) and spinal cord injury (Wrathall et al., 1994). For example, NBQX reduced cortical lesion volume and CA3 cell loss in rats subjected to lateral FPI (Bernert and Turski, 1996). A striking finding of this study was that NBQX also protected against CA3 cell loss when administered between 1 and 7 h post injury. Also, acute treatment with the AMPA/KA antagonist GYKI-52466 attenuated cognitive impairment induced by lateral FRI (Hylton et al., 1995). Although a number of studies indicate a limited role for AMPA/KA receptors in traumatic neuronal injury (Regan and Choi, 1994; Prehn et al., 1995; Mukhin et al., 1997b), the in vivo studies indicate that modulation of AMPA/KA receptors may have clinical potential.

Metabotropic Receptors and CNS/Neuronal Injury

The mGluRs have been shown to have a wide range of physiological roles, such as interactions with Ca^{2+} and K^+ channels, and regulation of ionotropic receptors (for review see Anwyl, 1999). Given that activation of the iGluRs, and in particular NMDA receptor activation, and subsequent Ca^{2+} influx, are known to be involved in neuronal injury, and because of the wide range of physiological roles and distribution of mGluRs throughout the brain, it was postulated that mGluRs would be involved in neuronal injury. The mGluR-mediated effects on high-voltage-activated (HVA) Ca^{2+} channels may influence neurotoxicity (Stefani et al., 1996). For example, Copani et al. (1995) report that both mGluR group II and III agonists and the HVA Ca^{2+} channel blocker nimodipine reduce β-amyloid induced toxicity in

TABLE 4.5   Animal Studies Using AMPA/KA Antagonists in Traumatic Brain Injury

Mechanism of Action	Compound	Injury Model	Outcome	References
AMPA/KA antagonists	NBQX	LFP	↓ Lesion volume ↓ Cell death	Bernert and Turski (1996)
	GYKI-52466	LFP	↑ Cognitive function	Hylton et al. (1995)

All studies were carried out in the rat model.
LFP, lateral fluid percussion.

cultured cerebellar granule cells. The interaction of mGluRs with K^+ channels also indicates a role for these receptors in neuronal injury. Activation of certain K^+ channels and subsequent efflux of K^+ has been suggested to underlie certain forms of neuronal apoptosis (Yu et al., 1997).

Some of the pathophysiological and neurodegenerative disorders that mGluRs may be involved in include epilepsy, cerebral ischemia (stroke), Huntington's chorea, Parkinson's disease, and Alzheimer's disease. MGluRs may be a potential target for drugs in the treatment of these disorders. One advantage of targeting mGluRs would be the fact that there should be minimal peripheral side effects as mGluRs are primarily localized in the CNS. Interference with mGluRs seems to have only a modest impact on fast excitatory synaptic transmission, which would also be an advantage for chronic therapies (Knöpfel et al., 1995; Pin and Duvoisin, 1995; Nicoletti et al., 1996; Toms et al., 1996; Anwyl, 1999; Hölscher et al., 1999).

Many of the early studies investigating the role of mGluR in neuronal injury involved the conformationally restricted glutamate analogue (1*S*,3*R*)-aminocyclo-pentane dicarboxylate (1*S*,3*R*-ACPD) or its racemic mixture, commonly referred to as *trans*-ACPD (tACPD). ACPD was one of the first agonists selective for mGluRs. In 1991, it was reported that 1*S*,3*R*-ACPD reduced the degeneration of cultured mouse cortical neurons produced by brief exposure to NMDA (Koh et al., 1991). 1*S*,3*R*-ACPD was subsequently shown to reduce NMDA-induced injury in mesen-cephalic neurons (Ambrosini et al., 1995), cultured rat cerebellar granule cells (Valerio et al., 1996), and rat hippocampal slices (Pizzi et al., 1996a). 1*S*,3*R*-ACPD was also found to counteract both Glu-induced and KA-induced neurotoxicity in cultured rat cerebellar granule cells (Pizzi et al., 1993, 1996b) by blocking the rise in intracellular Ca^{2+} caused by Glu or KA, through a mechanism involving protein kinase C (PKC; Pizzi et al., 1996b). The involvement of PKC in the neuroprotective action of 1*S*,3*R*-ACPD was further supported by the report that 1*S*,3*R*-ACPD protects against nitric oxide (NO)-induced toxicity via the modulation of PKC activity (Maiese et al., 1996).

However, several studies have indicated that ACPD can act as a powerful neurotoxic agent and neuroconvulsant. McDonald and Schoepp (1992) demon-strated that instrastriatal injections of 1*S*,3*R*-ACPD potentiated NMDA-mediated injury in 7-day-old rats in vivo, while the same group reported that higher doses of 1*S*,3*R*-ACPD alone can cause seizures and neurodegeneration in neonatal and adult rats (Sacann and Schoepp, 1992; McDonald et al., 1993; Schoepp et al., 1995). Brain injury was found to be dose dependent. More recently, it has also been reported that tACPD exacerbates posttraumatic injury in spinal cord white matter isolated from adult rats (Agrawal et al., 1998).

The contradictory results reported with ACPD are not surprising considering the lack of specificity of this agent. ACPD activates both the IP_3-linked group I receptors and the cAMP linked group II receptors (Pin and Duvoisin, 1995). The recent increase in the availability of mGluR ligands with greater specificity for the different mGluR groups and subtypes has helped clarify the role of each mGluR group in neuronal injury.

Group I mGluRs and Neuronal Injury. Striatal infusion of the endogenous NMDA receptor agonist quinolinic acid induces a loss of medium-sized spiny neurons, with relative sparing of interneurons, similar to that observed in the early phase of Huntington's chorea. It has been shown that local injection of (*S*)-4C3HPG, which acts as a competitive mGluR1 antagonist and an agonist at group II mGluRs (Watkins and Collingridge, 1994), protects striatal neurons from quinolinic acid-induced degeneration (Orlando et al., 1995). As these neurons express both mGluR5 and mGluR3, and given the mixed activity of (*S*)-4C3HPG, it is not possible to specify which group is involved. However, Buisson and Choi (1995) have reported that (*S*)-4C3HPG decreases lesions on the striatum induced by NMDA, in a cAMP-dependent manner, which suggests the involvement of group II receptors.

Whether group I receptor activation provides neuroprotection or induces injury seems to depend on the area of the brain, and the type of cell death (i.e., necrotic or apoptotic cell death) being studied. The specific group I agonist (*S*)-DHPG (Ito et al., 1995), was found to reduce the damage induced by oxygen–glucose deprivation, a well-studied model of necrotic cell death, in hippocampal slices in a PKC-dependent manner (Schroder et al., 1999). In the cerebellum, group I activation also appears to be neuroprotective. In cultured rat cerebellar granule cells, group I activation prevents toxicity induced by Glu or NMDA (Montoliu et al., 1997). The neuroprotective effect of tADA (*trans*-azatidine-2,4-dicarboxylic acid), which activates mGluR5 but not mGluR1 (Kozikowski et al., 1993), led the authors to conclude that group I neuroprotection may be mediated by mGluR5.

Group I mGluR activation also seems to be neuroprotective against apoptotic cell death. A recent study by Copani et al. (1998) shows that after 4 to 5 days in vitro, cerebellar granule cells grown in medium containing 10 mM K$^+$ undergo apoptosis. At this stage in development, mGluR5 expression begins to decline. Apoptotic cells were seen not to express the mGluR5 subtype, whereas induced overexpression of mGluR5 protected against apoptosis. The authors conclude that the decline in the expression of mGluR5 allows programmed cell death in cerebellar granule cells developing in culture. Also in rat cerebellar granule cells, group I activation has been shown to have a protective effect against apoptosis induced by *β*-amyloid, a protein that may play a role in the pathogenesis of Alzheimer's disease (Copani et al., 1995; Allen et al., 1999a), whereas blockade of group I mGluRs exacerbates cell death (Allen et al., 1999a). It has been suggested that this neuroprotective action may be mediated through modulation of intracellular Ca^{2+} homeostasis (Allen et al., 1999a). In rat cortical neuronal–glial cultures, the group I agonist (*S*)-DHPG significantly attenuates apoptotic cell death induced by both staurosporine, the nonspecific PKC inhibitor, and etoposide, an inhibitor of topoisomerase II. This effect was completely reversed by coapplication of the group I antagonist, AIDA (Allen and Faden, submitted).

In primary hippocampal cultures, (*S*)-DHPG has been reported to reduce NO-induced injury (Maiese and Vincent, 1999; Vincent et al., 1999). NO can induce apoptosis via activation of endonucleases that degrade DNA. Activation of the endonucleases is dependent on a decrease in intracellular pH caused by NO. Vincent et al. (1999) suggest that (*S*)-DHPG exerts its neuroprotective action by preventing the decrease in pH induced by NO, thereby preventing endonuclease activation and subsequent cell death. However, it should be noted that it has been reported that decreased cell death, induced by mechanical injury in cortical cultures, was observed under acidic conditions, whereas increased extracellular pH was associated with NMDA-dependent cell loss (Mukhin et al., 1998).

In contrast, in cortical and spinal cord neurons, group I activation seems to exacerbate necrotic neurotoxicity. In mouse cortical cultures mGluR group I agonists have been shown to amplify neuronal degeneration induced by a pulse of NMDA (Bruno et al., 1995b, 1999; Strasser et al., 1998). This proexcitotoxic effect of group I activation may be mediated in part by PKC activation (Bruno et al., 1995b) or by an enhancement of presynaptic Glu release (Strasser et al., 1998). This effect may also be mediated via mGluR1a activation, as LY367385, a potent and selective antagonist of mGluR1a, was neuroprotective in mouse cortical cultures exposed to an NMDA pulse (Bruno et al., 1999).

In rat mixed cortical/glial cultures, group I activation exacerbated injury induced by a specially designed in vitro punch injury model that induces delayed neuronal injury (Mukhin et al., 1996, 1997a, b). The exact mechanism of group I activation-induced exacerbation of injury has not been fully determined but appears to be mediated at least partly through NMDA modulation, as the NMDA antagonist MK801 partly reduced the DHPG-induced exacerbation of injury (Mukhin et al., 1997a). Such a modulation of NMDA receptors has been suggested to be through PKC activation and subsequent reduction of the Mg^{2+} block of NMDA receptors. However, other possible mechanisms, such as increased release of Ca^{2+} from intracellular stores via IP_3 activation, increased arachidonic acid production, or inactivation of cAMP cannot be ruled out (Mukhin et al., 1997a). It is likely that mGluR1 is involved in this exacerbation of injury, as antisense oligodeoxynucleotide (as-ODN) directed to mGluR1 reduced injury, while as-ODN directed to mGluR5 did not (Mukhin et al., 1996). Injury may also be exacerbated by activation of mGluR1 in mouse cortical cells (Bruno et al., 1999) and in isolated spinal cord segments (Agrawal et al., 1998), where mGluR1 immunoreactivity is present.

A small number of in vivo studies support a role for group I mGluR activation in neuronal injury (see Table 4.6). MCPG, a weak group I/II antagonist exhibiting greater antagonistic effects at mGluR1 than at mGluR5 (Brabet et al., 1995; Joly et al., 1995; Kingston et al., 1995) improves neurological recovery and postinjury behavioral deficits, and decreases CA1 pyramidal cell and ipsilateral hippocampal cell loss in vivo after lateral FPI when administered intracerebroventricularly, either 5 min before trauma (Gong et al., 1995) or 15 min before and 1 h after trauma (Mukhin et al., 1996). The potent and selective mGluR1a antagonist LY367385 was also seen to have significant neuroprotective effects when administered intrastriatally, in rats infused with NMDA into the caudate nucleus and in gerbils exposed to global ischemia (Bruno et al., 1999). The less specific mGluR1a and mGluR5 antagonist LY367366 also protected against injury under these conditions, but less efficaciously, implicating mGluR1a in the neurodegeneration (Bruno et al., 1999).

Group II mGluRs and Neuronal Injury. While there is some debate about the role of group I mGluRs in neuronal injury, there seems to be greater consensus in the literature with regard to the role of group II mGluR activation. Group II mGluR

TABLE 4.6 Animal Studies Using Metabotropic Glutamate Receptor Antagonists in Traumatic Brain Injury

Mechanism of Action	Compound	Injury Model	Outcome	References
Group I/II antagonist	MCPG	LFP	↑ Motor/cognitive function	Mukhin et al. (1996)
			↓ Cell death	Gong et al. (1995)
mGluR 1a/5 antagonist	LY367366	LFP	↓ Cell death	Bruno et al. (1999)
mGluR 1a antagonist	LY367385			
mGluR 2/3 agonist	LY354740	LFP	↑ Motor function	Allen et al. (1999b)

All studies were carried out in the rat model.
LFP, lateral fluid percussion.

activation generally reduces neuronal toxicity, both necrotic and apoptotic. However, Montoliu et al. (1997) report that group II activation with L-CCG-1 does not provide neuroprotection against glutamate-induced toxicity in primary cultures of cerebellar granule cells. DCG-IV, L-CCG-1, and 4C3HPG have been shown to attenuate toxicity induced by a pulse of NMDA, Glu, or KA in cultured mouse cortical neurons (Bruno et al., 1994, 1995a, 1996, 1997, 1998; Buisson and Choi, 1995), whereas activation of group II receptors with t-ACPD and L-CCG-1 protects against colchicine-induced apoptosis, possibly via both phosphoinositide activation of PKC and adenylyl cyclase inhibition (Kalda and Zharkovsky, 1999). Interestingly, the medium taken from pure astrocyte cultures pretreated for 2 to 20 h with DCG-IV, L-CCG-1, or 4C3HPG was found to be highly neuroprotective when transferred to mixed neuronal/glial cultures treated with NMDA (Bruno et al., 1997, 1998). Therefore, neuroprotection provided by group II mGluR activation may involve an interaction between glia and neurons, possibly by stimulating astrocytes to increase the formation and release of transforming growth factor β which in turn protects neighboring neurons from excitotoxic death (Bruno et al., 1998).

The problem with the three agonists mentioned (DCG-IV, L-CCG-1, and 4C3HPG) is that none of them is a selective group II agonist. DCG-IV also acts as an NMDA receptor agonist (Wilsch et al., 1994). L-CCG-1 at high concentrations has some activity at group I mGluRs (Nakagawa et al., 1990) and especially mGluR1 (Flor et al., 1996). L-CCG-1 also has some affinity for mGluR4a (Eriksen and Thompsen, 1996) and mGluR8 (Saugstad et al., 1997). 4C3HPG is also a group I antagonist with partial agonist activity at mGluR5 (Watkins and Collingridge, 1994). Recently, some more specific agents have been developed, such as 2R,4R-APDC, which has been shown to be a highly selective group II agonist with no activity at group I or II receptors (Monn et al., 1996); and LY354740, which has also been shown to be a highly selective group II agonist (Bond et al., 1997). Both of these agents have also been shown to attenuate neurotoxicity.

2R,4R-APDC protects against NMDA-induced toxicity in mouse mixed neuronal/glial cortical cultures (Battaglia et al., 1998), whereas a related compound, the amino derivative 1-amino-APDC, which acts as a partial agonist at group II receptors, also reduces NMDA-induced toxicity in mouse mixed neuronal/glial cortical cultures (Kozikowski et al., 1999). DCG-IV, LY354740 and 2R,4R-APDC have all been shown to reduce injury in rat mixed cortical neuronal/glial cell cultures injured with the in vitro punch trauma device (Allen et al., 1999b). In this model, it was found that the neuroprotective effect of group II receptor activation was additive to the effect of group I and NMDA receptor antagonism, suggesting that down-regulation of both the phosphoinositide and cAMP pathways is involved in providing neuroprotection. A role for cAMP is supported by the observation that 8-Br-cAMP, the cAMP analogue, exacerbated cell death, while intracellular cAMP levels increased following injury. It was also shown that treatment with the group II agonists caused a reduction in the posttraumatic Glu release. Reducing presynaptic glutamate *release* would be very beneficial, as it would be expected to limit both NMDA and group I mGluR activation, which have already been shown to contribute to posttraumatic cell death (Allen et al., 1999b).

Allen et al. (1999b) also performed in vivo studies to support the neuroprotective effects of group II mGluR activation (see Table 4.6). Treatment with LY354740, administered 30 min after trauma, significantly improved neurological recovery 14 days after the induction of lateral FPI in rats. The degree of protection provided by this agent was found to be comparable with that observed previously with competitive and noncompetitive NMDA antagonists in this model (Faden et al., 1989). This suggests that group II agonists may prove useful in clinical head injury management.

Group III mGluRs and Neuronal Injury. The fact that group III mGluRs share many physiological properties with group II mGluRs suggest that group III mGluRs would also be neuroprotective. Consistent with this hypothesis, a number of studies have demonstrated a neuroprotective action of mGluR III activation (see Table 4.6).

The specific group III agonist L-AP4 (Birse et al., 1993; Jane et al., 1994) reduces NMDA-induced excitotoxicity in mouse cerebellar granule cells (Lafon-Cazal et al., 1999) and in mouse cortical neurons (Bruno et al., 1996). Immunocytochemical analysis implicates mGluR7 in the cerebellar granule cells and mGluR4 in the cortical neurons (Bruno et al., 1996; Lafon-Cazal et al., 1999). L-AP4 has also been shown to reduce toxicity induced by NO in rat cortical cultures (Maiese et al., 1995) and in rat hippocampal cultures (Maiese et al., 1996), possibly through mGluR4-mediated protein kinase A (PKA) modulation. In the in vitro punch injury model described earlier, Faden et al. (1997) report that L-AP4 and L-SOP provide 30 percent neuroprotection in mixed rat cortical neuronal/glial cultures. The methyl derivatives of these compounds, MAP-4 and MSOP, respectively, two group III antagonists (Jane et al., 1994; Thomas et al., 1995), caused a significant exacerbation of traumatic injury. Basal cAMP levels were lower in the agonist-treated cells, suggesting a role for cAMP regulation in injury. However, the neuroprotective effect of the group III agonists was additive to the neuroprotection of MK801, which suggests that combined therapy may prove clinically useful. It was not determined which specific mGluR subtype might mediate this effect as mRNA for all four group III receptors was found in the cultures.

In conclusion, a large number of studies implicating the mGluRs in neuronal injury, both in vivo and in vitro, have been reviewed. The effect of group I mGluR activation seems to depend largely on whether necrotic or apoptotic injury has been induced, and also on the brain region being studied. For example, in cortical neurons, group I mGluR activation exacerbates necrotic injury and attenuates apoptotic cell death. Activation of both group II and III receptors reduces both types of neuronal injury. MGluR agonists or antagonists may prove useful in clinical treatments of TBI, possibly in combination with NMDA receptor antagonists. However, the contrasting effect of group I mGluR activation on necrotic versus apoptotic death brings into question the potential usefulness of group I specific compounds in the clinical setting.

EXTENT OF INVOLVEMENT OF GLUTAMATE IN HEAD TRAUMA

The overwhelming majority of the data unequivocally implicate Glu and all of its receptor subtypes in CNS injury. Not only are there changes in physiological measures (e.g., elevated Glu levels, altered Glu uptake, decreased receptor binding and protein levels), but the pharmacological studies demonstrate that manipulation of the different Glu receptors can either exacerbate or attenuate injury-induced pathology.

However, there has been considerable debate over the importance of Glu release in the pathophysiology of TBI and other types of CNS injury. EAA levels in the microdialysate of patients is sufficient to kill neurons in culture but not neurons in the intact rat brain (Bullock et al., 1999). Long periods of exposure at high levels (20 to 30 mM range) are needed to produce necrotic cell death in normal rats (Landolt and Bullock, 1993; Di et al., 1999). Although this might suggest that elevated Glu is not relevant to in vivo head injury, one must consider that the brain is in a compromised state following injury. One reason that Glu may not kill neurons in the normal brain is because of strong endogenous reuptake mechanisms that involve glial cells (Benveniste, 1991; Kimelberg and Norenberg, 1994). Glu exposure is much more neurotoxic in astrocyte-poor rat cell cultures than in astrocyte-rich cultures, demonstrating the importance of functional reuptake mechanisms that involve glia (Rosenberg et al., 1992). Glial cells are also perturbed following traumatic injury. For example, a distinct feature of TBI is reactive gliosis (Eddleston and Mucke, 1993; Kimelberg and Norenberg, 1994), which is characterized by marked increases in glial fibrillary acid protein (GFAP). Also, recent studies show postinjury decreases in uptake of Glu by astrocytes in culture at 1 and 24 h following traumatic injury (Bender and Norenberg, 1998). Decreases in protein expression of glial glutamate transporters (GLT1 and GLAST) are observed between 6 and 72 h after controlled cortical impact injury in the rat (Rao et al., 1998). Because endogenous Glu uptake mechanisms are disrupted following traumatic injury, there is potentially more Glu left in the extracellular space that can produce damage.

Benveniste (1991) thoroughly examined the issues surrounding the role of Glu excitotoxicity in cerebral ischemia, particularly assessment of postinsult levels of Glu in the interstitial space. She points out the importance of transforming data from dialysate levels to interstitial concentrations to provide better estimates of the "true" Glu levels. In addition, Benveniste (1991) suggests that tortuosity is likely an important factor in estimating Glu levels. Tortuosity refers to the contours that are inherent in the organization of the brain. The tucks and folds of the brain increase the surface area of the extracellular space and make it difficult to make precise measurements of substances present in the extracellular space. Not accounting for tortuosity may lead to an underestimation of the Glu levels present after insult. However, part of the problem is that the tortuosity factor is unknown. A recent study by Di et al. (1999) found that combining central FPI with an infusion of Glu produced a significantly larger lesion than either Glu exposure or TBI alone. These data indicate that shear impact of FPI further exacerbates the neurotoxicity produced by Glu release, suggesting a synergistic effect between Glu release and injury impact, and subsequently an important role for Glu in posttraumatic pathophysiology. Taken together, these studies highlight the continuing limitations in interpreting data on Glu levels and CNS insult. However, they also suggest that there may be underestimation of the levels of Glu in the extracellular space as well as the levels at which Glu can be neurotoxic.

Obrenovich and Urenjak (1997) also argue that excitotoxicity characterized by increases in extracellular Glu is unlikely to be a major contributor to injury mechanisms since Glu release is transient. Although injury-induced Glu release is transient in most experimental models, it appears to be sufficient to contribute to the disruption of important physiological and biochemical variables. Moreover, Glu changes occur in the context of tissue injury, which is associated with metabolic dysfunction.

It has been suggested that impaired metabolism contributes to a slow form of excitotoxicity, which may occur even with "physiological" concentrations of glutamate (Beal, 1995; Lancelot and Beal, 1998). Although this hypothesis was developed to explain excitotoxic mechanisms in chronic neurodegenerative diseases, it may also provide an explanation for the prolonged effectiveness of glutamate/glutamate receptor modulation. Thus it may be possible that under conditions of metabolic compromise, which is known to occur following traumatic CNS injury, even physiological levels of Glu may become neurotoxic, thereby continuing to contribute to posttraumatic injury even after the initial elevations in Glu have returned to baseline.

CLINICAL TRIALS

As reviewed above, many drugs that modulate Glu receptors have beneficial effects in experimental models of TBI. NMDA antagonists have been examined in clinical head injuries (see Chapters 19, 20, and 21). These include CGS-19755 (Selfotel),

CNS1102 (Cerestat), and Eliprodil (for a review, see Bullock et al., 1999). Improvements in outcome have been limited or restricted to selective subgroups of patients. CGS-19755 was reported to reduce intracranial pressure after severe brain injury, whereas Eliprodil was seen to produce better outcome in the "brain swelling" subgroup. Trials with CNS1102 (Cerestat) had to be terminated early due to high mortality in a parallel stroke trial; no benefits were observed prior to trial termination (Bullock et al., 1999).

There are several possible explanations for the discrepancy between the preclinical and clinical studies. These include issues related to the penetration of the drug into the CNS, the therapeutic window (i.e., timing of drug administration), the dosing regimen, and the heterogeneity of the head injury population (Doppenberg et al., 1997; Bullock et al., 1999). Clinical head injury includes complex pathological changes as secondary consequences of trauma, including hypoxia, ischemia, diffuse axonal injury, edema formation, and hematoma. Better stratification of patient populations may be helpful, as shown for other neuroprotective drugs (European Study Trial, 1994; Faden, 1996; Harders et al., 1996). Moreover, preclinical studies should better attempt to model clinically relevant issues such as therapeutic window, pharmacokinetics, and so on.

FUTURE DIRECTIONS

Although the role of Glu receptors in traumatic CNS injury has received considerable attention over the past two decades, much additional work is needed. First, it will be necessary to better characterize the role of specific Glu receptor subtypes in injury as well as subsequent downstream intracellular cascades. Second, it will be important to develop a deeper understanding of how metabolic compromise contributes to Glu-mediated toxicity. Finally, elucidating the final common pathways of posttraumatic cell death, both necrotic and apoptotic, should provide critical information for enhancing drug discovery aimed at modulating TBI.

ABBREVIATIONS

1-Amino-APDC	1-Aminopyrolidine dicarboxylate
1S,3R-ACPD	1S,3R-aminocyclopentane dicarboxylate
2R,4R-APDC	(2R,4R)-aminopyrolidine-2,4-dicarboxylate
3-NP	3-Nitropropionic acid
8-Br-cAMP	8-Bromo-cyclic adenosine monophosphate
AIDA	(R,S)-1-Aminoindan-1,5-dicarboxylic acid
AMPA	α-Amino-3-hydroxy-5-methyl-4-isoxazole propionate
APV	2-Amino-5-phosphovaleric acid
as-ODN	Antisense oligodeoxynucleotides

BBB	Blood–brain barrier
cAMP	Cyclic adenosine monophosphate
CNQX	6-cyano-7-nitroquinoxaline-2,3-dione
CNS	Central nervous system
CPP	3-(2-Carboxypiperizin-4-yl)-propyl-1-phosphonic acid
DCG-IV	$(2S,1'R,2'R,3'R)$-2-2',3'-dicarboxy cyclopropylglycine
DCS	D-Cycloserine
DHPG	3-5-Dihydroxyphenylglycine
EAA	Excitatory amino acid
FDA	Food and Drug Administration
FPI	Fluid percussion injury
GFAD	Glial fibrillary acid protein
Glu	L-Glutamate
HU-211	7-hydroxy-tetrahydrocannabinol 1,1-dimethylheptyl
HVA	High-voltage-activated
I2CA	Indole-2-carboxyiic acid
iGluR	Ionotropic glutamate receptor
IP$_3$	Inositol trisphosphate
KA	Kainate
KYN	Kynurenate
L-AP4	L-2-Amino-4-phosphonobutanoic acid
L-CCG-1	$(2S,1'S,2'S)$-2-Caroxypropylglycine
L-SOP	L-Serine-O-phosphate
MAP-4	α-Methyl-L-2-amino-4-phosphonobutanoic acid
MCPG	$(+)$-α-methyl-4-carboxyphenylglycine
mGluR	Metabotropic glutamate receptor
MK801	Dizocilpine maleate
MSOP	α-Methyl-O-phosphate
NBQX	2,3-Dihydroxy-6-nitro-7-sulfamoylbenzol
NMDA	N-Methol-D-aspartate
NO	Nitric oxide
ODC	Orrithine decarboxylase
PCP	Phencyclidine
PKA	Protein kinase A
PKC	Protein kinase C
PLA$_2$	Phospholipase A$_2$
PLC	Phospholipase C
(RS)-DHPG	(RS)-Dihydroxyphenylglycine

(*S*)-4C3HPG	(*S*)-4-Carboxy-3-hydroxyphenylglycine
SCI	Spinal cord injury
(*S*)-DHPG	(*S*)-Dihydroxyphenylglycine
tACPD	*Trans*-Aminocyclopentane dicarboxylate
tADA	*Trans*-Azetidine-2,4-dicarboxylic acid
TBI	Traumatic brain injury

REFERENCES

S. K. Agrawal, E. Theriault, and M. G. Fehlings, *J. Neurotrauma*, 15, 929–941 (1998).

J. W. Allen and A. I. Faden, *Cell Death Differ.*, 7, 70–476 (2000).

J. W. Allen, B. A. Eldadah, and A. I. Faden, *Neuropharmacology.*, 38, 1243–1252 (1999a).

J. W. Allen, S. A. Ivanova, L. Fan, M. G. Espey, A. S. Basile, and A. I. Faden, *J. Pharmacol. Exp. Ther.*, 290, 112–120 (1999b).

J. W. Allen, S. M. Knoblach, and A. I. Faden, *FASEB J.*, 13, 1875–1882 (1999).

A. Ambrosini, L. Bresciani, S. Fracchia, N. Brunello, and G. Racagni, *Mol. Pharmacol.*, 47, 1057–1064 (1995).

R. Anwyl, *Brain Res. Rev.*, 29(1), 83–120 (1999).

F. Bareyre, F. Wahl, T. K. McIntosh, and J. M. Stutzmann, *J. Neurotrauma*, 14, 839–849 (1997).

M. K. Baskaya, A. M. Rao, L. Puckett, M. R. Prasad, and R. J. Dempsey, *J. Neurotrauma*, 13, 85–92 (1996).

G. Battaglia, V. Bruno, R. B. Ngomba, R. Di Grezia, A. Copani, and F. Nicoletti, *Eur. J. Pharmacol.*, 356, 271–274 (1998).

M. F. Beal, *Ann Neurol.*, 38, 357–366 (1995).

A. S. Bender and M. D. Norenberg, *J. Neurotrauma*, 858 (1998).

H. Bernert and L. Turski, *Proc. Natl. Acad. Sci. USA*, 93, 5235–5240 (1996).

H. Benveniste, *Cerebrovasc. Brain Metab. Rev.*, 3, 213–245 (1991).

B. Bettler and C. Mulle, *Neuropharmacology*, 34, 123–139 (1995).

E. F. Birse, S. A. Eaton, D. E. Jane, P. L. St. J. Jones, R. H. P. Porter, P. C.-K. Pook, D. C. Sunter, P. M. Udvarhelyi, B. Wharton, P. J. Roberts, T. E. Salt, and J. C. Watkins, *Neuroscience*, 52, 481–488 (1993).

A. Bond, J. A. Monn, and D. Lodge, *Neuroreport.*, 8, 1463–1466 (1997).

I. Brabet, S. Mary, J. Bockaert, and J.-P. Pin, *Neuropharmacology*, 34, 895–903 (1995).

V. Bruno, A. Copani, G. Battaglia, R. Raffaele, H. Shinozaki, and F. Nicoletti, *Eur. J. Pharmacol.*, 256, 109–112(1994).

V. Bruno, G. Battaglia, C. Copani, R. G. Giffard, G. Raciti, R. Raffaele, H. Shinozaki, and F. Nicoletti, *Eur. J. Neurosci*, 7, 1906–1913 (1995a).

V. Bruno, A. Copani, T. Knöpfel, R. Kuhn, G. Casabona, P. Dell'Albani, D. F. Condorelli, and F. Nicoletti, *Neuropharmacology*, 34, 1089–1098 (1995b).

V. Bruno, A. Copani, L. Bonanno, T. Knöpfel, R. Huhn, P. J. Roberts, and F. Nicoletti, *Eur. J. Pharmacol.*, 310, 61–66 (1996).

V. Bruno, F. X. Sureda, M. Storto, G. Casabona, A. Caruso, T. Knöpfel, R. Kuhn, and F. Nicoletti, *J. Neurosci.*, 17, 1891–1897 (1997).

V. Bruno, G. Battaglia, G. Casabona, A. Copani, F. Caciagli, and F. Nicoletti, *J. Neurosci.*, 18, 9594–9600 (1998).

V. Bruno, G. Battaglia, A. Kingston, M. J. O'Neill, M. V. Catania, R. Di Grezia, and F. Nicoletti, *Neuropharmacology*, 38, 199–207 (1999).

A. Buisson and D. W. Choi, *Neuropharmacology*, 34, 1081–1087 (1995).

M. R. Bullock, B. G. Lyeth, and J. P. Muizelaar, *Neurosurgery*, 45, 207–220 (1999).

R. Bullock, D. I. Graham, S. Swanson, and J. McCulloch, *J. Cereb. Blood Flow Metab.*, 14, 466–471 (1994).

R. Bullock, A. Zauner, J. J. Woodward, J. Myseros, S. C. Choi, J. D. Ward, A. Marmarou, and H. F. Young, *J. Neurosurg.*, 89, 507–518 (1998).

D. W. Choi, *J. Neurobiol.*, 23, 1261–1276 (1992).

D. W. Choi, J. Y. Koh, and S. Peters, *J. Neurosci.*, 8, 185–196 (1988).

J. R. Cooper, F. E. Bloom, and R. H. Roth, *The Biochemical Basis of Neuropharmacology* 7th Edition, University Press, Oxford, New York, 1996.

A. Copani, V. Bruno, G. Battaglia, G. Leanza, R. Pellitteri, A. Russo, S. Stanzani, and F. Nicoletti, *Mol. Pharmacol.*, 47, 890–897 (1995).

A. Copani, G. Casabona, V. Bruno, A. Caruso, D. F. Condorelli, A. Messina, V. Di Giorgi Gerevini, J.-P. Pin, R. Kuhn, T. Knöpfel, and F. Nicoletti, *Eur. J. Neurosci.*, 10, 2173–2184 (1998).

S. W. D'Souza, S. E. McConnell, P. Slater, and A. J. Barson, *Arch. Dis. Child.*, 69, 212–215 (1993).

X. Di, J. Gordon, and R. Bullock, *J. Neurotrauma*, 16, 195–201 (1999).

E. M. R. Doppenberg, S. C. Choi, and M. R. Bullock, *Ann N.Y. Acad. Sci.*, 825, 305–322 (1997).

M. Eddleston and L. Mucke, *Neuroscience*, 54, 15–36 (1993).

E. F. Ellis, J. S. McKinney, K. A. Willoughby, S. Liang, and J. T. Povlishock, *J. Neurotrauma*, 12, 325–339 (1995).

L. Eriksen and C. Thompsen, *Br. J. Pharmacol.*, 116, 3279–3287 (1996).

European Study Group on Nimodipine in Severe Head Injury, *J. Neurosurg.*, 80, 797–804 (1994).

A. I. Faden, *J. Am. Med. Assoc.*, 276, 569–570 (1996).

A. I. Faden, M. M. Lemke, R. P. Simon, and L. J. Noble, *J. Neurotrauma*, 5, 27–37 (1988).

A. I. Faden, P. Demediuk, S. S. Panter, and R. Vink, *Science*, 244, 798–800 (1989).

A. I. Faden, S. A. Ivanova, A. G. Yakovlev, and A. G. Mukhin, *J. Neurotrauma*, 14, 885–895 (1997).

P. J. Flor, J. Gomeza, M. A. Jones, R. Khun, T. P. Pin, and T. Knöpfel, *J. Neurochem.*, 67(1), 58–63 (1996).

R. Gill, *Cerebrovasc. Brain Metab. Rev.*, 6, 225–256 (1994).

F. M. Golding and R. Vink, *Mol. Chem. Neuropathol.*, 24, 137–150 (1995).

Q. Z. Gong, T. M. Delahunty. R. J. Hamm, and B. C. Lyeth, *Neurosci. Lett.*, 203, 211–213 (1995).

S. H. Graham, J. Chen, J. Lan, J. Leach, and R. P. Simon, *J. Pharmacol. Exp. Ther.*, 269, 854–859 (1994).

S. D. Grossman, B. B. Wolfe, R. Yasuda, and J. R. Wrathall, *J. Neurosci.*, 19, 5711–5720 (1999).

B. J. Gwag, D. Lobner, J. Koh, M. B. Wie, and D. W. Choi, *Neuroscience.*, 68, 615–619 (1995).

S. S. Haghighi, G. C. Johnson, C. F. de Vergel, and B. J. Vergel-Rivas, *Neurol. Res.*, 18, 509–515 (1996).

R. J. Hamm, D. M. O'Dell, B. R. Pike, and B. C. Lyeth, *Cog. Brain Res.*, 1, 223–226 (1993).

A. Harders, A. Kakarieka, R. Braakman, and the German tSAH study Group, *J. Neurosurg.*, 85, 82–89 (1996).

R. L. Hayes, L. W. Jenkins, B. C. Lyeth, R. L. Balster, S. E. Robinson, G. L. Clifton, J. F. Stubbins, and H. F. Young, *J. Neurotrauma*, 5, 259–274 (1988).

D. L. Heath and R. Vink, *J. Neurotrauma*, 15, 183–189 (1998).

D. L. Heath and R. Vink, *J. Neurosurg.*, 90, 504–509 (1999).

R. R. Hicks, D. H. Smith, T. A. Gennarelli, and T. McIntosh, *Brain Res.*, 655, 91–96 (1994).

S. Hogg, C. Perron, P. Barnéoud, D. J. Sanger, and P. C. Moser, *J. Neurotrauma*, 15, 545–553 (1998).

C. Hölscher, J. Gigg, and S. M. O'Mara, *Neurosci. Biobehav. Rev.*, 23, 399–410 (1999).

C. Hylton, B. Penn, M. Voddi, D. Smith, R. Raghupathi, L. Tarnawa, T. Gennarelli and T. McIntosh, *J. Neurotrauma*, 12, 124 (1995).

I. Ito, A. Kohda, S. Tanabe, E. Hirose, M. Hayashi, S. Mitsunaga, and H. Sugiyama, *Neuroreport*, 3, 1013–1016 (1995).

D. E. Jane, P. L. St. J. Jones, P. C.-K. Pook, H.-W. Tse, and J. C. Watkins, *Br. J. Pharmacol.*, 112, 809–816 (1994).

C. Joly, J. Gomeza, I. Brabet, K. Curry, J. Bockaert, and J.-P. Pin, *J. Neurosci.*, 15, 3970–3981 (1995).

A. Kalda and A. Zharkovsky, *Neuroscience*, 92, 7–14 (1999).

Y. Katayama, D. P. Becker, T. Tamura, and D. A. Hovda, *J. Neurosurg.*, 73, 889–900 (1990).

T. Kawamata, Y. Katayama, D. A. Hovda, A. Yoshino, and D. P. Becker, *J. Cereb. Blood Flow Metab.*, 12, 12–24 (1992).

H. K. Kimelberg and M. D. Norenberg, in S. Salzman and A. I. Faden, Eds., *The Neurobiology of Central Nervous System Trauma*, Oxford University Press, Oxford, 1994.

A. E. Kingston, J. P. Burnett, N. C. Mayne, and D. Lodge, *Neuropharmacology*, 34, 887–894 (1995).

T. S. Knöpfel, R. Kuhn, and H. Allegier, *J. Med. Chem.*, 38, 1417–1426 (1995).

J. Y. Koh, E. Palmer, and C. Cotman, *Proc. Natl. Acad. Sci. USA*, 88, 9431–9435 (1991).

J. Kornhuber and M. Weller, *Biol. Psychiatry*, 41, 135–144 (1997).

A. P. Kozikowski, V. Tuckmantel, Y. Liao, H. Manev, S. Ikonomovic, and J. T. Wroblewski, *J. Med. Chem.*, 36, 2706–2708 (1993).

A. P. Kozikowski, G. L. Araldi, W. Tuckmantel, S. Pshenichkin, E. Surina, and J. T. Wroblewski, *Bioorg. Med. Chem. Lett.*, 9, 1721–1726 (1999).

S.-N. Kroppenstedt, G.-H. Schneider, U.-W. Thomale, and A. W. Unterberg, *J. Neurotrauma*, 15, 191–197 (1998).

M. Lafon-Cazal, L. Fagni, M. J. Guiraud, S. Mary, M. Lerner-Natoli, J.-P. Pin, R. Shigemoto, and J. Bockaert, *Eur. J. Neurosci.*, 11, 663–672 (1999).

F. Lancelot and M. F. Beal, *Prog Brain Res.*, 116, 331–347 (1998).

H. Landolt and R. Bullock, *J. Cereb. Blood Flow Metab.*, 13 (Suppl. 1), S644 (1993).

K. Maiese and A. M. Vincent, *Neurosci. Lett.*, 264, 17–20 (1999).

K. Maiese, R. Greenberg, L. Boccone, and M. Swiriduk, *Neurosci. Lett.*, 194, 173–176 (1995).

K. Maiese, M. Swiriduk, and M. TenBroeke, *J. Neurochem.*, 66, 2419–2428 (1996).

L. J. Martin, C. D. Blackstone, A. I. Levey, R. L. Huganir, and D. L. Price, *Neuroscience*, 53, 327–358 (1993).

M. Masu, Y. Tanabe, K. Tsuchida, R. Shigemoto, and S. Nakanishi, *Nature*, 349, 760–765 (1991).

J. W. McDonald and D. D. Schoepp, *Eur. J. Pharmacol.*, 215, 353–354 (1992).

J. W. McDonald, A. S. Fix, J. P. Tizzano, and D. D. Schoepp, *J. Neurosci.*, 13, 4445–4455 (1993).

T. K. McIntosh, A. I. Faden, I. Yamakami, and R. Vink, *J. Neurotrauma*, 5, 17–31 (1988).

T. K. McIntosh, R. Vink, H. Soares, R. L. Hayes, and R. Simon, *J. Neurotrauma*, 6, 247–259 (1989a).

T. K. McIntosh, R. Vink, I. Yamakami, and A. I. Faden, *Brain Res.*, 482, 252–260 (1989b).

T. K. McIntosh, R. Vink, H. Soares, R. L. Hayes, and R. Simon, *J. Neurochem.*, 55, 1170–1179 (1990).

T. K. McIntosh, D. H. Smith, M. Voddi, B. R. Perri, and J. M. Stutzmann, *J. Neurotrauma*, 13, 767–780 (1996).

T. K. McIntosh, M. Juhler, and T. Wieloch, *J. Neurotrauma*, 15, 731–769 (1998).

L. P. Miller, B. G. Lyeth, L. W. Jenkins, L. Oleniak, D. Panchision, R. J. Hamm, L. L. Phillips, C. E. Dixon, G. L. Clifton, and R. L. Hayes, *Brain Res.*, 526, 103–107 (1990).

D. Monaghan, R. J. Bridge, and C. W. Cotman, *Annu. Rev. Pharmacol. Toxicol.*, 29, 365–402 (1989).

J. A. Monn, M. J. Valli, B. G. Johnson, C. D. Salhoff, R. A. Wright, T. Howe, A. Bond, D. Lodge, L. A. Spangle, J. W. Paschal, J. B. Campbell, K. Griffey, J. P. Tizzano, and D. D. Schoepp, *J. Med. Chem.*, 39, 2990–3000 (1996).

C. Montoliu, M. Llansola, C. Cucurella, S. Grisolia, and V. Felipo, *J. Pharmacol. Exp. Ther.*, 281, 643–647 (1997).

H. Monyer, M. P. Goldberg, and D. W. Choi, *Brain Res.*, 483, 347–354 (1989).

J. H. Morrison, S. J. Siegel, A. H. Gazzaley, and G. W. Huntley, *Neuroscientist*, 2, 272–283 (1996).

A. Mukhin, L. Fan, and A. I. Faden, *J. Neurosci.*, 16, 6012–6020 (1996).

A. G. Mukhin, S. A. Ivanova, S. M. Knoblach, and A. I. Faden, *J. Neurotrauma*, 14, 651–663 (1997a).

A. G. Mukhin, S. A. Ivanova, and A. I. Faden, *Neuroreport*, 8, 2561–2566 (1997b).

A. G. Mukhin, S. A. Ivanova, J. W. Allen, and A. I. Faden, *J. Neurosci. Res.*, 51, 748–758 (1998).

Y. Nakagawa, K. Saitah, T. Ishihara, M. Ishida, and H. Shinozaki, *Eur. J. Pharmacol.*, 184, 205–206 (1990).

F. Nicoletti, V. Bruno, A. Copani, G. Casabona, and T. Knöpfel, *Trends Neurosci.*, 19, 267–271 (1996).

P. Nicotera and S. A. Lipton, *J. Cereb. Blood Flow Metab.*, 19, 583–590 (1999).

T. P. Obrenovich and J. Urenjak, *J. Neurotrauma*, 14, 677–698 (1997).

K. Okiyama, D. H. Smith, T. A. Gennarelli, R. P. Simon, M. Leach, and T. K. McIntosh, *J. Neurochem.*, 64, 802–809 (1995).

K. Okiyama, D. H. Smith, W. F. White, K. Richter, and T. K. McIntosh, *J. Neurotrauma*, 14, 211–222 (1997).

K. Okiyama, D. H. Smith, W. F. White, and T. K. McIntosh, *Brain Res.*, 792, 291–298 (1998).

J. W. Olney, J. Labruyere, and M. I. Price, *Science*, 244, 1360–1362 (1989).

L. R. Orlando, D. G. Standaert, J. B. Jr. Penney, and A. B. Young, *Neurosci. Lett.*, 202, 109–112 (1995).

S. S. Panler and A. I. Faden, *Neurosci. Lett.*, 136, 165–168 (1992).

J.-P. Pin and R. Duvoisin, *Neuropharmacology.*, 34, 1–26 (1995).

M. Pizzi, C. Fallacara, V. Arrighi, M. Memo, and P. F. Spamo, *J. Neurochem.*, 61, 683–689 (1993).

M. Pizzi, O. Consolandi, M. Memo, and P. F. Spano, *Eur. J. Neurosci.*, 8, 1516–1521 (1996a).

M. Pizzi, P. Galli, O. Consolandi, V. Arrighi, M. Memo, and P. F. Spano, *Mol. Pharmacol.*, 49, 586–594 (1996b).

J. H. M. Prehn, K. Lippert, and J. Krieglstein, *Eur. J. Pharmacol. Env. Toxicol. Pharmacol. Sec.*, 292, 179–189 (1995).

V. L. Rao, M. K. Baskaya, A. Dogan, J. D. Rothstein, and R. J. Dempsey, *J. Neurochem.*, 70, 2020–2027 (1998).

R. F. Regan and D. W. Choi, *Brain Res.*, 633, 236–242 (1994).

C. Riedel, W. Wetzel, and K. G. Reymann, *Prog. Neuro-Psychopharmacol. Psychiatry*, 20, 761–789 (1996).

P. A. Rosenberg, S. Amin, and M. Leitner, *J. Neurosci.*, 12, 56–61 (1992).

B. A. Rzigalinski, J. T. Weber, K. A. Willoughby, S. Liang, J. J. Woodward, and E. F. Ellis, *J. Neurotrauma*, 15, 894 (1998).

A. I. Sacaan and D. D. Schoep, *Neurosci. Lett.*, 139, 77–82 (1992).

J. A. Saugstad, J. M. Kinzie, M. M. Shinohara, T. P. Segerson, and G. L. Westbrook, *Mol. Pharmacol.*, 51, 119–125(1997).

D. D. Schoepp, J. Goldsworthy, B. G. Johnson, C. R. Salhoff, and S. R. Baker, *J. Neurochem.*, 63, 769–772 (1994).

D. D. Schoepp, J. P. Tizzano, R. A. Wright, and A. S. Fix, *Neurodegeneration*, 4, 71–80 (1995).

U. H. Schroder, T. Opitz, T. Jager, C. F. Sabelhaus, J. Breder, and K. G. Reymann, *Neuropharmacology*, 38, 209–216 (1999).

Y. Shapira, G. Yadid, S. Cotev, A. Niska, and E. Shohami, *J. Neurotrauma*, 7, 131–139 (1990).

R. Shigemoto, A. Kinoshita, E. Wada, S. Nomura, H. Ohishi, M. Takada, P. J. Flor, S. Nakanishi, and N. Mizuno, *J. Neurosci.*, 17, 7503–7522 (1997).

E. Shohami, M. Novikov, and R. Bass, *Brain Res.*, 674, 55–62 (1995).

E. Shohami, M. Novikov, and R. Mechaoulam, *J. Neurotrauma*, 10, 109–119 (1993).

E. Shohami, R. Gaillilly, R. Mecholaum, R. Bass, and T. Ben-Hur, *J. Neuroimmunol.*, 72, 169–177 (1997).

P. K. Sladeczek, J. P. Pin, M. Recasens, J. Bockaert, and S. Weiss, *Nature*, 317, 717–719 (1985).

D. H. Smith, K. Okiyama, T. A. Gennarelli, and T. K. McIntosh, *Neurosci. Lett.*, 157, 211–214 (1993a).

D. H. Smith, K. Okiyama, M. J. Thomas, and T. K. McIntosh, *J. Neurosci.*, 13, 5383–5392 (1993b).

D. H. Smith, B. R. Perri, R. Raghupathi, K. E. Saatman, and T. K. McIntosh, *Neurosci. Lett.*, 231, 135–138 (1997).

A. Stefani, A. Pisanin, N. B. Mercuri, and P. Calebresi, *Mol. Neurobiol.*, 13, 81–95 (1996).

U. Strasser, D. Lobner, M. M. Behrens, L. M. Canzoniero, and D. W. Choi, *Eur. J. Neurosci.*, 10, 2848–2855 (1998).

H. Sugiyama, I. Ito, and C. Hirono, *Neuron*, 3, 129–132 (1987).

F.-Y. Sun and A. I. Faden, *Brain Res.*, 666, 88–92 (1994).

F.-Y. Sun and A. I. Faden, *Brain Res.*, 673, 133–140 (1995a).

F.-Y. Sun and A. I. Faden, *Brain Res.*, 693, 163–168 (1995b).

M. D. Temple and R. J. Hamm, *Brain Res.*, 741, 246–251 (1996).

M. D. Temple, L. L. Phillips, R. J. Hamm, T. M. Delahunty, and B. G. Lyeth, *J. Neurotrauma*, 14, 766 (1997).

N. K. Thomas, D. E. Jane, H.-W. Tse, and J. C. Watkins, *Neuropharmacology*, 35, 637–642 (1995).

N. J. Toms, P. J. Roberts, T. E. Salt, and P. C. Staton, *Trends Pharmacol. Sci.*, 17, 429–435 (1996).

S. Toulmond, A. Serrano, J. Benavides, and B. Scatton, *Brain Res.*, 620, 32–41 (1993).

A. Valerio, A. Alberici, M. Paterlini, M. Grilli, P. Galli, M. Pizzi, M. Memo, and P. Spano, *Neuroreport*, 6, 1307–1321 (1995).

A. M. Vincent, M. TenBroeke, and K. Maiese, *Exp. Neurol.*, 155, 79–94 (1999).

M. D. Voddi, B. R. Perri, K. G. Perlman, D. H. Smith, M. Leach, and T. K. McIntosh, *J. Neurotrauma*, 12, 146 (1995).

F. Wahl, E. Renou, V. Mary, and J. M. Stutzmann, *Brain Res.*, 756, 247–255 (1997).

J. Watkins and G. L. Collingridge, *Trends Pharmacol. Sci.*, 15, 333–342 (1994).

J. C. Watkins, in A. P. Kozikowski and C. Barrionuevo, Eds., *Neurobiology of the NMDA Receptor: From Chemistry to the Clinic.* VCH, New York, 1991.

V. W. Wilsch, V. I. Pidoplichko, T. Opitz, H. Shinozaki, and K. Reymann, *Eur. J. Pharmacol.*, 262, 287–291 (1994).

E. H. F. Wong and J. A. Kemp, *Annu. Rev. Pharmacol. Toxicol.*, 31, 401–425 (1991).

J. R. Wrathall, D. Choiniere, and Y. D. Teng, *J. Neurosci.*, 14, 6598–6607 (1994).

M. Wyszynski, J. C. Valtschanoff, S. Naisbitt, A. W. Dunah, E. Kim, D. G. Standaert, R. Weinberg, and M. Sheng, *J. Neurosci.*, 19, 6528–6537 (1999).

S. P. Yu, C.-H. Yeh, S. L. Sensi, B. J. Gwag, L. M. T. Canzoniero, Z. B. Farhangrazi, H. S. Ying, M. Tian, L. L. Dugan, and D. W. Choi, *Science*, 278, 114–117 (1997).

C. Zhang, R. Raghupathi, K. E. Saatman, D. H. Smith, J. M. Stutzmann, F. Wahl, and T. K. McIntosh, *J. Neurosci. Res.*, 52, 342–349 (1998).

L. Zhang, B. A. Rzigalinski, E. F. Ellis, and L. S. Satin, *Science*, 274, 1921–1923 (1996).

CHAPTER 5

CHOLINERGIC RECEPTORS IN HEAD TRAUMA

BRUCE G. LYETH

Department of Neurological Surgery, University of California at Davis, Davis, California

INTRODUCTION

Traumatic brain injury (TBI) produces an acute elevation in the concentration of extracellular neurotransmitters including glutamate and acetylcholine (ACh). While the neurotoxic effects of glutamate have been the focus of receptor-mediated injury processes in TBI (see Chapter 4 for a review of this topic), there is considerable evidence that excessive activation of ACh receptors immediately after injury also contributes to receptor-mediated injury processes via a cholinergic-potentiated toxicity. Cholinergic activation contributes not only to elevated intracellular calcium but also to further depolarization, which recruits glutamate release thereby amplifying the toxic neuronal environment. Over time, ACh appears to play a biphasic role in TBI pathology in that the period of acute cholinergic activation or hyperfunction is followed by a period of chronic cholinergic insufficiency or hypofunction. The relatively long-lasting period of cholinergic hypofunction develops days after injury and may underlie aspects of cognitive morbidity associated with TBI. This biphasic shift in cholinergic activity after TBI has tremendous implications on the strategy for therapeutic application in the clinic related to ACh. The shift from cholinergic hyperfunction to hypofunction dictates diametrically opposed therapeutic interventions characterized by acute cholinergic receptor blockade followed by chronic enhancement of cholinergic receptor activation. Several lines of evidence are reviewed in the present chapter indicating that (1) the elevated levels of extracellular ACh impact upon the muscarinic cholinergic signal transduction pathways; (2) the initial activation of muscarinic cholinergic receptors after injury contributes to the state of traumatic unconsciousness; (3) the acute activation of muscarinic receptors

Head Trauma: Basic, Preclinical, and Clinical Directions, Edited by Leonard P. Miller and Ronald L. Hayes, Co-edited by Jennifer K. Newcomb
ISBN 0-471-36015-5 © 2001 John Wiley & Sons, Inc.

also contributes to the development of chronic morbidity; and (4) the chronic morbidity is due in part to a cholinergic insufficiency developing days after injury.

CHOLINERGIC RECEPTOR CLASSIFICATION

Acetylcholine receptors are dichotomized into muscarinic and nicotinic categories, with several subtypes within each category (Tables 5.1 and 5.2). Muscarinic receptors are metabotropic receptors coupled to membrane-bound G proteins and derive their name from the selective receptor agonist property of the alkaloid muscarine from the mushroom *Amanita muscaria*. Nicotinic receptors are ligand-gated ion channels and derive their name from the tobacco alkaloid nicotine, which is a selective agonist for these receptors.

Muscarinic receptors are abundant in the central nervous system (CNS) and play a dominant role in mediating the actions of ACh in the brain. ACh produces both excitation and inhibition in the brain by binding to a family of muscarinic receptor subtypes that are located both presynaptically and postsynaptically. The receptor consists of a protein with seven transmembrane domains. Each receptor subtype has unique amino acid sequences at the extracellular end loop and at the third intracellular loop, which appears to be responsible for the subtype differences in receptor–effector coupling specificity. There are five subtypes, M1 to M5, encoded by different genes, *m1* to *m5*.

The odd-numbered muscarinic subtypes (M1, M3, M5) are coupled by a G protein to phospholipase C (PLC). Activation by ACh (Figure 5.1) causes these muscarinic receptors to bind to and activate a trimeric G protein. The α subunit dissociates from the activated G protein and activates PLC. Activated PLC cleaves, through a process of hydrolysis, the membrane phospholipid phosphatidylinositol 4,5-bisphosphate (PIP_2) into the second messengers, inositol 1,4,5-trisphosphate (IP_3) and diacylglycerol (DAG). IP_3 contributes to increases in free intracellular calcium (Ca^{2+}) by releasing it from endoplasmic reticulum. DAG activates protein kinase C (PKC), which phosphorylates a number of neuronal ion channels, including the N-methyl-D-aspartate (NMDA) receptor–ion complex, thereby potentiating calcium entry through the NMDA channel. Activation of postsynaptic M1 and M3 receptor subtypes in the brain also mediates a slow neuronal excitability in part by inhibiting several potassium channels including a Ca^{2+}-regulated potassium current ($I_{K(ca)}$) and a potassium M-current ($I_{K(M)}$). The inhibition of the $I_{K(Ca)}$ and $I_{K(M)}$ tends to inhibit the after-hyperpolarization phase of the action potential and thereby increase cell excitability (Jones, 1993). Activation of muscarinic M1 and M3 subtypes does not directly lead to action potentials, but enhances the neurons' response to other excitatory input.

The even-numbered subtypes (M2, M4) are negatively coupled to adenylate cyclase. The M2 and M4 receptors also activate a G protein-gated inward rectifier potassium (K^+) current ($I_{K(IR)}$) channel, which mediates hyperpolarizing post-synaptic potentials and inhibition of neuronal firing (Doupnik et al., 1997). M2 and M4 are located primarily presynaptically where they function as "autoreceptors,"

TABLE 5.1 Muscarinic Acetylcholine Receptors

Subtype	G protein	K⁺ currents	Second Messenger	Antagonist	Agonists	Predominant CNS localization
M1	$G_{q/11}$	$\downarrow I_{K(M)}, I_{K(Ca)}$	$\uparrow IP_3/DAG$	Pirenzepine Dicyclomine Scopolamine	Muscarine Pilocarpine Oxotremorine	Hippocampus (CA1, DG), basal forebrain, olfactory tubercle and bulb, cortex
M2	G_i	$\uparrow I_{K(IR)}$	$\downarrow$ cAMP	AF-DX 116 Methoctramine Scopolamine	Same	Brain stem (pontine), olfactory tubercle and bulb, cortex
M3	$G_{q/11}$	$\downarrow I_{K(M)}$ and $I_{K(Ca)}$	$\uparrow IP_3/DAG$	4-DAMP Hexahydrosiladifenidol Scopolamine	Same	Hippocampus (CA1, DO), basal forebrain, olfactory tubercle and bulb, cortex
M4	G_i	$\uparrow I_{K(IR)}$	$\downarrow$ cAMP	Tropicamide Himbacine Scopolamine	Same	Hippocampus (CA1, DG), striatum, olfactory tubercle
M5	$G_{q/11}$		$\uparrow IP_3/DAG$	Scopolamine	Same	Extremely low levels and limited distribution

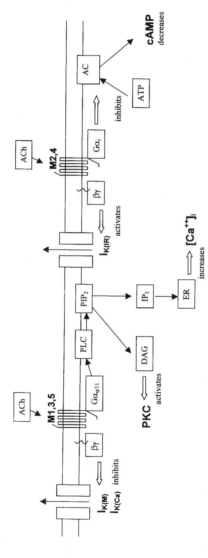

Figure 5.1 Intracellular signaling cascades associated with muscarinic receptor activation. Upon binding of an agonist to M1,3,5 receptors (which are generally located postsynaptically) the $\alpha_{q/11}$ subunit of the G protein dissociates from the $\beta\gamma$ subunit complex. The α subunit activates PLC causing the hydrolysis of PIP_2 into IP_3 and DAG. IP_3 causes the release Ca^{2+} from endoplasmic reticulum (ER) and elevation of the concentration of intracellular Ca^{2+} $[Ca^{2+}]_i$. DAG activates PKC, which phosphorylates a number of proteins including ion channels and the NMDA receptor complex. The $\beta\gamma$ G protein subunit inhibits both muscarinic ($I_{K(M)}$) and calcium-regulated ($I_{K(Ca)}$) potassium currents. Thus, the activation of M1,3,5 receptors is associated with depolarizing and excitatory modulation. Agonist binding to M2,4 receptors (generally located presynaptically) causes the G protein α_i subunit to inhibit adenylyl cyclase and thus decrease the production of cAMP. The $\beta\gamma$ G protein subunit inhibits an inwardly rectifying potassium current ($I_{K(IR)}$). During physiological conditions, activation of the ($I_{K(IR)}$) allows potassium current to flow outward and thus contributes to hyperpolarization (current flows inward only during artificial membrane hyperpolarization beyond the equilibrium potential for K^+ imposed by voltage clamp conditions). Thus, activation of M2,4 receptors is associated with hyperpolarizing and inhibitory modulation.

inhibiting the release of neurotransmitter. In cardiac tissue, the M2 receptor activates G protein-coupled potassium channels to hyperpolarize heart muscle and thereby slow the heart rate. Blocking the actions of endogenous ACh in cardiac tissue with atropine, a nonselective muscarinic antagonist, produce tachycardias.

The M1, M2, M3, and M4 subtypes are predominant in the brain. M1 receptor density is high in hippocampus (especially in CA1 and the dentate gyrus), basal forebrain, olfactory tubercle and bulb, and throughout the cortex. M1 receptor density is low in the diencephalon and superior colliculi, and extremely low in the rest of the brain stem (Cortes and Palacios, 1986; Adem et al., 1997). The M2 subtype is expressed at high levels in the pontine and relatively low levels in the rest of the brain stem and the basal forebrain. The M3 subtype has similar density distribution to M1 (Levey et al., 1994). However, M3 density is enriched relative to M1 receptors in diencephalic and brain stem regions (Zubieta and Frey, 1993). The M4 subtype density is high in the striatum and olfactory tubercle, intermediate in CA1 and the dentate gyrus, and of low density in CA3 and the frontal cortex (Jerusalinsky et al., 1998). The M5 subtype is expressed at extremely low levels and with a very limited distribution in the brain.

Nicotinic ACh receptors are membrane-bound protein complexes that form ligand-gated ion channels permeable to sodium (Na^+), K^+, and Ca^{2+} ions. Nicotinic receptors are categorized into four groups (see Table 5.2): neuronal, α-bungarotoxin-sensitive; neuronal, α-bungarotoxin-insensitive; ganglionic; and muscular, α-bungarotoxin-sensitive (Sargent, 1993). A recent study proposed a further subclassification scheme for neuronal nicotinic receptors with one α-bungarotoxin-sensitive subtype and three α-bungarotoxin-insensitive subtypes (Zoli et al., 1998). The structure of the nicotinic receptor consists of five subunits, each containing a structural motif of four transmembrane-spanning domains. Nine α subunits, three β subunits, one δ subunit, and one ε subunit have been cloned. Each receptor subtype contains two α subunits, which comprise binding sites for ACh molecules. Autoradiographic binding studies in brain tissue reveal the greatest density of neuronal nicotinic receptors in the thalamus and superior colliculus, moderate density in the cortex, striatum, and hippocampus, and very low density in the cerebellum (Horti et al., 1999). Very little research on the role of nicotinic receptors in brain injury pathophysiology has been performed.

Acute activation of cholinergic receptors contributes to the pathological cascades following TBI. There is a large and rapid release of extracellular ACh immediately after TBI that results in cholinergic receptor downregulation as well as alterations in muscarinic signal transduction processes. TBI-induced cholinergic receptor activation contributes to the phenomenon of traumatic unconsciousness and to more enduring deficits of motor and memory function. Evidence from other disciplines indicate that intense activation of cholinergic receptors can produce seizures and brain damage.

ACh Toxicity and Seizures

Olney and Ho (1970) coined the term "excitotoxicity" in describing the neurotoxic properties of excitatory amino acids, in particular glutamate and aspartate. It was

TABLE 5.2 Nicotinic Acetylcholine Receptors

Subtypes	Signal transduction	Selective antagonist	Agonist	Predominant CNS localization
Neuronal α-bungarotoxin-sensitive	Na^+, K^+, Ca^{2+} ions	Dihydro-β-erythroidine	Nicotine Dimethylphenylpiperazinium	Thalamus, superior colliculus, cortex, striatum, hippocampus
Neuronal α-bungarotoxin-insensitive	Na^+, K^+, Ca^{2+} ions	Methyllycaconitine	Nicotine Dimethylphenylpiperazinium	Thalamus, superior colliculus, cortex, striatum, hippocampus
N1 Muscular	Na^+, K^+, Ca^{2+} ions	D-Tubocurarine (competitive)	Nicotine	None
α-bungarotoxin-sensitive		Decamethonium	Phenyltrimethylammonium	
N2 Ganglionic	Na^+, K^+, Ca^{2+} ions	Trimethaphan (competitive) Hexamethonium (noncompetitive)	Nicotine Dimethylphenylpiperazinium	None

also Olney and colleagues (1983) who first described the potencies of cholinergic agents to induce brain damage in animals. Seizures and postsynaptic neuronal necrosis are produced by activation of cholinergic receptors by a variety of agents including cholinomimetics (e.g., oxytremorine, pilocarpine, carbachol) (Olney et al., 1983; Turski et al., 1983), acetylcholinesterase inhibitors (e.g., physostigmine, neostigmine) (Olney et al., 1983), and stimulation of ACh tracts (Sloviter, 1983; McGeer and McGeer, 1985). Olney and colleagues (1983) found that neither nicotine nor ACh injections into the amygdala produced brain damage. However, extensive neuronal damage was produced when ACh was coadministered with a very low dose of neostigmine, which alone did not produce any brain damage. These data indicated that the activation of muscarinic receptors in the limbic system could produce seizures and brain damage resembling that produced by status epilepticus. Furthermore, these data underscored the importance of acetylcholinesterase (AChE) in controlling the seizure potential of endogenous ACh. Olney and colleagues (1983) postulated that activation of cholinergic receptors initiates seizure activity and that the subsequent release of excitatory amino acids produced the neuronal damage at the foci of sustained limbic seizures. Later studies by Sloviter and Dempster (1985) demonstrated that intraventricular injections of ACh could produce body tremors and tonic-clonic convulsions that were of greater intensity than those produced by similar injections of glutamate or aspartate. However, if chloral hydrate was administered to prevent convulsions, intraventricular injections of ACh did not produce hippocampal neuronal cell loss, whereas glutamate and aspartate still produced cell loss. Thus, it appeared that ACh was not directly toxic to neurons. This was confirmed by subsequent studies indicating that the "cholinergic toxins" produce cell damage through the secondary release of glutamate and activation of NMDA and non-NMDA receptors (Lallement et al., 1993). Later studies confirmed that substantial glutamate is released following pilocarpine-induced seizures (Liu et al., 1997; Smolders et al., 1997). Other studies have shown that the NMDA antagonist TCP [N-(1-[2-thienyl]cyclohexyl)piperidine] or the AMPA (α-amino-3-hydroxy-5-methylisoxazole-4-propionic acid) antagonist NBQX (2,3-dihydroxy-6-nitro-7-sulfamoylbenzoquinoxaline) can significantly reduce soman-induced neuronal damage and dampen behavioral seizures (Lallement et al., 1993). Although some studies suggest that NMDA antagonists may block seizures (Ormandy et al., 1989), the stereotypic behavioral side effects of NMDA antagonists may confound the behavioral interpretation of cholinergic-induced limbic seizures by masking their behavioral manifestation. For example, rats treated with MK801 20 min prior to injection of pilocarpine exhibit electrographic seizure recordings of a similar magnitude and duration to those in rats treated with pilocarpine alone (Rice and DeLorenzo, 1998). However, blocking NMDA receptors during the seizure activity prevents the damaging consequences of pilocarpine-induced seizures. For example, CA1 neuronal cell loss, water maze deficits, and late-developing spontaneous recurring seizures are all prevented by pretreatment with MK801 even though pilocarpine-induced electrographic seizures are not eliminated or reduced (Rice and DeLorenzo, 1998; Rice et al., 1998). These studies suggest that intense activation of muscarinic receptors can drive limbic circuits to release excitotoxic levels of glutamate and it is glutamate receptor activation that produces the neuronal damage.

The acute elevations in extracellular ACh following TBI (described below) have the potential to initiate seizures and potentate brain damage. Posttraumatic seizures are sometimes observed within hours after severe human TBI (Elvidge, 1939) and electrographic evidence of seizures is sometimes observed in animal models of TBI (Bornstein, 1946; Dixon et al., 1987). The muscarinic antagonist atropine can abolish injury-induced electrographic seizure activity or prevent its development if administered within 30 min after TBI (Bornstein, 1946).

Extracellular Levels of ACh Increase Following TBI

Research as early as the 1940s indicated that the traumatically injured brain liberates significant amounts of ACh. These early experimental studies of traumatic brain injury used cats, dogs, and rats in various models of injury including air gun (Sachs, 1957) and mallet blow to the skull (Ruge, 1954) or hydraulic impacts directly to the cortex surface (Bornstein, 1946; Metz, 1971). ACh, measured with biological assays, increased within minutes after the injury and in some cases remained elevated for days (Bornstein, 1946; Sachs, 1957). These studies led to several uncontrolled clinical evaluations of anticholinergic treatments in head-injured patients (reviewed below).

Interest in the role of ACh in traumatic brain injury resurfaced in the 1980s and 1990s. The use of standardized, well-characterized animal models of TBI (fluid percussion, controlled cortical impact) along with advanced methods of sampling (microdialysis), detecting (gas chromatography), and quantifying ACh molecules confirmed and extended the findings of the earlier observations. Gorman and colleagues (1989) reported significant increases in hippocampal ACh at 5 min after central fluid percussion TBI in the rat using the microdialysis technique. Other studies measuring ACh concentrations in rat brain CSF following central fluid percussion reported significant 2-fold increases at 5 min (Lyeth et al., 1993) and 5-fold increases at 12 min post injury (Robinson et al., 1990a; Enters et al., 1992). The concentrations of ACh detected in ventricular CSF or in brain parenchyma by microdialysis may greatly underestimate the actual local synaptic concentrations of neurotransmitter available to activate ACh receptors. Synaptic concentrations of ACh are rapidly inactivated under normal conditions by AChE thereby ceasing further stimulation of ACh receptors. That measurable elevations of ACh can be detected at all after TBI suggests that extracellular synaptic concentration of ACh may have exceeded the inactivation capacity of AChE. Thus, the probability of a period of intense activation of cholinergic receptors is likely.

Receptor Binding Studies

Receptor binding alterations following TBI provide further evidence of the involvement of muscarinic receptors in TBI. As soon as one hour after central fluid percussion TBI there is a significant reduction in the affinity of receptors for the nonselective muscarinic antagonist, [^{3}H]QNB (quinuclidinylbenzilate) in the hippocampus and brain stem (Lyeth et al., 1994). This decrease in affinity suggests a downregulation in response to intense stimulation in regions particularly vulnerable to fluid percussion injury. For example, TBI disrupts performance on hippocampal-dependent spatial memory tasks (Lyeth et al., 1990; Hamm et al., 1992), blocks the induction of long-term potentiation (LTP) in the Schaeffer collateral CA1 system (Miyazaki et al., 1992; Reeves et al., 1995), and increases dorsal hippocampal CA1 pyramidal neuron vulnerability to a controlled posttraumatic ischemic insult (Jenkins et al., 1989). Brain stem sites also contribute to TBI pathophysiology. Activation of pontine cholinergic sites is implicated as a mechanism mediating traumatic unconsciousness following fluid percussion TBI (Hayes et al., 1984, 1986; Katayama et al., 1984) (see below). The rapid (1 h) decrease in affinity, which can occur rather quickly as a result of phosphorylation, is consistent with an acute, large release of ACh and subsequent excessive receptor stimulation.

In similar receptor binding studies performed at 15 days after TBI, affinity for [^{3}H]QNB was normal but a significant increase was detected in receptor number (B_{max}) in the hippocampus and cortex (Jiang et al., 1994). When animals were administered the nonselective muscarinic receptor antagonist scopolamine at the time of injury B_{max} values at 15 days post injury in the hippocampus and cortex did not differ from those in sham-injured rats (Jiang et al., 1994). This is consistent with other recent laboratory studies suggesting that brain cholinergic systems are altered weeks after fluid percussion TBI (see section below). Furthermore, preinjury administration of scopolamine normalized the alteration in receptor number at 15 days in both hippocampus and neocortex (Jiang et al., 1994). This finding is also congruent with laboratory studies indicating that acute intervention with anticholinergics can reduce behavioral morbidity days or even weeks after TBI (see below). These findings suggest that acute activation of muscarinic receptors soon after brain impact produces alterations in the function of brain cholinergic systems that can persist for weeks after injury.

Signal Transduction Alterations

The high levels of extracellular ACh following TBI would presumably lead to excessive activation of both muscarinic and nicotinic receptor signaling cascades, depending, of course, on regional localization of ACh release as well as regional distribution of ACh receptor subtypes. There is evidence for excessive PLC-coupled muscarinic receptor activation, but the evidence of c-AMP-coupled muscarinic receptor or nicotinic receptor activation has yet to be investigated. Wei and colleagues (1982) first reported PLC activation immediately following fluid percussion TBI in cats. Later studies in the rat lateral fluid percussion model found elevated levels of IP$_3$ at 5 min post injury in the ipsilateral hippocampus and for up to 20 min after injury in the ipsilateral cortex (Prasad et al., 1994). Subsequent studies measured the phosphodiestric breakdown of membrane PIP$_2$ following fluid percussion TBI in rats and found that concentrations of tissue PIP$_2$ were significantly decreased at times when DAG and free-fatty acids (FFA) were elevated (5 and

20 min post injury) (Dhillon et al., 1995). These findings provide compelling evidence that PIP_2 signal transduction pathways are activated after TBI and that the enhanced PLC-catalyzed phophodiesteric breakdown of PIP_2 is a mechanism of liberation of FFA after TBI. However, these studies did not determine whether muscarinic PLC-coupled receptors participated in the activation process. Later studies examining the link between muscarinic receptors and TBI-induced activation of the PLC signal transduction pathway reported that pharmacological blockade of muscarinic receptors with scopolamine at the time of injury significantly blunts the acute elevations in PIP_2 and FFA (Lyeth et al., 1996). This has important implications for pathological processes since the same dose of scopolamine also diminishes motor deficits (Lyeth et al., 1988b, 1992) and learning and memory deficits (Hamm et al., 1993) associated with experimental TBI (see below). However, the enhanced activation of the PLC signal transduction pathway is only partially blocked by scopolamine, suggesting that other PLC-coupled receptors (e.g., metabotrophic glutamate group I, histamine H1, serotonin 5-HT2, α1-adrenoreceptors) may also contribute to the TBI-induced cascade. Thus, TBI appears to cause a significant increase in the hydrolysis of membrane phospholipids that is, in part, attributed to the activation of muscarinic receptors. Regional increases in IP_3, DAG, and FFA occur within minutes after fluid percussion TBI in rats, providing strong biochemical evidence for a period of intense activation of PLC-coupled excitatory neurotransmitter receptors.

In pathological conditions involving elevations of glutamate and ACh (e.g., TBI), the activation of PLC-coupled cholinergic receptors may potentiate NMDA excitotoxicity. ACh initiates a long-lasting facilitation of the NMDA component of excitatory postsynaptic potentials (EPSP) in the rat hippocampus through the IP_3 pathway (Markram and Segal, 1990, 1992). In cultured rat hippocampal neurons, combined application of ACh and NMDA produces a much greater rise in intracellular free Ca^{2+} than the simple additive effects of either agent alone (Segal, 1992). By amplifying the NMDA component in EPSPs, ACh increases the probability and amplitude of long-term potentiation (Ito et al., 1988; Tanaka et al., 1989). Thus, the abrupt rise in extracellular levels of ACh and the subsequent activation of PLC-coupled muscarinic receptors following TBI is likely to produce a condition of "cholinergic-potentiated excitotoxicity."

A series of experiments by Delahunty and colleagues, using a "functional assay" of the muscarinic receptor-linked PLC–IP_3 signal transduction pathway, suggest that TBI acutely alters muscarinic receptor–effector coupling. This assay loads fresh brain tissue with [^{3}H]myoinositol, exposes the tissue homogenate to the muscarinic agonist carbachol, and then quantifies the radiolabeled inositol phosphate (IP) products of PIP_2 hydrolysis. At 1 h following central fluid percussion TBI, the production of IP in rat hippocampus in response to muscarinic receptor stimulation is enhanced by 60% over control after mild (Delahunty, 1992) and by 200% over control after moderate injury (Delahunty et al., 1995). This enhancement occurs even though at the same time muscarinic receptor affinity for [^{3}H]QNB is reduced (there was no change in B_{max}) (Lyeth et al., 1994). These data suggest that early after injury the traumatized brain produces a more intense second messenger signal in response to receptor activation; in essence, an amplification of the muscarinic receptor stimulated signal. The IP production remains enhanced by 25% at 15 days after moderate TBI (Delahunty et al., 1995), but this is likely due to an increase in muscarinic B_{max} at that time (Jiang et al., 1994). The apparent amplification of PLC-coupled muscarinic receptors at 1 h has important implications for secondary insults such as hypoxia or ischemia. Even a mild secondary insult involving release of ACh might have deleterious consequences from the amplified IP production (e.g., greater IP_3-evoked release of Ca^{2+} from endoplasmic reticulum). For example, Jenkins and colleagues (1989) demonstrated that a mild central fluid percussion TBI, when combined with a controlled mild transient forebrain ischemia one hour later, produces extensive CA1 neuronal cell death; a consequence that neither insult alone produces. Furthermore, combined pharmacological blockade of muscarinic and NMDA receptors during the TBI component in this model attenuates the increased sensitivity of the traumatized brain to delayed secondary ischemia (Jenkins et al., 1988).

Behavioral Studies

Ach and Traumatic Unconsciousness. Human TBI is often associated with a period of traumatic unconsciousness ranging from a brief loss of consciousness after concussive injury to extended periods of coma in severe head injury. Most animal models of TBI faithfully reproduce the transient loss of consciousness associated with concussion but fail to produce extended periods of coma (Gennarelli, 1994). Studies as early as the 1940s suggested that ACh liberated by TBI can influence traumatic unconsciousness. In case report laboratory studies, Bornstein (1946) found elevated levels of ACh in the cerebrospinal fluid (CSF) of cats and dogs that persisted for up to 48 h after TBI. In some cases, administration of atropine counteracted the stupor and loss of body tone associated with injury. Several lines of evidence suggest that activation of a cholinoceptive area located in the rostral pons contributes to components of behavioral suppression associated with transient unconsciousness following concussive brain injury (for detailed review, see Hayes et al., 1986). Hayes and Katayama performed a series of experiments systematically examining the relationship between ACh and traumatic unconsciousness. Fluid percussion TBI in the cat produced increased rates of local glucose utilization in regions within the dorsomedial pontine tegmentum, a cholinoceptive region, for at least 2 h immediately after trauma (Hayes et al., 1984). The turnover rate of ACh in the pons is transiently increased after low level concussion in the rat, also suggesting an acute activation of this region after TBI (Saija et al., 1988). Pharmacological activation of the dorsomedial pontine tegmentum in uninjured cats by bilateral microinjections of carbachol produced unconsciousness and EEG changes resembling those following fluid percussion TBI in the cat (Hayes et al., 1984; Katayama et al., 1984, 1985a,b). Systemic administrations or microinjections of atropine, but not mecamylamine (nicotinic antagonist) reversed the carbachol-induced behavioral suppression (Hayes et al., 1984; Katayama et al., 1984). Blocking action potentials and nerve conduction in that region with microinjections of the sodium channel blocker tetracaine failed to produce unconsciousness (Hayes et al., 1984). Thus, inactivation of this brain stem area does not produce unconsciousness. In TBI rats, the centrally acting muscarinic antagonists scopolamine or dicyclomine, but not the nicotinic antagonist mecamylamine, reduce the duration of traumatic unconsciousness associated with moderate fluid percussion TBI (Lyeth et al., 1988a; Robinson et al., 1990b). The above studies suggest that activation of brain stem cholinoceptive regions contributes to the behavioral suppression following concussive levels of TBI and that traumatic unconsciousness can be attenuated by pharmacotherapy.

Acute ACh Hyperfunction and Long-term Behavioral Deficits. Laboratory studies have also demonstrated that excessive activation of muscarinic cholinergic receptors significantly contributes to long-lasting functional deficits associated with experimental TBI in the rat. A single administration of the muscarinic antagonist scopolamine (1.0 mg/kg, i.p.) at the time of injury can significantly reduce motor deficits (Lyeth et al., 1988b, 1992; Robinson et al., 1990b) and memory deficits (Hamm et al., 1993) which typically last for days to weeks after fluid percussion TBI in the rat. However, if treatment with scopolamine is delayed until 30 min post injury, no reduction of behavioral deficits is observed (Lyeth et al., 1992). Further studies indicated that dicyclomine (1.0 or 10.0 mg/kg, i.p.), a selective M1 muscarinic antagonist administered prior to TBI, provided protection equal to that afforded by scopolamine (Robinson et al., 1990b), indicating the importance of PLC-coupled receptor activation in producing behavioral morbidity.

Depleting ACh stores prior to injury also reduces long-term behavioral deficits. For example, administration of hemicholinium-3 derivatives, which selectively deplete, either central stores of ACh or peripheral ACh concentrations, significantly reduces motor deficits following TBI in the rat (Robinson et al., 1990a). The protection afforded by peripheral depletion is likely due to reducing the availability of blood-borne concentrations of ACh to cross a compromised blood–brain barrier (Jiang et al., 1992). These studies suggest that a brief and transient period of excessive muscarinic receptor activation can contribute to relatively long-lasting behavioral deficits.

CHRONIC CHOLINERGIC HYPOFUNCTION

Hayes and colleagues (1989, 1992) first postulated that TBI produces biphasic effects on CNS excitability such that the mechanisms inducing chronic behavioral deficits may differ from the mechanisms maintaining them. Dixon and colleagues (1994a) elaborated on this concept and postulated that the immediate elevations in extracellular ACh and excessive stimulation of ACh receptors lasting for only minutes could subsequently produce chronic deficits in cholinergic neurotransmission lasting for weeks or months. There is now considerable evidence supporting the hypothesis that a chronic period of cholinergic hypofunction following TBI contributes to persistent deficits in memory.

Markers and Mechanisms of Cholinergic Dysfunction

Memory deficits are the most common and persistent sequelae of human TBI (Levin, 1985; Oddy et al., 1985) and are also a prominent feature of experimental TBI in animals (e.g., Lyeth et al., 1990; Smith et al., 1991, 1993; Hamm et al., 1992, 1993; Pierce et al., 1993). Since cholinergic pathways in the brain play an important role in learning and memory processes (Squire and Davis, 1981), it is likely that any TBI-induced alterations in cholinergic system integrity may contribute to the memory deficits associated with trauma. Dixon and colleagues (1994a) used a scopolamine pharmacological challenge to probe the general function of brain cholinergic systems after controlled cortical impact TBI in the rat. This methodology, which was originally used with human patients, administers a muscarinic antagonist at doses that do not significantly disrupt memory in normal persons, but produces profound memory deficits in patients with Alzheimer's (Sunderland et al., 1985, 1987) or Parkinson's diseases (Dubois et al., 1987). The scopolamine challenge also significantly exacerbates Morris water maze memory deficits 19 or 35 days after controlled cortical impact TBI in the rat; the same dose of scopolamine had no effect on sham-injured control animals (Dixon et al., 1994a, 1995a). The scopolamine challenge also revealed "covert deficits" by eliciting memory deficits at days 47 and 75 post injury when such deficits in TBI rats had spontaneously recovered (Dixon et al., 1995a). The enhanced vulnerability to memory disruption by blocking muscarinic receptors suggests that cholinergic-mediated memory function may be somehow disturbed in the traumatized brain even after spontaneous recovery has apparently occurred.

Neurochemical assessment of choline, the rate-limiting factor in ACh synthesis, revealed a significant decrease in hippocampal high-affinity choline uptake at 2 weeks after controlled cortical impact TBI in rats even though basal choline availability appeared normal (Dixon et al., 1994b). These data suggested that posttraumatic cholinergic deficits in memory might be associated with either a decreased ability of cholinergic neurons to take up choline and/or a loss of cholinergic neurons. Further studies by Dixon and colleagues (1995b, 1997a) measured basal and scopolamine-evoked release of ACh in the hippocampus and neocortex by microdialysis at 14 days after controlled cortical impact TBI in rats. Evoked release of ACh (by blocking presynaptic autoreceptors) was significantly reduced in TBI rats compared to sham-injured controls, while basal levels of ACh were unchanged.

Presynaptic alteration in the storage and release of ACh may also contribute to the cholinergic hypofunction after TBI. From 2 to 4 weeks after controlled cortical impact TBI there is a late-developing 40% to 50% increase in vesicular ACh transporter in rat dorsal hippocampus (Ciallella et al., 1998; Shao et al., 1999). The vesicular ACh transporter mediates accumulation of ACh into secretory vesicles and can be used as an indicator of ACh storage capacity. These studies also measured a concomitant decrease in M2 receptor protein. These changes may represent compensatory responses to cholinergic hypofunction by upregulating ACh storage capacity and downregulating inhibitory presynaptic autoreceptors.

Anatomical evidence also indicates chronic cholinergic dysfunction following experimental TBI. There is a significant loss of choline acetyltransferase (ChAT) immunoreactivity in the forebrain following both central (Schmidt and Grady, 1995) and lateral fluid percussion (Leonard et al., 1994; Gorman et al., 1996) as well as after controlled cortical impact (Dixon et al., 1997c). The basal forebrain projects to the hippocampal formation and is thought to play a major role in memory (Harrell et al., 1987). A postmortem human study reports a 50% reduction of ChAT activity in the temporal cortex after severe TBI suggesting a significant presynaptic abnormality of cholinergic neurotransmission (Dewar and Graham, 1996). Furthermore, central fluid percussion TBI in rats produces an up regulation of muscarinic receptors (increase in B_{max}) at 15 days after injury and may be a compensatory response to chronic loss of cholinergic tone after injury (Jiang et al., 1994). These data strongly indicate a chronic alteration in cholinergic function that, in some injury models, remains hidden or "covert" until challenged, since basal function may appear normal. TBI-induced alterations to the cholinergic system may include presynaptic cholinergic dysfunction, loss of cholinergic neurons, functional impairment of cholinergic terminals, or changes in ACh release mechanisms.

Treatment: AChE Inhibitors

A number of studies have examined the effects of delayed administration of cholinergic activity-enhancing agents targeted at the cholinergic hypofunction phase of TBI. These experiments have often used pharmaceuticals originally targeted to improve age-related cognitive deficits. One strategy employed to enhance cholinergic neurotransmission after TBI used AChE inhibitors. Tetrahydroamino-acridine (Tacrine[TM]), a reversible AChE inhibitor, administered daily starting at 24 h after central fluid percussion TBI, failed to improve Morris water maze performance (Pike et al., 1997a). The highest dosing (9 mg/kg per day) exacerbated maze deficits (measured by latency to find the goal platform), which may have been confounded by motor deficits since swim speeds were significantly reduced. Interestingly, Tacrine[TM] caused a dose-related impairment in maze performance in a concurrently run sham-injured group These negative observations result from several factors. The chronic prolongation of ACh activity in the synapse by an AChE inhibitor may result in prolonged tonic stimulation of postsynaptic receptors and subsequent receptor downregulation. The "nonspecific" nature of prolonging synaptic ACh activity may also compromise the intricate, endogenous patterning of ACh release that likely occurs with normal neuronal signaling.

In another series of experiments, a single subcutaneous bolus of ENA713, a brain-selective AChE inhibitor, administered up to 2 h after weight drop closed head injury in the rat reduced brain edema, disruption of the blood–brain barrier, and impairment of reflexes and motor function (Chen et al., 1998). A dose of ENA713 that inhibited approximately 50% of AChE in hippocampus and cortex provided the greatest degree of improvement in a composite neurological score when administered at 5 min after trauma and somewhat less improvement when administered at 60 or 120 min after trauma. These results seem contradictory to numerous other studies showing behavioral protection from administering muscarinic antagonists acutely after TBI. Interestingly, Chen and colleagues (1998) also included 5 min postinjury treatment groups of scopolamine (1 mg/kg) and mecamylamine (2.5 mg/kg). Scopolamine provided behavioral and edema efficacy equal to that of ENA713, while mecamylamine had no effect. The protective effects of cerebral hypothermia may have confounded the ENA713 treatment groups, since ENA713 decreased rectal body temperature by $2°C$. The protective effects of ENA713 may also act at a relatively later stage after TBI when the initial cholinergic hyperactivity has subsided, since the maximal AChE inhibition produced does not occur until 60 min after injection (Chen et al., 1998).

Treatment: ACh Synthesis Enhancement

A second strategy for enhancing cholinergic function chronically after TBI used cytidine diphosphorylcholine (CDP-choline), which indirectly stimulates the biosynthesis of ACh by providing additional choline. When administered daily for 18 days starting at 24 h after controlled cortical impact TBI, CDP-choline reduced Morris water maze deficits and attenuated the TBI-induced increased sensitivity to the memory-disrupting effects of the scopolamine challenge (Dixon et al., 1997b). This study also demonstrated that a single intraparenchymal injection of CDP-choline could increase extracellular levels of ACh in hippocampus and neocortex of the awake, freely moving rat. However, the beneficial effects of CDP-choline may be related to mechanisms other than cholinergic enhancement, since CDP-choline can help maintain cellular integrity by accelerating phospholipid membrane formation (Lopez-Coviella et al., 1995) and enhancing brain metabolism (Villa et al., 1993).

Treatment: Targeted Receptor Subtype Pharmacology

A third strategy for overcoming chronic cholinergic hypofunction targets pharmacological agonists or antagonists directed at specific muscarinic receptor subtypes. A study by Pike and Hamm (1995) reported that daily injections, starting at 24 h after TBI, of the selective M2 antagonist BIBN 99 attenuated Morris water maze deficits on days 11 to 15 in central fluid percussion TBI in rats. This protection was lost if the start of the BIBN 99 injection regimen was delayed until day 11 post injury. The selective blockade of M2 autoreceptors in these studies may have compensated the cholinergic hypofunction by amplifying existing signals in cholinergic pathways. This same research group tested a novel compound, LU 25-109-T, which is a partial M1 agonist that also has antagonist actions at presynaptic M2 autoreceptors (Pike and Hamm, 1997b). Daily subcutaneous administration of LU 25-109-T starting 24 h after central fluid percussion TBI significantly improved Morris water maze deficits measured on days 11 to 15 post injury. This same dosing regimen also attenuated the TBI-induced loss of ChAT immunoreactivity in the medial septal nucleus, diagonal band, and nucleus basalis magnocellularis (Pike and Hamm, 1997c). Parallel cresyl violet-stained sections indicated that the loss of ChAT immunoreactivity was not the result of a decrease in neuronal cell density. These results suggest that chronically increasing cholinergic tone after TBI may restore both cholinergic function and cognitive function.

ACh AND CEREBRAL ISCHEMIA

Cerebral ischemia shares some common mechanisms of injury with TBI and is often an accompanying insult in severe human head injury (Bouma et al., 1992). In the laboratory, transient forebrain ischemia also produces elevated levels of extracellular ACh in brain. Kumagae and Matsui (1991) reported that ACh levels rose 13-fold in extracellular microdialysate samples from rat hippocampus during four-vessel occlusion ischemia and remained elevated (3-fold) for 20 min after reperfusion. In contrast, brain tissue levels of ACh significantly decrease during ischemia (Kumagae and Matsui, 1991; Scremin and Jenden, 1991; Frolich et al., 1993; Kozuka, 1995) and remain decreased for short periods after reperfusion (Sadoshima et al., 1995; Bertrand et al., 1996). The increase in extracellular ACh during ischemia and concomitant decrease in tissue stores of ACh are consistent with a widespread synaptic release of ACh. A preliminary report using a rat model of subdural hematoma-induced ischemia found a significant reduction in cortical infarct volume when M1 receptors are blocked by dicyclomine administered 5 min after initiation of the insult (Jiang et al., 1998). While consistent with experimental TBI studies that provide protection with immediate muscarinic receptor blockade, the report of Jiang and colleagues (1998) appears to conflict with other reports of protection by an AChE inhibitor administered before or after cerebral ischemia (Tanaka et al., 1994, 1995).

CLINICAL STUDIES OF ACh IN BRAIN INJURY

Clinical research as early as the 1940s indicated that brain injury can liberate significant amounts of ACh into the CSF from moderately and severely head-injured patients (Cone et al., 1948; Tower and McEachern, 1949a,b; Sachs, 1957; Haber and Grossman, 1980). The reports suggested that the increased levels of ACh in CSF may in fact be injurious, since most often the more severely injured patients and/or those with poor clinical outcome had the highest levels of ACh. For example, two studies (Tower and McEachern 1949a; Haber and Grossman, 1980) reported that both depression of the EEG and a poor clinical state of the patient coincided with ACh in the CSF, while improvements of EEG and the clinical state paralleled the disappearance of ACh in the CSF. Sachs (1957) reported that ACh was present in the CSF during the first few days after severe head injury and disappeared as the patient recovered or stabilized neurologically.

The above observations led to several clinical administrations of anticholinergic drugs to block the suspected adverse effects of elevated ACh in the CSF. Clinical administration of atropine was reported to produce dramatic improvement in consciousness in certain patients ($n = 20$) comatose from head injury (Ward, 1950). A series of reports by Jenkner and Lechner (1954, 1955a,b) (total of 335 patients) found that various anticholinergic compounds (scopolamine, diethazine, biperiden hydrochloride) reduced or normalized pathological EEG in patients with head injuries ranging in magnitude from mild to severe. A much larger study

($n = 1700$) indicated that comatose, head-injured patients rapidly regained consciousness and that EEG improved or normalized soon after initiation of biperiden hydrochloride (Akineton[TM]) (Heppner and Diemath, 1958). It is important to note that data from these early clinical studies were not derived from randomized, prospective clinical trials and as such did not rigorously evaluate the effects of anticholinergic treatment. While these case reports only suggest a correlation between ACh in CSF and head injury severity and the possibility of protective effects of muscarinic antagonists, they have value in that they provide intriguing corroboration with the laboratory data reviewed above.

The cholinergic hypofunctional phase of TBI has also been treated clinically. In a preliminary study, CDP-choline or placebo was administered one month after mild or moderate closed head injury to a small group of patients ($n = 14$). The CDP-choline group experienced a significant reduction in postconcussional symptoms and a significant improvement in recognition memory compared to the placebo group (Levin, 1991). These findings suggest that CDP-choline might be effective in treating the sequelae of mild to moderate TBI pending replication in a larger group of patients.

SUMMARY

Cholinergic receptors play a biphasic role in the pathophysiology of TBI characterized by a shift from acute cholinergic hyperfunction to a chronic state of cholinergic hypofunction. Numerous studies have demonstrated that extracellular levels of ACh rapidly increase in the brain or CSF immediately after TBI in both man and animals. A second, diametrically opposed phase develops later and is characterized by a long-lasting period of cholinergic insufficiency (Fig. 5.2).

Activation of PLC-coupled muscarinic receptors (M1 and M3) increase intracellular free Ca^{2+} calcium via IP_3 and amplify the sensitivity of NMDA receptors. Activation of M1 and M3 receptors inhibits outward potassium currents (I_M and I_C), enhancing neuronal excitability. For at least one hour after TBI, there is an enhanced production of IP second messenger molecules that could amplify the effects of subsequent M1 and M3 receptor stimulation. Cholinergic-induced epilepsy studies suggests that the neurotoxicity associated with excessive cholinergic stimulation may actually be the result of indirect release of glutamate and subsequent excitotoxicity. Thus, the acute cholinergic hyperfunction immediately after TBI may produce a state of "cholinergic-potentiated excitotoxicity" that contributes to pathological changes and long-term behavioral morbidity. Trauma-induced cholinergic stimulation of muscarinic receptors in the brain stem pontine contributes to a period of traumatic unconsciousness immediately after injury. Administration of muscarinic antagonists at the time of injury attenuates both later developing behavioral morbidity as well as the immediate traumatic unconsciousness.

The acute cholinergic hyperfunction phase is followed by a chronic cholinergic hypofunction phase lasting for months in animal models. The cholinergic system is compromised by presynaptic decreases in synthesis, storage, and release of ACh,

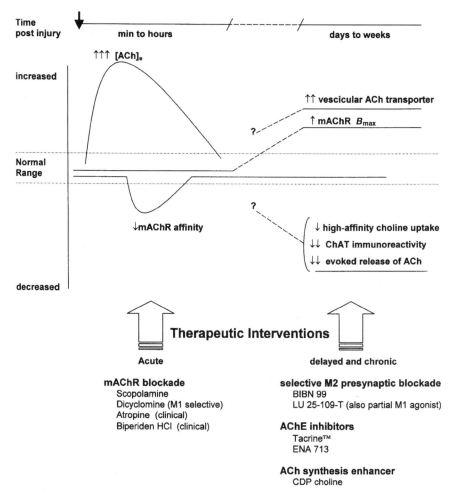

Figure 5.2 Time course of cholinergic hyperfunction/hypofunction asociated with TBI. An acute and transient period of cholinergic hyperfunction associated with elevated concentrations of extracellular acetylcholine ($[ACh]_e$) occurs within minutes to hours after TBI. Muscarinic ACh receptor (mAChR) affinity is decreased during this early period and is likely a compensatory response to excesssive receptor stimulation. A delayed and chronic period of cholinergic hypofunction associated with a general decreased availabilty of ACh for synaptic release develops days after injury and persists for weeks. An upregulation of mAChR number (B_{max}) and an increase in vesicular ACh transporter during this period are likely compensatory responses to reduced mAChR activation. The time course of transition from the hyperfunction period to the hypofunction period is not well established (denoted by the dashed line). Numerous therapeutic strategies have been targeted at the abnormalities in both the hyperfunction and hypofunction periods. $\uparrow$, $\uparrow\uparrow$, $\uparrow\uparrow\uparrow$ = relative magnitude of effect; ? = no data available during the acute period.

while postsynaptically there is a compensatory upregulation of receptors. Delayed treatments with AChE inhibitors, ACh synthesis enhancers, and targeted pre- and postsynaptic receptor pharmacology have all provided some reduction in cognitive deficits in animal models. The TBI-induced cholinergic shift from acute hypofunction to chronic hyperfunction necessitates diametrically opposed therapeutic interventions over time with administration of anticholinergic agents very early followed much later by cholinomimetic agents.

Clinical studies of ACh in TBI consist of case report observations, some dating back as far as 50 years. They report a large increase in ACh in the CSF that correlates with the magnitude of injury and the clinical state of the patient. Administration of antimuscarinic drugs appears to improve states of consciousness and clinical outcome. Although that data were not derived from randomized, prospective clinical trials, they still have value in that they corroborate later controlled laboratory data and thus may generate interest in future head injury clinical trials targeted at the cholinergic system.

FUTURE OF CHOLINERGIC RECEPTOR RESEARCH IN BRAIN INJURY

Several areas of research need more in exploration relation to cholinergic receptor-mediated brain injury. The role of acute nicotinic receptor activation during the cholinergic hyperfunction phase has not been systematically examined. This may be of particular relevance since nicotinic receptors are ionotropic, conducting Na^+, K^+, and Ca^{2+}. Thus, they have the potential to contribute to neuronal depolarization and increase intracellular free Ca^{2+}. Furthermore, our growing understanding of the complexity of neuronal nicotinic receptors resulting from different combinations of the α, β, δ, and ε subunits may uncover roles for these cholinergic receptors in TBI pathophysiology.

The possible interactions of muscarinic and NMDA receptor activation during the acute cholinergic hyperfunction phase needs further investigation. Basic questions of how M1 and M3 muscarinic receptor activation potentiates glutamate excitotoxicity remain to be sufficiently elucidated.

Further studies of ACh in ischemia are also warranted. Reports of extremely elevated extracellular ACh during and immediately after cerebral ischemia seem to conflict with other studies in which neuroprotection is afforded by preinjury administration of AChE inhibitors.

The large body of experimental literature demonstrating protection by early anticholinergic intervention, as well as similar results in clinical case reports, suggests that acute anticholinergic therapy should be considered for controlled clinical trials. Unfortunately, side effects of some muscarinic antagonists obtund certain clinical signs such as pupil diameter and also produce tachycardia. More selective drugs (e.g., selective M1 antagonists) may reduce certain of these unwanted effects. Finally, clinical pharmacotherapy during the chronic cholinergic hypofunction phase should be seriously considered. The rehabilitation medicine community might consider cholinergic-enhancing therapies for TBI survivors (e.g., CDP-choline or presynaptic autoreceptor antagonists), which may improve cognitive function with minimal adverse side effects.

ACKNOWLEDGMENT

This work was supported by grant NS 29995 from the National Institutes of Health.

ABBREVIATIONS

4-DAMP	4-Diphenylacetoxy-N-methylpiperidine
AC	Adenylyl cyclase
ACh	Acetylcholine
$[ACh]_e$	Extracellular concentration of acetylcholine
AChE	Acetylcholinesterase
AMPA	α-Amino-3-hydroxy-5-methylisoxazole-4-propionic acid
ATP	Adenosine 5'-triphosphate
B_{max}	Receptor number
$[Ca^{2+}]_i$	Intracellular concentration of calcium ions
cAMP	Cyclic adenosine 3',5'-monophosphate
CDP-choline	cytidine diphosphorylcholine
ChAT	Choline acetyltransferase
CNS	Central nervous system
CSF	Cerebrospinal fluid
DAG	Diacylglycerol
EEG	Electroencephalography
EPSP	Excitatory postsynaptic potentials
ER	Endoplasmic reticulum
FFA	Free fatty acids
G_α	α Subunit of G protein
$G_{\beta\gamma}$	$\beta\gamma$ Subunits of G protein
$I_{K(Ca)}$	Ca^{2+}-regulated potassium current
$I_{K(IR)}$	G protein-gated inward rectifier potassium current
$I_{K(M)}$	M-current potassium current
IP	Inositol phosphate
IP_3	Inositol 1,4,5-trisphosphate
LTP	Long-term potentiation
mAChR	Muscarinic acetylcholine receptor
NBQX	2,3-dihydroxy-6-nitro-7-sulfamoylbenzoquinoxaline
NMDA	N-methyl-D-aspartate

PIP$_2$	Phosphatidylinositol 4,5-bisphosphate
PKC	Protein kinase C
PLC	Phospholipase C
QNB	Quinuclidinylbenzilate
TBI	Traumatic brain injury
TCP	N-(1-[2-Thienyl]cyclohexyl)piperidine

REFERENCES

A. Adem, M. Jolkkonen, N. Bogdanovic, A. Islam, and E. Karlsson, *Brain Res. Bull.*, 44, 597–601 (1997).

N. Bertrand, H. Ishii, and M. Spatz, *Neurochem. Int.*, 28, 293–297 (1996).

M. B. Bornstein, *J Neurophysiol.*, 9, 349–366 (1946).

G. J. Bouma, J. P. Muizelaar, W. A. Stringer, S. C. Choi, P. Fatouros, and H. F. Young, *Neurosurg.*, 77, 360–368 (1992).

Y. Chen, E. Shohami, R. Bass, and M. Weinstock, *Brain Res.*, 784, 18–24 (1998).

J. R. Ciallella, H. Q. Yan, X. Ma, B. M. Wolfson, D. W. Marion, S. T. DeKosky, and C. E. Dixon, *Exp. Neurol.*, 152, 11–19 (1998).

W. V. Cone, D. B. Tower, and D. McEachern, *Trans. Am. Neurol. Assoc.*, 73, 59–63 (1948).

R. Cortes and J. M. Palacios, *Brain Res.*, 362, 227–238 (1986).

T. M. Delahunty, *Brain Res.*, 594, 307–310 (1992).

T. M. Delahunty, J. Y. Jiang, R. T. Black, and B. G. Lyeth, *Neurochem. Res.*, 20, 335–341 (1995).

D. Dewar and D. I. Graham, *J. Neurotrauma*, 13, 181–187 (1996).

H. S. Dhillon, T. Carbary, J. Dose, R. J. Dempsey, and M. R. Prasad, *Brain Res.*, 698, 100–106 (1995).

H. S. Dhillon, T. Carbary, J. Dose, R. J. Dempsey, and M. R. Prasad, *Brain Research*, 698, 100–106 (1995).

C. E. Dixon, B. G. Lyeth, J. T. Povlishock, R. L. Findling, A. Marmarou, H. F. Young, and R. L. Hayes, *J. Neurosurg.*, 67, 110–119 (1987).

C. E. Dixon, R. J. Hamm, W. C. Taft, and R. L. Hayes, *J. Neurotrauma*, 11(3), 275–287 (1994a).

C. E. Dixon, J. Bao, J. S. Bergmann, and K. M. Johnson, *Neurosci. Lett.*, 180, 127–130 (1994b).

C. E. Dixon, S. J. Liu, L. W. Jenkins, M. Bhattachargee, J. S. Whitson, K. Y. Yang, and R. L. Hayes, *Behav. Brain Res.*, 70, 125–131 (1995a).

C. E. Dixon, X. C. Bao, K. M. Johnson, K. Y. Yang, J. S. Whitson, G. L. Clifton, and R. L. Hayes, *Neurosci. Lett.*, 198, 111–114 (1995b).

C. E. Dixon, X. C. Ma, and D. W. Marion, *Brain Res.*, 749, 127–130 (1997a).

C. E. Dixon, X. Ma, and D. W. Marion, *J. Neurotrauma*, 14(3), 161–169 (1997b).

C. E. Dixon, P. Flinn, J. Bao, R. Venya, and R. L. Hayes, *Exp. Neurol.*, 146, 479–490 (1997c).

C. A. Doupnik, N. Davidson, H. A. Lester, and P. Kofuji, *Proc. Natl. Acad. Sci. USA*, 94, 10461–10466 (1997).

B. Dubois, F. Danzae, B. Pillon, G. Cusimano, F. Lhermitte, and Y. Agid, *Ann. Neurol.*, 22, 26–30 (1987).

A. R. Elvidge, *Trans. Am. Neurol. Assoc.*, 65, 125–129 (1939).

E. K. Enters, J. R. Pascua, K. P. McDowell, M. Z. Kapasi, J. T. Povlishock, and S. E. Robinson, *Brain Res.*, 576(2), 271–276 (1992).

L. Frolich, A. Dirr, P. Riederer, and S. Hoyer, *Neurochem. Res.*, 18, 1239–1244 (1993).

T. A. Gennarelli, *J. Neurotrauma*, 11(4), 357–368 (1994).

L. K. Gorman, K. Fu, D. A. Hovda, D. P. Becker, and Y. Katayama, *J. Neurotrauma*, 6, 203 (1989).

L. K. Gorman, K. Fu, D. A. Hovda, M. Murray, and R. J. Traysman, *J. Neurotrauma*, 13, 457–463 (1996).

B. Haber and R. G. Grossman, in J. H. Wood, Ed., *Neurobiology and Cerebrospinal Fluid*, Plenum Press, New York, 1980, pp. 345–350.

R. J. Hamm, M. O'Dell, B. R. Pike, and B. G. Lyeth, *J. Cogn. Brain Res.*, 1, 223–226 (1993).

R. J. Hamm, D. White-Gbadebo, B. G. Lyeth, L. W. Jenkins, and R. L. Hayes, *Neurosurgery*, 31, 1072–1078 (1992).

L. B. Harrell, T. S. Barlow, and D. Parsons, *Behav. Neurosci.*, 101, 644–652 (1987).

R. L. Hayes, L. W. Jenkins, and B. G. Lyeth, in Jane J. A., Anderson D. K., Tomer J. C., Young W. (Eds.). *Central Nervous System Trauma Status Report: 1991*, *J. Neurotrauma*, 9(Suppl. 1), S173–S187 (1992).

R. L. Hayes, C. M. Pechura, Y. Katayama, J. T. Povlishock, M. L. Giebel, and D. P. Becker, *Science*, 20, 301–303 (1984).

R. L. Hayes, H. H. Stonnington, B. G. Lyeth, C. E. Dixon, and T. Yamamoto, *Central Nervous System Trauma*, 3(2), 163–173 (1986).

R. L. Hayes, B. G. Lyeth, and L. W. Jenkins, in Levin H. S., Eisenberg H. I. M., Benton A. L., Eds, *Mild Head Injury*, Oxford University Press, New York, 1989, pp. 54–79.

F. Heppner and H. E. Diemath, *Monatsschrift fur Unfallheilkunde und Versicherungsmedizin*, 61, 257–265 (1958).

A. G. Horti, A. O. Koren, K. S. Lee, A. G. Mukhin, D. B. Vaupel, A. S. Kimes, M. Stratton, and E. D. London, *Nucl. Med Biol.*, 26, 175–182 (1999).

I. Ito, Y. Miura, and I. Kadokawa, *Can. J. Physiol. Pharmacol.*, 66, 1010–1016 (1988).

L. W. Jenkins, B. G. Lyeth, W. LeWelt, K. Moszynski, D. S. DeWitt, R. L. Balster, L. P. Miller, G. L. Clifton, H. F. Young, and R. L. Hayes, *J. Neurotrauma*, 5(4), 303–315 (1988).

L. W. Jenkins, K. Moszynski, B. G. Lyeth, W. LeWelt, D. S. DeWitt, A. Allen, C. E. Dixon, J. T. Povlishock, T. J. Majewski, G. L. Clifton, H. F. Young, D. P. Becker, and R. L. Hayes, *Brain Res.*, 477, 211–224 (1989).

F. L. Jenkner and H. Lechner, *Fortshritt Neurologie Psychiatrie*, 22, 270–276 (1954).

F. L. Jenkner and H. Lechner, *EEG Clin. Neurophysiol.*, 7, 303–305 (1955a).

F. L. Jenkner and H. Lechner, *Langenbecks Arch. u. Dtsch. Z. Chir.*, 280, 354–361 (1955b).

D. Jerusalinsky, E. Kornisiuk, P. Alfaro, J. Quillfeldt, M. Alonso, E. R. Verde, C. Cerveanansky, and A. Harvey, *Neuroreport*, 9, 1407–1411 (1998).

J. Y. Jiang, B. G. Lyeth, M. Z. Kapasi, L. W. Jenkins, and J. T. Povlishock, *Acta Neuropathol.*, 84, 495–500 (1992).

J. I. Jiang, B. G. Lyeth, T. M. Delahunty, L. L. Phillips, and R. J. Hamm, *Brain Res.*, 651, 123–128 (1994).

Z.-W. Jiang, Q.-Z. Gong, X. Di, and B. G. Lyeth, *J. Neurotrauma*, 15(10), 881 (1998).

S. V. P. Jones, *Life Sci.*, 52, 457–464 (1993).

Y. Katayama, D. S. DeWitt, D. P. Becker, and R. L. Hayes, *Brain Res.*, 296, 241–262 (1984).

Y. Katayama, D. P. Becker, and R. L. Hayes, *Brain Res.*, 33 5(2), 392–395 (1985a).

Y. Katayama, J. D. Glisson, D. P. Becker, and R. L. Hayes, *J. Neurosurg.*, 63, 97–105 (1985b).

Y. Katayama, S. Reuther, C. E. Dixon, D. P. Becker, and R. L. Hayes, *Brain Res.*, 334, 366–371 (1985c).

M. Kozuka, *Neurochem. Res.*, 20, 23–30 (1995).

Y. Kumagae and Y. Matsui, *J. Neurochem.*, 56, 1169–1173 (1991).

G. Lallement, I. S. Delamanche, I. Pernot-Marino, D. Baubichon, M. Denoyer, P. Carpentier, and G. Blanchet, *Brain Res.*, 618, 227–237 (1993).

J. R. Leonard, D. O. Maris, and M. S. Grady, *J. Neurotrauma*, 11, 379–392 (1994).

A. I. Levey, S. M. Edmunds, C. J. Heilman, T. J. Desmond, and K. A. Frey, *Neuroscience*, 63, 207–221 (1994).

H. S. Levin, in Becker, D. P. and Povlishock, J. T., Eds. *Central Nervous System Trauma Status Report*, NINCDS and NIH: Washington, D.C. 1985, pp. 281–299.

H. S. Levin, *J. Neurol. Sci.*, 103, S39–S42 (1991).

Z. Liu, C. E. Stafstrom, M. R. Sarkisian, Y. Yang, A. Hori, P. Tandon, and G. L. Holmes, *Neuroreport*, 8, 2019–2023 (1997).

I. Lopez-Coviella, J. Agut, V. Savci, J. A. Ortiz, and R. J. Wurtman, *J. Neurochem.*, 65, 889–894 (1995).

B. G. Lyeth, C. E. Dixon, R. J. Hamm, L. W. Jenkins, H. F. Young, H. H. Stonnington, and R. L. Hayes, *Brain Res.*, 448(1), 88–97 (1988a).

B. G. Lyeth, C. E. Dixon, L. W. Jenkins, R. J. Ham, A. Alberico, H. F. Young, H. H. Stonnington, and R. L. Hayes, *Brain Res.*, 452, 39–48 (1988b).

B. G. Lyeth, L. W. Jenkins, R. J. Hamm, C. E. Dixon, L. L. Phillips, G. L. Clifton, H. F. Young, and R. L. Hayes, *Brain Res.*, 526, 249–258 (1990).

B. G. Lyeth, J. Y. Jiang, S. E. Robinson, H. Guo, and L. W. Jenkins, *Mol. Chem. Neuropathol.*, 18, 247–256 (1993).

B. G. Lyeth, M. Ray, R. J. Hamm, J. Schnabel, J. J. Saady, A. Poklis, L. W. Jenkins, S. K. Gudeman, and R. L. Hayes, *Brain Res.*, 569, 281–286 (1992).

B. G. Lyeth, J. Y. Jiang, T. M. Delahunty, L. L. Phillips, and R. J. Hamm, *Brain Res.*, 640, 240–245 (1994).

B. G. Lyeth, Q.-Z. Gong, H. S. Dhillon, and M. R. Prasad, *Brain Res.*, 742, 63–70 (1996).

H. Markram and M. Segal, *J. Physiol.*, 427, 381–393 (1990).

H. Markram and M. Segal, *J. Physiol.*, 447, 5 13–533 (1992).

B. Metz, *J. Neurosurg.*, 35, 523–528 (1971).

E. McGeer and P. L. McGeer, *Can. J. Physiol. Pharmacol.*, 64, 363–368 (1985).

S. Miyazaki, Y. Katayama, B. G. Lyeth, L. W. Jenkins, D. S. DeWitt, S. J. Goldberg, P. G. Newlon, and R. L. Hayes, *Brain Res.*, 585, 335–339 (1992).

M. Oddy, T. Coughlan, A. Tyerman, and D. Jenkins, *J. Neurol. Neurosurg. Psychiatry*, 48, 564–568 (1985).

J. W. Olney and O. L. Ho, *Nature*, 227, 609–611 (1970).

J. W. Olney, T. de Gubareff, and J. Labruyere, *Nature*, 301, 520–522 (1983).

G. C. Ormandy, R. S. Jope, and O. S. Snead III, *Exp. Neurol.*, 106, 172–180 (1989).

J. E. S. Pierce, D. H. Smith, M. S. Eison, and T. K. McIntosh, *Brain Res.*, 624, 199–208 (1993).

B. R. Pike and R. J. Hamm, *Brain Res.*, 686, 37–43. (1995).

B. R. Pike, R. J. Hamm, M. D. Temple, D. L. Buck, and B. G. Lyeth, *J. Neurotrauma*, 14, 897–905 (1997a).

B. R. Pike and R. J. Hamm, *Pharmacol. Biochem. Behav.*, 57, 785–791 (1997b).

B. R. Pike and R. J. Hamm, *Exp. Neurol.*, 147, 55–65 (1997c).

M. R. Prasad, H. S. Dhillon, T. Carbary, R. J. Dempsey, and S. W. Scheff, *J. Neurochem.*, 63, 773–776 (1994).

I. M. Reeves, B. G. Lyeth, and J. T. Povlishock, *Exp. Brain Res.*, 106, 248–256 (1995).

A. C. Rice and R. J. DeLorenzo, *Brain Res.*, 782, 240–247 (1998).

A. C. Rice, C. L. Floyd, B. G. Lyeth, R. J. Hamm, and R. J. DeLorenzo, *Epilepsia*, 39(11), 1148–1157 (1998).

S. E. Robinson, R. M. Martin, T. R. Davis, C. A. Gyenes, J. E. Ryland, and E. K. Enters, *Brain Res.*, 509, 41–46 (1990a).

S. E. Robinson, S. D. Fox, M. Posner, R. M. Martin, T. R. Davis, H. Guo, and E. K. Enters, *Brain Res.*, 511, 141–148 (1990b).

D. Ruge, *J. Neurosurg.*, 11, 77–83 (1954).

E. Sachs Jr., *J. Neurosurg.*, 14, 22–27 (1957).

S. Sadoshima, S. Ibayashi, K. Fujii, T. Nagao, H. Sugimori, and M. Fujishima, *J. Cereb. Blood Flow Metab.*, 15, 845–851 (1995).

A. Saija, R. L. Hayes, B. G. Lyeth, C. E. Dixon, T. Yamamoto, and S. E. Robinson, *Brain Res.*, 452, 303–311 (1988).

P. Sargent, *Annu. Rev. Neurosci.*, 16, 403–443 (1993).

R. H. Schmidt and M. S. Grady, *J. Neurosurg.*, 83, 496–502 (1995).

O. U. Scremin and D. J. Jenden, *Stroke*, 22, 643–647 (1991).

M. Segal, *Brain Res.*, 587, 83–87 (1992).

L. Shao, J. R. Ciallella, H. Q. Yan, X. Ma, B. M. Wolfson, D. W. Marion, S. T. DeKosky, and C. E. Dixon, *J. Neurotrauma*, 16(7), 555–566 (1999).

R. S. Sloviter, *Brain Res. Bull.*, 10, 675–697 (1983).

R. S. Sloviter and D. W. Dempster, *Brain Res. Bull.*, 15, 39–60 (1985).

D. H. Smith, K. Okiyama, M. J. Thomas, B. Claussen, and T. K. McIntosh, *J. Neurotrauma*, 8, 259–269 (1991).

D. H. Smith, K. Okiyama, M. J. Thomas, and T. K. McIntosh, *J. Neurosci.*, 13, 5383–5392 (1993).

I. Smolders, G. M. Khan, J. Manil, G. Ebinger, and Y. Michotte, *Br. J. Pharmacol.*, 121, 1171–1179 (1997).

L. R. Squire and H. P. Davis, *Annu. Rev. Pharmacol. Toxicol.*, 21, 325–356 (1981).

I. Sunderland, P. Tariot, D. L. Murphy, H. Weingartner, E. A. Mueller, and R. M. Cohen, *Psychopharmacology (Berl.)*, 87, 247–249 (1985).

I. Sunderland, P. N. Tariot, R. M. Cohen, H. Weingartner, E. A. Mueller, and D. L. Murphy, *Arch. Gen. Psychiatry*, 44, 418–426 (1987).

Y. Tanaka, M. Sakurai, and S. Hayashi, *Neurosci. Lett.*, 98, 179–183 (1989).

K. Tanaka, N. Ogawa, K. Mizukawa, M. Asanuma, Y. Kondo, S. Nishibayashi, and A. Mori, *Neurochem. Res.*, 19(2), 117–122 (1994).

K. Tanaka, K. Mizukawa, N. Ogawa, and A. Mori, *Neurochem. Res.*, 20(6), 663–667 (1995).

D. B. Tower and D. McEachern, *Can. J. Res.*, 27, 105–119 (1949a).

D. B. Tower and D. McEachern, *Can. J. Res.*, 27, 120–131 (1949b).

W. A. Turski, S. J. Czuczwar, Z. Kleinrok, and L. Turski, *Experientia*, 39, 1408–1411 (1983).

R. F. Villa, F. Ingrao, G. Magri, A. Gorini, S. Reale, A. Costa, N. Ragusa, R. Avola, and A. Giuffrida-Stella, *Int. J. Dev. Neurosci.*, 11, 83–93 (1993).

A. Ward Jr., *J. Neurosurg.*, 7, 398–402 (1950).

B. P. Wei, R. G. Lamb, and H. A. Kontos, *J. Neurochem.*, 56, 695–698 (1982).

M. Zoli, C. Laena, M. R. Picciotto, and J. P. Changeux, *J. Neurosci.*, 18, 4461–4472 (1998).

J. K. Zubieta and K. A. Frey, *J. Pharmacol. Exp. Ther.*, 264, 415–422 (1993).

CHAPTER 6

ADENOSINE RECEPTOR ACTIVATION IN TRAUMATIC BRAIN INJURY

PATRICK M. KOCHANEK
Safar Center for Resuscitation Research, University of Pittsburgh, Pennsylvania

LEONARD P. MILLER
San Diego, California

INTRODUCTION

Adenosine receptor activation is a strategic approach for therapeutic intervention in brain injury based on a number of observations. These include (1) receptor-mediated attenuation of both excitotoxic and inflammatory events that contribute to the evolving injury process and (2) modulation of blood supply to the injured regions. Notably, adenosine functions as a tonically active neuromodulator in the CNS as evidenced by the stimulatory actions of adenosine receptor antagonists, such as theophylline and caffeine. In this regard, adenosine has been labeled as both the brain's neuroprotective agent (Rudolphi et al., 1992) and natural anticonvulsant (Dragunow et al., 1985). However, despite the knowledge of these beneficial events, to date no drug recruiting adenosine receptor activation has progressed into the clinic for either head trauma or brain ischemia. In fact, there are only a few drugs in various phases of clinical development that have emerged from a preclinical development program targeting this receptor. The present review will discuss the prevailing issues responsible, in part, for this lack of drugs targeting adenosine receptor activation in man. In addition, we will overview the current knowledge of adenosine receptor subtypes in the central nervous system (CNS), their distribution, second messenger systems, and how their function might contribute to the discovery of new and effective drugs for the clinical management of traumatic brain injury (TBI). We will also review research efforts to date on adenosine in preclinical TBI

Head Trauma: Basic, Preclinical, and Clinical Directions, Edited by Leonard P. Miller and Ronald L. Hayes, Co-edited by Jennifer K. Newcomb
ISBN 0-471-36015-5   © 2001 John Wiley & Sons, Inc.

models and present studies that add to the validation of this approach. Finally, we will describe the adenosine response to severe TBI in humans.

ADENOSINE RECEPTORS: OVERVIEW

To date, four adenosine receptor subtypes, labeled as A_1, A_{2a}, A_{2b} and A_3, have been classified based on ligand binding, signal transduction pathways, and molecular biology techniques (Table 6.1). Molecular cloning and sequencing studies show that adenosine receptors are part of the G protein-coupled receptor superfamily exhibiting the classical seven-transmembrane helix topology, an extracellular amino terminus, a cytoplasmic carboxy terminus with phosphorylation sites and a cytoplasmic domain with potential for interaction with G proteins (Linden et al., 1991). The effector systems initially identified for these receptors exhibited either an increase (A_{2a} and A_{2b}) or a decrease (A_1 and A_3) in intracellular cAMP levels. This classification has now expanded to include an increase in inositol trisphosphate (IP_3) (A_1 and A_3), K^+ conductance (A_1), and a decrease in Ca^{2+} flux (A_1) (Table 6.1). To date, potent and selective agonists for the A_1 (CCPA, ENBA, CPA, CHA, R-PIA), A_{2a} (CGS21680), and A_3 (2-Cl-IB-MECA) receptor subtypes have been identified (Fredholm, 1995). Pharmacological differentiation of A_{2a} and A_{2b} receptor subtypes remains a challenge for the future. These efforts will certainly be aided by access to cloned and expressed versions of these receptors in isolated cell systems.

Activation of adenosine receptors within the CNS leads to an array of functional responses that result in beneficial effects to compromised brain tissue (Fig. 6.1). In response to trauma or ischemia, intracellular adenosine levels increase dramatically due mainly to rapid metabolism of adenosine triphosphate (ATP) to support cell activities and maintain critical ion balance across membranes. This elevated adenosine is then rapidly exported from the cell via an equilibrative transport carrier system. Adenosine can also be formed extracellularly, although to a lesser extent, by ectonucleotidase-mediated breakdown of ATP co-released with other neurotransmitters (Dunwiddie et al., 1997). As extracellular adenosine levels rise to low nanomolar concentrations, A_1 receptors are activated to (1) presynaptically attenuate neurotransmitter release, (2) postsynaptically raise the threshold for membrane depolarization, and (3) hyperpolarize astrocyte cell membrane, which has been speculated to improve the uptake of excessive extracellular potassium and glutamate (Fig. 6.1). As adenosine levels further increase to low micromolar levels, A_2 receptors, located predominately within the vasculature, are activated, resulting in (4) smooth muscle relaxation and vasodilation leading to increased cerebral blood flow (CBF), thus augmenting nutrient supply, (5) inhibition of platelet aggregation, and (6) inhibition of neutrophil activation resulting in decreased adhesion to endothelial cells and subsequent capillary plugging and/or blood–brain barrier injury. These latter events are normal inflammatory responses to a number of identified physiological cues that, however, become adverse when they result in blockade of blood flow to the compromised region or injured vasculature. Of note,

Table 6.1 Features of Adenosine Receptor Subtypes[a]

Feature	Subtype			
	A_1	A_{2a}	A_{2b}	A_3
Amino acids	326	412	332	320
G protein coupling	Gi(1–3)/Go	Gs	Gs	Gi
Effector systems	Decrease cAMP Increase IP_3 Increase K^+ Decrease Ca^{2+}	Increase cAMP	Increase cAMP	Decrease cAMP
Agonists	CCPA > S(−)ENBA > CPA > CHA > R-PIA > 2CADO > NECA > S-PIA	NECA (1–20 nM) > CGS21680 > APEC	NECA (1–5 μM)	APNEA, IB-MECA, N^6-benzyl-NECA
Antagonists	XAC, CPT, CPX	XAC, CSC, KF17837, CGS15943	XAC, CPX, 8-PT, CGS15943	BW-A522
Distribution	Cortex, hippocampus cerebellum, testis, adipose tissue, heart, kidney	Striatum, nucleus accumbens, tuberculum olfactorium	Widely distributed	Testes, kidney, heart lung cortex, striatum hippocampus, olfactory

Source: Adapted from Fredholm et al. (1994a).

[a] Abbreviations: cAMP, cyclic adenosine monophosphate; IP_3, inositol trisphosphate; CCPA, 2-chlorocyclopentyladenosine; S(−)ENBA, endonorbornyladenosine; CPA, cyclopentyladenosine; CHA, cyclohexyladenosine; R-PIA, N^6-(R-phenylisopropyl)adenosine; 2CADO, 2-chloroadenosine; NECA, 5′-N-ethylcarboximidoadenosine; S-PIA, N^6-(S-phenylisopropyl)adenosine; CGS21680, 2-[p-(2-carbonylethyl)phenylethylamino]-5′-N-ethylcarboxyamidoadenosine; APNEA, N^6-2-(4-aminophenyl)-ethyladenosine; IB-MECA, N^6-(3-iodobenzyl)-5′-N-methylcarboxamidoadenosine; XAC, xanthine amino congener; CPT, cyclopentyltheophylline; CPX (DPCPX), 1,3-dipropyl-8-cyclopentylxanthine; CSC, 8-(3-chlorostyryl)caffeine; KF17837, CGS15943, 9-cloro-2-(2-furanyl)-5,6-dihydro[1,2,4)-triazolo[1,5]quinazolin-5-imine monomethanesulfonate; CGS1, 9-chloro-2-(2-furanyl)-5,6-dihydro-[1,2,4]-triazolo[1,5]quinazolin-5-imine monomethanesulfonate; 8-PT, 8-phenyltheophylline; BW-A522, 3-(3-iodo-4-aminobenzyl)-8-(4-oxyacetate)-1-propylxanthine.

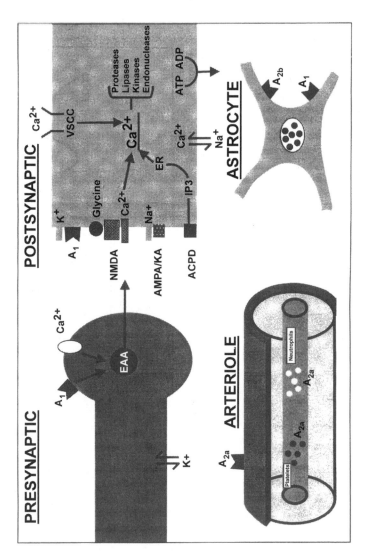

Figure 6.1 Sites of action of the various adenosine receptor subtypes within brain parenchyma and cerebrovasculature.

however, the consequences of adenosine-mediated inhibition of platelet aggregation on hemodynamics in TBI are presently unknown.

Adenosine Receptors: Subtypes

A_1 receptors are widely distributed throughout brain and peripheral tissues. Within the CNS, A_1 receptors are found predominantly in the hippocampus, neocortex, cerebellum, and striatum (Jarvis and Williams, 1990). Moreover, A_1 receptors are strategically located presynaptically to inhibit Ca^{2+} currents needed for transmitter release and postsynaptically to increase K^+ conductance resulting in membrane hyperpolarization (Dunwiddie, 1990). Consequently, adenosine acting through the A_1 receptor functions in a dual manner to inhibit the release of excitatory amino acids (EAAs) and to dampen EAA-mediated effects on postsynaptic membranes. These A_1 receptor-mediated processes are presumed to be responsible, for the most part, in the neuroprotection observed with the application of a number of A_1 agonists in ischemia and head trauma models that are reviewed in a subsequent section of this chapter. An alternative strategy for the development of new pharmacophores directed at the A_1 receptor would be to target a modulatory site located on the A_1 receptor complex that potentiates the effects of A_1 receptor activation. Viability of this latter approach was first identified with the drug PD81723, which has been shown to be effective as an allosteric enhancer in both binding and in vitro functional assays (Bruns and Fergus, 1990; Kollias-Baker et al., 1997). Other studies supporting this modulatory site approach include potentiation of the depressant action of adenosine on evoked responses in hippocampal slices (Janusz et al., 1991), depression of seizures in the same preparations (Janusz and Berman, 1993), and depression in peak ischemia-evoked level of glutamate release in rat cortex (Phillis et al., 1994a). However, to our knowledge, PD81723 or a similar compound has never been investigated in a preclinical head trauma model, possibly due to the failure of this compound to provide protection in a gerbil ischemia model when preadministered at three different doses (Cao and Phillis, 1995).

A_{2a} receptors are abundantly expressed in dopamine-rich regions of the brain such as the striatum but are present at low levels in other brain regions (Jarvis and Williams, 1989). In the striatum, in situ hybridization studies show that A_{2a} receptors are expressed in the medium spiny striatal GABAergic neurons, which also contain enkephalin and project to the external globus pallidus (Schiffmann et al., 1991). Mechanistically, several studies indicate that A_{2a} and D_2 receptors act in a mutually antagonistic manner and may have importance in the control of symptoms related to Parkinson's disease. With regard to neuroprotection, A_{2a} receptor activation on neurons may be detrimental since it appears to lead to enhanced ischemia-evoked EAA release. This conclusion was reached as the result of a number of different studies. In particular, application of two potent adenosine receptor agonists, cyclopentyladenosine (CPA) and 5'-N-ethyl carboximidoadenosine (NECA), directly into an ischemic region inhibited ischemic-evoked release of EAAs at low drug concentrations but not at high concentrations (Simpson et al., 1992). In the same study, sole application of the A_{2a} antagonist CGS15943 resulted in suppression of ischemia-evoked EAA release. It is of note that the influence of these various approaches to A_{2a} receptor intervention on the cerebrovasculature was not monitored in these studies. In an in vitro study utilizing hippocampal neuronal cell cultures, 3,7-dimethyl-1-propargylxanthine (DMPX), an A_2 receptor antagonist, potentiated the neuroprotective effect of adenosine (Sturm et al., 1993). In another study, CGS21680, a selective adenosine A_{2a} receptor agonist, when infused through a microdialysis probe placed in rat striatum, greatly enhanced extracellular glutamate levels (Popoli et al., 1995). More recent data show that brain injury induced by transient focal ischemia was attenuated in A_{2a} receptor-deficient mice (Chen et al., 1999). In summary, information to date supports the idea that endogenous adenosine, depending on its localized extracellular levels during the course of an ischemic insult, can have a beneficial effect by activating A_1 receptors to inhibit EAA-mediated release and responses, or an apparent detrimental effect by activation of neuronal A_{2a} receptors counteracting the positive influences of A_1 receptor activation.

A_{2b} receptors were first differentiated in radioligand binding studies by Bruns et al. (1986). These receptors exhibit a low affinity ($\approx 10\,\mu M$) for adenosine and are apparently distributed widely throughout the brain. While glial cells possess both A_1 and A_2 receptors (vanCalker et al., 1979), the most abundant receptor appears to be the A_{2b} subtype based, in particular, on studies utilizing the D384 astrocytoma cell line (Altiok et al., 1992). A_{2b} receptors on rat astrocytes in primary culture showed positive coupling to adenyl cyclase, which was unaffected by coactivation of A_1 receptors (Peakman and Hill, 1994). Additional studies revealed the presence of A_{2b} receptors on both type 1 and type 2 astrocyte-enriched cultures derived from neonatal rat forebrains (Peakman and Hill, 1996). The responses mediated by A_{2b} receptor activation on glial cells are modified in the short and long terms by inflammatory mediators (Fredholm and Altiok, 1994). Activation of A_{2b} receptors has been suggested to mediate both beneficial and detrimental responses during periods of tissue compromise. On the beneficial side, A_{2b} receptor activation could reduce the formation of free radicals from microglia (Benati et al., 1994). On the detrimental side, A_{2b} receptor activation could be involved in astroglial swelling during ischemia, thus contributing to brain edema. Overall, the functional significance of A_{2b} receptor activation or even inhibition during brain ischemia remains an unresolved issue open to future investigations.

A_3 receptors were initially discovered using standard molecular biology techniques (Zhou et al., 1992) and were shown to be highly concentrated in rat testes. Like A_1 receptors, A_3 receptors are linked to G_i protein and have been demonstrated to activate phospholipase C and the inositol phosphate pathway (Abbracchio et al., 1995) and to activate protein kinase C on presynaptic terminals (Macek et al., 1998). A differential distribution of A_3 receptors in mouse CNS was observed, with the highest density in the cerebellum and striatum but less so in the hippocampus (Jacobson et al., 1993). The first indication of a central effect of A_3 receptor activation was suggested when intraperitoneally injected IB-MECA [N^6-(3-iodobenzyl)-5'-N-methylcarboxamidoadenosine] induced behavioral depression in mice (Jacobson et al., 1993). Activation of A_3 receptors resulted in potentiation of

Ca^{2+} currents in an acutely dissociated hippocampal pyramidal neuron preparation (Fleming and Mogul, 1997), an increase in electrical excitability of hippocampal pyramidal neurons in a rat slice preparation (Fleming et al., 1997), and a progressive, dose-dependent increase in leukocyte adherence and venular fluorescein leakage in pial venular endothelium of anesthetized newborn pigs (Park et al., 1997). Acute treatment with the A_3 agonist IB-MECA resulted in impaired postischemic cerebral blood flow and increased mortality, and produced extensive hippocampal neuronal damage in the gerbil global ischemia (10 or 20 min) model (Von Lubitz et al., 1994). Acute administration of an A_3 antagonist, MRS1191, also in the gerbil model, resulted in pronounced improvement in a number of outcome measures: animal survival, hippocampal neuronal survival, MAP-2 preservation and NADPH-disphorase reaction product. To date, information on this adenosine receptor subtype would suggest benefits from the application of A_3 receptor antagonists in brain injury. However, future studies are certainly needed to delineate further the merits of this proposal.

ADENOSINE-REGULATING AGENTS

Although the merits of agonist-mediated activation of particular receptor subtypes have been addressed, there are numerous unfavorable side effects associated with this type of approach. In particular, systemic administration of A_1 receptor agonists results in profound hypotension, bradycardia, and heart block due to activation of adenosine receptors within the cardiovascular system (Mullane and Williams, 1990). Other documented side effects include marked sedation and hypothermia (Dunwiddie and Worth, 1982). On the other hand, an alternative strategy designed specifically to harness the neuroprotective effects of adenosine receptor activation is to potentiate endogenous adenosine in an event- and site-specific manner. This approach was originally described by Gruber and colleagues (1989) in their study with the prototypical adenosine-regulating agent (ARA) acadesine in heart ischemia. Acadesine potentiated endogenous adenosine levels during the ischemic insult but not under normoxic conditions. As illustrated in Figure 6.2, there are a number of pathways involved in the disposition of endogenous adenosine that can be targeted to potentiate levels of this autocoid. Enzymes and processes critical in the maintenance of flux through these pathways include adenosine kinase, adenosine deaminase, adenosine monophosphate deaminase, and adenosine transport.

Adenosine kinase (AK) (ATP : adenosine-5′-phosphotransferase: EC 2.7.1.20) catalyzes the conversion of adenosine to adenosine monophosphate (AMP). It is a cytosolic enzyme with a widespread distribution throughout different body tissues (Ho et al., 1968; Krenitsky et al., 1974) and is also generally distributed in both rodent and human central nervous systems. AK is a key enzyme regulating endogenous adenosine levels with a $K_m < 1\,\mu M$ for adenosine (Arch and Newsholme, 1978). A number of in vitro studies attest to the potentiation of adenosine levels in response to the application of specific AK inhibitors. While these studies have been reviewed (Miller, 1999), it is worthwhile noting the most elegant

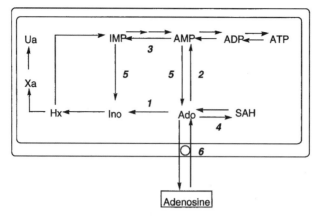

Figure 6.2   Enzymatic reactions involved in the metabolism of endogenous adenosine and its distribution across cell membranes. *1*, Adenosine deaminase; *2*, adenosine kinase; *3*, AMP deaminase; *4* SAH hydrolase; *5*, 5′-nucleotidase; *6*, adenosine transport. Ado, adenosine; SAH, *s*-adenosyl-homocysteine; IMP, inosine monophosphate; Ino, inosine; Ua, uric acid; Hx, hypoxanthine; Xa, xanthine.

experiments that were accomplished with the introduction of an AK inhibitor directly into the cytoplasm of individual CA1 pyrimidal neurons while monitoring presynaptic inhibition of excitatory transmission (Brundege and Dunwiddie, 1998). These experiments showed that AK predominantly influences adenosine levels such that inhibition of this enzyme results in a substantial release of adenosine into the extracellular milieu sufficient to inhibition neurotransmission. A number of in vivo studies revealed neuroprotective effects of peripherally administered AK inhibitors in rat focal stroke even when administered peristroke (Miller et al., 1996; Jiang et al., 1997). However, whether there are problems such as toxicity associated with this approach needs to be clarified based on the recent (1999) termination of AK programs for a new class of analgesics by both Abbott and Pfizer in partnership with Metabasis Therapeutics (San Diego).

Adenosine deaminase (ADA) (EC 3.5.4.4) catalyzes the deamination of adenosine to inosine and has been localized to brain capillary endothelial cells (Schrader et al., 1987) and neurons (Nagy et al., 1985) by immunohistochemical and radioligand binding techniques. ADA has a high K_m (50 µM) for adenosine and a relatively high V_{max}. Arch and Newsholme (1978) showed that in rat brain the K_m value of ADA for adenosine is 20-fold higher than that of AK, while the maximal activities (V_{max}) of these two enzymes are similar. Thus, under physiological conditions the velocity of ADA, which is operating well below saturation, is significantly lower than the velocity of AK. In vitro studies with inhibitors of ADA have, for the most part, been consistent with these observations in that inhibition of ADA resulted in no or modest changes in endogenous adenosine levels compared to results obtained with inhibitors of AK. These particular studies have been reviewed adequately elsewhere (Miller, 1999).

With regard to adenosine transport, at least six different nucleoside transporters have been identified (Cass, 1995). Briefly, these transporters have been characterized by a number of features, such as equilibrative (e) versus concentrative (c), sensitive (s), or insensitive (i) to inhibition by NBTI, Na^+ dependency, and substrate selectivity [i.e., purine selectivity (f), pyrimidine selectivity (t), and broad selectivity (b)]. In the central nervous system, the e transport systems appear to be the most abundant, although there also appears to be some cs-like transport. In a number of in vitro studies blockade of nucleoside transporter greatly potentiated the release of adenosine evoked by EAA receptor activation (Craig and White, 1993; Lobner and Choi, 1994) or oxygen–glucose deprivation and reduced epileptiform activity in human epileptogenic cortical slices (Kostopoulos et al., 1989). However, while a number of nucleoside transport inhibitors are available, such as dipyridamole, dilazep, propentofylline, and NBTI, some are nonspecific in their actions and all exhibit poor penetration across the blood–brain barrier (DeLeo et al., 1988).

Adenosine 5′-monophosphate deaminase (AMPDA) (EC 3.5.4.6) is a cytosolic enzyme that catalyzes the hydrolytic deamination of AMP to yield inosinic acid and ammonia. The K_m value of AMPDA for AMP is approximately 1 mM. Inhibition of AMPDA could lead to a shunting of AMP metabolism through 5′-nucleotidase, resulting in an augmentation of adenosine levels. However, testing of this hypothesis necessarily requires selective and potent inhibitors of AMPDA. In this regard, a recent report outlined a drug with a K_i of 3 nM for human erythrocytic AMPDA and selectivity ($>30,000$-fold using ADA from calf intestinal mucosa) (Kasibhatla et al., 1997). Availability and future application of this class of inhibitors to normal and ischemic tissue will, no doubt, help in the assessment of the importance of AMPDA as a potential target for enhancing endogenous adenosine levels within the CNS.

IN VIVO HEAD TRAUMA STUDIES

Unique Adenosine-Related Considerations in TBI

The role of adenosine in the evolution of secondary damage after experimental TBI has been the subject of limited study to date. This is in marked contrast to the panoply of studies investigating adenosine in experimental models of focal and global cerebral ischemia. Surprisingly, the limited amount of investigation of adenosine in experimental TBI has occurred despite the fact that previous studies have suggested an inadequate endogenous adenosine response to TBI, and a potential therapeutic benefit by augmenting this response. Despite the limited amount of information on the role of adenosine in experimental TBI, we have recently provided data on the endogenous adenosine response to CNS injury in adults and children with severe TBI. Before discussing these experimental and clinical studies, it is important to consider several unique aspects of experimental and clinical TBI.

Although TBI and cerebral ischemia (both focal and global) share many mechanisms, there are important differences between these insults. This is readily apparent when one considers an example such as the sources of the increase in interstitial concentration of the EAA glutamate after TBI versus ischemia. In ischemia, the increase in glutamate is generally attributed to presynaptic release and failure of reuptake (Obrenovitch and Richards, 1995). In contrast, after TBI, the increase results not only from these same two mechanisms but also from both the direct mechanical disruption of neurons—spilling their transmitters through micropores (Bullock et al., 1998) into the local milieu—and the passive movement of glutamate from blood to brain in the presence of an often severely damaged blood–brain barrier, which is particularly true early after the injury (Palmer et al., 1993a, b). These mechanistic differences between TBI and cerebral ischemia may translate into important therapeutic differences. For example, mild to moderate hypothermia attenuates EAA extracellular surge in cerebral ischemia (Busto et al., 1989). However, within a cerebral contusion, similar conditions of hypothermia fail to modify glutamate surges (Palmer et al., 1993b). The contribution of direct disruption of neurons and vasculature to the observed increases in brain interstitial levels of adenosine after experimental and clinical TBI remains to be determined. Similarly, the implications of these factors for therapeutic attempts to augment local adenosine concentration after TBI, though undefined, could be considerable.

A second potentially important difference between TBI and cerebral ischemia relates to the distribution of the selectively vulnerable cells after these two insults. In rodent models of experimental TBI, CA3 hippocampus and dentate hilus are the most vulnerable regions and frequently exhibit delayed neuronal death occurring over the span of 1 to 2 days (Lowenstein et al., 1992; Clark et al., 1997b). In contrast, CA1 hippocampus is selectively vulnerable in models of cerebral global ischemia (Brierley et al., 1973; Nitatori et al., 1995). In autopsy studies of humans who were victims of severe TBI, both CA1 and CA3 cell death are observed (Kotapka et al., 1992). Again, the ramifications of this important regional difference between traumatic and ischemic insults for adenosine-related therapeutic strategies remain to be determined.

Control of intracranial hypertension and secondary cerebral swelling, along with the prevention of cerebral herniation, is of fundamental importance to the clinical management of severe TBI. In contrast, these mechanisms are not believed to be viable therapeutic targets in the management of patients with global cerebral ischemic insults from cardiac arrest (Safar, 1986; Sarnaik et al., 1985) and they are, at best, controversial therapeutic targets in stroke (Schwab et al., 1998). Related to this issue, the cerebrovascular effects of adenosine mediated by A_{2a} receptor activation could have important effects on cerebral blood volume and thus intracranial dynamics.

Microscopic or gross cerebral hemorrhage is invariably seen in severe TBI, but is less common in stroke and rare in cardiac arrest. Antiplatelet effects of adenosine at the A_{2a} receptor could have added theoretical liabilities in severe TBI compared to ischemic insults. However, this remains to be determined even in experimental models. Unlike in cerebral ischemia, blood–brain barrier injury from direct vascular disruption is also almost uniformly seen in severe TBI in the experimental and clinical settings. This is particularly true early after cerebral contusion (Smith and Hall, 1996; Adelson et al., 1998). However, this may actually allow for the successful use in TBI of therapies (such as adenosine analogues or regulating agents) with limited blood–brain barrier permeability.

Although there are important differences between TBI, stroke, and cardiac arrest, it would be incorrect to underestimate the likely role for secondary cerebral ischemia in the evolution of secondary damage after experimental and clinical TBI. In both the lateral fluid percussion model (Yamakami and McIntosh, 1989) and the controlled cortical impact model (Cherian et al., 1994; Kochanek et al., 1995), cerebral hypoperfusion in and around the contusion site is invariably seen. Despite the fact that the extent of flow reduction is often less severe than that seen in the central core in models of focal cerebral ischemia, the marked excitotoxicity that is superimposed in the setting of focal contusion is suggested to produce important relative ischemia and energy failure (Hovda et al., 1995). Similarly, clinical studies have consistently reported marked hypoperfusion early after severe TBI (Marion et al., 1991; Bouma et al., 1992; Adelson et al., 1997). Based on the flow-promoting and antiexcitotoxic properties of adenosine, the combination of hypoperfusion and simultaneous hypermetabolism that occurs early after TBI represents a logical therapeutic target for an adenosine-based strategy. Depending on the severity of the insult, this early low-flow phase may progress into a state of normal, increased, or persistently reduced CBF during the period of delayed cerebral swelling that follows over hours and days. Adenosine may also play a role during the development of this secondary increase in CBF. In addition, secondary insults are common in patients with severe TBI and can include events such as hypoxemia at the injury scene from impact apnea or hemorrhage-induced hypotension from accompanying extra-cranial injuries. The role of adenosine and the possibility of augmenting adenosine in these settings are now areas of active investigation in experimental and clinical TBI.

Finally, as discussed in a number of reviews (Phillis, 1989; Miller and Hsu, 1992; Rudolphi et al., 1992; Geiger et al., 1997; Miller, 1999), studies of experimental cerebral ischemia and normal cerebrovascular physiology have defined important roles for adenosine in the regulation of CBF and metabolism and in neuroprotection. However, defining the role of adenosine in human cerebral ischemia (stroke and cardiac arrest) has lagged considerably behind. We and others studying TBI have taken advantage of opportunities to evaluate human biological fluids [cerebrospinal fluid (CSF) and cerebral dialysate fluid] and tissue (surgically removed contusion for therapeutic decompression). These samples are obtained as part of the standard of care of patients with severe TBI (Bullock et al., 1996) and are rarely available in clinical stroke or cardiac arrest. The use of ventricular catheters as standard of care in the management of intracranial hypertension in patients with severe TBI could also afford a unique opportunity for intracerebroventricular (ICV) drug delivery. These valuable tools provide a window of opportunity to study and treat the human condition that will be discussed.

Endogenous Adenosine Response to Experimental TBI

Although studies have been limited, there has been some investigations of the role of adenosine in three specific in vivo models of TBI in rodents; (1) weight drop, (2) lateral fluid percussion, and (3) controlled cortical impact. Using a weight drop model of cerebral contusion and cortical microdialysis, Nilsson and colleagues (1990) first showed that interstitial adenosine is increased immediately after injury to levels 50- to 100-fold greater than baseline. In that study, adenosine was not the focus of investigation, but represented one of a number of metabolites that were measured to characterize the metabolic pattern of energy failure in focal cerebral contusion in rats. Using the fluid percussion model of TBI in rats, Headrick et al. (1994) reported that brain interstitial concentration of adenosine was increased during the first hour after injury, peaking at 10 min. However, ATP depletion (assessed by phosphorus-31 nuclear magnetic resonance spectroscopy) peaked at 2 to 3 h. This suggested that the duration of the increase in brain interstitial levels of adenosine was shorter than the duration of energy failure after fluid percussion TBI, a finding similar to the report of Phillis et al. (1994b) in experimental focal cerebral ischemia, where marked increases in glutamate, but not adenosine, persist during reperfusion. These studies suggest that further augmenting the degree or duration of the increase in adenosine after TBI is a logical therapeutic strategy. Bell et al. (1998) measured interstitial brain adenosine, inosine, hypoxanthine, and cAMP levels in both contusion center and penumbra after controlled cortical impact in rats. Adenosine, inosine, and hypoxanthine were dramatically increased (16- to 85-fold) after injury versus sham in both contusion and penumbra. No changes were seen in cAMP. Adenosine levels peaked in the first 20 min and returned to near baseline by 40 min after injury. This suggested that ATP breakdown is a potential source of adenosine, while metabolism of cAMP does not appear to contribute importantly to the posttraumatic increase in adenosine levels. However, the contribution of direct cellular disruption and blood–brain barrier disruption to the increase in interstitial adenosine in the contusion is unclear. In addition, the duration of the posttraumatic increase in adenosine in this model was much shorter than the duration of hypoperfusion, again suggesting the possibility of an inadequate adenosine response, similar to that seen by Headrick et al. (1994) in fluid percussion injury. Finally, increases in adenosine in the dorsal hippocampus beneath the contusion site in the controlled cortical impact model (Robertson et al., 1998) also suggest a putative role for adenosine in attempting to defend injured brain because dorsal hippocampus is highly vulnerable penumbral region in the acute phase after experimental TBI. As previously discussed, hippocampal neurons reproducibly undergo delayed neuronal death in the controlled cortical impact and lateral fluid percussion models of TBI.

Adenosine-Related Therapies in Experimental TBI

To our knowledge, there have only been three published reports of adenosine-targeted therapy in the setting of experimental TBI. All three reports suggest a beneficial effect of the administration of adenosine analogues. Mitchell et al. (1995)

reported that trauma-induced neuronal death in rat cultured hippocampal neurons was attenuated by treatment with the A_1-receptor agonist cyclopentyladenosine (CPA). In that study, neuronal trauma was produced by mechanical disruption. Neuronal death was not blocked by MK-801, suggesting that traumatic cell death in culture may be mediated by multiple mechanisms that can be targeted by adenosine. Headrick et al. (1994), in the previously discussed study of adenosine and cerebral energetics after fluid percussion TBI in rats, also examined the effect of ICV administration of the adenosine analogue 2-chloroadenosine (0.5 or 2.5 nmol). Treatment with 2-chloroadenosine before injury improved energy failure. Further supporting this hypothesis, ICV administration of 2-chloroadenosine (versus vehicle) also improved functional outcome of the rats in this model. In a preliminary report (Robertson et al., 1999b) we studied the effect of parenchymal injection of 2-chloroadenosine (0.3 nmol) or saline vehicle into the lesion penumbra immediately after controlled cortical impact injury in rats. Using magnetic resonance imaging methods, cerebral blood flow and the in vivo spin–lattice relaxation time of tissue water (T_{1obs}, a putative marker of posttraumatic cerebral edema) were acquired in multiple regions of interest at about 3 to 4 h after injury. Treatment with 2-chloroadenosine produced a significant reduction in T_{1obs} (presumably edema) in hippocampus and cortex compared to vehicle treatment. However, CBF was not significantly increased in any region of interest by 2-chloroadenosine treatment. We speculated that this may have been due to reduced excitotoxicity early after injury conferred by treatment with the adenosine analogue. These results agree those of the prior report of Headrick et al. (1994) in fluid percussion injury.

Based on these initial data, it was unclear whether the failure of local injection of 2-chloroadenosine to increase CBF after TBI was due to the use of an inadequate dose or was related to the possibility that the cerebral vasculature at the contusion site was not responsive to 2-chloroadenosine after injury. To this end, we also investigated the effect of 2-chloroadenosine injection on CBF in normal rats (Kochanek et al., 2001). We tested the dose–response effect of cortical injection of 2-chloroadenosine (at 0.3, 6, or 12 nmol versus saline vehicle) on CBF assessed by perfusion MRI in pentobarbital-anesthetized rats. At a dose of 0.3 nmol, 2-chloroadenosine did not increase CBF. However, at doses of 6.0 or 12.0 nmol, regional and hemispheric increases in CBF (respectively) were observed. Remarkably, injection of 12 nmol of 2-chloroadenosine into parietal cortex produced a sustained 2-fold increase in CBF that involved the entire hemisphere ipsilateral to the injection. These data also suggest a possible explanation for our findings with a low dose (0.3 nmol) of 2-chloroadenosine in TBI. This dose was inadequate to increase CBF even in normal brain. Thus, the 5- to 10-fold selectivity of 2-chloroadenosine for the A_1 versus A_{2a} receptor (Ijzerman et al., 1994) may have resulted in a significant effect on T_{1obs} (reduction in edema) after TBI in the absence of an effect on CBF. We are currently studying the effect of higher doses of 2-chloroadenosine on posttraumatic CBF in our model. These preliminary data support the concept that augmentation of local adenosine concentration could influence both edema and CBF after TBI. These studies also raise the interesting possibility of the therapeutic use of local administration of adenosine analogues either directly into brain parenchyma near surgically resected contusions or into the CSF (via the ventricular catheter) in patients with severe TBI. Further studies in experimental models of TBI are needed, including investigation of the effects of these local approaches on intracranial pressure and on long-term functional outcome.

Remarkably, published studies on the effect of ADA or AK inhibitors, blockage of nucleoside transporters, or manipulation of the A_3 receptor in experimental TBI are lacking. This is in marked contrast to the large number of studies of agents targeting these pathways in cerebral ischemia. In a preliminary report, we examined the effect of the ADA inhibitor *erythro*-hydroxynonyladenine (EHNA) on interstitial brain concentration of adenosine and purine metabolites early after controlled cortical impact with a secondary hypoxemic insult in rats (Robertson et al., 1998). Brain interstitial concentration of adenosine was increased by only 17 % with this strategy, while inosine levels were more markedly reduced by EHNA. Brain interstitial inosine concentration was decreased 46 %. These results are similar to the limited ability of ADA inhibitors to augment local adenosine levels in cerebral ischemia (Sciotti and Van Wylen, 1993). Additional investigations of the effect of inhibitors of AK and nucleoside transporters and manipulation of the A_3 receptor are needed in experimental models of TBI.

Finally, a number of novel approaches have been developed that may facilitate our understanding of both the role of adenosine in the response to TBI and the efficacy of adenosine-based therapies. Nyce (1999) recently reported the successful use of antisense strategies targeting the A_1 receptor in a model of asthma. Local administration of the antisense was achieved by the inhaled route of administration. Local infusion of antisense into brain parenchyma was also described. The selectivity and surprising duration (6.8 days) of the therapeutic effect of this antisense approach to adenosine receptors are intriguing, particularly as it might be applied to down-regulate of the A_{2a} receptor in injured brain parenchyma. In addition, a variety of mutant mice have recently been developed for investigation of the role of adenosine (Ledent et al., 1997; Nyce, 1999). None has yet been studied in experimental TBI. Combination therapies may also represent an important potential avenue for the use of adenosine-related therapies in TBI. For example, pathological activation of acetylcholine muscarinic receptors uncouples adenosine neuronal inhibition in CA1 hippocampus (Worley et al., 1987). This suggests that the combination of muscarinic antagonists with A_1 receptor agonists may be even more beneficial than A_1 receptor agonists alone.

Endogenous Adenosine after Severe TBI in Humans

Severe TBI in humans affords a unique opportunity to study the endogenous role of adenosine in the injured brain at the bedside. We have taken advantage of the availability of both ventricular CSF and brain interstitial fluid (obtained from microdialysis samples) from adults with severe TBI. Similarly, we have recently quantified adenosine levels in CSF samples from infants and children with severe TBI.

To begin to define the role of adenosine in clinical TBI, Clark et al. (1997a) serially measured concentrations of adenosine in ventricular CSF collected in 67 samples from 13 adults during the initial 5 days after severe TBI (GCS ≤7). The possible association between adenosine and cerebral blood flow (xenon-133 method), cerebral metabolic rate for oxygen ($CMRO_2$), and arterial venous difference in oxygen content ($AVDO_2$), was also assessed in these patients. Control lumbar CSF samples were obtained from six nontraumatized, noninfected adult patients. To obtain clues as to both the possible source of adenosine and the underlying mechanisms behind the role of adenosine in delayed cerebral swelling, we also measured CSF lactate and cAMP levels in these samples. Our results showed that CSF adenosine concentration was strongly associated with death ($p < 0.001$) and was increased when $AVDO_2$ was ≤4 versus >4 vol%. Furthermore, CSF lactate concentration remained significantly increased (versus normal) until 5 days after TBI. cAMP concentration in CSF was not increased (versus control) at any time after TBI. The powerful association between CSF adenosine concentration and death (Fig. 6.3) and $AVDO_2$ (≤4 vol%, indicating uncoupling of oxidative metabolism and CBF), supports an important biological role for adenosine in human brain after severe TBI, presumably a failed attempt at neuroprotection in severely injured patients. As in the controlled cortical impact model studies, the low levels of cAMP in CSF observed in these patients, but persistently increased CSF lactate, suggest that adenosine is produced from ATP breakdown (resulting from either hyperglycolysis or occult ischemic foci). Adenosine is important in coupling CBF to

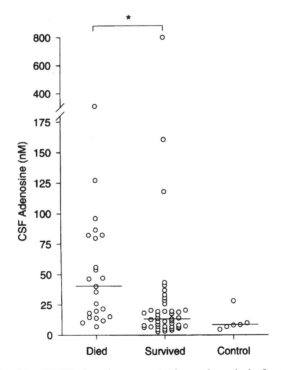

Figure 6.3 Relationship of CSF adenosine concentration and survival after severe TBI in humans. CSF samples ($n = 23$) were taken from the 4 patients who died and from the 44 patients who survived (*$p < 0.001$ nonsurvivors versus survivors, generalized multivariate model). Reprinted with permission, Clark et al. (1997a).

metabolic demands during functional activation (Dirnagl et al., 1994) and, as previously discussed, is a neuroprotectant when it is formed from the breakdown of ATP during ischemia. Based on the recent work of both Pellerin and Magistretti (1994) and Bergsneider et al. (1997), one possible explanation for the concurrent increase in CBF, reduction in $CMRO_2$, and increase in adenosine during the secondary cerebral swelling phase after TBI is that adenosine is participating in a coupled increase in CBF in response to increased cerebral glucose utilization (hyperglycolysis). This hyperglycolysis could be stimulated by glutamate, potassium, cytokines (TNF, IL-1), or arachidonic acid (AA) (Fig. 6.4) as suggested by Pellerin and Magistretti (1994). Thus, adenosine may facilitate both coupling of this response and inhibition of $CMRO_2$ during this phase. If the mechanism proposed in Figure 6.4 is correct, adenosine may be attempting to perform an endogenous neuroprotective role in the most severely injured patients. This hypothesis is supported by our subsequent clinical study described below.

Chesnut et al. (1993), in a seminal study, reported the association between secondary insults and poor outcome after TBI in humans. Gopinath et al. (1994) reported that even a single secondary insult [one episode of decreased jugular venous oxygen saturation ($SJVO_2$) to <50 percent] doubled mortality rate in patients after severe TBI. In an initial study examining the potential role of adenosine as an endogenous neuroprotectant in human TBI (Bell et al., 2001), we collaborated with the group of Dr. Claudia Robertson at the Baylor College of Medicine and hypothesized that brain interstitial adenosine and related purine metabolites would be increased during reductions in $SJVO_2$ in humans. We compared purine and lactate levels in six patients who suffered a $SJVO_2$ desaturation episode after severe TBI to evaluate the relationship between adenosine and increased glycolytic metabolism. Microdialysis samples were collected during periods of desaturation and normal $SJVO_2$ and levels of adenosine, inosine, hypoxanthine, xanthine, cAMP, and lactate

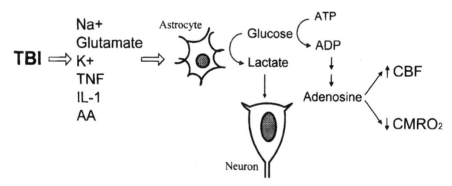

Figure 6.4 Schematic of the theoretical role that adenosine could be playing to defend the brain after TBI. Glycolysis in astrocytes in response to a variety of mediators produced or released after injury or secondary insults leads to adenosine production, which results in a reduction in metabolic demands and a compensatory increase in CBF.

were measured. Adenosine was increased 2.4-fold and xanthine was increased 3.9-fold during desaturations. Adenosine, xanthine, and hypoxanthine significantly correlated with lactate over both study periods. The marked increases in adenosine and xanthine, end products of ATP breakdown, in brain interstitial fluid during $SJVO_2$ desaturations are evidence for energy failure during these episodes. Correlation of these metabolites with lactate also supports this hypothesis and suggests that adenosine is increased during periods of enhanced glycolysis. These findings suggest that adenosine may play an important role in defending the brain during secondary insults after severe TBI in humans, and strongly support the investigation of agents augmenting local adenosine concentration in experimental TBI.

It is noteworthy to point out that the peak increases in brain interstitial levels of adenosine in humans (about 300 to 1000 nM) were only about 20 % as high as seen by Bell et al. (1998) in the injury penumbra of the rat model of controlled cortical impact. This may result from the fact that, in humans, the adenosine measurements were made at sites more remote from the injury than in the rat model. In addition, the measurements in humans were obtained during episodes of secondary insult hours or days after the injury—compared to the immediate postimpact measurements that were made in the rat. The large increases in brain interstitial levels of adenosine during secondary insults in humans suggest that adenosine's role as an endogenous neuroprotectant is operating during the subacute phase after the injury, even after the patient has been transferred from the emergency department to the intensive care unit. Thus, adenosine-targeted pharmacological strategies could have a broad temporal window of opportunity after TBI. However, it will be important to determine the quantitative contribution of adenosine to neuroprotection in both the immediate and delayed periods after TBI. It is also important to note that peak brain interstitial levels of adenosine after severe TBI with a secondary insult in humans (about 300 to 1000 nM) are about 5- to 10-fold higher than those seen in CSF from similar patients (about 30 to 200 nM).

Finally, Robertson et al. (1999a) recently reported the time course and magnitude of concentrations of adenosine in CSF from infants and children after severe TBI. Samples ($n = 304$) of ventricular CSF were collected from 27 pediatric patients during the first 7 days after severe TBI (GCS ≤ 7). Adenosine levels were markedly increased (about 10-fold) in CSF of these infants and children after severe TBI versus control and were independently associated with GCS ≤ 4—that is, the most severe injuries. Peak and mean CSF adenosine levels in adults and children were remarkably similar in magnitude after severe TBI (Clark et al., 1997a; Robertson et al., 1999a).

Taken as a whole, our clinical data suggest that there are marked increases in adenosine in CSF after severe TBI in humans. Association of adenosine with $AVDO_2 < 4$ supports the purported reduction in metabolism and increase in CBF in response to its local production. In addition, brain interstitial fluid levels of adenosine increase briskly during episodes of secondary insult in humans with severe TBI at the bedside in the neurointensive care unit. These exciting new data strongly support a role for adenosine in the endogenous response to human head injury.

CONCLUSION

In conclusion, we have presented the relative merits of adenosine receptor activation as a therapeutic target in head trauma. Receptor activation can be achieved by either agonist application or utilization of an adenosine-potentiating agent. The difficulties encountered with each approach are discussed in detail. Regardless, beneficial effects can be attained by adenosine receptor activation within brain parenchyma to attenuate excitotoxic mechanisms and/or within the cerebrovasculature to antagonize the pathoinflammatory segment of the ischemic cascade in addition to influencing beneficially localized CBF. To further support the therapeutic potential of adenosine receptor activation we have also summarized the studies to date in both animals and humans that address this potential. Overall, the results from these studies support the need to further explore the potential for adenosine receptor activation and how this approach could be utilized clinically in the management of head trauma patients.

ACKNOWLEDGMENT

We thank Dr. Larry Jenkins for his critical review of this chapter.

ABBREVIATIONS

AA	Arachidonic acid
ADA	Adenosine deaminase
AK	Adenosine kinase
AMP	Adenosine monophosphate
AMPDA	Adenosine 5′-monophosphate deaminase
ARA	Adenosine-regulating agent
ATP	Adenosine triphosphate
$AVDO_2$	Arterial venous difference in oxygen content
cAMP	Cyclic adenosine monophosphate
CBF	Cerebral blood flow
CCPA	2-Chlorocyclopentyladenosine
CHA	Cyclohexyladenosine
$CMRO_2$	Cerebral metabolic rate for oxygen
CNS	Central nervous system
CPA	Cyclopentyladenosine
CSF	Cerebrospinal fluid
DMPX	3,7-Dimethyl-1-propargylxanthine
EAA	Excitatory amino acid

EHNA	*Erythro*-hydroxynonyladenine
ENBA	*Endo*-norbornyladenosine
GCS	Glasgow coma scale
IB-MECA	N^6-(3-iodobenzyl)-5′-N-methylcarboxamidoadenosine
ICV	Intracerebroventricular
IP_3	Inositol trisphosphate
MAP	Microtubule-associated protein
NECA	5′-N-ethylcarboximidoadenosine
R-PIA	N^6-(R-phenylisopropyl)adenosine
$SJVO_2$	Jugular venous oxygen saturation
TBI	Traumatic brain injury
T_{1obs}	In vivo spin–lattice relaxation time of tissue water
NBTI	Nitrobenzylthioinosine

REFERENCES

M. P. Abbracchio, R. Brambilla, S. Ceruti, H. O. Kim, D. K. von Lubitz, K. A. Jacobson, and F. Cattabeni, *Mol. Pharmacol.*, 48, 1038–1045 (1995).

P. D. Adelson, B. Clyde, P. M. Kochanek, S. R. Wisniewski, D. W. Marino, and H. Yonas, *Pediatr. Neurosurg.*, 26, 200–207 (1997).

P. D. Adelson, M. Whalen, P. Robichaud, T. Carlos, and P. Kochanek, *Acta Neurochir. Suppl. (Wien)*, 71, 104–106 (1998).

N. Altiok, A. J. Balmforth, and B. B. Fredholm, *Acta Physiol. Scand.*, 144, 55–63 (1992).

J. R. S. Arch and E. A. Newsholme, *Biochem. J.*, 174, 965–977 (1978).

M. Bell, C. Robertson, P. Kochanek, J. Goodman, S. Gopinath, J. Carcillo, R. Clark, D. Marion, Z. Mi, and E. Jackson, *Crit. Care Med.*, in press, (2001).

M. J. Bell, P. M. Kochanek, J. A. Carcillo, Z. Mi, J. K, Schiding, S. R. Wisniewski, R. S. B. Clark, C. E. Dixon, D. W. Marion, and E. Jackson, *J. Neurotrauma*, 15, 163–170 (1998).

R. B. Benati, P. Schubert, G. Rothe, Rudolphi Gehrmann, K., G. Valet, and G. W. Dreutzberg, *J. Cereb. Blood Flow Metab.*, 14, 145–149 (1994).

M. Bergsneider, D. A. Hovda, E. Shalmon, D. F. Kelly, P. M. Vespa, N. A. Martin, M. E. Phelps, D. L. McArth, M. J. Caron, J. F. Kraus, and D. P. Becker, *J. Neurosurg.*, 86, 241–251 (1997).

G. J. Bouma, J. P. Muizelaar, W. A. Stringer, S. C. Choi, P. Fatouros, H. F. Young, *J. Neurosurg.*, 77, 360–368 (1992).

J. B. Brierley, B. S. Meldrum, and A. W. Brown, *Arch. Neurol.*, 29, 367–374 (1973).

J. M. Brundege and T. V. Dunwiddie, *Neuroreport*, 14, 3007–3011 (1998).

R. F. Bruns and J. H. Fergus, *Mol. Pharmacol.*, 38, 939–949 (1990).

R. F. Bruns, G. H. Lu, and T. A. Pugsley, *Mol. Pharmacol.*, 29, 331–346 (1986).

R. Bullock, R. M. Chesnut, G. Clifton, J. Ghajar, D. W. Marion, R. K. Narayan, D. W. Newell, L. Pitts, M. J. Rosner, and J. E. Wilberger, *J. Neurotrauma*, 13, 693–697 (1996).

R. Bullock, A. Zauner, J. J. Woodward, J. Myseros, S. C. Choi, J. D. Ward, A. Marmarou and H. F. Young, *Neurosurgery.*, 89, 507–518 (1998).

R. Busto, M. Y.-T. Globus, W. D. Dietrich, E. Martinez, I. Valdez, and M. D. Ginsberg, *Stroke*, 20, 904–909 (1989).

X. Cao and J. W. Phillis, *Gen. Pharmacol.*, 26, 1545–1548 (1995).

C. E. Cass, *Drug Transport in Antimicrobial and Anticancer Chemotherapy.* Marcel Dekker, New York, 1995, pp. 403–451.

J. F. Chen, Z. Huang, J. Ma, J. Zhu, R. Moratalla, D. Standaert, M. A. Moskowitz, J. S. Fink, and M. A Schwarzschild, *J. Neurosci.*, 19, 9192–9200 (1999).

L. Cherian, C. S. Robertson, C. F. Contant, and R. M. Bryan, *J. Neurotrauma*, 11, 573–585 (1994).

R. M. Chesnut, L. F. Marshall, M. R. Klauber, B. A. Blunt, N. Baldwin, H. M. Eisenberg, A. Marmarou, and M. A. Foulkes, *J. Trauma*, 34, 216–222 (1993).

R. S. Clark, J. A. Carcillo, P. M. Kochanek, W. D. Obrist, E. K. Jackson, Z. Mi, S. R. Wisniewski, Bell, and D. W. Marion, *Neurosurgery*, 41, 1284–1292 (1997a).

R. S. Clark, P. M. Kochanek, C. E. Dixon, M. Chen, D. W. Marion, S. Heineman, S. T. DeKosky and S. H. Gra, *J. Neurotrauma*, 14, 179–189 (1997b).

C. G. Craig and T. D. White, *J. Neurochem.*, 60, 1073–1080 (1993).

K. De Leo, P. Schubert, and G. W. Kreutzberg, *Neurosci. Lett.*, 84, 307–311 (1988).

U. Dirnagl, K. Niwa, U. Lindauer, and A. Villringer, *Am. J. Physiol.*, 267, H296–301 (1994).

M. Dragunow, G. V. Goddard, and R. Laverty, *Epilepsia*, 26, 480–487 (1985).

T. V. Dunwiddie, in *Adenosine and Adenosine Receptors*, Humana Press, Totowa, NJ, 1990, pp. 143–172.

T. V. Dunwiddie and T. Worth, *J. Pharmacol. Exp. Ther.*, 220, 70–76 (1982).

T. V. Dunwiddie, L. Diao, and W. R. J. Proctor, *Neuroscience*, 17, 7673–7682 (1997).

K. M. Fleming and D. J. Mogul, *Neuropharmacology*, 36, 353–362 (1997).

K. M. Fleming, T. Ji, and D. J. Mogul, *Soc. Neurosci.*, Abstr. 695.16 (1997).

B. B. Fredholm, *Pharmacol. Toxicol.*, 76, 228–239 (1995).

B. B. Fredholm, M. P. Abbracchio, G. Burnstock, J. W. Daly, T. K. Harden, K. A. Jacobson, P. Leff, and M. Williams, *Pharmacol. Rev.*, 46, 143–156 (1994).

B. B. Fredholm and N. Altiok, *Neurochem. Int.*, 25, 99–102 (1994).

J. D. Geiger, F. E. Parkinson, and E. A. Kowaluk, in K. A. Jacobson, and M. F. Jarvis, Eds., *Purinergic Approaches in Experimental Therapeutics*, Wiley-Liss, New York, pp. 55–84 (1997).

S. P. Gopinath, C. S. Robertson, C. F. Contant, C. Hayes, Z. Feldman, R. K. Narayan, and R. G. Grossman, *J. Neurol. Neurosurg. Psychiatry.*, 57, 717–723 (1994).

H. E. Gruber, M. E. Hoffer, D. R. McAllister, P. K. Laikind, T. A. Lane, G. W. Schmid-Schonbein, and R. L. Engler, *Circulation*, 80, 1400–1411 (1989).

J. P. Headrick, M. R. Bendall, A. I. Faden, and R. Vink, *J. Cereb. Blood Flow Metab.*, 14, 853–861 (1994).

D. H. W. Ho, J. K. Luce, and E. Frei III, *Biochem. Pharmacol.*, 17, 1025–1035 (1968).

D. A. Hovda, S. M. Lee, M. L. Smith, S. von Stuck, M. Bergsneider, D. Kelly, E. Shalmon, N. Martin, M. Caron, J. Mazziotta, M. Phelps, and D. P. Becker, *J. Neurotrauma*, 12, 903–906 (1995).

A. P. Ijzerman, J. K. von Frijtag, S. Vittori, et al., *Nucleos. Nucleot.*, 13, 2267–2281 (1994).

K. A. Jacobson, O. Nikodijevic, D. Shi, C. Gallo-Rodriguez, M. E. Olah, G. L. Stiles, and J. W. Daly, *FEBS Lett.*, 336, 57–60 (1993).

C. A. Janusz and R. F. Berman, *Brain Res.*, 619, 131–136 (1993).

C. A. Janusz, R. F. Bruns, and R. F. Berman, *Brain Res.*, 567, 181–187 (1991).

M. F. Jarvis and M. Williams, in *Adenosine and Adenosine Receptors*, Humana Press, Totowa, NJ, 1990, pp. 423–474.

M. F. Jarvis and M. Williams, *Eur. J. Pharmacol.*, 168, 243–246 (1989).

N. Jiang, E. A. Kowaluk, L. Chi-Hung, H. Mazdiyasni, and M. Chopp, *Eur. J. Pharmacol.*, 320, 131–137 (1997).

S. R. Kasibhatla, B. C. Bookser, G. Probst, J. R. Appleman, and M. D. Erion, *Medi 078, 214th ACS National Meeting, Las Vegas, Nevada*, September (1997).

P. M. Kochanek, D. Marion, W. Zhang, J. K. Schiding, M. White, A. Palmer, R. S. B. Clark, M. O'Mally, S. Styren, C. Ho, and S. DeKosky, *J. Neurotrauma*, 12, 1015–1025 (1995).

P. M. Kochanek, K. S. Hendrich, C. L, Robertson, D. S. Williams, J. A. Melick, C. Ho, D. W. Marion, E. K. Jackson, *Magn. Reson. Med.*, in press, (2001).

C. A. Kollias-Baker, J. Ruble, M. Jacobson, J. K. Harrison, M. Ozeck, J. C. Shryock, and L. Belardinelli, *J. Pharmacol. Exp. Ther.* 281, 761–768 (1997).

G. Kostopoulos, C. Drapeau, M. Avoli, A. Olivier, and J. G. Villemeure, *Neurosci. Lett.*, 106, 119–124 (1989).

M. J. Kotapka, D. I. Graham, J. H. Adams, and T. A. Gennarelli, *Acta Neuropathol.*, 83, 530–534 (1992).

T. A. Krenitsky, R. L. Miller, and J. A. Fyfe, *Biochem. Pharmacol.*, 23, 170–172 (1974).

C. Ledent, J.-M. Vaugeois, S. N. Schiffmann, T. Pedrazzini, M. El Yacoubi, J.-J. Vanderhaeghen, J. Costentin, J. K. Heath, G. Vassart, and M. Parmentier, *Nature*, 388, 674–678 (1997).

J. Linden, A. L. Tucker, and K. R. Lynch, *Trends Pharmacol. Sci.*, 12, 326–328 (1991).

D. Lobner and D. W. Choi, *Stroke*, 25, 2085–2090 (1994).

D. H. Lowenstein, M. J. Thomas, D. H. Smith, and T. K. McIntosh, *J. Neurosci.*, 12, 4846–4853 (1992).

T. A. Macek, H. Schaffhauser, and P. J. Conn, *J. Neurosci.*, 18, 6138–6146 (1998).

D. W. Marion, J. Darby, and H. Yonas, *J. Neurosurgery*, 74, 407–414 (1991).

L. P. Miller, *Stroke Therapy: Basic, Preclinical and Clinical Directions*, Wiley-Liss, Inc., New York, 1999, pp. 131–156.

L. P. Miller and C. Hsu, *J. Neurotrauma*, 9, S563–S577 (1992).

L. P. Miller, L. A. Jelovich, L. Yao, J. DaRe, B. Ugarkar, and A. C. Foster, *Neurosci. Lett.*, 220, 73–76 (1996).

H. L. Mitchell, W. A. Frisella, R. W. Brooker, and K.-W. Yoon, *Neurosurgery*, 36, 1003–1008 (1995).

K. M. Mullane and M. Williams, in *Adenosine and Adenosine Receptors*, Humana Press, Totowa, NJ, 1990, pp. 289–334.

J. I. Nagy, J. D. Geiger, and P. E. Daddona, *Neurosci. Lett.*, 55, 47–53 (1985).

P. Nilsson, L. Hillered, U. Ponten, and U. Ungerstedt, *J. Cereb. Blood Flow Metab.*, 10, 631–637 (1990).

T. Nitatori, N. Sato, S. Waguri, Y. Karasawa, H. Araki, K. Shibanai, E. Kominami, and Y. Uchiyama, *J. Neurosci.*, 15, 1001–1011 (1995).

J. W. Nyce, *Trends Pharmacol. Sci.*, 20, 79–83 (1999).

T. P. Obrenovitch and D. A. Richards, *Cerebrovasc. Brain Metab. Rev.*, 7, 1–54 (1995).

A. M. Palmer, D. W. Marion, M. L. Botscheller, P. E. Swedlow, S. D. Styren, and S. T. DeKosky, *J. Neurochem.*, 61, 2015–2024, (1993a).

A. M. Palmer, D. W. Marion, M. L. Botscheller, and E. E. Redd, *J. Neurotrauma*, 10, 363–372 (1993b).

T. S. Park, J. W. Beetsch, E. R. Gonzales, A. R. Shah, and J. M. Gidday, *Soc. Neurosci.*, A744.5 (1997).

M. C. Peakman and S. J. Hill, *Br. J. Pharmacol.*, 111, 191–198 (1994).

M. C. Peakman and S. J. Hill, *Eur. J. Pharmacol.*, 306, 281–289 (1996).

L. Pellerin and P. J. Magistretti, *Proc. Natl. Acad. Sci. USA*, 91, 10625–10629 (1994).

J. W. Phillis, *Cerebrovasc. Brain Metab. Rev.*, 1, 26–54 (1989).

J. W. Phillis, M. Smith-Barbour, L. M. Perkins, and M. H. O'Regan, *Brain Res. Bull.*, 34, 457–466 (1994a).

J. W. Phillis, M. Smith-Barbour, M. H. O'Regan, and L. M. Perkins, *Neurochem. Res.*, 19, 1125–1130 (1994b).

P. Popoli, P. Betto, R. Reggio, and G. Ricciarello, *Eur. J. Pharmacol.*, 287, 215–217 (1995).

C. L. Robertson, P. M. Kochanek, E. A. Jackson, Z. Mi, S. R. Wisniewski, J. K. Schiding, J. A. Melick, and J. A. Carcillo, *J. Neurotrauma*, 15, 893 Abstract (1998).

C. L. Robertson, M. J. Bell, P. M. Kochanek, P. D. Adelson, R. Ruppel, S. R. Wisniewski, X. Mi, K. Janesko, R. S. B. Clark, and E. K. Jackson, *J. Neurotrauma*, (Abstract) (1999a).

C. L. Robertson, K. S. Hendrich, P. M. Kochanek, E. K. Jackson, J. A. Melick, S. H. Graham, D. W. Marion, D. S. Williams, and C. Ho, *Proc. Int. Soc. Magn. Reson. Med.*, 7, 896 Abstract (1999b).

K. A. Rudolphi, P. Schubert, F. E. Parkinson, and B. B. Fredholm, *Cereb. Brain Metab. Rev.*, 4, 346–369 (1992).

P. Safar, *Circulation*, 74: IV, 138–153 (1986).

A. P. Sarnaik, G. Preston, M. Lieh-Lai, and A. B. Eisenbrey, *Crit. Care Med.*, 13, 224 (1985).

S. N. Schiffmann, O. Jacobs, and J. J. Vanderhaeghen, *J. Neurochem.*, 57, 1062–1067 (1991).

W. P. Schrader, C. A. West, and N. L. Strominger, *J. Histochem. Cytochem.*, 35, 443–451 (1987).

S. Schwab, T. Steiner, A. Ashcoff, S. Schwarz, H. H. Steiner, O. Jansen, and W. Hacke, *Stroke*, 29, 1888–1893 (1998).

V. M. Sciotti and D. G. Van Wylen, *J. Cereb. Blood Flow Metab.*, 13, 201–207 (1993).

R. E. Simpson, M. H. O'Regan, L. M. Perkins, and J. W. Phillis, *J. Neurochem.*, 58, 1683–1690 (1992).

S. L. Smith and E. D. Hall, *J. Neurotrauma*, 13, 1–9 (1996).

C. D. Sturm, W. A. Frisella, and K.-W. Yoon, *J. Neurosurg.*, 79, 111–115 (1993).

D. VanCalker, M. Muller, and B. Hamprecht, *J. Neurochem.*, 3, 300–315 (1979).

D. K. Von Lubitz, R. C. Lin, P. Popik, M. F. Carter, and K. A. Jacobson, *Eur. J. Pharmacol.*, 263, 59–67 (1994).

P. F. Worley, J. M. Baraban, M. McCarren, S. H. Snyder, B. E. Alger, *Proc. Natl. Acad. Sci. USA*, 84, 3467–3471 (1987).

I. Yamakami and T. K. McIntosh, *J. Cereb. Blood Flow Metab.*, 9, 117–124 (1989).

Q. Y. Zhou, C. Li, M. E. Olah, R. A. Johnson, G. L. Stiles, and O. Civelli, *Proc. Natl. Acad. Sci. USA*, 89, 7432–7436 (1992).

CHAPTER 7

GROWTH FACTORS

SETH P. FINKLESTEIN* and ANDRONIKI PLOMARITOGLOU

CNS Growth Factor Laboratory* and Department of Neurology, Massachusetts General Hospital, Harvard Medical School, Boston, Massachusetts

INTRODUCTION

Growth factors are natural polypeptides exerting important roles on multiple cell processes in the body. The first growth factor discovered, nerve growth factor (NGF), was identified more than 50 years ago. Since then, many more have been identified, and grouped into "superfamilies" by virtue of sequence homologies. Many of these factors have been found to act in the central nervous system: those having effects on neurons are termed "neurotrophic," and those having effects on glial cells or blood vessels may be termed "gliotrophic" or "angiogenic," respectively. Working through high-affinity cell surface receptors, growth factors provoke a cascade of signal transduction leading to new gene expression and protein synthesis, resulting in cell survival, proliferation, and differentiation. Growth factors play an important role as signaling molecules during brain development and in response to injury.

GROWTH FACTORS: FAMILIES, DISTRIBUTION, RECEPTORS, EFFECTS

History

In the late nineteenth and early twentieth centuries, Forsmann and Ramon y Cajal hypothesized that there must be a "neurotrophic" stimulus that provokes neuronal outgrowth (Forsmann, 1898; Cajal, 1928). In 1934, Hamburger found hypoplasia of neurons innervating the wing of the chick embryo, after wing bud extirpation (Levi-

Head Trauma:, *Preclinical, and Clinical Directions*, Edited by Leonard P. Miller and Ronald L. Hayes, Co-edited by Jennifer K. Newcomb
ISBN 0-471-36015-5 © 2001 John Wiley & Sons, Inc.

Montalcini, 1987). In 1948, Bueker found that mouse-sarcoma tissue grafts favored sensory nerve growth in recipient chick embryos (Levi-Montalcini, 1987). His results led Levi-Montalcini and Hamburger to identify a soluble agent responsible for neuronal outgrowth and differentiation. With the collaboration of Cohen, the first growth factor, nerve growth (NGF) factor, was identified from mouse-sarcoma tissue, and later from snake venom and from mouse submandibular salivary glands (Levi-Montalcini, 1987). In 1971, the sequencing of the mouse submandibular NGF was achieved (Levi-Montalcini, 1987). Since then, many more polypeptides with growth factor properties have been identified.

2.1 Neurotrophins

The neurotrophin family consists of nerve growth factor (NGF), brain-derived neurotrophic factor (BDNF), neurotrophin-3 (NT-3), and neurotrophin-4/5 (NT-4/5) (Chen and Finklestein, 1998). NGF is a 26 kDa homodimer isolated in two distinct forms: the first, named 7S because of its molecular size, is a high-molecular-weight complex containing two copies of each of three subunits (α, β, γ), and the second, 2.5S, is indistinguishable from the β subunit of the 7S NGF. The three subunits of 7S NGF have a noncovalent interaction, which is affected by pH and concentration. BDNF is a 13 kDa monomer, and shares a 50 percent sequence homology with NGF (Leibrock et al., 1989). NT-3 is a small basic protein, homologous to BDNF. NT-4 and NT-5 are highly homologous and probably represent the same biological molecule (Apfel, 1997).

NGF binds to two membrane-associated receptors: trkA, a high-affinity tyrosine kinase receptor; and p75, a low-affinity receptor (Meakin et al., 1992; Chao, 1994). The signal transduction pathway of the trkA receptor involves activation of the phosphatidylinositol (PI) 3-kinase, phospholipase C-γ, and mitogen-activated kinase pathways, among others (Mocchetti and Wrathall, 1995). The p75 receptor activates the sphyngomyelin pathway, among others (Dobrowsky et al., 1994). NGF activity generally results from coactivation of the trkA and p75 receptors. BDNF and NT-3 bind with high affinity to trkB and trkC receptors, respectively (Lamballe et al., 1991; Squinto et al., 1991; Chao, 1992). NT-4/5 also binds to the trkB receptor (Klein et al., 1992).

NGF and its high-affinity receptor (trkA) are localized in several regions of the mature mammalian brain, including the basal forebrain, septum, nucleus of the diagonal band of Broca, nucleus basalis of Meynert, hippocampus, olfactory bulb, and neocortex, especially in cholinergic neurons and their terminals (Korsching et al., 1985; Richardson et al., 1986; Nishio et al., 1994). The p75 receptor appears to be more widely distributed, and is also found in hypothalamic nuclei, cerebellar Purkinje cells, nucleus ambiguus, and hypoglossal and trigeminal nuclei in the brain stem (Koh et al., 1989; Yan and Johnson, 1989). Secreted NGF is taken up by axons and is transported retrogradely to neuronal cell bodies (Seiler and Schwab, 1984; Korsching et al., 1985). In the CNS, BDNF is found mainly in cortex, striatum, hippocampus, cerebellum, and spinal cord (Hofer et al., 1990). NT-3 is localized in cerebellum, olfactory bulb, septum, and hippocampus (Berlove and Finklestein, 1993; Katoh-Semba et al., 1996).

NGF supports the survival, outgrowth, and differentiation of brain cholinergic neurons (Hefti, 1986; Williams et al., 1986; Tuszynski et al., 1990). NGF also modifies neuropeptide levels and acts as a chemoattractant of microglia and macrophages in the adult brain (Lindsay and Harmar, 1989; Gilad and Gilad, 1995). BDNF promotes the survival of septal cholinergic neurons, ventral mesencephalic dopaminergic neurons, and retinal ganglion cells (Alderson et al., 1990; Hyman et al., 1991). It induces branching and lengthening of GABAergic neuronal axons, and the formation of excitatory and inhibitory synapses in the developing hippocampus (Vicario-Abejon et al., 1998). BDNF also protects dopaminergic neurons against the neurotoxicity of 1-methyl-4-phenyl-1,2,3,6-tetrahydropyridine (MPTP) by reducing cellular oxidative stress in mesencephalic cell cultures (Spina et al., 1992). NT-3 enhances the survival and outgrowth of striatal and hippocampal neurons, and promotes the survival of oligodendrocyte precursors (Morfini et al., 1994; Bertollini et al., 1997). NT-4/5 enhances the survival of cortical, hippocampal, and cerebellar neurons (Cheng et al., 1994; Gao et al., 1995).

All neurotrophins are expressed during brain development. NGF levels increase in cortex and hippocampus, decrease in cerebellum, and remain unchanged in brain stem and diencephalon during the first postnatal month in rats (Sakamoto et al., 1998). Later, with aging, NGF levels decrease in cortex, but remain unchanged in hippocampus and cerebellum (Katoh-Semba et al., 1998). During development from fetal to adult rat brain, NT-3 and BDNF have a reciprocal pattern of expression; NT-3 is highly expressed in the immature areas of the CNS and its expression decreases with maturation, whereas BDNF levels are low in these immature regions and increase significantly with maturation (Maisonpierre et al., 1990; Berlove and Finklestein, 1993). NT-3 levels appear to increase in cortex, decrease in cerebellum, and remain unchanged in hippocampus in aging rats, whereas BDNF levels increase in hippocampus and decrease in cortex, striatum, and cerebellum during aging (Katoh-Semba et al., 1998). NT-4/5 is strongly expressed in the embryonic brain, but decreases significantly postnatally (Zhang et al., 1999).

Fibroblast Growth Factors

The fibroblast growth factor (FGF) family consists of more than 20 proteins that are derivatives of a common ancestral gene, including acidic FGF (aFGF, FGF-1), basic FGF (bFGF, FGF-2), int-2, and HST/k-FGF, among others. These proteins share a 35 percent to 80 percent homology of a common 125-amino-acid sequence (Thomas, 1993a). Acidic and basic FGF, 16 kDa and 18 kDa polypeptides, respectively, were the first identified and are most thoroughly studied. These proteins are products of two different genes, located on chromosomes 5 and 4, respectively (Jaye et al., 1986; Mergia et al., 1986). They have a 55 percent sequence homology and the same tertiary folding pattern (Esch et al., 1986; Zhu et al. 1991). Both acidic FGF and basic FGF lack a leader sequence and are not freely secreted from cells (Abraham et al., 1986; Forough et al., 1993; D'Amore, 1990; Mignatti et al., 1992).

All members of the FGF family bind to heparin, reflecting binding to heparan sulfate proteoglycan in the extracellular matrix. FGFs also bind to a family of membrane-bound tyrosine kinase receptors, FGFRs. There are at least four different FGFRs, with numerous splice variants possible. The extracellular matrix may be considered the "low-affinity" FGF receptor, whereas the FGFRs are "high-affinity" receptors (Thomas, 1993b; Roghani et al., 1994; Mocchetti and Wrathall, 1995).

FGFs are found in the mature mammalian brain. Basic FGF is widely distributed in the cortex, hippocampus, hypothalamus, and brain stem of the rat brain, among other regions (Emoto et al., 1989). It is localized in astrocytes, endothelia, and some brain neuronal populations (Woodward et al., 1992). Acidic FGF is found in the brain stem, and at lower levels in the cortex, cerebellum, striatum, and hippocampus of the rat brain (Ishikawa et al., 1991). Acidic FGF appears to be localized largely in neurons (Stock et al., 1992). High-affinity FGF receptors are widely localized in the rodent brain (Wanaka et al., 1990).

FGFs are multipotential growth factors, promoting the survival and outgrowth of a wide variety of CNS neurons, as well as glial and endothelial cell survival and proliferation. FGFs promote axonal outgrowth from neurons. They also protect neurons against a variety of toxins and insults, including excitatory amino acids, free radicals, anoxia, hypoglycemia, and nitric oxide. Basic FGF is also a potent vasodilator, working through upregulation of endothelial nitric oxide synthase (eNOS) on cerebral endothelial cells (Freese et al., 1992; Finklestein et al., 1993; Regli et al., 1994; Rosenblatt et al., 1994; Nakao et al., 1996; Fagan et al., 1997; Kawamata et al., 1997).

The expression of acidic FGF and basic FGF is upregulated during brain development. These factors induce mitosis of cells of the embryonic mesoderm and neuroectoderm, including neuroblasts, astrocytes, fibroblasts, and vascular endothelial cells (Gospodarowicz et al., 1987; Perraud et al., 1988; Caday et al., 1990). Basic FGF (FGF-2) also promotes the proliferation of neural progenitor cells and their differentiation into neurons in the developing and mature rat brain (Palmer et al., 1999). FGF-4 has similar effects (Ray et al., 1997). In the developing rat brain, basic FGF and its high-affinity receptors are expressed in several brain regions including the hippocampus, occipital cortex, inferior colliculus, cerebellum, and brain stem. Basic FGF and FGFR-2 expression vary between different regions and increase gradually postnatally, whereas FGFR-1 expression shows little variation between brain regions (El-Husseini et al., 1994). Basic FGF and FGFR-1 are expressed in cortical neurons, and in the basement membranes of the cortical capillary endothelia of the developing brain in the human fetus (Gonzalez et al., 1996). Acidic FGF is expressed in neurons of cortex, cerebellum, hippocampus, substantia nigra, and locus ceruleus of the developing rat brain (Wilcox and Unnerstall, 1991).

Insulin-like Growth Factor (IGF) Family

The IGF family includes insulin, and IGF-1 and IGF-2, two structurally related peptides of 7.6 and 7.4 kDa, respectively (Ibelgaufts, 1995a). There are two types of receptors, a tyrosine kinase receptor for insulin and IGF-1, and a high-affinity cation-independent mannose 6-phosphate receptor for IGF-2; both have a cysteine-rich extracellular domain (LeRoith et al., 1993). Six IGF-binding proteins (IGFBPs) have been identified (Chen and Finklestein, 1998). These serve to transport IGF-1 and -2 to their receptors and modulate their interactions.

Insulin is localized largely in the hypothalamus and olfactory bulb, whereas IGF-1 and -2 have a more widespread distribution, including hippocampus, cerebral cortex, cerebellum, and brain stem in the rat brain. IGF-1 and -2 are also expressed in the choroid plexuses of the rat brain (Bach et al., 1991; Bondy et al., 1992; Kar et al., 1993). IGF receptors are found in all of the above regions. Most IGFBPs are found in meninges, ependyma, choroid plexus, and cerebral cortex of the rodent brain. Cells expressing IGF-1 are mainly neurons, and to a lesser extent endothelial and glial cells, whereas only glial cells express IGF-2 (Garcia-Segura et al., 1997; Walter et al., 1997, 1999; Niblock et al., 1998).

IGF-1 and IGF-2 induce survival and outgrowth in several neuronal types. IGF-1 and -2 promote cell proliferation and differentiation of mesencephalic dopaminergic, septal, and pontine cholinergic neurons in culture (Knusel et al., 1990; Cheng and Mattson, 1992). IGF-1 induces axonal sprouting in the oxytocinergic neurons of the magnocellular neurosecretory system in the hypothalamus of adult rats, and dendrite branching of pyramidal cells of rat primary somatosensory cortex (Zhou et al., 1999; Niblock et al., 2000). IGF-1 increases the number of neurons of the medullary nuclei, and promotes neuritic outgrowth in the medulla of transgenic mice over-expressing IGF-1 (Dentremont et al., 1999). Overexpression of IGFBP-1 impairs brain development (Ni et al., 1997).

Insulin promotes axonal growth in fetal rat brain neuron cultures (Schechter et al., 1999). During development, IGF-1 promotes myelination and increases the number of oligodendrocytes in the anterior medullary velum of the postnatal rat brain (Goddard et al., 1999). IGF-1 and IGF-2 stimulate proliferation of neuronal precursor cells in cultures of fetal rat brain (Nielsen et al., 1991). IGF-1 is expressed mainly in neurons of several brain regions of the developing brain, whereas IGF-2 is expressed mainly in mesenchymal and neural crest origin cells (D'Ercole et al., 1996; Sherrard et al., 1997). During development, IGF-1 mRNA levels remain relatively stable postnatally, whereas IGF-1 protein levels appear to decrease in rat brain with aging (Niblock et al., 1998; Sonntag et al., 1999). IGFBPs are differentially expressed in developing oligodendrocytes and astrocytes in rat central nervous system, and their expression has regional and developmental specificity (Cheng et al., 1996; D'Ercole et al., 1996; Mewar and McMorris, 1997).

Epidermal Growth Factor Family

Epidermal growth factor (EGF) and transforming growth factor-α (TGF-α) belong to the same superfamily. The mature form of EGF is a 53-amino-acid single-chain polypeptide; TGF-α is a 50-amino-acid polypeptide, having a 30 percent sequence homology with EGF (Morrison, 1993). Heparin-binding EGF-like factor (HB-EGF) is an 86-amino-acid protein, also a member of the same superfamily, which shares 40 percent sequence homology with EGF and TGF (Ibelgaufts, 1995b). EGF, TGF-α and HB-EGF bind to the same high-affinity tyrosine kinase receptor, a 170 kDa glycoprotein (Puolakkainen and Twardzik, 1993a; Ibelgaufts, 1995b).

In mouse and rat, EGF and TGF-α mRNAs are localized widely throughout the brain, in both neurons and glia; TGF-α is significantly more abundant than EGF, of which the latter has highest concentrations in the cerebellum, the olfactory bulb, and the hypothalamus (Lazar and Blum, 1992; Seroogy et al., 1993). In the rat brain, HB-EGF mRNA and protein are expressed in various brain regions, most strongly in the cerebellum, the olfactory bulb, the hippocampus, and the cerebral cortex. Cells expressing HB-EGF are neurons and interfascicular glial cells (Hayase et al., 1998). EGF receptors are largely located on neurons in the rat as well as the human brain, and especially in the cerebral cortex, the cerebellar Purkinje cells, and the hippocampus (Gomez-Pinilla et al., 1988; Werner et al., 1988; Tucker et al., 1993).

In vitro studies have shown that EGF promotes the survival and outgrowth of embryonic and neonatal neurons in several regions of the rat brain, such as dopaminergic and GABAergic mecencephalic neurons, and cerebellar neurons (Morrison et al., 1988; Kornblum et al., 1990; Casper et al., 1994).

In vitro studies have shown that both EGF and TGF-α are active mitogens in the developing brain and promote the proliferation of brain progenitor cells (Mahanthappa and Schwarting, 1993; Kitchens et al., 1994).

Transforming Growth Factor-β (TGF-β) Family

The TGF-β family contains TGF-β isoforms 1 to 3 that are found in the mammalian CNS, as well as other structurally related factors, including the bone morphogenetic protein (BMP) subfamily (Ibelgaufts, 1995c). TGF-β is a homodimeric 24 kDa polypeptide, comprised of two identical 112-amino acid chains (Puolakkainen and Twardzik, 1993b). There are four classes of high-affinity TGF-β receptors, which are serine/threonine kinase receptors (Kolodziejczyk and Hall, 1996; Massague, 1998; Wrana, 1998).

In adult rat brain, TGF-β2 and TGF-β3 mRNAs are expressed in several regions, including cerebral cortex, hippocampus, striatum, cerebellum, and brain stem. TGF-β isoform 1 is localized in the meninges and the choroid plexus, whereas isoforms 2 and 3 are more present in cerebral cortical layers II, III, V, in hippocampus, amygdala, hypothalamus, and brain stem; cells expressing TGF-β in these regions are mainly neurons, and in the white matter areas are astrocytes (Unsicker et al., 1991). TGF-β receptor type II mRNA is found in the cortex, the brain stem, the cerebellum, and the hippocampus (Bottner et al., 1996). In normal human brain tissue, TGF-β isoforms are localized in ramified microglia and, more specifically, TGF-β2 and TGF-β3 in neurons of the gray matter. TGF-β receptor type I and TGF-β receptor type II are expressed on endothelial cells, astrocytes, microglia, and neurons (De Groot et al., 1999).

In vitro, TGF-β influences the regulation of brain endothelial tissue plasminogen activator and anticoagulant thrombomodulin by astrocytes, and increases the survival and outgrowth of several CNS neuronal types (Ishihara et al., 1994; Buisson et al., 1998; Tran et al., 1999).

TGF-βs regulate the development and differentiation of serotoninergic neurons of the raphe in the rat embryonic brain (Galter et al., 1999). In vitro, bone morphogenetic proteins promote the differentiation of cortical oligodendroglial and astroglial progenitor cells into astrocytes and suppress differentiation into oligodendroglial cells (Mabie et al., 1997). TGF-β2 regulates cerebellar granule cell proliferation and maturation in the developing rat brain (Kane et al., 1996). Many of the TGF-β family receptors are expressed in the neuroepithelium in the rat embryonic brain. Interestingly, TGF-β receptor type I but not type II receptor is found in the cerebral cortex in the mice developing brain (Soderstrom et al., 1996; Tomoda et al., 1996).

Ciliary Neurotrophic Factor (CNTF)

Ciliary neurotrophic factor, a 20.4 kDa protein structurally similar to some hematopoietic cytokines, was originally purified from chick ocular tissue (Barbin et al., 1984; Bazan, 1991). CNTF binds to high-affinity CNTF receptors that have two components, gp130 and LIF-receptor-b moieties (Davis et al., 1993). These receptors are structurally related to IL-6 receptors (Hall and Rao, 1992). CNTF and its receptors are expressed throughout the CNS, including the hippocampus, the cerebral cortex, the cerebellum, the dentate gyrus, the olfactory bulb, and the locus caeruleus in the rat brain. Cells expressing CNTF are both neurons and glia (Henderson et al., 1994; Kirsch and Hofmann, 1994; Seniuk-Tatton et al., 1995; Watanabe et al., 1996).

In vitro studies have shown that CNTF is a trophic factor for central nervous system neurons, including ciliary ganglionic, cholinergic, and GABAergic neurons of the adult rat brain (Ip et al., 1991; Levison et al., 1998). CNTF promotes the survival effect of BDNF and NT-4/5 on cholinergic neurons in the rat brain (Hashimoto et al., 1999). In vivo studies have shown that CNTF promotes the expression of the IGF type I receptor and FGF receptor 1 mRNAs in adult rat brain oligodendrocytes, and induces astrocyte hypertrophy and phenotypic changes in the striatum of the rat brain (Jiang et al., 1999; Lisovoski et al., 1997). CNTF appears to play an important role in the survival, and differentiation of these neurons during development. During the early postnatal stage, CNTF receptor is diffusely identified in the rat brain, whereas in adults it is significantly reduced except for the cortex and the olfactory bulb (Stockli et al., 1989; Ip et al., 1991; Kirsch and Hofmann, 1994; Larkfors et al., 1994; MacLennan et al., 1994).

Table 7.1 summarizes the localization and effects on neurons of representative members of growth factor families.

Table 7.1   Polypeptide Growth Factor Families

Family	Factor	Localization (Major Areas)	Effects on Neurons
Neurotrophins	NGF	Neocortex, basal forebrain, septum, hippocampus, cerebellum, olfactory bulb	Survival, outgrowth, differentiation
	BDNF	Cortex, striatum, hippocampus, cerebellum	Survival, outgrowth, synapses formation
	NT-3	Septum, hippocampus, cerebellum, olfactory bulb	Survival, outgrowth
Fibroblast growth factors (FGFs)	Acidic FGF	Cortex, hippocampus, hypothalamus, brain stem	Survival, outgrowth, neuroprotection, mitogenic activity, progenitor cell proliferation
	Basic FGF	Cortex, striatum, hippocampus, cerebellum, brain stem	
Insulin-like growth factors (IGFs)	IGF-1, -2	Cortex, hippocampus, cerebellum, brain stem, choroid plexus	Survival, differentiation, proliferation of precursors, myelination, outgrowth
Epidermal growth factor (EGF)	EGF	Hypothalamus, cerebellum, olfactory bulb, cortex, striatum, brain stem	Survival, outgrowth, mitogenic activity
	TGF-α	Cortex, striatum, hypothalamus, cerebellum, olfactory bulb, caudate, dentate gyrus, brain stem	Mitogenic activity
	HB-EGF	Cortex, hippocampus, cerebellum, olfactory bulb	Progenitor proliferation, survival
Transforming growth factor-β (TGF-β)	TGF-β	Cortex, striatum, hippocampus, cerebellum, brain stem, hypothalamus, amygdala	Survival, outgrowth, proliferation, maturation
Ciliary neuronotrophic factor (CNTF)	CNTF	Cortex, hippocampus, cerebellum, olfactory bulb, dentate gyrus	Survival, differentiation

EXPRESSION OF GROWTH FACTORS FOLLOWING BRAIN INJURY

Following head trauma, brain injury may vary from a reversible functional alteration such as seen in concussion to severe structural brain damage. In this latter instance, a cascade of biochemical, metabolic, physiological, and anatomical changes take place, including release of excitatory amino acids and oxygen free radicals, invasion of inflammatory cells, and increased expression of cytokines and growth factors (Berlove and Finklestein, 1993; White and Krause, 1993). In addition, secondary physiological and pathological changes may occur, including cerebral ischemia, edema, hydrocephalus, and seizures. A number of animal models have been devised to investigate head injury and its potential treatments. These models include direct weight drop, pneumatic, or fluid percussion injury to the exposed skull, dura, or brain, as well as models of direct mechanical or electrolytic lesions of the brain. Some models result in focal cortical lesions with variable involvement of deeper structures (e.g. hippocampus), whereas other models result in a diffuse axonal injury.

Neurotrophins

Animal Studies. Following unilateral or bilateral pneumatic percussion injury to the rat cortex, NGF mRNA levels increase 5- to 6-fold both in injured and adjacent cortex, peaking at 24 h and declining by 36 to 72 h after injury (DeKosky et al., 1994; Oyesiku et al., 1999). NGF protein levels in similar models increase 2- to 4-fold, peaking at 3 to 7 days in tissue surrounding focal cortical contusions. High-affinity NGF receptor (trkA) mRNA levels are upregulated in adjacent uninjured cortex at 12 to 36 h after injury.

Following bilateral pneumatic percussion injury to the rat cortex, BDNF mRNA levels increase in injured and adjacent tissue, peaking at 12 h after injury and declining thereafter (Oyesiku et al., 1999). In situ hybridization studies show that BDNF mRNA is increased in superficial cortical layers surrounding focal cortical contusions by 3 h after injury (Hicks et al., 1999). Moreover, BDNF mRNA levels also increase in regions distant from focal contusions, including piriform cortex and hippocampus (Hicks et al., 1997, 1999). High-affinity BDNF receptor (trkB) mRNA levels appear to decrease in injured cortex, but increase in adjacent noninjured cortex and hippocampus at 12 to 72 h after injury (Hicks et al., 1999; Oyesiku et al., 1999). In contrast to BDNF mRNA expression, NT3 mRNA expression decreases in hippocampus following focal parieto-occipital contusion (Hicks et al., 1997).

Human Studies. NGF protein levels are elevated in the CSF of patients with closed head trauma. In a study of 22 patients with closed head injury, NGF levels were measured in the CSF every three days for three weeks. CSF NGF levels were elevated in 14 patients, peaking during the first four days after the injury. NGF levels were correlated to the severity of injury, as assessed by clinical rating scales (Kossmann et al., 1996). CSF NGF levels in these patients were also correlated with CSF IL-6 and IL-8 levels (Kossmann et al., 1996, 1997).

Fibroblast Growth Factors

Animal Studies. Most studies have examined the expression of basic fibroblast growth factor (bFGF, FGF-2) following experimental brain injury. Following focal mechanical (aspiration or knife cut) injury to the rat cerebral cortex, bFGF mRNA levels increase within 4 h and peak within 3 to 7 days in tissue surrounding wounds. Increases in bFGF mRNA levels subside within 14 days following injury. bFGF mRNA levels are also increased in hippocampi following focal or diffuse brain injury (Frautschy et al., 1991; Logan et al., 1992a; Yang and Cui, 1998).

Increased bFGF protein levels follow increased bFGF mRNA levels in tissue surrounding focal brain wounds, and in the hippocampus following diffuse brain injury. Cells expressing bFGF mRNA and protein include macrophages, microglia, neurons, astrocytes, and endothelial cells. Early on (1 to 3 days), bFGF is expressed primarily in macrophages and microglia. Later, most bFGF expressing cells are astrocytes (Frautschy et al., 1991; Logan et al., 1992a; Yang and Cui, 1998). Levels of the bFGF receptor (flg) and its mRNA increase at 24 to 48 h in tissue surrounding focal brain wounds and peak at 10 to 14 days after injury. bFGF receptors are expressed in astrocytes, neurons, and endothelial cells (Reilly and Kumari, 1996).

Human Studies. FGF activity appears to be increased in CSF of patients with brain trauma. CSF from two patients with brain injury, collected at 24 h after injury, was added to cultures of PC-12 and NR-119 cells. NR-119 cells respond to NGF only, whereas PC-12 cells respond to both NGF and bFGF with neurite outgrowth. The patients' CSF promoted neurite outgrowth in both cell types. Outgrowth was blocked by anti-NGF sera in NR-119 cells, but not in PC-12 cells, suggesting the presence of non-NGF neurotrophic activity, possibly bFGF (Patterson et al., 1993).

Insulin-like Growth Factors

Animal Studies. Following unilateral direct injury to the rat cortex or overlying dura, IGF-1 mRNA levels increase 5-fold within and adjacent to injured tissue, peaking between 3 to 7 days, and declining by 10 days post injury. Increased expression of IGF-1 mRNA is identified in neurons, astrocytes, and endothelial cells in injured tissue (Sandberg-Nordquist et al., 1996; Walter et al., 1997). IGF-1 protein levels increase in macrophages and endothelial cells within 24 h and in neurons, astrocytes, and microglia within 3 days, peaking within 5 to 7 days after injury (Walter et al., 1997).

Following unilateral injury to the rat cortex or overlying dura, IGF-2 mRNA levels increase in tissue adjacent to injury, especially in astrocytes forming the glia limitans (Walter et al., 1999). Correspondingly, IGF-2 protein levels increase in astrocytes, as well as in some macrophages, microglia, and neurons surrounding focal brain wounds, peaking at 5 to 7 days after injury. IGF-2 protein levels also increase in the CSF (Walter et al., 1999). IGF-1R levels also increase in tissue surrounding focal brain wounds, especially in endothelial cells, neurons, astrocytes, and macrophages, peaking at 5 to 7 days after injury (Walter et al., 1997). IGF-2R levels increase in similar fashion, and remain persistently elevated in astrocytes of the glia limitans for up to 12 days after injury (Walter et al., 1999).

Transforming Growth Factors

Animal Studies. Following focal injury to the rat brain, TGF-β1 mRNA and protein levels increase in tissue adjacent to lesions within one day, peaking at 2 to 4 days, and declining after 7 days. Cells expressing TGFβ1 include macrophages, microglia, astrocytes, and endothelial cells (Logan et al., 1992b).

Human Studies. TGF-β1 levels are increased in the CSF of patients with severe traumatic brain injury at one day after injury (Morganti-Kossmann et al., 1999). However, there appears to be no direct correlation between the magnitude of TGF-β1 elevation and the severity of injury.

Ciliary Neurotrophic Growth Factor

Animal Studies. In a model of bilateral pneumatic compression injury to the rat cortex, CNTF mRNA levels increase 3-fold in injured tissue at 24 to 36 h after injury. In a model of direct unilateral injury to the rat cortex and hippocampus, CNTF protein levels increase in injured tissue at 3 to 7 days after injury. The cells expressing CNTF are astrocytes (Lee et al., 1997; Oyesiku et al., 1999).

Following bilateral or unilateral cortical injury, CNTF receptor mRNA levels decrease in injured and adjacent tissue during the first day after injury (Lee et al., 1997; Oyesiku et al., 1999). In situ hybridization studies show that after cortical injury, CNTF receptor mRNA expression is complex in the hippocampus, decreasing in neurons of the granular layer of the dentate gyrus and increasing in astrocytes of the outer molecular layer (Lee et al., 1997).

Table 7.2 and Figure 7.1 summarize the expression of growth factors in head trauma.

ADMINISTRATION OF GROWTH FACTORS TO INTACT AND INJURED BRAIN

Neurotrophins

Animal Studies. In the intact rat brain, continuous intraventricular infusion of NGF (25 μg to 100 μg) over two weeks results in an increase of choline acetyltransferase (ChAT) activity in septohippocampal cholinergic neurons that is sustained for at least one week after the end of the infusion (Vantini et al., 1990). Following transection of the fimbria fornix in the rat brain, immunohistochemical and morphometric studies show degeneration of cholinergic neurons in the medial septum and diagonal band of Broca.

Table 7.2 Expression of Growth Factors in Head Trauma

Family	Factor		Time of Peak	Animal Studies		Human Studies
				Injured Tissue	Adjacent Non-injured Tissue	CSF
Neurotrophins	NGF	mRNA	24 h	↑	↑	↑
		Protein	3–7 days			
Fibroblast growth factor (FGF)	BDNF	mRNA	12 h	↑	↑	
	bFGF	mRNA	3–7 days	↑	↑	↑
		Protein				
Insulin-like growth factors (IGF)	IGF-1	mRNA	3–7 days			
		Protein				
	IGF-2	Protein	5–7 days	↑	↑	
		Protein				
Transforming growth factor (TGF-β)	TGF-β	mRNA	2–4 days		↑	↑
		Protein				
Ciliary neuronotropic factor (CNTF)	CNTF	mRNA	36 h	↑[a]		
		Protein	7 days			

[a]Following bilateral pneumatic compression injury, whereas following direct brain injury levels of CNTF receptor decrease within and adjacent to injured tissue.

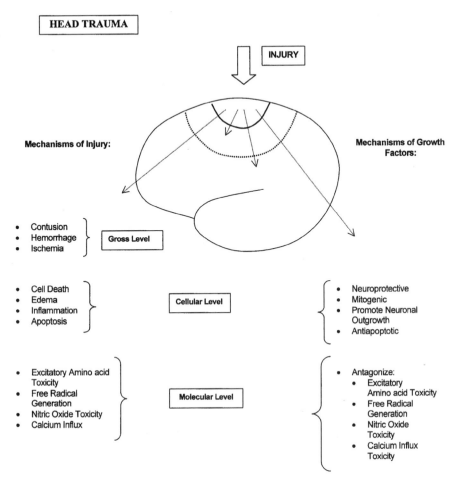

Figure 7.1   Schematic summary of the mechanisms of brain injury during head trauma, and the mechanisms of action of growth factors that result in neurotrophic effects in the injured brain.

Continuous intraventricular infusion of NGF (1 µg/week) starting 3 days before the injury, and continuing for 14 days, reverses this neuronal loss (Williams et al., 1986). Following fimbria fornix lesions in *Macaca fascicularis* monkeys, immuno-histochemical studies show that continuous intraventricular infusion of NGF (0.45 µg/h for 4 weeks), results in increased survival of cholinergic neurons in basal forebrain and increased axonal sprouting of surviving neurons (Tuszynski et al., 1990).

Following unilateral pneumatic brain injury to the rat cortex, continuous intraventricular infusion of NGF (0.3 µg/day for 1 week) improves spatial memory performance but not motor performance. Immunohistochemical studies in these rats show that the posttraumatic reduction in the number and crosssectional area of ChAT-positive septal neurons is completely prevented by NGF infusion (Dixon et al., 1997).

Following unilateral transection of the fimbria in the rat brain, immunohisto-chemical studies show that intraseptal BDNF infusion (12 μg/day for 2 weeks), preserves 60% of the medial septal ChAT neurons at the site of the injury, compared to 44% of ChAT neurons preserved after intraventricular BDNF infusion, and 28% of ChAT neurons preserved in vehicle-infused animals (Morse et al., 1993).

Human Studies. To date, the only studies of neurotrophin administration in humans have been done on patients with Alzheimer's disease and amyotrophic lateral schlerosis (ALS). NGF has been infused intraventricularly in three patients with Alzheimer's disease for three months. In two patients continuous infusions of a total of 6.6 mg of NGF were given, and in the third patient a total of 0.5 mg in three short periods was given. Minimal cognitive improvement was obtained, but significant side effects consisted of dose-related back pain, which occurred in all three patients, and weight loss, which occurred in the two patients who received 6.6 mg of NGF (Eriksdotter Jonhagen et al., 1998).

In a randomized, placebo-controlled, double-blind phase III trial of subcutaneous administration of BDNF in patients with ALS, no overall efficacy was seen in patient survival, although in post hoc analysis a subgroup of patients with early respiratory compromise seemed to benefit. The study duration was 9 months and there were three treatment arms: 25 μg/kg per day, 100 μg/kg per day, and placebo. No major side effects were seen with BDNF treatment in this study (The BDNF Study Group, 1999).

Fibroblast Growth Factors

Animal Studies. In the intact rat brain, intracortical infusion of a single dose of bFGF (4.0 ng) elevates GFAP mRNA levels within 3 days, increases the number of GFAP-positive astrocytes at 3 days, and increases the length and number of astrocytic processes by 7 days (Eclancher et al., 1996). Following direct mechanical injury to rat brain, immediate intralesional administration of bFGF (2 to 200 mg) increases GFAP mRNA levels 6-fold by 3 days post infusion, and promotes astrocyte hypertrophy, macrophage proliferation, and an increase in terminal astrocyte branching in the injured tissue. By 20 days post infusion, reactive gliosis is noticed (Menon and Landerholm, 1994; Eclancher et al., 1996). Following fluid percussion injury to rat brain, intravenous administration of bFGF (45 μg/kg per h beginning at 30 min and lasting for 3 h after injury) results in a significant reduction in the volume of focal contusion and in the number of necrotic cortical neurons (Dietrich et al., 1996). Delayed intralesional administration of bFGF, starting at 24 h after fluid percussion injury in rat brain, attenuates cognitive dysfunction. When given at this later time point, bFGF does not reduce contusion volume, but there is a trend of increased astrocytosis in the injured cortex (McDermott et al., 1997).

Human Studies. Human studies of the administration of bFGF in head injury have not yet been done, but studies of bFGF in stroke have been undertaken. In spite of initial studies showing safety, a large-scale North American study showed that a dose of 5 to 10 mg of bFGF given intravenously over 8 h was too high, causing unacceptable side effects (Clark et al., 2000). On the other hand, doses of 5 to 10 mg given intravenously over 24 h were safe in a European trial (Bogousslavsky et al., 2000). Moreover, an interim analysis of this trial showed some trends toward efficacy.

Insulin-like Growth Factors

Animal Studies. In a study of fluid percussion brain injury in rats, subcutaneous administration of IGF-1, 1.0 mg/kg twice daily or 4.0 mg/kg per day infused continuously for 14 days, both starting 15 min after injury, results in the attenuation of sensorimotor deficits and enhanced memory and learning of visuospatial tasks (Saatman et al., 1997).

Human Studies. A phase II open-label prospective randomized study to assess the safety and efficacy of intravenous administration of recombinant human IGF-I (rh-IGF-I) was conducted on patients with closed head injury. Within 72 h after injury, patients with moderate to severe head injury received rh-IGF-I in a continuous infusion of 0.01 mg/kg per h for 14 days. At the end of 14 days, clinical outcome scales and metabolical parameters were assessed. There was a positive trend on improvement of neurological outcome, and on better nutritional outcome in the group of patients who received rh-IGF-I. No serious life-threatening events were noted (Hatton et al., 1997).

Ciliary Neurotrophic Factor

Animal Studies. Intralesional administration of CNTF (1.0 μL containing 100 ng) at the time of injury in a model of cortical brain injury in rats resulted in upregulation of GFAP mRNA within 10 h in gray and subcortical white matter, normalizing after 72 h, whereas vimentin (another glial marker) mRNA levels increased by 24 h, peaking at 48 h and remaining elevated at 72 h, mainly in the subcortical white matter. Immunohistochemical and morphological studies show that GFAP and vimentin protein levels are increased at 48 h in the gray and subcortical white matter, and show astrocyte hypertrophy in the injected hemisphere (Levison et al., 1996; Hudgins and Levison, 1998).

Human Studies. To date, no studies of CNTF administration have been done in patients with head injury. However, clinical trials have been conducted in patients with ALS. These trials failed to show benefit, and CNTF treatment was associated with significant side effects, including stomatitis, cough, asthenia, and anti-rhCTNF antibody formation, causing some patients to withdraw from the study (ALS CNTF Treatment Study Group, 1996).

CONCLUSION

In summary, the available data demonstrate a complex pattern of changes of growth factor expression after brain trauma. In particular, the expression of many growth factors and their receptors increase in tissue directly affected by and surrounding focal brain wounds. Many questions remain to be resolved about the role of endogenous growth factor expression after brain injury. Do growth factors participate in the processes of cell survival versus cell death after injury? Do growth factors contribute to repair and recovery processes following injury, including neuronal sprouting and new synapse formation? If so, what is the relative contribution of each factor to these processes? How do factors interact? What are the molecular (i.e., signal transduction) mechanisms by which growth factors exert their effects in the injured brain?

The answers to such questions may lead to the eventual application of growth factors as molecular treatments for brain injury, both as agents to enhance cell survival following acute injury and as agents to enhance recovery and repair processes in chronic brain injury. Advances in recombinant DNA technology and protein chemistry have made possible the commercial synthesis of large amounts of pharmaceutical-grade growth factors. Moreover, based on understanding of ligand–receptor interactions, it is possible to design and synthesize small-molecule "growth factor-mimetic" compounds that more easily cross the blood–brain barrier. Finally, growth factors may find a useful role as adjunct treatments to be given in combination with promising cell-based (including stem cell) treatments for brain injury.

ABBREVIATIONS

ALS	Amyotrophic lateral schlerosis
NGF	Nerve growth factor
BDNF	Brain-derived neurotrophic factor
NT-3	Neurotrophin-3
NT-4/5	Neurotrophin-4/5
aFGF	Acidic fibroblast growth factor
bFGF	Basic fibroblast growth factor
IGF	Insulin-like growth factor
EGF	Epidermal growth factor
TGF-α	Transforming growth factor-α
HB-EGF	Heparin binding EGF-like factor
TGF-β	Transforming growth factor-β
BMP	Bone morphogenetic protein
OP-1	Osteogenic protein-1

CNTF	Ciliary Neurotrophic Factor
MPTP	1-Methyl-4-phenyl-1,2,3,6-tetrahydropyridine
FGFR	Fibroblast growth factor receptor
eNOS	Endothelial nitric oxide synthase
IGFBP	IGF-binding protein
CNS	Central nervous system
ChAT	Choline acetyltransferase
GFAP	Glial fibrillary acidic protein

REFERENCES

J. A. Abraham, J. L. Whang, A. Tumolo, A. Mergia, J. Friedman, D. Gospodarowicz, and J. C. Fiddes, *EMBO J.*, 5, 2523–2528 (1986).

R. F. Alderson, A. L. Alterman, Y. A. Barde, and R. M. Lindsay, *Neuron*, 5, 297–306 (1990).

ALS CNTF Treatment Study Group, *Neurology*, 46, 1244–1249 (1996).

S. C. Apfel. *Clinical Applications of Neurotrophic Factors*, Lippincott-Raven, Philadelphia, 1997, p. 20.

M. A. Bach, Z. Shen-Orr, W. L. Lowe Jr., C. T. Roberts Jr., and D. LeRoith, *Brain Res. Mol. Brain Res.*, 10, 43–48 (1991).

G. Barbin, M. Manthorpe, and S. Varon, *J. Neurochem.*, **43**, 1468–1478 (1984).

J. F. Bazan, *Neuron*, 7, 197–208 (1991).

D. J. Berlove and S. P. Finklestein, "Growth factors and brain injury," in T. W. Moody, Ed., *Growth Factors, Peptides and Receptors*, Plenum Press, New York, 1993, pp. 137–147.

L. Bertollini, M. T. Ciotti, E. Cherubini, and A. Cattaneo, *Brain Res.*, 746, 19–24 (1997).

J. Bogousslavski, G. A. Donnan, C. Fieschi, M. Kaste, J.-M. Orgozozo, A. Chamorro, and S. J. Victor for the European Australian Fiblast (Trafermin) in Acute Stroke Group, *Cerebrovasc. Dis.*, 10(S2), 1–116 (2000).

C. Bondy, H. Werner, C. T. Roberts, Jr., and D. LeRoith, *Neuroscience*, 46, 909–923 (1992).

M. Bottner, K. Unsicker, and C. Suter-Crazzolara, *Neuroreport*, 7, 2903–2907 (1996).

A. Buisson, O. Nicole, F. Docagne, H. Sartelet, E. T. Mackenzie, and D. Vivien, *FASEB J.*, 12, 1683–1691 (1998).

C. G. Caday, M. Klagsbrun, P. J. Fanning, A. Mirzabegian, and S. P. Finklestein, *Brain Res. Dev. Brain Res.*, 52, 241–246 (1990).

S. R. Cajal, *Degeneration and regeneration of the nervous system*. Translated by Raoul M. May, Oxford University Press, London, 1928.

D. Casper, G. J. Roboz, and M. Blum, *J. Neurochem.*, 62, 2166–2177 (1994).

M. V. Chao, *Neuron*, 9, 583–593 (1992).

M. V. Chao, *J. Neurobiol.*, 25, 1373–1385 (1994).

K. E. Chen and S. P. Finklestein, "Ischemic Stroke: From Basic Mechanisms to New Drug Development," in C. Y. Hsu, Ed., *Monographs in Clinical Neuroscience*, Vol. 16, Basel, Karger, 1998, pp. 116–126.

B. Cheng and M. P. Mattson, *J. Neurosci.*, 12, 1558–1566 (1992).

B. Cheng, Y. Goodman, J. G. Begley, and M. P. Mattson, *Brain Res.*, 650, 331–335 (1994).

H. L. Cheng, K. A. Sullivan, and E. L. Feldman, *Brain Res. Dev. Brain Res.*, 92, 211–218 (1996).

W. M. Clark, J. D. Schim, S. E. Kasner, S. J. Victor, and the Fiblast Stroke Study Investigators, *Neurology*, 54 (Suppl. 3), A88 (2000).

P. A. D'Amore, *Cancer Metastasis Rev.*, 9, 227–238 (1990).

S. Davis, T. H. Aldrich, N. Stahl, L. Pan, T. Taga, T. Kishimoto, N. Y. Ip, and G. D. Yancopoulos, *Science*, 260, 1805–1808 (1993).

C. J. De Groot, L. Montagne, A. D. Barten, P. Sminia, and P. Van Der Valk, *J. Neuropathol. Exp. Neurol.*, 58, 174–187 (1999).

S. T. DeKosky, J. R. Goss, P. D. Miller, S. D. Styren, P. M. Kochanek, and D. Marion, *Exp. Neurol.*, 130, 173–177 (1994).

K. D. Dentremont, P. Ye, A. J. D'Ercole, and J. R. O'Kusky, *Brain Res. Dev. Brain Res.*, 114, 135–141 (1999).

A. J. D'Ercole, P. Ye, A. S. Calikoglu, and G. Gutierrez-Ospina, *Mol. Neurobiol.*, 13, 227–255 (1996).

W. D. Dietrich, O. Alonso, R. Busto, and S. P. Finklestein, *J. Neurotrauma*, 13, 309–316 (1996).

C. E. Dixon, B. G. Lyeth, J. T. Povlishock, R. L. Findling, R. J. Hamm, A. Marmarou, H. F. Young, and R. L. Hayes, *J. Neurosurg.*, 67, 110–119 (1997).

R. T. Dobrowsky, M. H. Werner, A. M. Castellino, M. V. Chao, and Y. A. Hannun, *Science*, 265, 1596–1599 (1994).

F. Eclancher, P. Kehrli, G. Labourdette, and M. Sensenbrenner, *Brain Res.*, 737, 201–214 (1996).

A. el-D. El-Husseini, J. A. Paterson, and R. P. Shiu, *Mol. Cell Endocrinol.*, 104, 191–200 (1994).

N. Emoto, A. M. Gonzalez, P. A. Walicke, E. Wada, D. M. Simmons, S. Shimasaki, and A. Baird, *Growth Factors*, 2, 21–29 (1989).

M. Eriksdotter Jonhagen, A. Nordberg, K. Amberla, L. Backman, T. Ebendal, B. Meyerson, L. Olson, A. Seiger, M. Shigeta, E. Theodorsson, M. Viitanen, B. Winblad, and L. O. Wahlund, *Dement. Geriatr. Cogn. Disord.*, 9, 246–257 (1998).

F. Esch, A. Baird, N. Ling, N. Ueno, F. Hill, L. Denoroy, R. Klepper, D. Gospodarowicz, P. Bohlen, and R. Guillemin, *Proc. Natl. Acad. Sci. USA*, 82, 6507–6511 (1986).

S. P. Finklestein, A. Kemmou, C. G. Caday, and D. J. Berlove, *Stroke*, 24 (12 Suppl.), I141–143 (1993).

R. Forough, Z. Xi, M. MacPhee, S. Friedman, K. A. Engleka, T. Sayers, R. H. Wiltrout, and T. Maciag, *J. Biol. Chem.*, 268, 2960–2968 (1993).

J. Forsmann, *Beitr. Path. Anat. Allg. Path.*, 24, 56–100 (1898).

S. A. Frautschy, P. A. Walicke, and A. Baird, *Brain Res.*, 553, 291–299 (1991).

A. Freese, S. P. Finklestein, and M. Difiglia, *Brain Res.*, 575, 351–355 (1992).

D. Galter, M. Bottner, and K. Unsicker, *J. Neurosci. Res.*, 56, 531–538 (1999).

W. Q. Gao, J. L. Zheng, and M. Karihaloo, *J. Neurosci.*, 15, 2656–2667 (1995).

L. M. Garcia-Segura, J. R. Rodriguez, and I. Torres-Aleman, *J. Neurocytol.*, 26, 479–490 (1997).

G. M. Gilad and V. H. Gilad, *J. Neurosci. Res.*, 41, 594–602 (1995).

D. R. Goddard, M. Berry, and A. M. Butt, *J. Neurosci. Res.*, 57, 74–85 (1999).

F. Gomez-Pinilla, D. J. Knauer, and M. Nieto-Sampedro, *Brain Res.*, 438, 385–390 (1988).

A. M. Gonzalez, D. J. Hill, A. Logan, P. A. Maher, and A. Baird, *Pediatr. Res.*, 39, 375–385 (1996).

D. Gospodarowicz, G. Neufeld, and L. Schweigerer, *J. Cell Physiol. Suppl.* (Suppl. 5), 15–26 (1987).

C. E. Gross, M. M. Bednar, D. B. Howard, and M. B. Sporn, *Stroke*, 24, 558–562 (1993).

A. K. Hall and M. S. Rao, *Trends Neurosci.*, 15, 35–37 (1992).

Y. Hashimoto, Y. Abiru, C. Nishio, H. Hatanaka, *Brain Res. Dev. Brain Res.*, 115, 25–32 (1999).

J. Hatton, R. P. Rapp, K. A. Kudsk, R. O. Brown, M. S. Luer, J. G. Bukar, S. A. Chen, C. J. McClain, N. Gesundheit, R. J. Dempsey, and B. Young, *J. Neurosurg.*, 86, 779–786 (1997).

Y. Hayase, S. Higashiyama, M. Sasahara, S. Amano, T. Nakagawa, N. Taniguchi, and F. Hazama, *Brain Res.*, 784, 163–178 (1998).

F. Hefti, *J. Neurosci.*, 6, 2155–2162 (1986).

J. T. Henderson, N. A. Seniuk, and J. C. Roder, *Brain Res. Mol. Brain Res.*, 22, 151–165 (1994).

R. R. Hicks, S. Numan, H. S. Dhillon, M. R. Prasad, and K. B. Seroogy, *Brain Res. Mol. Brain Res.*, 48, 401–406 (1997).

R. R. Hicks, C. Li, L. Zhang, H. S. Dhillon, M. R. Prasad, and K. B. Seroogy, *J. Neurotrauma*, 16, 501–510 (1999).

M. Hofer, S. R. Pagliusi, A. Hohn, J. Leibrock, and Y. A. Barde, *EMBO J.*, 9, 2459–2464 (1990).

S. N. Hudgins and S. W. Levison, *Exp. Neurol.*, 150, 171–182 (1998).

C. Hyman, M. Hofer, Y. A. Barde, M. Juhasz, G. D. Yancopoulos, and S. P. Squinto, *Nature*, 350, 230–232 (1991).

H. Ibelgaufts, *Dictionary of Cytokines*, Verlagsgesellschaft mbH, Weinheim, 1995a, pp. 356–357.

H. Ibelgaufts, *Dictionary of Cytokines*, Verlagsgesellschaft mbH, Weinheim, 1995b, p. 307.

H. Ibelgaufts, *Dictionary of Cytokines*, Verlagsgesellschaft mbH, Weinheim, 1995c, pp. 96–97.

N. Y. Ip, Y. P. Li, I. van de Stadt, N. Panayotatos, R. F. Alderson, and R. M. Lindsay, *J. Neurosci.*, 11, 3124–3134 (1991).

A. Ishihara, H. Saito, and K. Abe, *Brain Res.*, 639, 21–25 (1994).

R. Ishikawa, K. Nishikori, and S. Furukawa, *J. Neurochem.*, 56, 836–841 (1991).

M. Jaye, R. Howk, W. Burgess, G. A. Ricca, I. M. Chiu, M. W. Ravera, S. J. O'Brien, W. S. Modi, T. Maciag, and W. N. Drohan, *Science*, 233, 541–545 (1986).

F. Jiang, S. W. Levison, and T. L. Wood, *J. Neurosci. Res.*, 57, 447–457 (1999).

C. J. Kane, G. J. Brown, and K. D. Phelan, *Brain Res. Dev. Brain Res.*, 96, 46–51 (1996).

S. Kar, J. G. Chabot, and R. Quirion, *Comp. Neurol.*, 333, 375–397 (1993).

R. Katoh-Semba, Y. Kaisho, A. Shintani, M. Nagahama, and K. Kato, *J. Neurochem.*, 66, 330–337 (1996).

R. Katoh-Semba, R. Semba, I. K. Takeuchi, and K. Kato, *Neurosci. Res.*, 31, 227–234 (1998).

T. Kawamata, D. W. Dietrich, T. Schallert, J. E. Gotts, R. R. Cocke, L. I. Benowitz, and S. P. Finklestein, *Proc. Natl. Acad. Sci. USA*, 94, 8179–8184 (1997).

T. Kawamata, J. Ren, T. C. K. Chan, M. Charette, and S. P. Finklestein, *Neuroreport*, 9, 1441–1445 (1998).

M. Kirsch and H. D. Hofmann, *Neurosci. Lett.*, 180, 163–166 (1994).

D. L. Kitchens, E. Y. Snyder, and D. I. Gottlieb, *J. Neurobiol.*, 35, 797–807 (1994).

R. Klein, F. Lamballe, S. Bryant, and M. Barbacid, *Neuron*, 8, 947–956 (1992).

B. Knusel, P. P. Michel, J. S. Schwaber, and F. Hefti, *J. Neurosci.*, 10, 558–570 (1990).

S. Koh, G. A. Oyler, and G. A. Higgins, *Exp. Neurol.*, 106, 209–221 (1989).

S. M. Kolodziejczyk and B. K. Hall, *Biochem. Cell Biol.*, 74, 299–314 (1996).

H. I. Kornblum, H. K. Raymon, R. S. Morrison, K. P. Cavanaugh, R. A. Bradshaw, and F. M. Leslie, *Brain Res.*, 535, 255–263 (1990).

S. Korsching, G. Auburger, R. Heumann, J. Scott, and H. Thoenen, *EMBO J.*, 4, 1389–1393 (1985).

T. Kossmann, V. Hans, H. G. Imhof, O. Trentz, and M. C. Morganti-Kossmann, *Brain Res.*, 713, 143–152 (1996).

T. Kossmann, P. F. Stahel, P. M. Lenzlinger, H. Redl, R. W. Dubs, O. Trentz, G. Schlag, and M. C. Morganti-Kossmann, *J. Cereb. Blood Flow Metab.*, 17, 280–289 (1997).

F. Lamballe, R. Klein, and M. Barbacid, *Cell*, 66, 967–979 (1991).

L. Larkfors, R. M. Lindsay, and R. F. Alderson, *Eur. J. Neurosci.*, 6, 1015–1025 (1994).

L. M. Lazar and M. Blum, *J. Neurosci.*, 12, 1688–1697 (1992).

M. Y. Lee, T. Deller, M. Kirsch, M. Frotscher, and H. D. Hofmann, *J. Neurosci.*, 17, 1137–1146 (1997).

J. Leibrock, F. Lottspeich, A. Hohn, M. Hofer, B. Hengerer, P. Masiakowski, H. Thoenen, and Y. A. Barde, *Nature*, 341, 149–152 (1989).

D. LeRoith, C. T. Roberts, Jr., H. Werner, C. Bondy, M. Raizada, and M. L. Adamo, "Insulin-like Growth Factors in the Brain," in S. E. Loughlin and J. H. Fallon, Eds., *Neurotrophic Factors*, Academic Press, Inc., San Diego, 1993, p. 399.

R. Levi-Montalcini, *Science*, 237, 1154–1162 (1987).

S. W. Levison, M. H. Ducceschi, G. M. Young, and T. L. Wood, *Exp. Neurol.*, 141, 256–268 (1996).

S. W. Levison, S. N. Hudgins, and J. L. Crawford, *Brain Res.*, 803, 189–193 (1998).

R. M. Lindsay and A. J. Harmar, *Nature*, 337, 362–364 (1989).

F. Lisovoski, S. Akli, E. Peltekian, E. Vigne, G. Haase, M. Perricaudet, P. A. Dreyfus, A. Kahn, and M. Peschanski, *J. Neurosci.*, 17, 7228–7236 (1997).

A. Logan, S. A. Frautschy, A. M. Gonzales, and A. Baird, *J. Neurosci.*, 12, 3828–3837 (1992a).

A. Logan, S. A. Frautschy, A. M. Gonzales, M. B. Sporn, and A. Baird, *Brain Res.*, 587, 215–225 (1992b).

P. C. Mabie, M. F. Mehler, R. Marmur, A. Papavasiliou, Q. Song, and J. A. Kessler, *J. Neurosci.*, 17, 4112–4120 (1997).

A. J. MacLennan, A. A. Gaskin, and D. C. Lado, *Brain Res. Mol. Brain Res.*, 25, 251–256 (1994).

N. K. Mahanthappa and G. A. Schwarting, *Neuron*, 10, 293–305 (1993).

P. C. MaisonPierre, L. Belluscio, B. Friedman, R. F. Alderson, S. J. Wiegand, M. E. Furth, R. M. Lindsay, and G. D. Yancopoulos, *Neuron*, 5, 501–509 (1990).

J. Massague, *Annu. Rev. Biochem.*, 67, 753–791 (1998).

K. L. McDermott, R. Raghupathi, S. C. Fernandez, K. E. Saatman, A. A. Protter, S. P. Finklestein, G. Sinson, D. H. Smith, and T. K. McIntosh, *J. Neurotrauma*, 14, 191–200 (1997).

S. O. Meakin, U. Suter, C. C. Drinkwater, A. A. Welcher, and E. M. Shooter, *Proc. Natl. Acad. Sci. USA*, 89, 2374–2378 (1992).

V. K. Menon and T. E. Landerholm, *Exp. Neurol.*, 129, 142–154 (1994).

A. Mergia, R. Eddy, J. A. Abraham, J. C. Fiddes, and T. B. Shows, *Biochem. Biophys. Res. Commun.*, 138, 644–651 (1986).

R. Mewar and F. A. McMorris, *J. Neurosci. Res.*, 50, 721–728 (1997).

P. Mignatti, T. Morimoto, and D. B. Rifkin, *J. Cell Physiol.*, 151, 81–93 (1992).

I. Moccheti and J. R. Wrathall, *J. Neurotrauma*, 12, 853–870 (1995).

G. Morfini, M. C. DiTella, F. Feiguin, N. Carri, and A. Caceres, *J. Neurosci. Res.*, 39, 219–232 (1994).

M. C. Morganti-Kossmann, V. H. Hans, P. M. Lenzlinger, R. Dubs, E. Ludwig, O. Trentz, and T. Kossmann, *J. Neurotrauma*, 16, 617–628 (1999).

R. Morrison, "Epidermal Growth Factor: Structure, Expression, and Functions in the Central Nervous System," in S. E. Loughlin and J. H. Fallon, Eds., *Neurotrophic Factors*, Academic Press, Inc., San Diego, 1993, p. 340.

R. S. Morrison, R. F. Keating, and J. R. Moskal, *J. Neurosci. Res.*, 21, 71–79 (1988).

J. K. Morse, S. J. Wiegand, K. Anderson, Y. You, N. Cai. J. Carnahan, J. Miller, P. S. DiStefano, C. A. Altar, R. M. Lindsay, et al., *J. Neurosci.*, 13, 4146–4156 (1993).

N. Nakao, P. Odin, O. Lindvall, and P. Brundin, *Exp. Neurol.*, 138, 144–157 (1996).

W. Ni, K. Rajkumar, J. I. Nagy, and L. J. Murphy, *Brain Res.*, 769, 97–107 (1997).

M. M. Niblock, J. K. Brunso-Bechtold, C. D. Lynch, R. L. Ingram, T. McShane, and W. E. Sonntag, *Brain Res.*, 804, 79–86 (1998).

M. M. Niblock, J. K. Brunso-Bechtold, and D. R. Riddle, *J. Neurosci.*, 20, 4165–4176 (2000).

F. C. Nielson, E. Wang, and S. Gammeltoft, *J. Neurochem.*, 56, 12–21 (1991).

T. Nishio, S. Furukawa, I. Akiguchi, N. Oka, K. Ohnishi, H. Tomimoto, S. Nakamura, and J. Kimura, *Neuroscience*, 60, 67–84 (1994).

N. M. Oyesiku, C. O. Evans, S. Houston, R. S. Darrell, J. S. Smith, Z. L. Fulop, C. E. Dixon, and D. G. Stein, *Brain Res.*, 833, 161–172 (1999).

T. D. Palmer, E. A. Markakis, A. R. Willhoite, F. Safar, and F. H. Gage, *J. Neurosci.*, 19, 8487–8497 (1999).

S. L. Patterson, M. S. Grady, and M. Bothwell, *Brain Res.*, 605, 43–49 (1993).

F. Perraud, G. Labourdette, M. Miehe, C. Loret, and M. Sensenbrenner, *J. Neurosci. Res.*, 20, 1–11 (1988).

J. H. Prehn, C. Backhauss, and J. Krieglstein, *J. Cereb. Blood Flow Metab.*, 13, 521–525 (1993).

P. Puolakkainen and D. R. Twardzik, "Transforming Growth Factors," in S. E. Loughlin and J. H. Fallon, Eds., *Neurotrophic Factors*, Academic Press, Inc., San Diego, 1993a, p. 365.

P. Puolakkainen and D. R. Twardzik, "Transforming Growth Factors," in S. E. Loughlin and J. H. Fallon, Eds., *Neurotrophic Factors*, Academic Press, Inc., San Diego, 1993b, p. 371.

J. Ray, A. Baird, and F. H. Gage, *Proc. Natl. Acad. Sci. USA*, 94, 7047–7052 (1997).

L. Regli, R. E. Anderson, and F. B. Meyer, *Brain Res.*, 665, 155–157 (1994).

J. F. Reilly and V. G. Kumari, *Exp. Neurol.*, 140, 139–150 (1996).

P. M. Richardson, V. M. Issa, and R. J. Riopelle, *J. Neurosci.*, 6, 2312–2321 (1986).

M. Roghani, A. Mansukhani, P. Dell'Era, P. Bellosta, C. Basilico, D. B. Rifkin, and D. Moscatelli, *J. Biol. Chem.*, 269, 3976–3984 (1994).

S. Rosenblatt, K. Irikura, C. G. Caday, S. P. Finklestein, and M. A. Moskowitz, *J. Cereb. Blood Flow Metab.*, 14, 70–74.

K. E. Saatman, P. C. Contreras, D. H. Smith, R. Raghupathi, K. L. McDermott, S. C. Fernandez, K. L. Sanderson, M. Voddi, and T. K. McIntosh, *Exp. Neurol.*, 147, 418–427 (1997).

H. Sakamoto, H. Kuzuya, M. Tamaru, S. Sugimoto, J. Shimizu, M. Fukushima, T. Yazaki, T. Yamazaki, Y. Nagata, *Neurochem. Res.*, 23, 115–120 (1998).

A. C. Sandberg Nordqvist, H. von Holst, S. Holmin, V. R. Sara, B. M. Bellander, and M. Schalling, *Brain Res. Mol. Brain Res.*, 38, 285–293 (1996).

R. Schechter, M. Abboud, and G. Johnson, *Brain Res. Dev. Brain Res.*, 116, 159–167 (1999).

M. Seiler and M. E. Schwab, *Brain Res.*, 300, 33–39 (1984).

N. A. Seniuk-Tatton, J. T. Henderson, and J. C. Roder, *J. Neurosci. Res.*, 41, 663–676 (1995).

K. B. Seroogy, K. H. Lundgren, D. C. Lee, K. M. Guthrie, and C. M. Gall, *J. Neurochem.*, 60, 1777–1782 (1993).

R. M. Sherrard, N. A. Richardson, and V. R. Sara, *Brain Res. Dev. Brain Res.*, 98, 102–113 (1997).

S. Soderstrom, H. Bengtsson, and T. Ebendal, *Cell Tissue Res.*, 286, 269–279 (1996).

W. E. Sonntag, C. D. Lynch, S. A. Bennett, A. S. Khan, P. L. Thornton, P. T. Cooney, R. L. Ingram, T. McShane, and J. K. Brunso-Bechtold, *Neuroscience*, 88, 269–279 (1999).

M. B. Spina, S. P. Squinto, J. Miller, R. M. Lindsay, and C. Hyman, *J. Neurochem.*, 59, 99–106 (1992).

S. P. Squinto, T. N. Stitt, T. H. Aldrich, S. M. Bianco, C. Radziejewski, D. J. Glass, P. Masiakowski, M. E. Furth, D. M. Valenzuela, et al., *Cell*, 65, 885–893 (1991).

A. Stock, K. Kuzis, W. R. Woodward, R. Nishi, and F. P. Eckenstein, *J. Neurosci.*, 12, 4688–4700 (1992).

K. A. Stockli, F. Lottspeich, M. Sendtner, P. Masiakowski, P. Carroll, R. Gotz, D. Lindholm, and H. Theonen, *Nature*, 342, 920–923 (1989).

T. Tomoda, T. Shirasawa, Y. I. Yahagi, K. Ishii, H. Takagi, Y. Furiya, K. I. Arai, H. Mori, and M. A. Muramatsu, *Dev. Biol.*, 179, 79–90 (1996).

The BDNF Study Group, *Neurology*, 52, 1427–1433 (1999).

K. A. Thomas, "Fibroblast Growth Factors,' in S. E. Loughlin and J. H. Fallon, Eds., *Neurotrophic Factors*, Academic Press, Inc., San Diego, 1993a, pp. 288–291.

K. A. Thomas, "Fibroblast Growth Factors,' in S. E. Loughlin and J. H. Fallon, Eds., *Neurotrophic Factors*, Academic Press, Inc., San Diego, 1993b, pp. 292–294.

N. D. Tran, J. Correale, S. S. Schreiber, and M. Fisher, *Stroke*, 30, 1671–1678 (1999).

M. S. Tucker, I. Khan, R. Fuchs-Young, S. Price, T. L. Steininger, G. Greene, B. H. Wainer, and M. R. Rosner, *Brain Res.*, 631, 65–71 (1993).

M. H. Tuszynski, H. S. U, D. G. Amaral, and F. H. Gage, *J. Neurosci.*, 10, 3604–3614 (1990).

K. Unsicker, K. C. Flanders, D. S. Cissel, R. Lafyatis, and M. B. Sporn, *Neuroscience*, 44, 613–625 (1991).

G. Vantini, M. Fusco, N. Schiavo, M. Gradkowska, M. Zaremba, A. Leon, and B. Oderfeld-Nowak, *Acta Neurobiol. Exp. (Warsz)*, 50, 323–331 (1990).

C. Vicario-Abejon, C. Collin, R. D. McKay, and M. Segal, *J. Neurosci.*, 18, 7256–7271 (1998).

H. J. Walter, M. Berry, D. J. Hill, S. Cwyfan-Hughes, J. M. Holly, and A. Logan, *Endocrinology*, 140, 520–532 (1999).

H. J. Walter, M. Berry, D. J. Hill, and A. Logan, *Endocrinology*, 138, 3024–3034 (1997).

A. Wanaka, E. M. Johnson, Jr., and J. Milbrandt, *Neuron*, 5, 267–281 (1990).

D. Watanabe, R. Yoshimura, M. Khalil, K. Yoshida, T. Kishimoto, T. Taga, and H. Kiyama, *Eur. J. Neurosci.*, 8, 1630–1640, (1996).

M. H. Werner, L. B. Nanney, C. M. Stoscheck, and L. E. King, *J. Histochem. Cytochem.*, 36, 81–86 (1988).

B. C. White, G. S. Krause, *Ann. Emerg. Med.*, 22, 970–979 (1993).

B. J. Wilcox and J. R. Unnerstall, *Neuron*, 6, 397–409 (1991).

L. R. Williams, S. Varon, G. M. Peterson, K. Wictorin, W. Fischer, A. Bjorklund, and F. H. Gage, *Proc. Natl. Acad. Sci. USA*, 83, 9231–9235 (1986).

W. R. Woodward, R. Nichi, C. K. Meshul, T. E. Williams, M. Coulombe, and F. P. Eckenstein, *J. Neurosci.*, 12, 142–152 (1992).

J. L. Wrana, *Miner. Electrolyte Metab.*, 24, 120–130 (1998).

Q. Yan and E. M. Johnson, Jr., *J. Comp. Neurol.*, 290, 585–598 (1989).

S. Y. Yang and J. Z. Cui, *J. Neurosurg.*, 89, 297–302 (1998).

S. H. Zhang, X. F. Zhou, Y. S. Deng, and R. A. Rush, *J. Neurosci. Methods*, 89, 69–74 (1999).

X. Zhou, J. P. Herman, and C. M. Paden, *Exp. Neurol.*, 159, 419–432 (1999).

X. Zhu, H. Komiya, A. Chirino, S. Faham, G. M. Fox, T. Arakawa, B. T. Hsu, and D. C. Rees, *Science*, 251, 90–93 (1991).

CHAPTER 8

THE INFLAMMATORY RESPONSE AS A THERAPEUTIC TARGET IN TRAUMATIC BRAIN INJURY

PATRICK M. KOCHANEK[1,4], MICHAEL J. WHALEN[1], TIMOTHY M. CARLOS[2], ROBERT S. B. CLARK[1,4], C. EDWARD DIXON[3], STEVEN T. DeKOSKY[5], and DONALD W. MARION[3]

Departments of [1]Anesthesiology and Critical Care Medicine, [2]Medicine, [3]Neurological Surgery, [4]Pediatrics, and [5]Psychiatry and Neurology, University of Pittsburgh, Pittsburgh, Pennsylvania

INTRODUCTION

Despite its importance as a public health problem, the mainstay of treatment of traumatic brain injury remains supportive care. A large number of cellular, molecular and biochemical cascades have been suggested to contribute to the evolution of secondary damage after the primary traumatic event; however, the quantitative contribution of each of these cascades remains to be determined. One such cascade that has been touted to contribute importantly to the evolution of secondary damage is the local inflammatory response in the injured brain. Although the brain has traditionally been considered to be immunologically privileged, and unlikely to be influenced by aspects of the inflammatory process, a large body of recent data suggests that there is a marked local inflammatory response to injury, and that selected aspects of this response amplify the secondary damage.

The inflammatory response to traumatic brain injury is highly complex and involves both local and systemic events. These events have acute, subacute, and chronic components. Further complicating this situation is the fact that both deleterious and beneficial aspects of the inflammatory response appear to play roles in both the local and systemic compartments. This chapter will focus on

Head Trauma: Basic, Preclinical, and Clinical Directions, Edited by Leonard P. Miller and Ronald L. Hayes, Co-edited by Jennifer K. Newcomb
ISBN 0-471-36015-5 © 2001 John Wiley & Sons, Inc.

selected aspects of the local acute inflammatory response to traumatic brain injury—specifically, those that represent putative targets for anti-inflammatory therapy. Studies addressing the use of therapeutic approaches directed toward interleukin-1β (IL-1β), tumor necrosis factor α (TNF-α), IL-10, and neutrophils will be reviewed. Studies carried out both in experimental models of traumatic brain injury and in patients with severe head injury are reviewed and discussed. In selected cases, we also incorporate into this review important findings in other forms of central nervous system injury, such as spinal cord injury and, rarely, cerebral ischemia. A comprehensive review of the inflammatory response to cerebral ischemia was recently published (Barone and Feuerstein, 1999).

INTERLEUKIN-1β

A role for the proinflammatory cytokine IL-1β in traumatic brain injury was suggested by Giulian and Lachman as early as 1985. Reports from several laboratories demonstrated increases in IL-1β activity in the initial 72 h after focal experimental trauma in rat brain (Nieto-Sampedro and Berman, 1987; Woodroofe et al., 1991). These initial reports describing increases in IL-1β activity, assessed by bioassay, were subsequently confirmed by a number of studies examining expression of IL-1β mRNA (Yan et al., 1992; Fan et al., 1995; Goss et al., 1995). In these studies, early induction of IL-1β gene expression—between one and six hours after injury—was observed (Fan et al., 1995; Goss et al., 1995). Although the specific cellular sources of the IL-1β produced in brain in response to traumatic injury remain to be definitively identified, astrocytes, activated microglia, neurons, macrophages, and vascular endothelium have been implicated (Tchelingerian et al., 1996; Gourin and Shackford, 1997; Sanderson et al., 1999).

Putative detrimental effects of the proinflammatory cytokine IL-1β in the evolution of central nervous system damage include upregulation of intercellular adhesion molecule-1 (ICAM-1) on brain microvessels—with subsequent infiltration of inflammatory leukocytes (Yang et al., 1999), augmentation of excitotoxic injury (Rothwell and Relton, 1993), upregulation of the inducible form of nitric oxide synthase (Kilbourn et al., 1990; Clark et al., 1996), and upregulation of amyloid precursor protein expression (Pierce et al., 1996; Sheng et al., 1996).

Remarkably, an increase in IL-1β in human cerebrospinal fluid (CSF) of adult victims of severe traumatic brain injury was demonstrated (versus age-matched controls) well over ten years ago by McClain et al. (1987). Serial CSF samples were assessed after drainage from an indwelling ventricular catheter. Consistently with a potential role for IL-1β in the evolution of tissue damage in human head injury, Clark et al. (1999) studied western analysis of brain samples resected from patients with refractory intracranial hypertension secondary to severe cerebral contusion. In these samples, IL-1β-converting enzyme (ICE) was consistent activated, as evidenced by specific cleavage. In contrast, ICE activation was not detected in brain samples from patients that died of noncentral nervous system etiologies

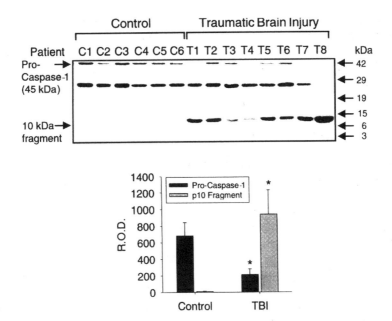

Figure 8.1 Evidence for activation of interleukin-1-converting enzyme (ICE, procaspase-1) in cerebral contusions resected from adult patients with severe traumatic brain injury and refractory intracranial hypertension. Western analysis demonstrating cleavage of the intact 45 kDa procaspase-1 to the 10 kDa fragment in each of eight victims of severe traumatic brain injury but in none of six control brain samples from patients who died of noncentral nervous system causes. Contusions were resected at a variety of times after injury depending on clinical indication. Reprinted with permission from Clark et al. (1999). ROD = relative optical density.

(Fig. 8.1). These studies strongly support the rapid production of IL-1β in the traumatically injured brain in both experimental models and the human condition.

Two studies in experimental models of traumatic brain injury suggest important therapeutic potential for inhibiting the effects of IL-1β. Toulmond and Rothwell (1995) studied the effect of recombinant human IL-1 receptor antagonist protein (rhIL-1ra) on histological damage after fluid percussion injury in rats. Serial intracerebroventricular injections of rhIL-1ra administered over 48 h beginning 15 min after injury significantly reduced the amount of histological damage assessed at either 72 h or 7 days. The therapeutic window for this effect appeared to be at least 4 h. Sanderson et al. (1999) studied the effect of systemic administration of rhIL-1ra, again in fluid percussion injury in rats. A seven-day subcutaneous infusion beginning 15 min after injury reduced damage in CA3, dentate, and cortex and improved cognitive function assessed by Morris water maze testing. However, despite beneficial effects on histopathology and cognition, high doses of rhIL-1ra actually worsened motor function assessed at one week after injury. Although therapies specifically targeting IL-1β after traumatic brain injury have not been tested in the clinic, Marion et al. (1997) demonstrated that transient, moderate hypothermia both improves clinical outcome and markedly reduces CSF levels of IL-1β after severe traumatic brain injury in patients. This result is similar to the attenuation of IL-1β mRNA by hypothermia reported by Goss et al. (1995) in the rat model of controlled cortical impact injury. To our knowledge, neither rhIL-1ra nor ICE inhibitors have been tested in human head injury.

TUMOR NECROSIS FACTOR-α

Production of TNF-α after experimental traumatic brain injury in rats was first demonstrated by Taupin et al. (1993). TNF-α levels peaked in the initial 8 h after fluid percussion and returned to baseline by 18 h. Shohami et al. (1994) also demonstrated increases in TNF-α activity as early as 1 h after closed head injury. TNF-α peaked at 4 h and decreased thereafter. Rapid production of TNF-α and mRNA for TNF-α was subsequently confirmed by a number of investigators, again using the fluid percussion model (Fan et al., 1996; Kita et al., 1997; Knoblach et al., 1999). The cellular sources of TNF-α in the injured brain remain to be completely elucidated; however, neurons, glia, and microvessels appear to be an important source, particularly early after injury (Feuerstein et al., 1994; Tchelingerian et al., 1996; Kita et al., 1997; Knoblach et al., 1999). Delayed increases in TNF-α immunoreactivity have been demonstrated in rat brain as long as three months after focal cerebral contusion (Holmin and Mathiesen, 1999).

Clinical reports of increases in TNF-α in CSF or brain tissue after human head injury are less common than for IL-1β. Kossmann et al. (1996) reported multiple peaks in CSF TNF-α in a study of 36 adults with severe head injury. However, increases in CSF TNF-α were variably observed, and nine of the patients showed no increase versus normal controls. Similar results were reported in CSF and plasma from head-injured patients by Ross et al. (1994). Gourin and Shackford (1997) reported the ex vivo production of TNF-α by human cerebral microvascular endothelium at 8 and 24 h after in vivo percussion injury.

Several therapeutic strategies have been used to inhibit the production or effects of TNF-α in experimental traumatic brain injury. Shohami et al. (1996) demonstrated a reduction in posttraumatic cerebral edema and blood–brain barrier injury, along with improved motor function and hippocampal neuronal survival in rats treated with either pentoxifylline to attenuate TNF-α production or TNF-binding protein after closed head injury. These agents were administered immediately after the injury. Similar beneficial findings by this group were also reported after treatment with dexabinol (HU-211), a synthetic cannabinoid that is a posttranscriptional inhibitor of TNF-α production. Carter et al. (1999) demonstrated that inhibitors of extracellular signal-regulated kinases (Erk) and p38 kinases resulted in dramatic reductions in endotoxin-induced TNF-α production in macrophages outside of the CNS. To our knowledge, such an approach has not been tested in experimental traumatic brain injury. Finally, Xu et al. (1998) demonstrated that methylpredisolone reduced TNF-α expression by 55 percent and nuclear factor kappa-B (NF-κB) activation. However, despite the therapeutic promise of strategies targeting TNF-α

immediately after injury, some caution is suggested based on the study of traumatic brain injury in TNF-α knockout mice. Scherbel et al. (1999) demonstrated improved functional outcome early after fluid percussion injury in TNF-α knockout mice; however, after the initial week after injury, functional outcome was actually worse than in wild-type mice subjected to an identical injury. In addition, ultimate lesion volume after injury was larger in TNF-α knockouts versus wild-type. Sullivan et al. (1999) reported similar exacerbation of damage in mice deficient in the p55 and p75 TNF-α receptors. Reduction of NF-κB-dependent expression of endogenous neuroprotectant gene products, such as manganese superoxide dismutase, was suggested to contribute to the overall detrimental effect that was observed. To our knowledge, there have been no published reports of the effect of therapies targeting TNF-α in human head injury.

INTERLEUKIN-10

Interleukin-10 (IL-10) is a potent anti-inflammatory cytokine. Outside of the central nervous system, IL-10 inhibits a variety of macrophage responses including synthesis of cytokines, adhesion molecules, chemokines, and reactive oxygen species (Bethea et al., 1999). IL-10 mediates these effects through both STAT-3- and NF-κB-mediated effects (Romano et al., 1996; O'Farrell et al., 1998). IL-10 reduces the antigen-presenting capacity of astrocytes and microglia, and also reduces TNF-α production by astrocytes. Also relevant to the central nervous system, IL-10 potently inhibits inflammatory cell infiltration in experimental pneumococcal meningitis.

Clinical reports of increases in IL-10 after traumatic brain injury are limited. Bell et al. (1997) reported increases in IL-10 in CSF of children with severe traumatic brain injury compared to those seen in controls. However, the increases in IL-10 were to a concentration of approximately 50 pg/mL, well below the ng/mL concentrations of IL-6 seen in this same patient population (Fig. 8.2). Increases in CSF IL-10 were associated both with age less than 4 years and mortality. Correlation with young age often reflects very severe injury since infants with severe traumatic brain injury are frequently victims of child abuse. Shimonkevitz et al. (1999) reported transient increases in IL-10 in serum of adults with severe traumatic brain injury, and peripheral blood monocytes were suggested as one potential source.

Two recent reports suggest potential efficacy of either local or systemic administration of IL-10 in experimental central nervous system injury. Knoblach and Faden (1998) demonstrated that intravenous administration of IL-10 (100 μg) 30 min before and 1 h after fluid percussion injury in rats improved functional outcome at both one and two weeks. In contrast, postinjury treatment with either local or intraventricular administration was only transiently effective or ineffective, respectively. More promising results with the postinsult administration of IL-10 were reported by Bethea et al. (1999) in experimental spinal cord injury. A single 5 μg dose of IL-10 administered 30 min after the insult reduced early postinsult TNF-α production and improved long-term motor function in a rat model of spinal cord

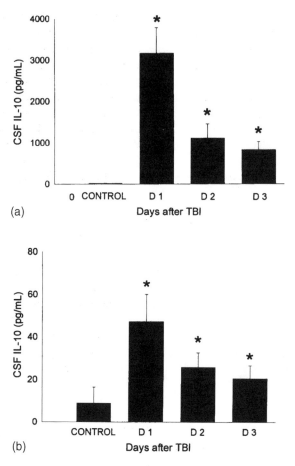

Figure 8.2 (a) IL-6 and (b) IL-10 concentration in cerebrospinal fluid (CSF) of infants and children with severe traumatic brain injury. A large increase in CSF IL-6 is seen in the initial three days after injury. A significant, albeit smaller, increase in CSF concentration of the anti-inflammatory cytokine IL-10 was also noted. Reprinted with permission from Bell et al. (1997).

injury. Curiously, however, multiple doses of IL-10 were ineffective (Fig. 8.3). IL-10 was also protective in a rat model of excitotoxic spinal cord injury (Brewer et al., 1999). Finally, Dietrich et al. (1999) reported a particularly beneficial effect of the combination of transient mild hypothermia and IL-10 administration after forebrain ischemia in rats. Although similar studies have not been carried out in experimental traumatic brain injury, the powerful beneficial effect of hypothermia in experimental and clinical traumatic brain injury suggests that this is an interesting combination for future evaluation (Marion et al., 1997).

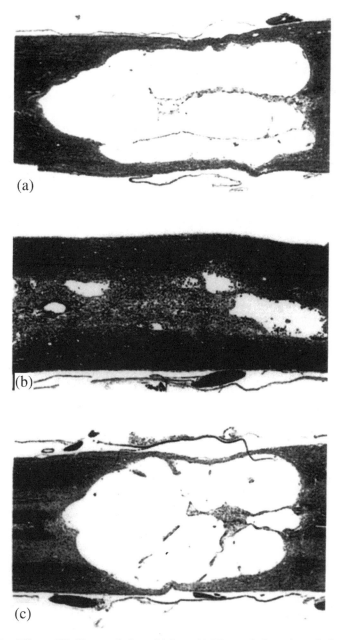

Figure 8.3   Effect of IL-10 on spinal cord injury. (a) Histopathology through the epicenter two months after injury in a vehicle-treated rat. (b,c) Histopathology from rats treated with a single dose of IL-10 or two doses, respectively. A marked beneficial effect of a single dose was demonstrated. Reprinted with permission from Bethea et al. (1999).

NEUTROPHILS

A robust accumulation of neutrophils has been demonstrated to occur after experimental traumatic brain injury produced by weight drop, controlled cortical impact injury, and fluid percussion injury (Schoettle et al., 1990; Clark et al., 1994; Soares et al., 1995). In all of these models, neutrophil accumulation begins in the initial four hours after the injury and peaks between approximately 8 and 24 h (Fig. 8.4). Recent studies by our group (Adelson et al., 1998) directly compared the amount of neutrophil accumulation in immature rats subjected either to a focal contusion produced by controlled cortical impact or to a diffuse injury produced by a modification of the Marmarou closed head weight drop model (Adelson et al., 1996). Both models produce a functional deficit on behavioral testing of the rats; however, only the controlled cortical impact model produces an area of necrosis and neuronal death. Neutrophil accumulation was completely dependent on the production of a contusion, suggesting the possibility that tissue necrosis was an important factor in stimulating neutrophil influx. Supporting the extrapolation of this finding from experimental traumatic brain injury to the clinical condition, Holmin et al. (1998) reported significant neutrophil accumulation in cerebral contusions resected from patients with severe head injury.

A variety of anti-inflammatory strategies can successfully inhibit neutrophil influx after experimental traumatic brain injury including inhibitors of Mac-1 (Clark et al., 1996), complement activation (Kaczorowski et al., 1995), or ICAM-1 (Carlos et al., 1997). Clinical assessments of CSF from both adult and pediatric patients after head

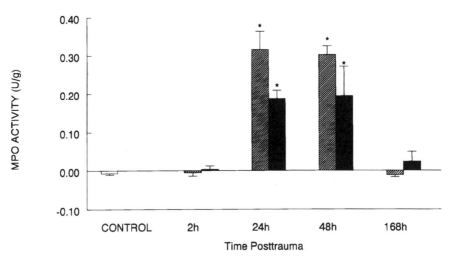

Figure 8.4 Time course of neutrophil accumulation after experimental traumatic brain injury in rats induced by either weight drop (cross-hatched bars) or controlled cortical impact (solid bars). Neutrophil accumulation, as quantified by the tissue myeloperoxidase assay, was increased early after injury, peaking at 24 h post trauma in both insults. Reprinted from Clark et al. (1994).

injury have demonstrated significant increases of soluble forms of both ICAM-1 and other molecules involved in leukocyte trafficking including P- and E-selectin and interleukin-8 (Kossmann et al., 1997; Pleines et al., 1998; Whalen et al., 1998, 2000b). These studies again suggest a linkage between bench and bedside for these inflammatory mechanisms.

Neutrophils release a variety of products that may mediate secondary injury such as superoxide anion, myeloperoxidase, elastase, cathepsins, and arachidonic acid metabolites (Jochum et al., 1993). A putative role for neutrophil-mediated secondary damage is also suggested to occur by vascular plugging with expansion of the ischemic penumbra (Hallenbeck et al., 1986). However, a number of studies have now failed to confirm an important role for neutrophils in the evolution of secondary damage after experimental traumatic brain injury. Schurer (1990) demonstrated that neutrophil deletion with anti-neutrophil antiserum actually exacerbated the development of posttraumatic cerebral edema after cryogenic injury in rats. Whalen et al. (1999a) reported that neutrophil depletion with a specific anti-neutrophil monoclonal antibody (RP-3) failed to attenuate blood–brain barrier injury after controlled cortical impact trauma in rats. In fact, the time courses of blood–brain barrier permeability and neutrophil accumulation were remarkably divergent—recovery of the blood–brain barrier was occurring during the period of peak neutrophil accumulation. Similarly, Uhl et al. (1994) demonstrated that neutrophil depletion with vinblastine sulfate failed to attenuate posttraumatic cerebral edema at 24 h after focal cerebral contusion in rats. There appear to be important differences between focal cerebral ischemia and experimental traumatic brain injury regarding the role of neutrophils and related adhesion molecules such as ICAM-1. For example, in focal cerebral ischemia/reperfusion in the rat, Soriano et al. (1996) demonstrated that infarct volume was dramatically attenuated in mice deficient in ICAM-1. In contrast, Whalen et al. (1999b) demonstrated that ICAM-1 deficient mice demonstrated histological and functional outcome after controlled cortical impact injury similar to injured wild-type controls. In addition, posttraumatic neutrophil accumulation was not inhibited by the ICAM-1 deficiency. More recently, Whalen et al. (2000a) demonstrated that mice deficient in both ICAM-1 and P-selectin exhibit a reduction in posttraumatic cerebral edema versus wild-type controls at 24 h after controlled cortical impact. However, there was no difference between groups in functional outcome, lesion volume, or posttraumatic neutrophil accumulation. This suggests a possible effect of P-selectin or ICAM-1 on posttraumatic edema that is independent of neutrophil accumulation.

Based on these studies, there has not been a great deal of interest in moving forward with anti-neutrophil strategies in human head injury. In addition, the failure of a monoclonal antibody targeting ICAM-1 in a clinical stroke trial has also contributed to the lack of enthusiasm for this approach. Indeed, it is well known that although patients with severe head injury exhibit a local inflammatory response that may contribute to secondary damage, the local inflammatory response to injury is occurring despite systemic immunosuppression—particularly of cell-mediated immunity (Hoyt et al., 1990; Quattrochi et al., 1991). This prompted a recent feasibility trial of treatment of patients with severe head injury with granulocyte colony-stimulating factor (GCSF), a cytokine that increases circulating absolute neutrophil count (Heard et al., 1998). Treatment with GCSF increased circulating absolute neutrophil count in these patients and reduced the incidence of bacteremia (defined as a positive blood culture) compared to treatment with vehicle. However, additional studies are needed to determine whether increasing circulating absolute neutrophil count adversely effects the injured brain. Preliminary studies in our rat model of controlled cortical impact indicate that a 10-fold increase in absolute neutrophil count did not exacerbate posttraumatic cerebral edema versus vehicle-treated controls (Whalen et al., 2000c).

BENEFICIAL ASPECTS OF THE LOCAL INFLAMMATORY RESPONSE

This chapter has focused on the potential therapeutic value of inhibiting selected aspects of the inflammatory response to traumatic brain injury. However, recently it has become clear that there are a number of beneficial aspects of the local inflammatory response to traumatic brain injury (Goss et al., 1995; DeKosky et al., 1996; Mattson, 1997). The best-described beneficial effect is mediated by the coupling of cytokine production to the elaboration of neurotrophils, presumably serving either an antiapoptotic or regenerative role. This concept is supported for IL-1β by studies in experimental models of traumatic brain injury (Goss et al., 1995; DeKosky et al., 1996) and for IL-8 in the clinical condition (Kossmann et al., 1997). Thus, inhibiting selected aspects of acute inflammation could be associated with a trade-off (Goss et al., 1995).

CONCLUSIONS

Evidence has been presented confirming the occurrence of a robust acute inflammatory response to traumatic brain injury both in contemporary experimental models in rodents and in the human condition. Laboratory studies suggest that therapies targeting the inhibition of proinflammatory cytokines such as TNFα or IL-1β early after injury have potential merit. Similarly, augmentation of the effect of the anti-inflammatory cytokine IL-10 also appears to have therapeutic promise. Based on studies in either models of cerebral ischemia or models outside of the central nervous system, additional potential strategies for future testing include inhibitors of p38 or STAT kinases, inhibition of NF-κB activation, or inhibitors of ICE. Finally, it is clear that there are putative detrimental effects of inhibiting either local or systemic inflammation. As discussed, the local inflammatory response is coupled to neurotrophin production and inhibiting this could have deleterious consequences. Also, in the complex clinical environment, the systemic consequences of anti-inflammatory therapies on infection risk may outweigh benefit. These must be carefully assessed in both the experimental and clinical conditions prior to proceeding with large randomized controlled trials of any strategy targeting the inflammatory response to traumatic brain injury.

ACKNOWLEDGMENT

This work is supported by grant NS30318 from NINDS/NIH.

ABBREVIATIONS

CSF	Cerebral spinal fluid
Erk	Extracellular signal-regulated kinase
GCSF	Granulocyte colony-stimulating factor
HU-211	Dexabinol
ICAM-1	Intercellular adhesion molecule-1
ICE	IL-1β-converting enzyme
IL-1β	Interleukin-1β
NF-κB	Nuclear factor kappa B
rh1L-1ra	Recombinant human IL-1 receptor antagonist protein
TNF-α	Tumor necrosis factor-α

REFERENCES

P. D. Adelson, R. J. Robichaud, R. L. Hamilton, and P. M. Kochanek, *J. Neurosurg.*, 85, 877–884 (1996).

P. D. Adelson, M. Whalen, P. Robichaud, T. Carlos, and P. Kochanek, *Acta Neurochir. Suppl. (Wien)*, 71, 104–106 (1998).

F. C. Barone and G. Z. Feuerstein, *J. Cereb. Blood Flow Metab.* 19, 819–834 (1999).

M. J. Bell, P. M. Kochanek, L. A. Doughty, J. A. Carcillo, P. D. Adelson, R. S. B. Clark, S. R. Wisniewski, M. J. Whalen, and S. T. DeKosky, *J. Neurotrauma* 14, 451–457 (1997).

J. R. Bethea, H. Nagashima, M. C. Acosta, C. Briceno, F. Gomez, A. E. Marcillo, K. Loor, J. Green, and W. D. Dietrich, *J. Neurotrauma*, 16, 851–863 (1999).

K. L. Brewer, J. R. Bethea, and R. P. Yezierski, *Exp. Neurol.*, 159, 484–493 (1999).

T. M. Carlos, R. S. B. Clark, D. Franicola-Higgins, J. K. Schiding, and P. M. Kochanek, *J. Leukoc. Biol.*, 61, 279–285 (1997).

A. B. Carter, M. M. Monick, and G. W. Hunninglake, *Am. J. Respir. Cell Mol. Biol.*, 20, 751–758 (1999).

R. S. B. Clark, J. K. Schiding, S. L. Kaczorowski, D. W. Marion, and P. M. Kochanek, *J. Neurotrauma*, 11, 499–506 (1994).

R. S. B. Clark, T. M. Carlos, J. K. Schiding, M. Bree, L. A. Fireman, S. T. DeKosky, and P. M. Kochanek, *J. Neurotrauma* 13, 333–341 (1996).

R. S. B. Clark, P. M. Kochanek, M. Chen, S. C. Watkins, D. W. Marion, J. Chen, R. L. Hamilton, J. E. Loeffert, and S. H. Graham, *FASEB J.*, 13, 813–821 (1999).

S. T. DeKosky, S. D. Styren, M. E. O'Malley, J. R. Goss, P. M. Kochanek, D. Marion, C. H. Evans, and P. D. Robbins, *Ann. Neurol.*, 39, 123–127 (1996).

W. D. Dietrich, R. Busto, and J. R. Bethea, *Exp. Neurol.*, 158, 444–450 (1999).

L. Fan, P. R. Young, F. C. Barone, G. Z. Feuerstein, D. H. Smith, and T. K. McIntosh, *Brain Res. Mol. Brain Res.*, 30, 125–130 (1995).

L. Fan, P. R. Young, F. C. Barone, G. Z. Feuerstein, D. H. Smith, and T. K. McIntosh, *Brain Res. Mol. Brain Res.*, 36, 287–291 (1996).

G. Z. Feuerstein, T. Liu, and F. C. Barone, *Cerebrovasc. Brain Metab. Rev.*, 6, 341–360 (1994).

D. Giulian and L. Lachman, *Science*, 228, 497–498 (1985).

J. R. Gross, S. D. Styren, P. D. Miller, P. M. Kochanek, A. M. Palmer, D. W. Marion, and S. T. DeKosky, *J. Neurotrauma*, 12, 159–167 (1995).

C. G. Gourin and S. R. Shackford, *J. Trauma*, 42, 1101–1107 (1997).

J. M. Hallenbeck, A. J. Dutka, T. Tanishima, P. M. Kochanek, K. K. Kumaroo, C. B. Thompson, T. P. Obrenovitch, and T. J. Contreras, *Stroke*, 17, 246–253 (1986).

S. O. Heard, M. P. Fink, R. L. Gamelli, J. S. Solomkin, M. Joshi, A. L. Trask, T. C. Fabian, L. D. Hudson, K. B. Gerold, E. D. Logan, and The Filgrastim Study Group, *Crit. Care Med.*, 26, 748–754 (1998).

S. Holmin and T. Mathieson, *Neuroreport*, 10, 1889–1891 (1999).

S. Holmin, J. Söderlund, P. Biberfeld, and T. Mathieson, *Neurosurgery*, 42, 291–299 (1998).

D. B. Hoyt, N. Ozkan, J. F. Hansbrough, L. Marshall, and M. van Berkum-Clark, *J. Trauma*, 30, 759–767 (1990).

M. Jochum, W. Machleidt, H. Neuhof, and H. Fritz, Proteinases, in G. Schlag and H. Redl, Eds., *Pathophysiology of Shock, Sepsis, and Organ Failure*, Springer-Verlag, Berlin, 1993, pp. 46–60.

S. L. Kaczorowski, J. K. Schiding, C. A. Toth, and P. M. Kochanek, *J. Cereb. Blood Flow Metab.*, 15, 860–864 (1995).

R. G. Kilbourn, S. S. Gross, A. Jubran, J. Adams, O. W. Griffith, R. Levi, and R. F. Lodato, *Proc. Natl. Acad. Sci. USA*, 87, 3629–3632 (1990).

T. Kita, L. Liu, N. Tanaka, and Y. Kinoshita, *Int. J. Legal Med.*, 110, 305–311 (1997).

S. M. Knoblach and A. I. Faden, *Exp. Neurol.*, 153, 143–151 (1998).

S. M. Knoblach, L. Fan, and A. I. Faden, *J. Neuroimmunol.*, 95, 115–125 (1999).

T. Kossmann, V. H. J. Hans, P. M. Lenzlinger, E. Csuka, P. F. Stahel, O. Trentz, M. C. Morganti-Kossmann, Analysis of Immune Mediator Production following Traumatic Brain Injury, in G. Schlag, H. Redl, and D. Traber, Eds., *Shock, Sepsis, and Organ Failure*, Springer-Verlag, Berlin, 1996, pp. 263–304.

T. Kossmann, P. F. Stahel, P. M. Lenzlinger, H. Redl, R. W. Dubs, O. Trentz, G. Schlag, and M. C. Morganti-Kossmann, *J. Cereb. Blood Flow Metab.*, 17, 280–289 (1997).

D. W. Marion, L. E. Penrod, S. F. Kelsey, W. D. Obrist, P. M. Kochanek, A. M. Palmer, S. R. Wisniewski, and S. T. DeKosky, *N. Engl. J. Med.*, 336, 540–546 (1997).

M. P. Mattson, *Neurosci. Biobehav. Rev.*, 21, 193–206 (1997).

C. J. McClain, D. Cohen, L. Ott, C. A. Dinarello, and B. Young, *J. Lab. Clin. Med.*, 110, 48–54 (1987).

M. Nieto-Sampredro and M. A. Berman, *J. Neurosci. Res.*, 17, 214–219 (1987).

A. M. O'Farrell, Y. Liu, K. W. Moore, and A. L. Mui, *EMBO J.*, 17, 1006–1018 (1998).

J. E. Pierce, J. Q. Trojanowski, D. I. Graham, D. H. Smith, and T. K. McIntosh, *J. Neurosci.*, 16, 1083–1090 (1996).

U. E. Pleines, J. F. Stover, T. Kossmann, O. Trentz, and M. C. Morganti-Kossmann, *J. Neurotrauma*, 15, 399–409 (1998).

K. B. Quattrocchi, E. H. Frank, C. H. Miller, A. Amin, B. W. Issel, and F. C. Wagner, *J. Neurosurg.*, 75, 766–773 (1991).

M. F. Romano, A. Lamberti, A. Petrella, R. Bisogni, P. F. Tassone, S. Formisano, S. Venuta, and M. C. Turco, *J. Immunol.*, 156, 2119–2123 (1996).

S. A. Ross, M. I. Halliday, G. C. Campbell, D. P. Byrnes, and B. J. Rowlands, *Br. J. Neurosurg.*, 8, 419–425 (1994).

N. J. Rothwell and J. K. Relton, *Neurosci. Biobehav. Rev.*, 17, 217–227 (1993).

K. L. Sanderson, R. Raghupathi, K. E. Saatman, D. Martin, G. Miller, and T. K. McIntosh, *J. Cereb. Blood Flow Metab.*, 19, 1118–1125 (1999).

U. Scherbel, R. Raghupathi, M. Nakamura, K. E. Saatman, J. Q. Trojanowski, E. Neugebauer, M. W. Marino, and T. K. McIntosh, *Proc. Natl. Acad. Sci. USA*, 96, 8721–8726 (1999).

R. J. Schoettle, P. M. Kochanek, M. J. Magargee, M. W. Uhl, and E. M. Nemoto, *J. Neurotrauma*, 7, 207–217 (1990).

L. Schurer, U. Prugner, O. Kempski, K.-E. Arfors, and A. Baethmann, *Acta Neurochir.*, S51, 49–51 (1990).

J. G. Sheng, K. Ito, R. D. Skinner, R. E. Mrak, C. R. Rovnaghi, L. J. Van Eldik, and W. S. Griffin, *Neurobiol. Aging*, 17, 761–766 (1996).

R. Shimonkevitz, D. Bar-Or, L. Harris, K. Dole, L. McLaughlin, and R. Yukl, *Shock*, 12, 10–16 (1999).

E. Shohami, M. Novikov, R. Bass, A. Yamin, and R. Gallily, *J. Cereb. Blood Flow Metab.*, 14, 615–619 (1994).

E. Shohami, R. Bass, D. Wallach, A. Yamin, and R. Gallily, *J. Cereb. Blood Flow Metab.*, 16, 378–384 (1996).

H. D. Soares, R. R. Hicks, D. Smith, and T. K. McIntosh, *J. Neurosci.*, 15, 8223–8233 (1995).

S. G. Soriano, S. A. Lipton, Y. F. Wang, M. Xiao, T. A. Springer, J.-C. Gutierrez-Ramos, and P. R. Hickey, *Ann. Neurol.*, 39, 618–624 (1996).

P. G. Sullivan, A. J. Bruce-Keller, A. G. Rabchevsky, S. Christakos, D. K. St. Clair, M. P. Mattson, and S. W. Scheff, *J. Neurosci.*, 19, 6248–6256 (1999).

V. Taupin, S. Toulmond, A. Serrano, J. Benavides, and F. Zavala, *J. Neuroimmunol.*, 42, 177–185 (1993).

J. L. Tchelingerian, F. Le Saux, and C. Jacque, *J. Neurosci. Res.*, 43, 99–106 (1996).

S. Toulmond and N. J. Rothwell, *Brain Res.*, 671, 261–266 (1995).

M. W. Uhl, K. V. Biagas, P. D. Grundl, M. A. Barmada, J. K. Schiding, E. M. Nemoto, and P. M. Kochanek, *J. Neurotrauma*, 11, 303–315 (1994).

M. J. Whalen, T. M. Carlos, P. M. Kochanek, M. J. Bell, S. R. Wisniewski, J. Carcillo, and P. D. Adelson, *J. Neurotrauma*, 15, 777–787 (1998).

M. J. Whalen, T. M. Carlos, P. M. Kochanek, R. S. Clark, S. Heineman, J. K. Schiding, D. Franicola, F. Memarzadeh, W. Lo, D. W. Marion, and S. T. DeKosky, *J. Neurotrauma*, 16, 583–594 (1999a).

M. J. Whalen, T. M. Carlos, C. E. Dixon, S. R. Wisnlewski, J. K. Schiding, R. S. B. Clark, E. Baum, D. W. Marion, and P. M. Kochaneck, *J. Neurotrauma*, 16, 299–309 (1999b).

M. J. Whalen, T. M. Carlos, C. E. Dixon, P. Robichaud, R. S. B. Clark, D. W. Marion, and P. M. Kochanek, *J. Leuk. Biol.*, 67, 160–168 (2000a).

M. J. Whalen, T. M. Carlos, P. M. Kochanek, S. R. Wisniewski, M. J. Bell, R. S. B. Clark, S. T. DeKosky, and P. D. Adelson, *Crit. Care Med.*, 28, 929–934 (2000b).

M. J. Whalen, T. M. Carlos, S. R. Wisniewski, R. S. B. Clark, J. Melick, D. W. Marion, and P. M. Kochaneck, *Crit. Care Med.*, 28, 3710–3717 (2000c).

M. N. Woodroofe, G. S. Sarna, M. Wadhwa, G. M. Hayes, A. J. Loughlin, A. Tinker, and M. L. Cuzner, *J. Neuroimmunol.*, 33, 227–236 (1991).

J. Xu, G. Fan, S. Chen, Y. Wu, X. M. Xu, and C. Y. Hsu, *Brain Res. Mol. Brain Res.*, 59, 135–142 (1998).

H. Q. Yan, M. A. Banos, P. Herregodts, R. Hooghe, and E. L. Hooghe-Peters, *Eur. J. Immunol.*, 22, 2963–2971 (1992).

G.-Y. Yang, G. P. Schielke, C. Gong, Y. Mao, H.-L. Ge, X.-H. Liu, and A. L. Betz, *J. Cereb. Blood Flow Metab.*, 19, 1109–1117 (1999).

CHAPTER 9

CONTRIBUTION OF IONIC ALTERATIONS TO METABOLIC DYSFUNCTION FOLLOWING TRAUMATIC BRAIN INJURY

AMIR SAMII, AMY H. MOORE, CHRISTOPHER C. GIZA, AND DAVID A. HOVDA

Neurotrauma Laboratory, Division of Neurosurgery, UCLA School of Medicine, Los Angeles, California

INTRODUCTION

Traumatic brain injury (TBI) induces numerous pathophysiological events that may lead to cell vulnerability and functional deficits. One of the characteristics that has been shown both in animal models and in humans following head injury is a distinct profile of change in cerebral metabolism and blood flow. Although described in greater detail later in this chapter, the trauma-induced metabolic cascade is characterized as an acute period of hyperglycolysis followed by a chronic state of metabolic depression, which coincides with behavioral deficits. In addition, cerebral blood flow is reduced following injury, suggesting a compromise of substrate delivery and metabolic coupling.

It has been estimated that the average adult human brain consumes approximately 4×10^{21} molecules of ATP per minute, or nearly 20 percent of all energy produced in the body (Sokoloff, 1960). The brain, in contrast to other organs with high energy production (i.e., heart, kidney) does not perform mechanical or osmotic work. Thus, it is assumed that the predominant role for energy formed from the metabolism of glucose, the main energy substrate in the brain, is to maintain ATP-driven ionic pumps that preserve the ionic homeostasis. Although the mechanisms for the postinjury metabolic changes are not fully understood, they may be related to the disruption of ionic equilibrium reported after TBI. This chapter gives a systematic

Head Trauma: Basic, Preclinical, and Clinical Directions, Edited by Leonard P. Miller and Ronald L. Hayes, Co-edited by Jennifer K. Newcomb
ISBN 0-471-36015-5 © 2001 John Wiley & Sons, Inc.

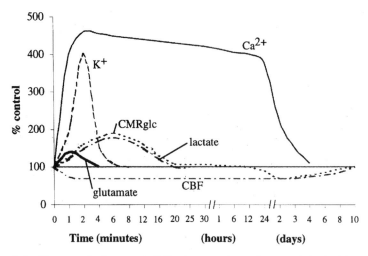

Figure 9.1   Neurometabolic cascade following experimental traumatic brain injury in the rat.

overview of ionic fluxes following experimental TBI and their potential role in posttrauma metabolic dysfunction (Fig. 9.1).

ACUTE METABOLIC AND IONIC RESPONSES TO TRAUMATIC BRAIN INJURY

Several experimental animal models of brain injury have shown that rates of cerebral glucose utilization increase dramatically following the insult. The perturbation of ionic gradients across the neuronal cell membrane (from action potentials, seizures, spreading depression, etc.) activates energy-dependent ionic pumps (Bull et al., 1973; Lewis and Schuetle, 1975; Lothman et al., 1975; Mayevsky et al., 1974; Rosenthal et al., 1979), which results in an increase in glucose utilization. Applying 2-[^{14}C]deoxyglucose (2DG) autoradiography, rates of cerebral glucose metabolism immediately increased by < 75 percent and remained at this level for 30 min after fluid percussion injury (FPI) in rat. This elevation in metabolism was observed in regions ipsilateral to the site of injury, including the cortex and hippocampus. A similar magnitude of increased glucose utilization was seen up to 4 h following controlled cortical impact (CCI) (Samii et al., 1998).

Since rates of cerebral oxidative metabolism are presumed to be at or near maximum levels (Bennett and Rose, 1992), the heightened rates of glucose metabolism indicate an increase in glycolysis to meet the immediate energy demand of the cell. This sudden increase in energy metabolism has been shown to produce a decline in high-energy phosphates (ATP), which disinhibits anaerobic metabolism (Racker et al., 1983; Rose et al., 1964). One natural consequence of the increase in anaerobic metabolism would be the accumulation of lactate and the development of intracellular acidosis (Becker, 1985; Yang et al., 1985).

Cerebral lactic acidosis is a frequent finding in severe head injury in patients (DeSalles et al., 1986; Jaggi et al., 1990; Robertson et al., 1987). Posttraumatic cerebral lactate production is evidenced by an acute and prolonged increase in cerebrospinal fluid (CSF) lactate, and a negative arteriovenous difference in lactate content (higher jugular venous than arterial concentration) (DeSalles et al., 1987; Hotson et al., 1973; Robertson et al., 1987).

Previous observations indicate that lactate clearly increases in cerebrospinal fluid as well as in brain tissue during the initial 60 min following mild to moderate fluid percussion injury in rat (Choi, 1992; Inao et al., 1988; Yang et al., 1985). Severe fluid percussion injury causes progressive, longer-lasting lactate accumulation, presumably because of cell disruption (Inao et al., 1988). Recently two important papers have been published addressing the changes in extracellular lactate following experimental TBI. Using a weight drop model in rats Nilsson and colleagues

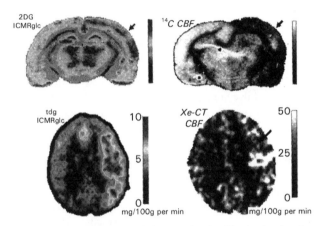

Figure 9.2 Posttraumatic hyperglycolysis is associated with a reduction in cerebral blood flow in both rats and humans. The top row illustrates two studies done in rats within the first hour following a lateral fluid percussion brain injury (arrow). Both images are coronal autoradiographs through the middle of the thalamus and dorsal hippocampus. The left image illustrates hyperglycolysis on the side of the injury utilizing deoxy-D-[^{14}C]glucose autoradiography. The right image illustrates the reduction of cerebral blood flow using [^{14}C]iodoantipyrine autoradiography on the same side exhibiting hyperglycolysis [see Hovda, (1996) for review]. The bottom row confirms these experimental findings in human traumatic brain injury using deoxy-D-[^{18}F]glucose positron emission tomography (left) and xenon computer tomography (right). These human brain images were obtained during the first few days following traumatic brain injury (pedestrian versus automobile) in which the patient endured an epidural hematoma, which was surgically removed. The images are axial sections with the front of the brain at the top and the injured side oriented to be the same as that in the animal study. Taken just superior to the thalamus, the images illustrate hyperglycolysis on the right side of the left image involving most of the cerebral cortex. However, as can be seen in the right image, there are areas of reduced cerebral blood flow (see arrow) indicating that, although the demands for glucose metabolism are high, the cerebral blood flow appears to be compromised.

demonstrated that there was a 4- to 5-fold increase in the dialysate concentration of lactate, which did not return to normal levels until 80 min after the insult (Nilsson et al., 1990, 1993). When the severity of the injury was increased, a more pronounced elevation of lactate (approximately 7-fold) was exhibited that did not return to normal levels until after two hours. This increase in extracellular lactate concentration is thought to be due to a combination of an increase in energy demand from injury-induced ionic changes and a concomitant decrease in cerebral blood flow.

Acutely, increased energy demand required to reestablish the ionic equilibrium occurs in the setting of a potential restriction in substrate delivery (Fig. 9.2). This mismatch between metabolism and blood flow may be critical in the restoration of ionic homeostasis and compromise cellular recovery. Since the ionic perturbation following TBI is initially illustrated by the profile of potassium efflux, the role of this ion on cellular metabolism will be examined.

POTASSIUM

Several earlier studies have indicated that a massive increase in extracellular potassium concentration $[K^+]_e$ occurs in response to experimental traumatic brain or spinal cord injury (Hubschmann and Kornhauser, 1983; Takahashi et al., 1981; Young et al., 1982). As described following fluid-percussion injury in the rat, this increase peaks by 2 min and returns to normal concentration by 5 min post insult (Isacson et al., 1984).

Nonspecific breakdown of the plasma membrane may explain an increase in $[K^+]_e$, particularly in regions of the brain subjected to localized contusions (Takahashi et al., 1981; Young et al., 1982) or intracerebral hemorrhages (Hubschmann et al., 1983). However, an increase in $[K^+]_e$ has also been reported following concussive brain injury (Katayama et al., 1990; Takahashi et al., 1981), which, although it transmits a mechanical stress to wide areas of the brain, does not result in overt morphological damage. This increase in $[K^+]_e$ following concussive brain injury could be explained in terms of a K^+ flux through voltage-gated K^+ channels associated with neuronal discharges (Fig. 9.3), since deformation of neural tissue alone can produce sufficient depolarization resulting in neuronal firing (Julian and Goldman, 1962). Several lines of evidence suggest that intense neuronal discharge occurs at the initial moment following concussive brain injury (Hayes et al., 1988; Walker et al., 1944). Additional support for depolarization-induced K^+ release is found in experiments that demonstrate the attenuation of K^+ flux associated with mild (but not severe) concussion with tetrodotoxin administered via microdialysis (Katayama et al., 1990).

Another possible explanation for the increase in $[K^+]_e$ is due to an opening of ligand-gated ion channels as a result of an indiscriminate release of neurotransmitters. Among the various neurotransmitters, the excitatory amino acids (EAAs), especially glutamate, appear to be the most likely candidates to produce such a large ionic flux (Cotman and Iverson, 1987; Hablitz and Langmoen, 1982; Mayer and

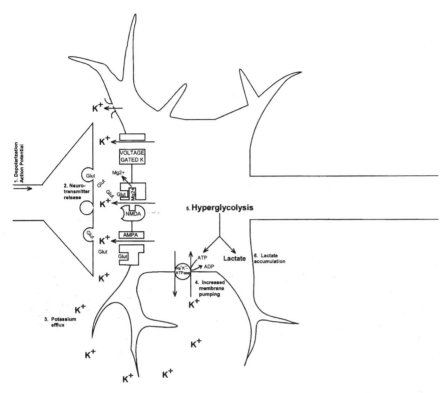

Figure 9.3 Potassium cascade after traumatic brain injury. (1) Mechanical stresses trigger membrane depolarization and action potential propagation. (2) Excitatory neurotransmitters are released. (3) Potassium exits the neuron via membrane disruption, voltage-gated K^+ channels, AMPA receptors, and NMDA receptors. The latter two are activated by the excitatory neurotransmitter glutamate. (4) Na^+-K^+-ATPase activity increases in an attempt to restore membrane potential. This creates a significant energy demand. (5) Glycolysis is increased to meet the elevated ATP requirements. (6) Lactate accumulates as a product of glycolysis (Giza and Hovda, 2000).

Westbrook, 1987). EAAs activate kainate and AMPA receptors opening channels permeable to both sodium and potassium. In addition, EAAs stimulate N-methyl-D-aspartate (NMDA) receptors opening channels permeable to calcium as well as sodium and potassium (Cotman and Iverson, 1987; Hablitz and Langmoen, 1982; Mayer and Westbrook, 1987). The level of EAA glutamate was seen to increase in conjunction with the increase in K^+ following fluid percussion brain injury (Katayama et al., 1990). Furthermore, administering (in situ) the EAA blocker kynurenic acid greatly reduces injury-induced increase in $[K^+]_e$ (Katayama et al., 1990).

The brain usually possesses a powerful mechanism for the uptake of elevated $[K^+]_e$ (Heinemann and Lux, 1977; Katzman, 1976; Orkand, 1980), primarily by glial cells (Ballanyi et al., 1987; Kuffler, 1967; Paulson and Newman, 1987). These mechanisms are effective enough to rapidly balance any $[K^+]_e$ increase resulting from neuronal discharges and to maintain $[K^+]_e$ below a limit ranging from 6 to 10 mM (Heinemann and Lux, 1977; Hotson et al., 1973; Moody et al., 1974; Sypert and Ward, 1974). Even in abnormal states of neuronal discharge, such as seizure activity (Moody et al., 1974; Sypert et al., 1974) or postconcussive injury (mild) (Katayama et al., 1990), the small increase in $[K^+]_e$, is likely to stay below the physiological ceiling of $[K^+]_e$ (approximately 10 mM). However, it has been shown that severe concussive injury induces an increase in $[K^+]_e$, (Katayama et al., 1990) that is 70 percent of the maximum level attained in ischemia (80 mM) (Astrup et al., 1980; Hansen, 1977, 1978), indicating that the physiological ceiling of $[K^+]$ is surpassed. In addition, impaired glial uptake following TBI (D'Ambrosio et al., 1999) may contribute to the elevated and sustained levels of extracellular K^+.

Previous research has shown that neurons are vulnerable to increased $[K^+]$, which leads to increased neuronal excitability (Ballanyi et al., 1987; R. D'Ambrosio et al., 1999), leading to additional release of EAAs and further efflux of $[K^+]_e$. As demonstrated in the cortex following electrical stimulation, increase of $[K^+]$ due to neuronal discharges elicits another massive depolarization and further increase in $[K^+]_e$ followed by a period of hyperpolarization and reduced neuronal function, termed "spreading depression" (Nicholson and Kraig, 1981; Prince et al., 1973; Somjen et al., 1985; Sugaya et al., 1975; Van Harreveld, 1978).

There are, in fact, a number of similarities between the large $[K^+]_e$ increase following severe concussive brain injury (Katayama et al., 1990) and spreading depression (Nicholson and Kraig, 1981). For example, spreading depression propagates, even in the presence of tetrodotoxin (TTX) (Sugaya et al., 1975; Tobiasz and Nicholson, 1982) much faster than by simple diffusion of K^+ and is dependent on the presence of Ca^{2+} (Nicholson and Kraig, 1981; Van Harreveld, 1978). Although the $[K^+]_e$ increase following concussive brain injury occurs simultaneously in wide areas of the brain (DeSalles et al., 1986; Katayama et al., 1988; Takahashi et al., 1981; Tsubokawa, 1983), in contrast to a true "spreading" depression, the underlying mechanism(s) may be similar. From the work of Katayama et al. (1990), it appears that in concussive brain injury $[K^+]_e$ initially increases due to sudden intense neuronal discharges. Thus, when the level of $[K^+]_e$ surpasses the physiological ceiling, neurotransmitters are rapidly released, resulting in much greater K^+ flux. The large postconcussive increase in $[K^+]_e$ is resistant to (in situ) administration of TTX (Katayama et al., 1990). Therefore, this $[K^+]_e$ efflux is likely due to neurotransmitter release from adjacent brain regions, employing mechanisms similar to the propagation of spreading depression.

To examine the relationship between K^+ flux and hyperglycolysis, studies observed posttraumatic metabolism following the administration of EAA antagonists or a Ca^{2+} channel blocker (Kawamata et al., 1990; 1992). Significant reductions in the hyperglycolytic effect were seen with the application of APV, (2-amino-5-phosphoralenic acid), an NMDA-channel blocker, and CNQX, (6-cyano-7-nitroquinoxaline-2,3-dione), non-NMDA channel blocker, with no differences in the injury-induced metabolic change following cobalt, a Ca^{2+} channel blocker. More specifically, APV had a greater attenuating effect on the posttraumatic hyperglycolysis compared to CNQX, suggesting the critical role of the NMDA receptor in the increased energy demand reported after TBI. Application of kynurenic acid, a general EAA-antagonist, also prevented the injury-induced increase in lactate (Kawamata et al., 1995). Additional studies in lesioned animals support the role of glutamate in posttraumatic hyperglycolysis (Yoshino et al., 1992). In animals in which the CA3 region of the ipsilateral hippocampus was lesioned, removing glutamatergic input to the CA1 area, FPI induced an acute increase in the cerebral metabolic rate for glucose (CMRglc) in the ipsilateral cortex but with no increase observed in the CA1 region of the hippocampus.

Thus, the acute ionic flux of K^+ appears to be mediated through the NMDA channel. This immediate flux induces an increase in energy demand, which leads to greater rates of glycolysis with a concomitant accumulation of lactate. By attenuating the release of K^+ through blockade of the NMDA ionophore or removal of glutamatergic afferents, this posttraumatic hyperglycolysis and lactate accumulation can be diminished.

CHRONIC METABOLIC AND IONIC RESPONSES TO TRAUMATIC BRAIN INJURY

After the initial increase in cerebral metabolism, rates of glucose utilization significantly fall at 6 h following fluid percussion injury in the adult rat relative to controls and remain decreased for 5 to 10 days following the insult (Yoshino et al., 1991). Although this state of metabolic depression has been reported in other experimental models of brain injury, its mechanism and function are not fully understood.

Additional research has suggested that the duration of depressed rates of glucose metabolism represents diminished oxidative metabolism and, thus, impaired ATP production at the level of the mitochondria. Measurement of cytochrome oxidase histochemistry following TBI in rat indicates a significant decrease in relative oxidative capacity in the cortex at one day following the injury which recovered by day 2 (Hovda et al., 1991). Interestingly, this depressed state of oxidative metabolism returned at day 3 post injury, was maximal at day 5, and returned to control levels by 10 days after the insult. Since mitochondrial function is sensitive to ionic changes, this biphasic response in oxidative metabolism may be due to the long-term effects of injury-induced ionic perturbations, namely, by calcium (Ca^{2+}) and magnesium (Mg^{2+}).

CALCIUM

As mentioned above, the TBI-induced acute neuronal depolarization leads to the indiscriminate release of neurotransmitters. Excitatory amino acids, specifically glutamate, open ligand-gated channels that are permeable to Ca^{2+}. Recently, a number of studies have demonstrated an increase of intracellular calcium following various experimental TBI models (Fineman et al., 1993; Nadler et al., 1995; Nilsson et al., 1996; Xiong et al., 1997). As described after fluid percussion injury in the adult rat, $^{45}Ca^{2+}$ accumulation is diffusely elevated for up to 4 days in the ipsilateral cortex, hippocampus, striatum and thalamus (Fineman et al., 1993).

In recent work, we have reported the efficacy of a N-type calcium channel blocker (SNX-111) in reducing calcium accumulation following a lateral fluid percussion injury using $^{45}Ca^{2+}$ autoradiography (Samii et al., 1999). Given that SNX-111 is a potent N-type calcium channel blocker (Abe et al., 1986; Dooley et al., 1987; Koyano et al., 1987; Sano et al., 1987), the protective effect demonstrated in experimental brain injury could be attributed to a reduced the total stimulation of NMDA receptors due to inhibition of neurotransmitter release. Supporting this hypothesis, others (Takizawa, 1995) have demonstrated that SNX-111 significantly reduced the total amount of extracellular glutamate (from 44.2 μM to 21.4 μM) in an in vivo ischemia model in the rat.

While it may seem intuitive that the post-TBI increase in $[Ca^{2+}]_i$ is due to influx via the NMDA receptor, studies with NMDA receptor antagonists have been inconclusive. Nilsson et al. (1996) showed no reduction of $^{45}Ca^{2+}$ accumulation following a weight drop brain injury when injured animals were treated with the NMDA receptor antagonist MK-801. However, treatment with HU-211, a synthetic cannabinoid with pharmacological properties characteristic of an NMDA receptor blocker without any cannabimimetic effects, did significantly reduce $^{45}Ca^{2+}$ signal after experimental TBI (Nadler et al., 1995).

In general, this movement of calcium into the intracellular space has been interpreted as a reliable marker for impending cell death. Cell death associated with an increase in intracellular calcium has been attributed to a number of different mechanisms (Verity, 1992; Tymianski and Tator, 1996). For example, increased intracellular calcium can contribute to the overstimulation of phospholipases (Farooqui and Horrocks, 1991), plasmalogenase, calpains (Kampfl et al., 1997; Roberts-Lewis and Siman, 1993), protein kinases (Verity, 1992), guanylate cyclase (Carter et al., 1987), nitride oxide synthetase, calcineurins, and endonucleases. The downstream consequences of these cellular changes include the overproduction of toxic reaction products (such as free radicals) (Schmidley, 1990; Siesjo, 1992), major alterations in cytoskeletal organization (Bignami and Clark, 1987; Iwasaki et al., 1987), and activation of apoptotic genetic signals (Morgan and Curran, 1986).

Although not always resulting in cellular death, increases in intracellular calcium concentration may promote a state of diminished oxidative metabolism in the mitochondria (Fig. 9.4), leading to cell vulnerability. Investigators have recently suggested that calcium disrupts mitochondrial functioning by compromising the metabolic machinery of the cell to such an extent that any secondary metabolic demand or challenge cannot be met, resulting in energy failure (Xiong et al., 1977). By using a fura-2 fluorescent assay in isolated forebrain mitochondria, these investigators have recently demonstrated that intramitochondrial Ca^{2+} was significantly increased primarily on the side ipsilateral to injury following a controlled cortical impact. The increase in Ca^{2+} lasted up to two weeks after injury. In addition, the same group showed that by using a selective N-type calcium channel blocker, the respiratory chain-linked functions of the mitochondria were improved when

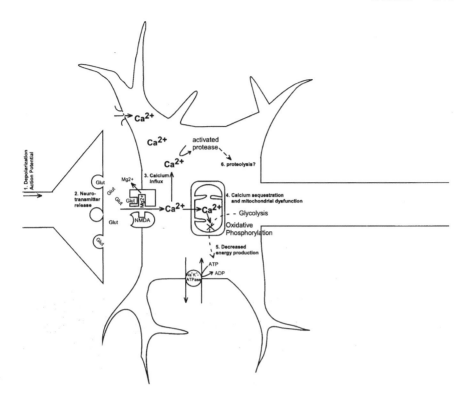

Figure 9.4   Calcium cascade after traumatic brain injury. (1) Mechanical stresses trigger membrane depolarization, action potential propagation and (2) excitatory neurotransmitter release, as in Fig. 9.2. (3) Activation of the NMDA receptor channel allows entry of calcium. (4) Excess intracellular calcium is sequestered in the mitochondria and can lead to metabolic dysfunction. (5) Impairment of mitochondrial oxidative metabolism results in decreased ATP production, with less energy to drive the Na^+-K^+-ATPase. (6) Additionally, intracellular calcium may activate proteases that degrade cellular proteins (Giza and Hovda, 2000).

compared with untreated animals after TBI (Verweij et al., 1997). They extended this study and reported that isolated mitochondria from resected tissue of a small group of head-injured patients showed lower respiratory rates than did nontrauma neurosurgical patients.

To elucidate the specific effect of calcium on the mitochondria, Schinder et al. (1996) found that calcium overloading, induced by glutamate, led to changes in mitochondrial membrane potential that were correlated with neuronal death in cultured rat hippocampus cells. This excitotoxic sequence may be initiated by the opening of the mitochondrial transition pore, increasing the permeability to small ions. This effect could be blocked by the addition of cyclosporin, which inhibits the mitochondrial permeability transition pore and, thus, stabilizes the mitochondrial membrane potential (Gunter et al., 1994).

MAGNESIUM

Several studies have stated that experimental TBI causes an immediate substantial decline in brain intracellular free and total Mg^{2+} concentration that lasts for up to four days following TBI (Heath et al., 1996; Vink et al., 1987, 1988a). Ionized and total blood magnesium has also been shown to be significantly lowered following TBI (Altura et al., 1995; Bareyre et al., 1999a; Heath and Vink, 1998). Using ^{31}P magnetic resonance spectroscopy to determine the intracellular free Mg^{2+} concentration prior to and following fluid percussion-induced TBI in rats, Vink and colleagues (Vink et al., 1987) showed that free Mg^{2+} declined by 70 percent in the injured cortex within the first hour and remained decreased at 3 h post injury. In a subsequent study, the same group reported that this injury-induced rapid decrease in intracellular free Mg^{2+} was significantly correlated with the severity of injury (Vink et al., 1988a). Demonstrating this result clinically, Memon et al. (1995) reported that acute head trauma was associated with graded deficits in serum Mg^{2+} (up to 62 percent, mean = 25 percent) in humans, which were related to severity of injury based on CT scans and other diagnostic parameters.

It has been suggested that an injury-induced decrease in oxidative capacity following TBI is related to the reduction in the cellular bioenergetic state. This reduction in the bioenergetic state is partly due to the loss of intracellular magnesium (Mg^{2+}) which decreases the cell's capacity for oxidative phosphorylation (Vink et al., 1988b, 1994). Presence of Mg^{2+} on a number of membrane binding sites is necessary in order to maintain the impermeability of the mitochondrial inner membrane (Binet and Volfin, 1975) and the functional integrity of the ATPase (Ebel and Gunther, 1980) (Fig. 9.5). Consequently, even though respiratory chain activity may be largely unaffected by an injury-induced decrease in intracellular Mg^{2+}, mitochondrial respiration may become uncoupled. In agreement with this possibility, the decrease in cytosolic phosphorylation potential is linearly correlated with the decline in intracellular free Mg^{2+} concentration across different levels of FP injury severity (Vink et al., 1988b). Hence, exposure to massive ionic disturbances during injury will likely lead to mitochondria that are compromised in their ability to respond to any further disruption inherently associated with secondary injury.

In addition to its impact on the bioenergetic state, it has been proposed that Mg^{2+} plays a pivotal role in determining the extent of excitotoxic damage following TBI, since changes in intra- and extracellular Mg^{2+} concentrations seem to directly affect the opening and closing of Na^+ and Ca^{2+} ion channels (Fagg and Langthorne, 1985; Johnson and Ascher, 1991).

Overall, there is much evidence to support the notion that there is a close correlation between decline in Mg^{2+} and consequences of TBI, such ss behavioral abnormalities, impaired cognitive performance, and brain edema (Emerson and Vink, 1992; Heath and Vink, 1998; McIntosh et al., 1988). In the same line, therapeutic attempts to replace Mg^{2+} loss showed promising effects (Bareyre et al., 1999; Feldman et al., 1996; Heath and Vink, 1997, 1999; McIntosh et al., 1989).

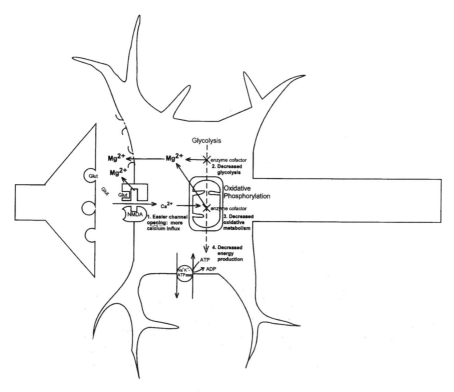

Figure 9.5 Magnesium cascade after traumatic brain injury. (1) Intracellular magnesium levels fall after injury, resulting in loss of the voltage block on the NMDA receptor channel, allowing greater calcium influx. (2) Magnesium is a necessary cofactor for glycolytic and oxidative enzymes, and a decrease in the available magnesium inhibits both glycolysis and (3) oxidative phosphorylation. (4) In turn, there is a decrease in the production of ATP and an overall reduction in the cell's bioenergetic state (Giza and Hovda, 2000).

SUMMARY

It is now clear that in both experimental and clinical studies the ionic cascade induced by TBI has numerous consequences related to a cellular metabolic crisis (Fig. 9.4). Cells that are not biomechanically and irreversibly damaged exist in a vulnerable state for an extended period of time. The degree to which this state of metabolic crisis participates in secondary injury is only now beginning to be appreciated. The extent to which this metabolic dysfunction affects the rate or degree of recovery of function has yet to be determined.

ACKNOWLEDGMENT

This research was supported by grants NS 30308 and NS 27544, and the Lind Lawrence Foundation.

ABBREVIATIONS

AMPA	α-Amino-3-hydroxy-5-methyl-4-isoxazole propionic acid
APV	2-Amino-5-phosphovaleric acid
ATP	Adenosine triphosphate
CCI	Controlled cortical impact
CMRglc	Cerebral metabolic rate for glucose
CNQX	6-Cyano-7-nitroquinoxaline-2,3-dione
CSF	Cerebrospinal fluid
2DG	2-Deoxyglucose
EAA	Excitatory amino acid
FPI	Fluid percussion injury
NMDA	N-methyl-D-aspartate
$[K^+]_e$	Extracellular concentration of potassium
TTX	Tetrodotoxin
TBI	Traumatic brain injury

REFERENCES

T. Abe, K. Koyano, H. Saisu, Y. Nishiuchi, and S. Sakakibara, *Neurosci. Lett.*, 71, 203–208 (1986).

B. M. Altura, Z. S. Memon, B. T. Altura, and R. Q. Cracco, *Alcohol*, 12, 433–437 (1995).

J. Astrup, S. Rehncrona, and B. K. Siesjo, *Brain Res.*, 199, 161–174 (1980).

K. Ballanyi, P. Grafe, and G. ten Bruggencate, *J. Physiol. (Lond.)*, 382, 159–174 (1987).

F. M. Bareyre, K. E. Saatman, M. A. Helfaer, G. Sinson, J. D. Weisser, A. L. Brown, and T. K. McIntosh, *J. Neurochem.*, 73, 271–280 (1999a).

D. P. Becker, "Brain Acidosis in Head Injury: A Clinical Trial," in D. P. Becker and J. T. Povlishock, Eds., *Central Nervous System Trauma Status Report – 1985*, Byrd Press, Richmond, 1985, pp. 229–242.

M. C. Bennett and G. M. Rose, *Behav. Neur. Biol.*, 58, 72–75 (1992).

A. Bignami and K. Clark, *Brain Res.*, 409, 143–145 (1987).

A. Binet and P. Volfin, *Arch. Biochem. Biophys.*, 170, 576–586 (1975).

S. Bröcher, A. Artola, and W. Singer, *Proc. Natl. Acad. Sci. USA*, 89, 123–127 (1992).

R. J. Bull and J. T. Cummins, *J. Neurochem.*, 21, 923–937 (1973).

C. J. Carter, F. Noel, and B. Scatton, *J. Neurochem.*, 49, 195–200 (1987).

C. W. Cotman and L. L. Iverson, *Trends Neurosci.*, 263–265 (1987).

R. D'Ambrosio, D. O. Mavis, M. S. Grady, H. R. Winn, and D. Janigro, *J. Neurosci.*, 19(18), 8152–8162 (1999).

A. A. DeSalles, L. W. Jenkins, R. L. Anderson, J. Opokuedusei, A. Marmarou, and R. L. Hayes, *Soc. Neurosci.*, (12), 967 (1986).

A. A. DeSalles, H. A. Kontos, J. D. Ward, A. Marmarou, and D. P. Becker, *Neurosurgery*, 20, 297–301 (1987).

D. J. Dooley, A. Lupp, and G. Hertting, *Naunyn. Schmiedebergs Arch. Pharmacol.*, 336, 467–470 (1987).

H. Ebel and T. Gunther, *J. Clin. Chem. Clin. Biochem.* 18, 257–270 (1980).

C. S. Emerson and R. Vink, *Neuroreport*, 3, 957–960 (1992).

G. E. Fagg and T. H. Lanthorn, *Br. J. Pharmacol.*, 86, 743–751 (1985).

A. A. Farooqui and L. A. Horrocks, *Brain Res. Brain Res. Rev.*, 16, 171–181 (1991).

Z. Feldman, B. Gurevitch, A. A. Artru, A. Oppenheim, E. Shohami, E. Reichenthal, and Y. Shapira, *J. Neurosurg.*, 85, 131–137 (1996).

I. Fineman, D. A. Hovda, M. Smith, A. Yoshino, and D. P. Becker, *Brain Res.*, 624, 94–102 (1993).

C. C. Giza and D. A. Hovda, "Ionic and Metabolic Consequences of Concussion," in R. C. Cantu, Ed., *Neurologic Athletic Head and Spine Injuries*, Saunders, 2000, pp. 83–89.

T. E. Gunter, K. K. Gunter, S. S. Sheu, and C. E. Gavin, *Am. J. Physiol.*, 267, C313–C339 (1994).

J. J. Hablitz and I. A. Langmoen, *J. Physiol. (Lond.)*, 325, 317–331 (1982).

A. J. Hansen, *Acta Physiol. Scand.*, 99, 412–420 (1977).

A. J. Hansen, *Acta Physiol. Scand.*, 102, 324–329 (1978).

R. L. Hayes, Y. Katayama, H. F. Young, and J. G. Dunbar, *Brain Inj.*, 2, 31–49 (1988).

D. L. Heath and R. Vink, *Brain Res.*, 738, 150–153 (1996).

D. L. Heath and R. Vink, *Neurosci. Lett.*, 228, 175–178 (1997).

D. L. Heath and R. Vink, *Scand. J. Clin. Lab. Invest.*, 58, 161–166 (1998).

D. L. Heath and R. Vink, *J. Pharmacol. Exp. Ther.*, 288, 1311–1316 (1999).

U. Heinemann and H. D. Lux, *Brain Res.*, 120, 231–249 (1977).

J. R. Hotson, G. W. Sypert, and A. A. J. Ward, *Exp. Neurol.*, 38, 20–26 (1973).

D. A. Hovda, A. Yoshino, T. Kawamata, Y. Katayama, and D. P. Becker, *Brain Res.*, 567, 1–10 (1991).

D. A. Hovda, "Metabolic Dysfunction," in R. K. Narayan, J. E. Wilberger and J. T. Povlishock, Eds., *Neurotrauma*, McGraw-Hill, New York, 1996, pp. 1459–1478.

O. R. Hubschmann and D. Kornhauser, *J. Neurosurg.*, 59, 289–293 (1983).

S. Inao, A. Marmarou, G. D. Clarke, B. J. Andersen, P. P. Fatouros, and H. F. Young, *J. Neurosurg.*, 69, 736–744 (1988).

O. Isacson, P. Brundin, P. A. T. Kelly, F. H. Gage, and A. Bjorklund, *Nature*, 311, 458–460 (1984).

Y. Iwasaki, H. Yamamoto, H. Iizuka, T. Yamamoto, and H. Konno, *Brain Res.*, 406, 99–104 (1987).

J. L. Jaggi, W. D. Obrist, T. A. Gennarelli, and T. W. Langfitt, *J. Neurosurg.*, 72, 176–182 (1990).

J. W. Johnson and P. Ascher, "Dual Block by Mg^{2+} of the NMDA Activated Channel," in P. Strata and E. Carbone, Eds., Mg^{2+} *and Excitable Membranes*, Springer-Verlag, Berlin, 1991, pp. 105–118.

F. J. Julian and D. E. Goldman, *J. Gen. Physiol.*, 297 (1962).

A. Kampfl, R. M. Posmantur, X. Zhao, E. Schmutzhard, G. L. Clifton, and R. L. Hayes, *J. Neurotrauma*, 14, 121–134 (1997).

Y. Katayama. D. P. Becker, T. Tamura, and D. A. Hovda, *J. Neurosurg.*, 73, 889–900 (1990).

Y. Katayama, M. Cheung, L. K. Gorman, T. Tamura, and D. P. Becker, *Soc. Neurosci.* (14), 1154 (1988).

R. Katzman, *Fed. Proc.*, 35, 1244–1247 (1976).

T. Kawamata, D. A. Hovda, and A. Yoshino et al., *Soc. Neurosci.*, (abstract), 16, 778 (1990).

T. Kawamata, Y. Katayama, and D. A. Hovda et al., *J. Cereb. Blood Flow Metab.*, 12, 12–24 (1992).

T. Kawamata, Y. Katayama, D. A. Hovda, A. Yoshino, and D. P. Becker, *Brain Res.*, 674, 196–204 (1995).

K. Koyano, T. Abe, Y. Nichiuchi, and S. Sakakibara, *Eur. J. Pharmacol.*, 135, 337–343 (1987).

S. W. Kuffler, *Proc. R. Soc. Lond. B Biol. Sci.*, 168, 1–21 (1967).

D. V. Lewis and W. H. Schuette, *J. Neurophysiol.*, 38, 405–417 (1975).

E. Lothman, J. Lamanna, G. Cordingley. M. Rosenthal, and G. Somjen, *Brain Res.*, 88, 15–36 (1975).

M. L. Mayer and G. L. Westbrook, *Trends Neurosci.*, 59–61 (1987).

A. Mayevsky and B. Chance, *Brain Res.*, 65, 529–533 (1974).

T. K. McIntosh, A. I. Faden, M. R. Bendall, and R. Vink, *J. Neurochem.*, 49, 1530–1540 (1987).

T. K. McIntosh, A. I. Faden, I. Yamakami, and R. Vink, *J. Neurotrauma*, 5, 17–31 (1988).

T. K. McIntosh, R. Vink, I. Yamakami, and A. I. Faden, *Brain Res.*, 482, 252–260 (1989).

Z. I. Memon, B. T. Altura, J. L. Benjamin, R. Q. Cracco, and B. M. Altura, *Scand. J. Clin. Lab. Invest.*, 55, 671–677 (1995).

W. J. Moody, K. J. Futamachi, and D. A. Prince, *Exp. Neurol.*, 42, 248–263 (1974).

J. I. Morgan and T. Curran, *Nature.*, 322, 552–555 (1986).

V. Nadler, A. Biegon, E. Beit-Yannai, J. Adamchik, and E. Shohami, *Brain Res.*, 685, 1–11 (1995).

C. Nicholson and R. P. Kraig, "The Behavior of Extracellular Ions During Spreading Depression," in T. Zeuthen, Ed., *The Application of Ion-Sensitive Electrodes*, Elsevier, New York, 1981, pp. 217–238.

P. Nilsson, L. Hillered, U. Ponten, and U. Ungerstedt, *J. Cereb. Blood Flow Metab.*, 10, 631–637 (1990).

P. Nilsson, L. Hillered, Y. Olsson, M. J. Sheardown, and A. J. Hansen, *J. Cereb. Blood Flow Metab.*, 13, 183–192 (1993).

P. Nilsson, H. Laursen, L. Hillered, and A. J. Hansen, *J. Cereb. Blood Flow Metab.*, 16, 262–270 (1996).

R. K. Orkand, *Fed. Proc.*, 39, 1515–1518 (1980).

O. B. Paulson and E. A. Newman, *Science*, 237, 896–898 (1987).

D. A. Prince, H. D. Lux, and E. Neher, *Brain Res.*, 50, 489–495 (1973).

E. Racker, J. H. Johnson, and M. T. Blackwell, *J. Biol. Chem.*, 258, 3702–3705 (1983).

J. P. Rauschecker, M. W. von Grunau, and C. Poulin, *Exp. Brain Res.*, 67, 100–112 (1987).

J. M. Roberts-Lewis and R. Siman, *Ann. N.Y. Acad. Sci.*, 679, 78–86 (1993).

C. S. Robertson, R. G. Grossman, J. C. Goodman, and R. K. Narayan, *J. Neurosurg.*, 67, 361–368 (1987).

I. A. Rose, J. V. B. Warms, and D. M. O'Dell, *Biochem. Biophys. Res. Commun.*, 33–37 (1964).

M. Rosenthal, J. Lamanna, S. Yamada, W. Younts, and G. Somjen, *Brain Res.*, 162, 113–127 (1979).

A Samii, S. M. Lee, and D. A. Hovda, *J. Neurotrauma*, 15(10), 894 (1998).

A. Samii, H. Badie, K. Fu, R. R. Luther, and D. A. Hovda, *J. Neurotrauma*, 16(10), 879–892 (1999).

K. Sano, K. Enomoto, and T. Maeno, *Eur. J. Pharmacol.*, 141, 235–241 (1987).

A. F. Schinder, E. C. Olson, N. C. Spitzer, and M. Montal, *J. Neurosci.*, 16, 6125–6133 (1996).

J. W. Schmidley, *Stroke*, 21, 1086–1090 (1990).

B. K. Siesjo, *J. Neurosurg.*, 77, 337–354 (1992).

L. Sokoloff, "Local Cerebral Circulation at Rest and During Altered Cerebral Activity Induced by Anesthesia or Visual Stimulation," in S. S. Kety and J. Elkes, Eds., *The Regional Chemistry, Physiology and Pharmacology of the Nervous System*, Pergamon Press, Oxford, 1960, pp. 107–117.

G. G. Somjen, J. L. Giacchino, *J. Neurophysiol.*, 53, 1098–1108 (1985).

E. Sugaya, M. Takato, and Y. Noda, *J. Neurophysiol.*, 38, 822–841 (1975).

G. W. Sypert and A. A. J. Ward, *Exp. Neurol.*, 45, 19–41 (1974).

H. Takahashi, S. Manaka, and K. Sano, *J. Neurosurg.*, 55, 708–717 (1981).

S. Takizawa, *J. Cereb. Blood Flow Metab.*, 15, 611–618 (1995).

C. Tobiasz and C. Nicholson, *Brain Res.*, 241, 329–333 (1982).

T. Tsubokawa, *No Shinkei Geka*, 11, 563–573 (1983).

M. Tymianski and C. H. Tator, *Neurosurgery*, 38, 1176–1195 (1996).

A. Van Harreveld, *J. Neurobiol.*, 9, 419–431 (1978).

M. A. Verity, *Neurotoxicology*, 13, 139–147 (1992).

B. H. Verweij, J. P. Muizelaar, F. C. Vinas, P. L. Peterson, Y. Xiong, and C. P. Lee, *Neurol. Res.*, 19, 334–339 (1997).

R. Vink, T. K. McIntosh, P. Demediuk, and A. I. Faden, *Biochem. Biophys. Res. Commun.*, 149, 594–599 (1987).

R. Vink, T. K. McIntosh, P. Demediuk, M. W. Weiner, and A. I. Faden, *J. Biol. Chem.*, 263, 757–761 (1988a).

R. Vink, A. I. Faden, and T. K. McIntosh, *J. Neurotrauma*, 5, 315–330 (1988b).

R. Vink, E. M. Golding, and J. P. Headrick, *J. Neurotrauma*, 11, 265–274 (1994).

A. E. Walker, J. J. Kolloros, and T. J. Case, *J. Neurosurg.*, 103 (1944).

Y. Xiong, Q. Gu, P. L. Peterson, J. P. Muizelaar, and C. P. Lee, *J. Neurotrauma*, 14, 23–34 (1997).

M. S. Yang, D. S. DeWitt, D. P. Becker, and R. L. Hayes, *J. Neurosurg.*, 63, 617–621 (1985).

A. Yoshino, D. A. Hovda, T. Kawamata, Y. Katayama, and D. P. Becker, *Brain Res.* 561(1), 106–119 (1991).

A Yoshino, D. A. Hovda, Y. Katayama, T. Kawamata, and D. P. Becker, *J. Cereb. Blood Flow Metab.*, 12(6), 996–1006 (1992).

CHAPTER 10

CONTRIBUTIONS OF CALPAINS AND CASPASES TO CELL DEATH FOLLOWING TRAUMATIC BRAIN INJURY

R. L. HAYES, B. R. PIKE, AND S. M. DeFORD
University of Florida Brain Institute, Department of Neuroscience, Center for
Traumatic Brain Injury Studies, Gainseville, Florida

J. K. NEWCOMB
University of Texas-Houston Health Science Center, Department of Neurosurgery,
Vivian L. Smith Center for Neurologic Research, Houston, Texas

INTRODUCTION

The molecular events occurring after traumatic brain injury are just beginning to be understood. Recent studies have implicated loss of intracellular calcium homeostasis in delayed neuronal cell damage and cell death following a number of central nervous system (CNS) injuries. Several studies have reported that neuronal calcium overload is a reliable feature of experimental traumatic brain injury (TBI) (Nadler et al., 1995) and cerebral ischemia (Siesjoe and Bengtsson, 1989) in vivo. This calcium overload may be triggered by several mechanisms including brief (6 to 10 min) potassium depolarization (Katayama et al., 1990; Nilsson et al., 1993) and excessive exposure to certain excitatory amino acids (Faden et al., 1989; Hayes et al., 1992). Elevated neuronal calcium levels activate a number of calcium-dependent enzymes such as phospholipases (Nishida et al., 1994), kinases (Yang et al., 1994), phosphatases (Morioka et al., 1992), and proteases (Bartus et al., 1994; Posmantur et al., 1994), all of which can modulate post-TBI cytoskeletal protein loss.

Although the relative contribution of various calcium-regulated processes to neuronal cytoskeleton damage has not been established, recent evidence has clearly

Head Trauma:, Preclinical, and Clinical Directions, Edited by Leonard P. Miller and Ronald L. Hayes,
Co-edited by Jennifer K. Newcomb
ISBN 0-471-36015-5 © 2001 John Wiley & Sons, Inc.

implicated the pathological activation of calpains (Melloni and Pontremoli, 1989) and caspases as a major biochemical event in the pathology of CNS insult (for review see Kampfl et al., 1997; Wang and Yuen, 1994; Yuen and Wang, 1996). Calpains have been implicated in CNS damage after traumatic brain injury (Kampfl et al., 1997; Newcomb et al., 1997; Pike et al., 1998a; Posmantur et al., 1997a; Saatman et al., 1996b), spinal cord injury (Banik et al., 1997), and cerebral ischemia in vivo (Hong et al., 1994; Roberts-Lewis et al., 1994). Although the calpains are generally thought to be associated with necrotic cell death, mounting evidence now indicates a role for calpains in apoptotic cell death as well (Nath et al., 1996b; Pike et al., 1998b). Caspase-3 is regarded as a critical executioner of apoptosis in several in vitro cell culture systems (Nicholson and Thornberry, 1997), and caspase-3 activation has been observed in vivo after TBI (Beer et al., 2000; Clark et al., 1999, 2000; Pike et al., 1998a; Yakovlev et al., 1997) and cerebral ischemia (Namura et al., 1998). Thus, calpain and caspase-3 responses to brain injury have received a great deal of attention. The significant progress being made in understanding the contributions of calpains and caspases to cell injury/death is discussed in this chapter.

IMPLICATIONS FOR CELL INJURY

Calpain Biochemistry

Calpains are calcium-activated, neutral cysteine proteases. The calpain family can be divided into two groups on the basis of distribution of ubiquitously expressed and tissue-specific calpains (Sorimachi et al., 1994). Currently, two major isoenzymes of calpain are known to exist in the CNS system, μ-calpain and m-calpain (for review see Saido et al., 1994; Sorimachi et al., 1994). μ-Calpain has micromolar sensitivity to calcium and is located primarily in the neuronal soma and dendrites and less abundantly in axons and glia (Hamakubo et al., 1986; Perlmutter et al., 1990). m-Calpain has a millimolar sensitivity to calcium activation and is prominently located in glia, with low levels also found in axons (Hamakubo et al., 1986), as well as being a possible constituent of myelin (Li and Banik, 1995). Structurally, calpain contains a large calcium-dependent catalytic subunit (80 kDa) and a smaller regulatory subunit (30 kDa). The catalytic subunit contains four complexes that can bind calcium. An important event in the intramolecular activation of μ-calpain seems to be subunit autolysis. In the presence of sufficient calcium, autolysis of the catalytic 80 kDa subunit to a 76 kDa subunit occurs, as well as autolysis of the 30 kDa regulatory subunit to a 19 kDa isoform. Substrate cleavage follows the autolysis of the catalytic and regulating subunits (Saido et al., 1994). Calpain has relative selectivity for proteolysis of a subset of cellular proteins. These include cytoskeletal proteins (e.g., neurofilaments, microtubule-associated protein 2, spectrin, tau), calmodulin-binding proteins (e.g., G proteins), enzymes involved in signal transduction (e.g., protein kinase C, phosphatases calcineurin, phospholipases such as phospholipase C), membrane proteins (e.g., receptors), and transcription factors (e.g., Fos, Jun; for review see Saido et al., 1994).

Although much is known about the structural and enzymological properties of μ-calpain and m-calpain, the normal physiological functions of calpain in vivo are not clearly understood. For example, a clear discrepancy exists in the in vitro calcium requirement of calpain and the physiological intracellular calcium-concentration. As mentioned earlier, in vitro substrate proteolysis by μ-calpain requires more than 10^{-6} M of calcium, whereas the intracellular calcium concentration usually fluctuates between 10^{-8} and 10^{-6} M. However, recent research has provided evidence that the sensitivities of both μ-calpain and m-calpain to calcium are increased by calpain autolysis and interaction with membrane phospholipids (Saido et al., 1992b, 1994), suggesting a physiological role of calpain. For example, recent reports emphasized the importance of calpain in neuronal differentiation (Hirai et al., 1991), physiological cytoskeletal protein turnover (Giancotti et al., 1992), and long-term potentiation (del Cerro et al., 1990).

PATHOLOGICAL CONSEQUENCES OF CALPAIN ACTIVATION FOLLOWING ACUTE BRAIN INJURY

Pathological consequences of TBI-related calpain activation may include modulation of post-TBI cytoskeletal protein loss (Bartus et al., 1994; Posmantur et al., 1994). The neurocytoskeleton is a dynamic structure involved in intracellular transport (e.g., organelles, vesicles) as well as maintaining cellular shape, intracellular space, and membrane stability. Integrity of the cytoskeleton is essential for cell survival and function. Possible functional consequences of neuronal cytoskeletal loss could involve disturbances of axonal transport, structural integrity, and neuronal cell death, resulting in cognitive/behavioral deficits (see Fig. 10.1).

Microfilaments, intermediate filaments, and microtubules comprise the neurocytoskeleton. The major function of microtubules is the transport of intracellular proteins and organelles by ATP-dependent transport mechanisms involving kinesin and dynein motor systems. Microtubules consist of α- and β-tubulin subunit heterodimers aligned in a linear fashion with cross-linking microtubule-associated proteins (MAPs). The α and β tubulins are found throughout the neuron, whereas subclassifications of microtubules containing specific MAPs may be highly localized to dendritic (MAP-2) or axonal (tau) environments. Microfilaments, approximately 8 nm in diameter, are formed in the presence of ATP. Their functions include growth cone motility, endocytosis and exocytosis, synaptical vesicle release, and adhesion of various microfilament lattices with the plasma membrane. In addition to actin, other important microfilament proteins include the spectrins (Dhermy, 1991) and synapsin.

MAP-2 (280 kDa) is the most abundant MAP in the brain (Johnson and Jope, 1992). MAP-2 contains phosphorylation sites for multiple kinases, including protein kinases A and C, calmodulin II, and growth factor-sensitive MAP kinase (Johnson and Jope, 1992). Taft et al. (1992, 1993) documented profound enduring

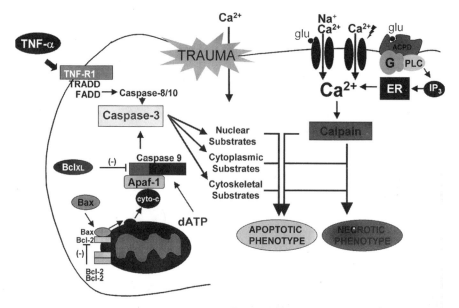

Figure 10.1   Summary of calpain and caspase-3 pathways mediating expression of apoptotic and/or necrotic cell death phenotypes. Traumatic brain injury can result in increased levels of TNF-α which bind to TNF-α-receptor 1 (TNF-R1). TNF-R1, when activated, couples to TNF-α-associated death domain protein (TRADD). TRADD can interact with another adaptor protein, FADD. A TRADD–FADD–caspase-8/10 interaction produces the autolytic activation of caspase-8/10, which in turn processes and activates caspase-3. Mitochondrially related events can also trigger caspase-3 activation. Three protein factors are necessary for caspase-3 activation: Apaf-1, cytochrome c, and the unactivated caspase-9 precursor. The unactivated caspase-9 precursor binds to Apaf-1 and this binding is dependent upon cytochrome c and dATP. This complex subsequently cleaves and activates caspase-3. Overexpression of Bcl-2 or its close family member BclXL blocks release of cytochrome c from mitochondria. In addition, Bcl-2 or related proteins could directly interact with Apaf-1. Bax is a mitochondrially mediated promoter of cell death unless it is bound either by Bcl-2 or Bcl-x_L. Calpain requires increased levels of cytosolic calcium for its activation. Increased levels of calcium could be produced by stimulation of glutamate receptors gating calcium input from the extracellular space or release of calcium from intracellular stores in the endoplasmic reticulum (ER).

hippocampal MAP-2 loss following mild fluid percussive injury in the absence of cell death. Significant decrease in MAP-2 has been noted as early as 15 min, peaking by 3 h in the cortex and 48 h post injury in the rat hippocampus (Posmantur et al., 1996a,b). Alteration in MAP-2 may occur through several mechanisms, including receptor-mediated modification, signal transduction systems, and Ca^{2+}-mediated enzymes (e.g., proteases).

Johnson et al. (1991) reported high sensitivity of MAP-2 to degradation, particularly by calpains. Ca^{2+}-dependent release of calpains has been shown to increase following TBI promoting calpain-modulated MAP-2 degradation (Kampfl et al., 1996b). Detailed studies by Hayes and colleagues have shown that cysteine proteases in particular are highly involved in the breakdown of cytoskeletal proteins following experimental brain injury (Posmantur et al., 1998) and that inhibitors of these proteases are protective (Kampfl et al., 1996b). Specifically, calpain-mediated proteolysis increased significantly in the cortex, hippocampus, and thalamus for up to two weeks, while caspase-3-mediated proteolysis was only evident in hippocampal and striatal tissue early (hours) after experimental TBI (Pike et al., 1998b).

Within the intermediate filament family are the neurofilaments (NF) triplet proteins including heavy ($\sim$200 kDa), middle ($\sim$150 kDa), and light ($\sim$68 kDa) molecular weight proteins (Allende et al., 1989). NFs function as the primary intermediate filaments of the neuronal cytoarchitecture, remaining relatively stable unlike the more dynamic microtubules (Kampfl et al., 1997; Shaw, 1986). Depending on their phosphorylation state, NFs are abundantly found in axons and dendrites (Shaw, 1986), regulating axonal caliber as well as intracellular structure and spacing. NFs are comprised of functional domains distinct to each of the triplet proteins. The phosphorylated carboxyl terminus of NF 150 and of NF 200 forms a sidearm domain that extends laterally from the adjoined amino-terminal α-helical rod domains. The degree of sidearm extension and charge is believed to partially modulate interfilament distance, and thus axonal caliber. Whitson et al. (1995) reported Ca^{2+}-dependent decreased phosphorylated and nonphosphorylated NF following brief K^+ depolarization.

Cytoskeletal alterations after experimental brain injury have pointed to the likelihood of calpain-mediated proteolysis. Preferred substrates for calpains include the cytoskeletal proteins spectrin (Harris et al., 1988; Roberts-Lewis et al., 1994), MAP-2 (Johnson et al., 1991), and NF proteins (Kamakura et al., 1985; Nixon and Sihag, 1991). Increased degradation of MAP-2 (Blomgren et al., 1995), the NF triplet proteins (Kaku et al., 1993), and spectrin (Bartus et al., 1995a; Hong et al., 1994) has been reported in cerebral ischemia. In addition, loss of MAP-2 (Posmantur et al., 1996b; Taft et al., 1992, 1993), NF 68, and NF 200 (Posmantur et al., 1994, 1997a) has been reported following TBI in vivo.

Prominent dendritic cytoskeletal proteolysis of MAP-2, presumably caused by calpain activation, has been described in cerebral ischemia (Kitagawa et al., 1989) in vivo. In addition, recent reports provide evidence that TBI can produce significant proteolysis of dendritic MAP-2 (Hicks et al., 1995; Posmantur et al., 1996b; Taft et al., 1992, 1993), NF 68, and NF 200 (Posmantur et al., 1996a) proteins in the absence of marked axonal changes, especially within the first 24 h after injury. Importantly, immunohistochemical investigations of calpain-specific breakdown products to brain spectrin have provided evidence for calpain overactivation in apical dendrites following cerebral ischemia (Roberts-Lewis et al., 1994) and TBI (Saatman et al., 1996b) in vivo. Moreover, in a recent TBI study the accumulation of calpain-mediated α-spectrin breakdown products in dendrites was observed primarily at the site of contusion and, to a lesser extent, in areas distal to the site of contusion (Newcomb et al., 1997).

While studies investigating cytoskeletal protein levels following CNS insult show degradation, these findings provide only indirect evidence for calpain activation, since cytoskeletal protein degradation may be at least partially attributable to proteases other than calpain. Protease inhibitors that block calpains have thus been used to provide more direct evidence of calpain activation in experimental brain injury. These inhibitors have been shown to be neuroprotective in cerebral ischemia (Bartus et al., 1994, 1995; Hong et al., 1994) and TBI (Posmantur et al., 1997a; Saatman et al., 1996a) in vivo models of acute CNS injury (Brorson et al., 1995; George et al., 1995; Kampfl et al., 1995, 1996a). Because none of these inhibitors is solely selective for calpains and detailed dose–response analyses were not conducted (Wang and Yuen, 1994), these data have provided relatively indirect evidence for calpain activation after TBI and cerebral ischemia.

The presence of breakdown products of cytoskeletal proteins has also historically been used as an indirect marker of calpain activity. Importantly, TBI has been shown to be associated with the loss of NF 68 and the appearance of low-molecular-weight (LMW) immunopositive breakdown products characteristic of calpain proteolysis (Posmantur et al., 1994). Interestingly, the action of calpain on NF proteins produces similar LMW immunopositive cleavage products of 57 kDa and 53 kDa for in vivo studies (Schlaepfer et al., 1985). Although other proteases can potentially produce immunopositive neurofilaments fragments, such as cathepsins B and D, trypsin, and α-chymotrypsin, the molecular weights of the proteolytic fragments are substantially lower or higher (Kamakura et al., 1985) and do not resemble the pattern observed following TBI. Recent in vitro digestion studies have also confirmed that only μ-calpain and m-calpain contribute to the presence of LMW 53 kDa and 57 kDa NF 68 breakdown products detected in post-TBI samples. Cathepsin B, cathepsin D, and caspase-3 failed to produce either the 53 kDa or 57 kDa NF breakdown products (Posmantur et al., 1997c).

More direct evidence that calpain is activated in neurons following experimental brain injury has been shown by the use of antibodies that react specifically to calpain-mediated breakdown products of cytoskeletal proteins. These studies included calpain-specific breakdown products to spectrin (Roberts-Lewis et al., 1994; Saido et al., 1993b). In recent reports, increased immunoreactivity for calpain-degraded α-spectrin has been shown in animal models of TBI (Kampfl et al., 1996b; Newcomb et al., 1997; Posmantur et al., 1997a; Saatman et al., 1996b) and cerebral ischemia (Roberts-Lewis et al., 1994; Saido et al., 1993b) in vivo.

Subunit autolysis seems to be an important early event in the intramolecular activation process of μ-calpain. Importantly, the ratio of the activated, autolyzed 76 kDa isoform to the 80 kDa precursor form has been shown to be an indicator for μ-calpain activity in vivo and in vitro (Ostwald et al., 1994). Autolysis of μ-calpain has been described in animal models of global cerebral ischemia (Neumar et al., 1996) and chronic hypoxia (Ostwald et al., 1994). In addition, a recent report described this autolytic event in an animal model of experimental TBI (Kampfl et al., 1996b). Using western blotting, these authors described increased calpain activation in cortical samples ipsilateral to the injury site at 15 min up to 12 h post injury. Although some reports have suggested that μ-calpain does not require autolysis for activation (Zhang et al., 1996; Guttmann et al., 1997), Kampfl and colleagues reported that autolysis of μ-calpain was temporally correlated with the appearance of calpain-mediated breakdown products to α-spectrin.

In addition to the several lines of indirect evidence for the role of calpain in pathological responses to TBI, Zhao and colleagues (1997a) have reported increases in both μ-calpain and m-calpain activity following TBI using casein zymography. Casein zymography is a technique employing denaturing casein-containing poly-acrylamide gels that makes possible differential and concurrent measurements of activity of both major calpain isoforms from in vivo tissue. Previous efforts to examine calpain activity from in vivo homogenates were hampered by the presence of the endogenous inhibitor calpastatin, a problem that casein zymography circumvents. Casein zymography showed that TBI increased μ-calpain and m-calpain activity as early as 15 min after injury. This increase persisted for as long as 24 h post injury. Although increased μ-calpain activity was associated with translocation of this isoform from the cytosol to the membrane, increased m-calpain activity remained in the cytosol. In addition, increased μ-calpain and m-calpain activity measured by casein zymography was found in both the ipsilateral (site of impact) and contralateral (an area outside of direct contusion) cortices. This evidence suggests calpain activity following TBI may not be restricted to sites of contusion but may represent a more global response to injury (Zhao et al., 1997a). Lastly, a follow-up report by Zhao and colleagues (1997b) has also demonstrated that strict control of pH is an important consideration in calpain assessments from TBI samples. μ-Calpain activity following cortical impact was detected between pH 7.0 and pH 8.0, with pH 7.5 being optimal. However, m-calpain activity was readily detected only between pH values of 7.2 and 7.4, with pH 7.3 producing the most prominent proteolytic activity.

The occurrence of early extensive dendritic damage following TBI (Posmantur et al., 1996a) might be due to the electrophysiological properties specific to dendrites. Dendritic processes (pyramidal apical dendrites) contain several low-voltage calcium and sodium channels and consequently may be more likely to open after TBI (Regehr and Tank, 1994). Thus, the electrophysiological properties of dendrites can potentially yield immediate focal alterations in intracellular Ca^{2+} homeostasis at sites of ion entry. Electrophysiological studies examining long-term potentiation following TBI (Miyazaki et al., 1992; Reeves et al., 1995) also support impaired dendritic functioning as inferred by decreased efficacy of synaptic transmission. In contrast, axons within white-matter tracts (i.e., corpus callosum) propagate neuronal transmission primarily by opening and closing of Na^+ and K^+ channels, suggesting that axons are less likely to experience large, immediate changes in calcium homeostasis after neuronal excitation. The potentially less stable Ca^{2+} environment within dendrites may lead to an increased pattern of Ca^{2+}-mediated protease activation compared with that observed within axons.

While recent research has provided clear evidence that dendritic cytoskeletal derangements following cerebral ischemia and TBI may be due to overactivation of calpain (discussed earlier), the role of calpain in induction of axonal cytoskeletal derangements following brain injuries in vivo is less well documented (Povlishock and Christman, 1995). Calcium-activated neutral protease neurofilament degradation has been reported in association with Wallerian degeneration (Schlaepfer et al., 1985), and past reports have provided some evidence that calpain activation can contribute to axonal damage following TBI. For example, calpain-degraded spectrin is found in axons within 15 to 90 min post TBI (Buki et al., 2000; Saatman et al., 1996b). A recent report has also shown delayed proteolysis of α-spectrin in the corpus callosum at 24 h following injury (Newcomb et al., 1997), in contrast to the rapid accumulation of calpain-mediated breakdown products in dendrites and soma. In addition, inhibitors of calpain (and other proteases) have been reported to attenuate axonal damage following brain injury in vivo (Posmantur et al., 1997a) and in vitro (George et al., 1995; also see Kampfl et al., 1996a). However, some papers have suggested that calpain activation may not be a likely mediator of cytoskeletal damage to axons following traumatic brain injury in vivo (Pettus et al., 1994; Yaghmai and Povlishock, 1992). These scientists have suggested that localized intraaxonal changes in cytoskeletal alignment lead to impairment in an anterograde transport, resulting in axonal swelling and eventual disconnection (Pettus et al., 1994; Povlishock et al., 1996; Yaghmai and Povlishock, 1992).

While the reason for discrepancies in the role of calpain in axonal injury following TBI is not entirely clear, it may be possible that these discrepant observations may be linked, in part, to the injury sustained at the moment of impact by individual axons. Those cases in which calpain-mediated proteolysis has been implicated appear to involve the most severe end of the injury spectrum involving axonal change occurring in relation to areas of focal contusion or tissue damage. In contrast, sites sustaining less severe injury do not seem to show calpain-mediated change (Saatman et al., 1996b). Support for this premise is also found in a recent communication (Povlishock et al., 1996) reporting that in animals subjected to severe injury a subpopulation of axons showed cytoskeletal changes reminiscent of calcium-mediated proteolysis, which, as such, involved frank degradation of the cytoskeleton. On the other hand, in the same animal, sites showing less dramatic injury revealed more subtle intraaxonal changes involving the misalignment and compaction of neurofilaments, which morphologically were inconsistent with a calpain-mediated proteolysis. Collectively, these findings suggest that the pathobiology of traumatically induced injury may be complex and may involve different initiating pathologies other than calpain-mediated proteolysis. In fact, recent data indicate that TBI can dephosphorylate neurofilaments proteins, an event that could disturb the assembly state of neurofilaments (Posmantur et al., 1997b,c; 2000).

Caspase-3 Biochemistry. Caspase-3, a 32 kDa cytoplasmic protein, is processed to two subunits, p17 and p12, which form the active enzyme complex (Nicholson et al., 1995). Caspase-3 has a conserved pentapeptide active site, QACXG (where X is R, Q, or G), common for the caspase family, and a preference for proteins that contain a DXXD (P_4–P_1) peptide region (for review see Fraser and Evan, 1997). There are at least 11 different caspases that may participate in apoptotic cascades (Fraser and Evan, 1997). Caspase-3 is usually viewed as the effector caspase whose activity can be modulated by other caspases (e.g., caspase-8, caspase-9; also see Fig. 10.1). Activated caspase-3 can proteolytically cleave a number of important intracellular, membrane, and nuclear proteins (Nicholson et al., 1995). Preferred substrates of caspase-3 include poly(ADP-ribose) polymerase (PARP;

Lazebnik et al., 1994; Nicholson et al., 1995), α-spectrin (Martin et al., 1995; Nath et al., 1996), sterol regulatory element-binding proteins, and calpastatin (Wang, 2000).

Relative Contribution of Calpain and Caspase to Cell Death Following TBI

Much current research focuses on the relative contributions of calpains and caspases to expression of necrotic and apoptotic cell death phenotypes. Early reports identifying apoptosis following TBI were restricted to hallmark features of apoptosis (Kerr and Harmon, 1991) including nuclear chromatin condensation, DNA laddering, and positive TUNEL staining (Colicos and Dash, 1996). Proteolytic cleavage of intracellular, membrane, and nuclear proteins can facilitate cell death during apoptosis (Nicholson et al., 1995). A recent study has implicated increased caspase-3 activity following TBI in areas that contain DNA laddering and positive TUNEL staining such as the hippocampus and the cortex (Yakovlev et al., 1997).

However, previous investigations examining activation of caspase-3 after experimental TBI in vivo, although important, have provided limited information regarding the pathological role of caspase-3 in TBI. These studies have focused on (1) detection of caspase-3 mRNA levels using semiquantitative RT-PCR and/or in situ hybridization (Yakovlev et al., 1997); (2) measurement of caspase-3 protease activity in brain lysate via the cleavage of a fluorogenic substrate in the presence and absence of caspase inhibitors (Yakovlev et al., 1997); and (3) degradation of putative caspase-3 substrates, including poly(ADP-ribose) polymerase (LaPlaca et al., 1999) and DNA fragmentation factor (DFF; Zhang et al., 1999). Although these studies have provided critical information regarding caspase-3 activation after TBI, important interpretational caveats remain as these studies provide only indirect evidence of caspase-3 activation because degradation of PARP and DFF may be at least partially attributable to proteases other than caspase-3 (Liu et al., 1999).

To our knowledge, only four recent studies provided direct evidence for caspase-3 activation following TBI in vivo. First, Clark et al. (1999) demonstrated cleavage of caspase-3 to its p18 and p12 subunits after TBI in humans. However, this study was limited in terms of injury magnitudes, time points of sample collection, and proper controls. Second, and as discussed above, our own laboratory (Pike et al., 1998b) showed increased proteolysis of α-spectrin to a 120 kDa breakdown product, mediated by caspase-3 activation, after cortical impact injury in the rat. However, our experiments did not investigate cell subtype distribution of activated caspase-3 following TBI in vivo. Third, Clark et al. (2000) demonstrated increased expression of the caspase-3 p12 subunit following experimental TBI in rats. However, this study did not investigate a thorough time course of caspase-3 activation following TBI. Moreover, the latter study, similarly to the study of Pike et al. (1998b), did not examine the cell subtype distribution of activated caspase-3 after TBI. Fourth, in the most recent study to examine caspase-3 activation directly, Beer and colleagues (2000) used an antibody against an activated isoform of caspase-3 to demonstrate activation in injured cortex after cortical impact TBI in rats. Importantly, this study was the first to examine which cell subtypes showed caspase-3 activation. Caspase-3 was activated in neurons, astrocytes, and oligodendrocytes after TBI (Beer et al., 2000).

While an increasing number of investigations have now documented apoptotic cell death and caspase-3 activation in various models of TBI, elusive but important questions remain to be addressed. Is caspase-3 activation and apoptotic cell death in TBI necessarily pathological? Might apoptotic cell death serve an important role in removing dysfunctional CNS cells from the brain parenchyma? These questions remain unanswered, but at least two studies to date have examined the effects of caspase-3 inhibition on behavioral outcome in experimental models of TBI and have reported equivocal results. For example, although Yakovlev et al. (1997) have shown that a relatively specific tetrapeptide inhibitor of caspase-3, z-DEVD-fmk, attenuates neurological recovery after fluid percussion-induced TBI, a subsequent study by Clark et al. (2000) failed to show improved behavioral outcome after cortical impact-induced TBI with the same inhibitor. Interestingly however, the latter study revealed reduced hemispheric contusion volume and hippocampal tissue loss following cortical impact injury. Therefore, the effect of specific caspase-3 inhibitors on neuronal and/or glial protection and concurrent behavioral outcome after TBI remains to be further elucidated.

However, the role of calpain as a contributing protease in apoptotic cell death cannot be excluded since it has been shown that calpain may increase in different models of apoptosis and in different cell types (Nath et al., 1996). A report from Pike et al. (1997) has provided the first systematic in vivo comparison of the contributions of caspase-3 and calpain proteolysis to TBI pathology using α-spectrin. α-Spectrin can be differentially cleaved by both caspase-3 and calpain to yield unique breakdown products, which include a calpain-specific 145 kDa fragment (Harris et al., 1988; Kevin K. W. Wang, personal communication) and a caspase-3-specific 120 kDa fragment (Nath et al., 1996a; Wang et al., 1997). Immunoblots from the study revealed regionally and temporally distinct patterns of calpain- and/or caspase-3–α-spectrin-mediated proteolysis following TBI (Pike et al., 1997). Findings include the rapid and sustained accumulation of the calpain-specific 145 kDa α-spectrin breakdown product (SBDP) in cortical regions from 3 h to 5 days post TBI in the absence of any significant accumulation of the caspase-3-specific 120 kDa SBDP. However, in the hippocampus there was a rapid and brief appearance of the 120 kDa SBDP from 15 min to 6 h post TBI, followed by a delayed and prolonged accumulation of the 145 kDa SBDP from 15 min to 7 days. Interestingly, in the striatum the caspase-mediate proteolysis predominated from 3 h to 2 days post TBI. In summary, in regions of overt necrosis such as the cortex, calpain-mediated proteolysis appears to be the primary proteolytic event. However, in other brain regions such as the hippocampus, an area that contains both necrotic and apoptotic cell death, there is evidence for both calpain and caspase-3 proteolysis. Lastly, there are select regions in the brain, such as the striatum, that contain predominantly caspase-3-mediated proteolysis. Further study is needed to better understand the role of these proteases in both necrotic and apoptotic cell death following TBI.

Although calpain or caspase-3 protease activation is widely reported after CNS injury, few investigations have assessed concurrent activation of these proteases

(Buki et al., 2000; Nath et al., 1996a,b; Pike et al., 1998b). In addition, TBI results in calpain and caspase-3 activation and necrotic and apoptotic cell death. Because calpains are associated with necrotic and apoptotic cell death while caspase-3 is associated only with apoptotic cell death, elucidation of the relative contribution of these two protease families to cell death after CNS injury is important.

Because calpain and caspase-3 activation occurs under similar CNS pathological conditions and process, many of the same substrates, calpain, and caspase-3 may interact and mediate the expression of apoptotic cell death phenotypes following acute CNS trauma. For example, both calpain and caspase-3 proteolyse proteins that may be responsible for the morphological alterations observed during apoptosis, including α-spectrin (Nath et al., 1996a,b; Wang et al., 1998), β-spectrin (Wang et al., 1998), tau (Canu et al., 1998), and actin (Wang, 2000). Recently, calpain was shown to cleave PARP, the best-known caspase-3 substrate (McGinnis et al., 1999). Other common substrates include CaM-kinase II and IV and amyloid precursor protein (Wang, 2000). Interactions between calpain and caspase-3 are further supported by recent reports of caspase-3-mediated proteolysis of calpastatin, calpain's endogenous inhibitor (Porn-Ares et al., 1998; Wang et al., 1998). Calpain-mediated proteolysis of caspase-3 and caspase-9 has also been detected, but in these studies proteolysis failed to produce active subunits and did not affect caspases' ability to interact with its substrates (McGinnis et al., 1999; Wolf et al., 1999). In contrast, a recent study reported that calpain-mediated proteolysis of caspase-9 produced a cleavage product unable to activate caspase-3, suggesting that calpain may negatively regulate caspase proteolysis and apoptosis by inactivating upstream caspases (Chua et al., 2000). Finally, both caspase-dependent calpain activation (Wood and Newcomb, 1999) and calpain-dependent caspase activation (Waterhouse et al., 1998; Wolf et al., 1999) have been documented. These data strengthen the theory of an interaction between calpain and caspase-3. In spite of this evidence, few studies have examined calpain and caspase-3 activity concurrently in in vivo (Buki et al., 2000; Pike et al., 1998a,b) or in vitro (Nath et al., 1996a; Pike et al., 1998a,b; Zhao et al., 1999, 2000) models of CNS injury.

Although beyond the scope of this chapter, other proteolytic processes can contribute to neuronal cell damage following TBI. These include the lysosomal cathepsin proteases (for review, see Katunuma, 1994), the proteosome or multi-catalytic proteases complex (MPC) pathway (Argiles and Lopez-Soriano, 1996), and matrix metalloproteinases (Rosenberg, 1995). Future challenges lie in establishing new lines of evidence for the potential role of these still relatively unexamined proteases in TBI.

Interactions between Calpain and Caspase-3 in Apoptosis

The prominent coexpression of calpain and caspase-3 activation suggests there may be opportunities for interaction between these two pathways. Calpain and caspase-3 share a variety of substrates that are proteolysed during apoptosis (Wang, 2000). Moreover, these proteases cleave proteins important to each other's regulation (i.e., caspase-3-mediated proteolysis of calpastatin, calpain-mediated proteolysis of pro-caspase-3 and pro-caspase-9) (McGinnis et al., 1999; Wang et al., 1998; Wolf et al., 1999). In addition, the contribution of calpain to the expression of apoptotic cell death phenotypes following a CNS injury is further supported. Additional evidence for calpain's involvement in apoptotic cell death in CNS injury is provided by recent studies examining in vivo traumatic brain injury. Calpain-mediated, but not caspase-3-mediated breakdown products were detected in the injured cortex following injury, a site associated with prominent apoptotic cell death (Newcomb et al., 1999; Pike et al., 1998a). In addition, Namura and colleagues reported that ~50 percent of TUNEL-positive cells failed to show caspase-3 activation (Namura et al., 1998). These data suggest that other proteases, such as calpain, are involved in the apoptotic changes observed following injury.

For instance, Hayes and colleagues have demonstrated that both calpains and caspase-3 protease contribute to apoptotic cell death in staurosporine-induced apoptosis (Pike et al., 1998b), whereas calpain but not caspase-3 contributes to maitotoxin-induced necrotic cell death in septohippocampal primary cell cultures (Zhao et al., 1999). Hayes and colleagues have recently reported apoptotic cell death (Newcomb et al., 1999) and independent or concurrent activation of calpains and caspase-3 proteases (Pike et al., 1998a) in various brain regions following lateral cortical impact TBI in rodents.

THERAPEUTIC OPPORTUNITY FOR PROTEASE INHIBITION

The involvement of proteases in pathological states is of particular clinical interest because further research may eventually lead to therapeutic applications. Yakovlev et al. (1997) and Clark et al. (2000) demonstrated protective effects of caspase inhibition on apoptosis. Additionally, Yakovlev et al. reported behavioral protection from TBI-induced deficits. Calpain activation has been inferred in acute derangements of neuronal structure and function following CNS injury (discussed earlier). In particular, proteolytic modification of neuronal cytoskeletal proteins, one of the most extensively studied substrates of calpain proteolysis, is likely to produce profound morphological and functional changes in neurons.

Past studies have consistently documented the efficacy of protease inhibitors in attenuating excitotoxic-induced cytoskeletal damage (for reviews, see Wang and Yuen, 1994; Bartus et al., 1994a,b 1995b; Yuen and Wang, 1996). It has been reported that administration of E-64c, an expoxysuccinyl peptide, attenuates the loss of MAP-2 in an animal model of focal cerebral ischemia (Inuzuka et al., 1990a). Further, Lee and colleagues (1991) reported that a cysteine protease inhibitor, leupeptin, reduced the degradation of spectrin in a hippocampal slice model of hypoxic/anoxic injury. Lastly, a recent report has provided evidence that MDL28170, a peptide aldehyde inhibitor, reduces the accumulation of spectrin breakdown products following cerebral ischemia in vivo (Hong et al., 1994) and excitotoxic damage in vitro (Brorson et al., 1995). Calpain inhibitors have been shown to be neuroprotective in cerebral ischemia (Bartus et al., 1994, 1995; Hong et al., 1994) and TBI (Posmantur et al., 1997a; Saatman et al., 1996a) as well as in vitro models of acute CNS injury (Brorson et al., 1995; George et al., 1995; Kampfl et al., 1996a).

From a therapeutic perspective, protease inhibitors may have several advantages over other more conventional targets such as ion channel blockers and glutamate antagonists, since calpain proteolysis represents a later component of a pathway mediating cell death initiated by excitotoxicity and elevated calcium levels. Therefore, one notable advantage of calpain as a therapeutic target is that antagonism of increased calpain activation may provide a longer window of opportunity for protection of neurons after the initiation of the neuronal injury. Importantly, recent reports have provided evidence that delayed antagonism of calpain up to 3 h following injury can still reduce neuronal damage in vivo (Bartus et al., 1994) and in vitro (Brorson et al., 1995). In addition, studies of calpain-mediated breakdown products of spectrin (Kampfl et al., 1996a; Posmantur et al., 1997a; Saatman et al., 1996b) following TBI and cerebral ischemia (Bartus et al., 1995a) and studies of μ-calpain autolysis (Kampfl et al., 1996b) have provided congruent evidence that calpain is upregulated for at least 24 h post injury. Although the temporal parameters (e.g., time of initiation and duration of treatment following injury) for treatment with calpain inhibitors have yet to be defined, these data suggest that the window of opportunity for calpain inhibitors is at least several hours. Equally important, these studies suggest that the duration of administration (or biological activity) of calpain inhibitors could critically influence the therapeutic efficacy of such agents.

In addition, several in vitro studies have demonstrated protective effects of other peptide aldehyde calpain inhibitors, including calpain inhibitors 1 and 2, against cytoskeletal protein loss (George et al., 1995; Kampfl et al., 1996a). Calpain inhibitor administration (calpain inhibitor AK 295) has also proven to significantly reduce infarct volume in an animal model of cerebral ischemia (Bartus et al., 1994) and to attenuate motor and cognitive deficits following TBI (Saatman et al., 1996a) in vivo. A recent report also provided evidence that calpain inhibitor 2 administration specifically reduces calpain-induced cytoskeletal protein loss and contusion volume after cortical impact injury (Posmantur et al., 1997a). Importantly, this study also demonstrated morphological preservation of dendritic and axonal structures post TBI.

Although the potential clinical utility of calpain inhibitors seems well established, a number of important considerations remain to be addressed. The need to determine the therapeutic window and optimal duration of administration has been mentioned already. The need for relatively specific calpain inhibitors may be greater in laboratory than in clinical applications. In fact, the ability of calpain inhibitors to reduce the activity of other proteases may provide additional protection, assuming that issues of toxicity are adequately addressed. Since calpain is a potential mediator of coagulation (see Saido et al., 1993a,b), care must be used in the prolonged administration of calpain inhibitors to traumatized patients. Lastly, many in vivo studies to date, including those of Posmantur et al. (1997a), Bartus et al. (1994) and Saatman et al. (1996a), administered calpain inhibitors via the carotid artery, an administration technique not readily applicable to humans. However, other reports have provided evidence that intravenous application of MDL 28170 significantly reduced spectrin degradation in an animal model of cerebral ischemia (Hong et al., 1994).

SUMMARY AND CONCLUSIONS

In summary, a number of lines of evidence strongly support the hypothesis that calpain activation and proteolysis of cytoskeletal substrates are important pathological components of traumatic brain injury. However, we currently do not have detailed information on factors that could modulate calpain activity following traumatic insults. For example, future studies need to focus on the role of membrane phospholipids and endogenous inhibitors such as calpastatin in determining calpain proteolysis. Systematic comparisons of the contributions of proteases, particularly calpain and caspase-3, will importantly enhance therapeutic options available to treat brain injury.

Finally, while calpain and caspase inhibitors may be potential therapeutic agents for treatment of brain injury, important preclinical questions must be addressed, including optimal doses, times, and durations of administration. The development of more specific inhibitors that could be administered by clinically practical routes, such as intravenous administration, would also represent an important clinical advance. Finally, although calpain inhibitors would be expected to have few side effects since calpain has low basal activity levels, future in vivo studies must carefully investigate the potential for undesirable side effects including inhibition of clotting (Saido et al., 1993a).

ACKNOWLEDGMENTS

This work was supported by NIH grants R01 NS21458-15 and R01 NS40182; US Army grant DAMD17-99-1-9565; University of Pittsburgh/Navy Project 99083106.

ABBREVIATIONS

CNS	Central nervous system
MAP-2	Microtubule-associated protein 2
MPC	Multicatalytic protease complex
NF	Neurofilament
PARP	Poly(ADP-ribose) polymerase
TBI	Traumatic brain injury
TUNEL	Terminal deoxynucleotidyl transferase-mediated biotinylated dUTP nick end labeling
LTP	Long-term potentiation
ATP	Adenosine triphosphate

LMW   Low-molecular weight
RT-PCR Reverse transcriptase polymerase chain reaction

REFERENCES

M. L. Allende, R. Y. Krauss, C. Tremblay, J. Alvarez, and N. C. Inestrosa, *J. Neurosci. Res.*, 22, 130–133 (1989).

J. Argiles and J. L. Lopez-Soriano, *Trends Pharmacol. Sci.*, 17, 222–226 (1996).

N. L. Banik, E. L. Hogan, J. M. Powers, and L. Whetstine, *Neurochem. Res.*, 7, 1465–1475 (1982).

N. L. Banik, D. C. Matzelle, G. Gantt-Wilfor, A. Osborne, and E. L. Hogan, *Brain Res.* 752(1–2), 301–306 (1997).

E. T. Bartus, N. J. Hayward, P. H. Elliot, S. D. Sawyer, K. L. Baker, P. L. Dean, A. Akiyama, J. A. Straub, S. L. Hargeson, A. Li, et al., *Stroke*, 25(11), 2265–2270 (1994a).

R. T. Bartus, K. L. Baker, A. D. Heiser, S. D. Sawyer, R. L. Dean, P. H. Elliot, and J. A. Straub, *J. Cereb. Blood Flow Metab.*, 14(4), 537–544 (1994b).

E. T. Bartus, R. L. Dean, K. Cavanaugh, D. Eveleth, D. L. Carriero, and G. Lynch, *J. Cereb. Blood Flow Metab.*, 15(6), 969–979 (1995a).

R. T. Bartus, P. H. Elliot, N. J. Hayward, R. L. Dean, S. Harbesson, J. A. Straub, Z. Li, and J. C. Powers, *Neurol. Res.*, 17(4), 249–258 (1995b).

R. Beer, G. Granz, A. Srinivasan, R. L. Hayes, B. R. Pike, X. Zhao, E. Schmutuzhard, W. Poewe, and A. Kampfl, *J. Neurochem.*, 75(3), 1264–1273 (2000).

K. Blomgren, A. McRae, L. Bona, T. C. Saido, J.-L. Karlson, and H. Hagberg, *Brain Res.*, 684, 136–142 (1995).

J. R. Brorson, C. J. Marcucilli, and R. J. Miller, *Stroke*, 26, 1259–1267 (1995).

A. Buki, D. O. Okonkwo, K. K. W. Wang, and J. T. Povlishock, *J. Neurosci.*, 20(8), 2825–2834 (2000).

N. Canu, L. Dus, C. Barbatu, M. T. Ciotti, C. Brancolini, A. M. Rinaldi, M. Novak, A. Cattaneo, A. Bradbury, P. Calissano, *J. Neurosci.*, 18(18), 7061–7074 (1998).

D. W. Choi, M. A. Maulucci-Gedde, and A. R. Kriegstein, *J. Neurosci.*, 7, 357–368 (1997).

B. T. Chua, K. Guo, and P. Li, *J. Biol. Chem.*, 275, 5131–5135 (2000).

R. S. Clark, P. M. Kochanek, M. Chen, S. C. Watkins, D. W. Marion, J. Chen, R. L. Hamilton, J. E. Loeffert, and S. H. Graham, *FASEB J.*, 13(8), 813–821 (1999).

R. S. Clark, P. M. Kochanek, S. C. Watkins, M. Chen, C. E. Dixon, N. A. Seidberg, J. Melick, J. E. Loeffert, P. D. Nathaniel, K. L. Jin, and S. H. Graham, *J. Neurochem.*, 74(2), 740–753 (2000).

M. A. Colicos and P. K. Dash, *Brain Res.*, 739, 120–131 (1996).

S. del Cerro, J. Larson, M. W. Oliver, and G. Lynch, *Brain Res.*, 530, 91–95 (1990).

D. Dhermy, *Biol. Cell*, 71, 249–254 (1991).

B. A. Eldadah, A. G. Yakovlev, and A. I. Faden, *Nucleic Acids Res.*, 24, 4092–4093 (1996).

A. L. Faden, P. Demediuk, S. S. Panter, and R. Vink, *Science*, 244, 798–800 (1989).

I. Fineman, D. Hovda, M. Smith, A. Yoshino, and D. Becker, *Brain Res.*, 624, 94–102 (1993).

A. Fraser and G. Evan, *Cell*, 85, 781–784 (1997).

E. B. George, J. D. Glass, and J. W. Griffin, *J. Neurosci.*, 15, 6445–6452 (1995).

F. G. Giancotti, M. A. Stepp, S. Suzuki, E. Engvall, and E. Ruoslahti, *J. Cell Biol.*, 118, 951–955 (1992).

R. P. Guttmann, J. S. Elce, P. D. Bell, J. C. Isbell, and G. V. Johnson, *J. Biol. Chem.*, 272, 2005–2012 (1997).

T. Hamakubo, R. Kannagi, T. Murachi, and A. Matus, *J. Neurosci.*, 6, 3103–3111 (1986).

A. S. Harris, D. E. Croall, and J. S. Morrow, *J. Biol. Chem.*, 263, 15754–15761 (1988).

R. L. Hayes, L. K. W. Jenkins, and B. G. Lyeth, *J. Neurotrauma*, 9, 173–187 (1992).

R. R. Hicks, D. H. Smith, T. K. McIntosh, *Brain Res.*, 678(1–2), 151–160 (1995).

S. Hirai, H. Kawasaki, M. Yaniv, and K. Suzuki, *FEBS Lett.*, 287, 57–61 (1991).

S. C. Hong, Y. Goto, G. Lanzino, S. Soleau, N. F. Kassell, and K. S. Lee, *Stroke*, 25, 663–669 (1994).

T. Inuzuka, A. Tamura, S. Shuzo, T. Kirino, I. Toyoshima, and Y. Miyatake, *Brain Res.*, 526, 177–179 (1990a).

T. Inuzuka, A. Tamura, S. Sato, T. Kirino, I. Toyoshima, and T. Miyatake, *Stroke*, 21, 917–922 (1990b).

E. M. Johnson, L. J. S. Greenlund, P. T. Akins, and C. Y. Hsu, *J. Neurotrauma*, 12, 843–852 (1995).

G. V. Johnson and R. Jope, *J. Neurosci. Res.*, 33(4), 505–512 (1992).

G. V. W. Johnson, J. M. Litersky, and R. S. Jope, *J. Neurochem.*, 56, 1630–1638 (1991).

Y. Kaku, Y. Yonekawa, T. Tsukahara, N. Ogata, T. Kimura, and T. Taniguchi, *J. Cereb. Blood Flow Metab.*, 13, 402–408 (1993).

K. Kamakura, S. Ishiura, K. Susuki, H. Sugita, and F. Takaku, *J. Neurosci. Res.*, 13, 391–403 (1985).

A. Kampfl, S. J. Whitson, X. Zhao, R. Posmantur, G. L. Clifton, and R. L. Hayes, *Neurosci. Lett.*, 194, 149–152 (1995).

A. Kampfl, X. Zhao, S. J. Whitson, R. Posmantur, C. E. Dixon, K. Yang, G. L. Clifton, and R. L. Hayes, *Eur. J. Neurosci.*, 8, 344–352 (1996a).

A. Kampfl, R. Posmantur, R. Nixon, F. Grynspan, X. Zhao, S. J. Liu, J. Newcomb, G. L. Clifton, and R. Hayes, *J. Neurochem.*, 67, 1575–1583 (1996b).

A. Kampfl, R. M. Posmantur, X. Zhao, E. Schmutzhard, G. L. Clifton, and R. L. Hayes, *J. Neurotrauma*, 14(3), 121–134 (1997).

Y. Katayama, D. P. Becker, T. Tamura, and D. A. Hovda, *J. Neurosurg.*, 73, 889–900 (1990).

N. Katunuma, Participation of Lysosomal Cathepsins in Antigen Processing and Bone Absorption, in N. Katunuma, K. Suzuki, J. Travis, and H. Fritz, Eds., *Biological Functions of Proteases and Inhibitors*, Japan Scientific Press, 1994, pp. 3–22.

J. F. R. Kerr and B. V. Harmon, Definition and Incidence of Apoptosis: An Historical Perspective of Apoptosis, in L. D. Tomei and F. O. Capo. Eds., *The Molecular Basis of Cell Death*, Cold Spring Harbor, NY, Cold Spring Harbor, Laboratory Press, 1991, p. 5.

K. Kitagawa, M. Matsumoto, M. Niinobe, K. Mikoshiba, R. Hata, H. Ueda, N. Handa, R. Fukunaga, Y. Isaka, K. Kimura, et al., *Neuroscience*, 31(2), 401–411 (1989).

M. C. LaPlaca, R. Raghupathi, A. Verma, A. A. Pieper, K. E. Saatman, S. H. Snyder, and T. McIntosh, *J. Neurochem.*, 73(1), 205–213 (1999).

Y. A. Lazebnik, S. H. Kaufman, S. Desnoyers, G. G. Poirier, and W. C. Earnshaw, *Nature*, 371, 346–247 (1994).

K. S. Lee, S. Frank, P. Vanderklish, A. Arai, and G. Lynch, *Proc. Natl. Acad. Sci. USA*, 88, 7233–7237 (1991).

Z. Li and N. L. Banik, *Brain Res.*, 697, 112–121 (1995).

B. Liu, M. Fang, M. Schmidt, Y. Lu, J. Mendelsohn, and Z. Fan, *Br. J. Cancer*, 82(12), 1991–1999 (1999).

S. J. Martin, G. A. O'Brien, W. K. Nishioka, A. J. McLahon, T. Mahboubin, T. C. Saido, and D. Green, *J. Biol. Chem.*, 270, 6425–6428 (1995).

K. M. McGinnis, M. E. Gnegy, Y. H. Park, N. Mukerjee, and K. K. Wang, *Biochem. Biophys. Res. Commun.*, 263(1), 94–99 (1999).

E. Melloni and S. Pontremoli, *Trends Neurosci.*, 12, 438–444 (1989).

S. Miyazaki, Y. Katayama, B. G. Lyeth, and R. L. Hayes, *Brain Res.*, 585, 335–339 (1992).

M. Morioka, K. Fukunaga, S. Yasugawa, S. Nagahiro, Y. Ushio, and E. Miyamoto, *J. Neurochem.*, 58, 1798–1809 (1992).

V. Nadler, A. Biegon, E. Beti-Yannai, J. Adamchik, and E. Shohami, *Brain Res.*, 685, 1–11 (1995).

S. Namura, J. Zhu, K. Fink, M. Endres, A. Srinivasan, K. J. Tomaselli, J. Yuan, and M. A. Moskowitz, *J. Neurosci.*, 18(10) 3659–3688 (1998).

R. Nath, K. J. Kaser, K. McGinnis, R. Nadimpalli, D. Stafford, and K. K. Wang, *Neuroreport*, 8(1), 249–255 (1996a).

R. Nath, K. Raser, D. Stafford, I. Hajimohammadreza, A. Posner, H. Allen, R. V. Talanian, P. W. Yuen, B. Gilbertson, and K. K. Wang, *Biochem. J.*, 319, 683–690 (1996b).

R. W. Neumar, S. M. Hagle, D. J. DeGarcia, G. S. Krause, and B. C. White, *J. Neurochem.*, 66, 421–424 (1996).

J. K. Neucomb, S. J. Liu, A. Kampfl, X. Zhao, R. Posmantur, G. L. Clifton, and R. L. Hayes, *J. Neurotrauma*, 6, 369–383 (1997).

J. K. Newcomb, X. Zhao, B. R. Pike, and R. L. Hayes, *Exp. Neurol.*, 158, 76–88 (1999).

D. W. Nicholson and N. A. Thornberry, *Trends Biochem. Sci.*, 22, 299–306 (1997).

D. W. Nicholson, A. N. Ambereen, N. A. Thornberry, J. P. Vallancourt, et al., *Nature*, 376, 37–43 (1995).

P. Nilsson, L. Hillered, Y. Olsson, M. J. Sheardown, and A. J. Hansen, *J. Cereb. Blood Flow Metab.*, 13, 183–192 (1993).

A. Nishida, K. Emoto, M. Shimizu, T. Uozumi, and S. Yamawaki, *Stroke*, 25, 1247–1251 (1994).

R. A. Nixon and C. A. Marotta, *J. Neurochem.*, 43, 507–516 (1984).

R. A. Nixon and R. K. Sihag, *Trends Neurosci.*, 14, 501–506 (1991).

K. Ostwald, M. Hayashi, M. Nakamura, and S. Kawashima, *J. Neurochem.*, 63, 1069–1076 (1994).

L. S. Perlmutter, C. Gall, M. Baudry, and G. Lynch, *J. Comp. Neurol.*, 296, 269–276 (1990).

E. H. Pettus, C. W. Christman, M. L. Giebel, and J. T. Povlishock, *J. Neurotrauma*, 11, 507–521 (1994).

B. R. Pike, X. Zhao, K. K. W. Wang, S. J. Liu, J. Newcomb, T. Gegeny, R. M. Posmantur, G. L. Clifton, and R. L. Hayes, *Soc. Neurosci.*, 23, 2194 (1997).

B. R. Pike, X. Zhao, J. K. Newcomb, R. M. Posmantur, K. K. W. Wang, and R. L. Hayes, *Neuroreport*, 9, 2437–2442 (1998a).

B. R. Pike, X. Zhao, J. K. Newcomb, K. K. W. Wang, R. M. Posmantur, and R. L. Hayes, *J. Neurosci. Res.*, 52, 505–520 (1998b).

M. I. Porn-Ares, A. Samali, and S. Orrenius, *Cell Death Differ.*, 5(12), 1028–1033 (1998).

R. Posmantur, R. L. Hayes, C. E. Dixon, and W. C. Taft, *J. Neurotrauma*, 11, 533–545 (1994).

R. M. Posmantur, A. Kampfl, S. J. Liu, K. Heck, W. C. Taft, G. L. Clifton, and R. L. Hayes, *J. Neuropathol. Exp. Neurol.*, 55, 68–90 (1996a).

R. Posmantur, A. Kampfl, W. C. Taft, M. Bhattacharjee, C. E. Dixon, J. Bao, and R. L. Hayes, *J. Neurotrauma*, 13, 125–137 (1996b).

R. Posmantur, A. Kampfl, R. Siman, S. J. Liu, X. Zhao, G. L. Clifton, and R. L. Hayes, *Neuroscience*, 77, 875–888 (1997a).

R. M. Posmantur, K. McGinnis, R. Nadimpalli, R. B. Gilbertsen, and K. Wang, *J. Neurochem.*, 68, 2328–2337 (1997b).

R. M. Posmantur, X. Zhao, A. Kampfl, G. L. Clifton, and R. L. Hayes, *Neurochem. Res.*, 23(10), 1265–1276 (1998).

R. M. Posmantur, J. K. Newcomb, A. Kampfl, and R. L. Hayes, *Exp. Neurol.*, 16(1), 15–26 (2000).

J. T. Povlishock and C. W. Christman, *J. Neurotrauma*, 12, 555–564 (1995).

J. T. Povlishock, A. Marmarou, T. McIntosh, J. Q. Trojanowski, and J. Moroi, *J. Neuropathol. Exp. Neurol.*, 56, 347–359 (1996).

T. M. Reeves, B. G. Lyeth, and J. T. Povlishock, *Exp. Brain Res.*, 106, 248–256 (1995).

W. G. Regehr and D. W. Tank, *Curr. Opin. Neurobiol.*, 4, 373–382 (1994).

J. M. Roberts-Lewis, M. J. Savage, V. R. Marcy, L. R. Pinsker, and R. Siman, *J. Neurosci.*, 14, 3934–3944 (1994).

G. Rosenberg, *J. Neurotrauma*, 12, 833–840 (1995).

K. E. Saatman, H. Murai, R. T. Bartus, D. H. Smith, N. H. Hayward, B. R. Perri, and T. K. McIntosh, *Proc. Natl. Acad. Sci. USA*, 93, 3428–3433 (1996a).

K. E. Saatman, D. Bozyczko-Coyne, V. Marcy, R. Siman, and T. K. McIntosh, *J. Neuropathol. Exp. Neurol.*, 55, 850–860 (1996b).

T. C. Saido, S. Nagao, M. Shiramine, M. Tsukaguchi, H. Sorimachi, H. Murofuchsi, T. Tsuchchiya, H. Ito, and K. Suzuki, *J. Biochem.*, 111, 81–86 (1992a).

T. C. Saido, M. Shubata, T. Takenawa, H. Murofush, and K. Suzuki, *J. Biol. Chem.*, 264, 24585–24590 (1992b).

T. C. Saido, H. Suzuki, H. Yamazaki, K. Tanoue, and K. Suzuki, *J. Biol. Chem.*, 268, 7422–7426 (1993a).

T. C. Saido, M. Yokota, S. Nagao, et al., *J. Biol. Chem.*, 33, 25239–25243 (1993b).

T. C. Saido, H. Sorimachi, and K. Suzuki, *FASEB J.*, 8, 814–822 (1994).

W. W. Schlaepfer, C. Lee, V. W. Lee, and U. J. Zimmerman, *J. Neurochem.*, 44, 502–509 (1985).

G. Shaw, *Bioessays*, 4, 161–166 (1986).

B. K. Siesjoe and F. Bengtsson, *J. Cereb. Blood Flow Metab.*, 9, 127–140 (1989).

H. Sorimachi, T. C. Saido, and K. Suzuki, *FEBS Lett.*, 343, 1–5 (1994).

W. C. Taft, K. Yang, C. E. Dixon, and R. L. Hayes, *J. Neurotrauma*, 9, 281–290 (1992).

W. C. Taft, K. Yang, C. E. Dixon, G. L. Clifton, and R. L. Hayes, *J. Cereb. Blood Flow Metab.*, 13, 796–802 (1993).

D. Tang and V. J. Kidd, *J. Biol. Chem.*, 273(44), 28549–28552 (1998).

K. K. Wang, *Trends Neurosci.*, 23(2), 59 (2000).

K. K. Wang, R. Posmantur, P. Nath, K. McGinnis, M. Whitton, R. V. Talanian, S. B. Glantz, and J. S. Morrow, *J. Biol. Chem.*, 273(35), 22490–22497 (1998).

K. K. W. Wang and P. Yuen, *Adv. Pharmacol.*, 37, 117–152 (1997).

K. K. W. Wang and P.-W. Yuen, *Trends Pharmacol. Sci.*, 15, 412–419 (1994).

N. J. Waterhouse, D. M. Finucane, D. R. Green, J. S. Elce, S. Kumar, E. S. Alnemri, G. Litwack, K. Khanna, M. F. Lavin, and D. J. Watters, *Cell Death Differ.*, 5(12), 1051–1061 (1998).

J. S. Whitson, A. Kampfl., X. Zhao, and R. L. Hayes, *Neurosci. Lett.*, 197, 159–163 (1995).

B. B. Wolf, J. C. Goldstein, H. R. Stennicke, et al., *Blood*, 94, 1683–1692 (1999).

D. E. Wood and E. W. Newcomb, *J. Biol. Chem.*, 274(12) 8309–8315 (1999).

A. Yaghmai and J. Povlishock, *J. Neuropathol. Exp. Neurol.*, 51, 158–176 (1992).

A. G. Yakovlev, S. M. Knoblach, L. Fan, G. B. Fox, R. Goodnight, and A. I. Faden, *J. Neurosci.*, 17, 7415–7424 (1997).

K. Y. Yang, W. C. Taft, C. E. Dixon, R. K. Yu, and R. L. Hayes, *J. Neurotrauma*, 11, 523–532 (1994).

P. Yuen and K. K. W. Wang, *Exp. Opin. Invest. Drugs*, 5, 1291–1304 (1996).

C. Zhang, R. Raghupathi, K. E. Saatman, M. C. LaPlaca, and T. K. McIntosh, *J. Neurochem.*, 73(4), 1650–1659 (1999).

W. Zhang, R. D. Lane, and R. L. Mellgran, *J. Biol. Chem.*, 271, 18825–18830 (1996).

X. Zhao, R. Posmantur, A. Kampfl, S. J. Liu, K. K. W. Wang, J. K. Newcomb, B. Pike, G. L. Clifton, and R. L. Hayes, *J. Cereb. Blood Flow Metab.*, 18(2), 161–167 (1998).

X. Zhao, R. Posmantur, K. K. W. Wang, B. Pike, J. K. Newcomb, and R. L. Hayes, *Neurosci. Lett.*, 247, 53–57 (1997b).

X. Zhao, B. R. Pike, J. K. Newcomb, K. K. W. Wang, R. M. Posmantur, and R. L. Hayes, *Neurochem. Res.*, 24(3), 371–382 (1999).

X. Zhao, J. K. Newcomb, B. R. Pike, K. K. Wang, D. d'Avella, and R. L. Hayes, *J. Cereb. Blood Flow Metab.*, 20(3), 550–562 (2000).

CHAPTER 11

APOPTOSIS AND DNA DAMAGE IN HEAD TRAUMA

RAMESH RAGHUPATHI

Department of Neurosurgery, University of Pennsylvania School of Medicine, and
Veterans Administration Medical Center, Philadelphia, Pennsylvania

INTRODUCTION

The spectrum of pathologies associated with human traumatic brain injury (TBI)
includes focal contusions in the gray matter and diffuse injuries to axons in the white
matter (Adams et al., 1985; Kotapka et al., 1992; Ross et al., 1993; Gennarelli et al.,
1998). It has been suggested that these pathologies may be a consequence of the
biomechanics of the impact; that is, focal injuries occur due to contact forces to the
head, while diffuse injuries occur as a result of noncontact, rotational forces to the
brain (Meaney et al., 1995). Focal and diffuse traumatic brain injuries are associated
with neuronal and oligodendroglial cell death, respectively (Fig. 11.1). In addition to
the necrosis (typically observed in pathological disease states), it is becoming
increasingly evident that both neurons and oligodendrocytes may undergo a more
controlled death program (apoptosis) following clinical and experimental brain
trauma. While multiple intracellular pathways are affected following a traumatic
insult to the brain (McIntosh et al., 1998), it is unclear if cell death in central nervous
system (CNS) injury follows the same pattern of initiation–commitment–execution
stages that has been extensively characterized in models of developmental neuronal
death (Oppenheim, 1991). Among the various pathways that lead to apoptotic cell
death, damage to nuclear DNA (i.e., DNA strand breaks) has been suggested to be
one initiating factor (Vamvakas et al., 1997). In addition to reviewing the state of the
current literature describing the patterns of apoptotic cell death following TBI in
humans and animals, this chapter also discusses the many pathways that lead to

Head Trauma: Basic, Preclinical, and Clinical Directions, Edited by Leonard P. Miller and
Ronald L. Hayes, Co-edited by Jennifer K. Newcomb
ISBN 0-471-36015-5   © 2001 John Wiley & Sons, Inc.

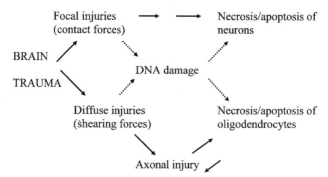

Figure 11.1 Focal and diffuse types of brain trauma result in death of neurons and oligodendrocytes, respectively. Apoptosis may be one component of traumatic neural cell death, which may, in part, be mediated by oxidative damage to nuclear DNA. Dotted lines represent putative mechanisms underlying the pathological changes.

trauma-induced apoptosis, with a particular focus on mechanisms leading to damage of nuclear DNA.

NECROSIS VERSUS APOPTOSIS IN THE NERVOUS SYSTEM

Pathological cell death in the nervous system, such as that observed following acute neurologic insults including hypoxia–ischemia, seizures, or trauma, has long been associated with a necrotic morphology. At the level of the individual cell, necrosis is characterized by mitochondrial swelling, nuclear pyknosis, karyorrhexis (chromatin fragmentation), and disruption of the plasma membrane, leading to complete cellular disintegration (Lo et al., 1995). These morphological changes are accompanied by biochemical events such as irreversible mitochondrial dysfunction (and a concomitant loss of ATP), and a profound disruption of ionic homeostasis. In contrast to necrosis, a cell undergoing apoptosis is characterized by uniform internucleosomal DNA fragmentation, nuclear shrinkage, chromatin compaction and fragmentation, as well as cytoplasm condensation and disintegration. In the later stages of apoptosis, the cell surface membrane undergoes blebbing and breaks down into spherical apoptotic bodies, which appear to be quickly absorbed via phagocytosis by surrounding cells (Lo et al., 1995). While certain morphological features such as nuclear condensation and plasma membrane disruption appear to be associated with both apoptotic and necrotic cell death, the point at which they occur during the process of cell death is an important difference. Thus, necrosis is accompanied by an early disruption of the plasma membrane, which is followed by nuclear pyknosis and karyorrhexis, whereas during apoptosis the plasma membrane remains viable until a very late stage. At the level of the tissue, entire masses of cells undergo necrosis, which is accompanied by a massive influx of inflammatory phagocytic cells that serve to lyse and remove cell debris. In contrast, apoptosis may occur in isolated

TABLE 11.1   Necrosis Versus Apoptosis in the Nervous System

Necrosis	Apoptosis
Plasma membrane disruption occurs early	Plasma membrane remains intact until the late stages of death, at which time blebbing occurs
Nucleus undergoes pyknosis	Nucleus undergoes pyknosis
Chromatin fragments, and DNA is randomly degraded	Chromatin condenses, and DNA fragments into regular 180 to 200-base-pair pieces
Mitochondria swell, and lose ability to synthesize ATP	Mitochondria may remain intact, and accumulate around the nucleus. ATP production is not affected
Masses of cells undergo death, leading to a massive immune/inflammatory response in surrounding "healthy" tissue	Isolated cells can undergo death, and dying/dead cells are phagocytosed by neighboring macrophages to prevent an inflammatory response

cells, which are immediately phagocytosed by adjacent cells or macrophages, thereby avoiding an inflammatory response. These differences are itemized in Table 11.1.

Apoptosis has also been considered the morphological manifestation of programmed cell death (PCD), and has typically been associated with the formation of the normal CNS during development as well as for the maintenance of homeostasis (Oppenheim, 1991). Over the last decade, increasing evidence suggests that neural cell apoptosis may significantly contribute to the pathology of neurodegenerative diseases such as Alzheimer's, Parkinson's, and Huntington's diseases, and amyotrophic lateral sclerosis (Yoshiyama et al., 1994; Portera et al., 1995; Smale et al., 1995; Mochizuki et al., 1996). Recently, apoptotic neurons have also been identified following acute neurologic insults in man such as stroke, and brain and spinal cord trauma (Emery et al., 1998; Love et al., 1998; Clark et al., 1999). That neuronal and glial apoptosis is associated with pathological diseases of the adult CNS has been confirmed using animal models of these neurodegenerative diseases, stroke, and CNS trauma (Portera et al., 1995; Rink et al., 1995; Crowe et al., 1997; Conti et al., 1998; Shaikh et al., 1998).

DIFFERENTIATING NECROSIS FROM APOPTOSIS IN TISSUE SECTIONS

The dramatically different morphologies of dying cells described above allow for the clear identification of apoptosis and necrosis using electron microscopy, and this technique remains the most reliable method to determine the mode of cell death. Although the biochemical and histological techniques have been utilized to detect apoptosis, one must exercise caution during interpretations of these observations.

One biochemical hallmark of apoptosis is internucleosomal DNA fragmentation, which results in a regular banding pattern of nuclear DNA in agarose gels, each band separated by 180 to 200 base pairs (Lo et al., 1995). In contrast, necrosis results in a smear of DNA fragments, which are produced as a result of random degradation of chromatin. Apoptotic chromatin cleavage occurs as a result of activation of nuclear endonucleases (Zakeri et al., 1993), and enzymatic techniques allow for the in situ labeling of the newly formed 3'-hydroxyl end of the DNA (Gavrieli et al., 1992). Terminal deoxynucleotidyl transferase-mediated nick end-labeling (TUNEL) has been widely used to visualize apoptotic cells containing fragmented DNA in tissue sections. However, TUNEL results must be interpreted cautiously because DNA degradation leading to the formation of free 3'-hydroxyl groups can occur in the late phases of necrosis. Consequently, identification of apoptotic cells using light microscopy must be based on stringent morphological evaluation of chromatin margination, and nuclear and cytoplasmic condensation within TUNEL(+) cells (Charriaut-Marlangue and Ben-Ari, 1995; Conti et al., 1998). Other techniques utilize the compaction of nuclear chromatin, which leads to an increase in the fluorescence of the dye, bis-benzamide (Hoechst 33342), to detect apoptosis, or the appearance of phosphatidylserine in the outer leaflet of the plasma membrane, which occurs due to a loss of plasma membrane asymmetry (van Engeland et al., 1998).

PATHOLOGY OF TBI IN HUMANS AND ANIMALS

Traumatic brain injury (TBI) in humans results in neuronal loss in the cortex, hippocampus, cerebellum, and thalamus (Adams et al., 1985; Kotapka et al., 1992; Ross et al., 1993), patterns that have been replicated in animal models (Gennarelli, 1994; Povlishock et al., 1994). The depth and extent of contusions in various parts of the injured human brain have been quantitatively evaluated (Adams et al., 1985), and bilateral loss of hippocampal neurons has been observed in 85% of fatal head injury cases as early as 48 h following the trauma (Kotapka et al., 1992). In the early posttraumatic period (hours to days), injured neurons in contusions appear swollen, but over time (days to weeks), appear shrunken and eosinophilic, with pyknosis of the nuclei (Cervos-Navarro and Lafuente, 1991).

In experimental models of brain injury in the rat, neuronal degeneration is evident in the injured cortex and hippocampus in the acute period (minutes to hours) (Sutton et al., 1993; Dietrich et al., 1994; Hicks et al., 1996). Electron-microscopic analysis of these degenerating neurons revealed a general swollen appearance, with swollen mitochondria, vacuolated cytoplasm, and pyknotic nuclei (Sutton et al., 1993; Dietrich et al., 1994), suggestive of necrosis. Interestingly, observations of a time-dependent increase in the volume of the cortical lesion, and the presence of degenerating (dystrophic) neurons in the chronic posttraumatic period, have led to the suggestion that delayed or chronic neuronal degeneration may be a significant component of posttraumatic pathology (Dietrich et al., 1994; Colicos et al., 1996; Hicks et al., 1996; Bramlett et al., 1997). Injury to the white matter is characterized by the widespread distribution of injured axons, which, in the acute posttraumatic stage, appear as swollen fibers containing accumulated cytoskeletal proteins (Gennarelli et al., 1998). Over time, these swollen axons eventually undergo complete axotomy (Wallerian degeneration) (Povlishock et al., 1992), a process that is associated with death of oligodendrocytes (Beattie et al., 1998). Traumatic oligodendrocyte death may also be induced by the reactive microglia and astrocytes present in the white matter (Crowe et al., 1997; Shuman et al., 1997; Gennarelli et al., 1998).

EVIDENCE FOR NEURAL APOPTOSIS IN TBI

In the first report describing the presence of apoptotic cells in the setting of experimental brain trauma, Rink and co-workers observed that in the hours to days (12 h to 3 days) following lateral fluid-percussion brain injury in the rat, a small but significant number of injured neurons in the cortex and hippocampus of the rat exhibited TUNEL reactivity (Rink et al., 1995). Two types of TUNEL(+) cells were identified: type I which were neuron-like, with diffuse TUNEL reactivity throughout the cell, and type II, which were compact and spherical and were intensely TUNEL(+). Using electron microscopy, these authors reported that while type I cells were vacuolated and necrotic, type II cells exhibited signs of classical apoptosis (Rink et al., 1995). These initial observations of trauma-induced neuronal apoptosis were confirmed by a number of investigators using different models of TBI. Apoptotic neurons were observed in the cortex and hippocampus following controlled cortical impact brain injury in rats and mice (Colicos and Dash, 1996; Clark et al., 1997; Yakovlev et al., 1997; Fox et al., 1998; Kaya et al., 1999; Newcomb et al., 1999). In addition to TUNEL, the bis-benzamide dye has also been utilized to demonstrate posttraumatic apoptotic nuclear condensation in neurons in injured brain regions (Clark et al., 1997; Yakovlev et al., 1997; Fox et al., 1998; Newcomb et al., 1999). Using the lateral fluid-percussion brain injury model, Conti and co-workers (1998) extended the initial observations of Rink et al., to demonstrate that there was a biphasic increase (at 24 h and 1 week post injury) in the number of apoptotic cells in the cortex. In addition, apoptotic neurons were present in the injured thalamus, but did not appear until 1 week post-injury, suggestive of a delayed pattern of apoptosis (Conti et al., 1998). In contrast to lateral fluid-percussion brain injury, neuronal apoptosis following controlled cortical impact brain injury in rats was restricted to the impacted cortex, and was maximal at 24 h post injury (Clark et al., 1997; Newcomb et al., 1999). At more severe levels of impact, neuronal apoptosis was observed in the hippocampus (Colicos and Dash, 1996; Kaya et al., 1999). Moreover, few apoptotic neurons were observed in any region of the brain at 2 weeks post injury (Colicos and Dash, 1996; Newcomb et al., 1999). In addition to neurons, oligodendrocytes (in the white matter) and astrocytes appear to undergo apoptosis following experimental TBI (Conti et al., 1998; Newcomb et al., 1999). That neural cell apoptosis contributes to the pathology of TBI was confirmed by the presence of TUNEL(+) neurons and oligodendrocytes in human head-injured tissue (Smith et al., 2000; Clark et al., 1999).

CELLULAR MECHANISMS UNDERLYING APOPTOTIC CELL DEATH IN TBI

It has been suggested that calcium-mediated mechanisms were the "final common pathway leading to cell death" following CNS injury (Young, 1992). Recent data suggest low $[Ca]_i$ leads to apoptosis, whereas high $[Ca]_i$ induces necrosis (Gwag et al., 1999). Although increases in intracellular calcium have been demonstrated following experimental TBI (Shapira et al., 1989; Fineman et al., 1993; Nilsson et al., 1996), the state of the current literature would suggest that a more complicated scenario is likely, involving altered anti- and pro-cell death signaling pathways (Pettman and Henderson, 1998) (Fig. 11.2). For example, the death-inducing activity of members of the Bcl-2 family (Bax, Bad, Bid, Bcl-x_S) appears to be in a dynamic equilibrium with their survival-promoting cognates
(Bcl-2, Bcl-x_L) (Merry and Korsmeyer, 1997). As a result of these shifts in intracellular levels of Bcl-2 family proteins, the death-inducing cysteine proteases, caspases, are activated (Thornberry and Lazebnik, 1998). Disruption of the balance between mitogen-activated protein kinase (MAPK)-mediated intracellular signaling pathways may also control the fate of the cell. Activation of c-Jun N-terminal kinase (JNK) or p38MAPK may lead to cell death, while extracellular signal-regulated kinase (ERK1/2) and Akt kinase are critical regulators of cell survival (Xia et al., 1995).

Although originally characterized as genes that are associated with developmental cell death, recent evidence suggests that the Bcl-2 family of genes may participate in both apoptotic and necrotic cell death following a pathological insult (Bredesen, 1995). Neurotoxin- or ischemia-mediated apoptotic death was preceded by increased Bax mRNA and protein, and decreased expression of Bcl-2 in cells that are destined to die (Gillardon et al., 1995, 1996; Krajewski et al., 1995), while an increase in Bcl-2 immunoreactivity was observed in neurons, glia, and endothelial cells that survived focal ischemic injury (Chen et al., 1995). Similarly, increased expression of

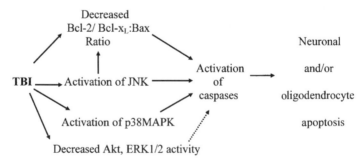

Figure 11.2 Activation of multiple cell death pathways following traumatic brain injury. Neural cell death can be a result of decreased activity of survival-promoting factors, or conversely, activation of death-inducing factors. In addition, it is also likely that there may be cell type-specific differences in cell death pathways.

Bcl-2 has been observed in neurons that survive the traumatic insult in the rat and in brain-injured humans (Clark et al., 1997, 1999), while Bax was observed to translocate to the nucleus of apoptotic cells following experimental brain injury (Kaya et al., 1999). That Bcl-2 may participate in neuronal cell death following TBI was further supported by recent observations that transgenic mice overexpressing the human Bcl-2 protein exhibited significantly less neuronal loss in the injured cortex and hippocampus following experimental TBI (Raghupathi et al., 1998; Nakamura et al., 1999). Bcl-2 family members may control cell death by regulating the release of cytochrome *c* from the mitochondria (Kluck et al., 1997; Yang et al., 1997b; Jurgensmeier et al., 1998) (see Chapter 11). Once in the cytosol, cytochrome *c* aids in the activation of caspases, a phenomenon that is associated with neuronal and oligodendroglial cell death resulting from multiple kinds of stimuli such as growth factor deprivation, hypoxia, free radical generation, ionizing radiation, and ischemia (Chen et al., 1998; Namura et al., 1998; Nath et al., 1998; Park et al., 1998; Gu et al., 1999). The current hypothesis regarding the mechanism(s) by which caspases kill cells is that caspases cleave multiple proteins, the sum of which leads to cell death (Thornberry and Lazebnik, 1998) (see Chapter 10). For instance, caspases may cleave antiapoptotic regulators such as the inhibitor of the nuclease response for DNA fragmentation, as well as cytoskeletal proteins (e.g., spectrin and actin), resulting in the disassembly of the dying cell (Li et al., 1997; LeBlanc, 1998). Activation of caspase-3 has been reported in injured cerebral cortex in the acute period following experimental (Yakovlev et al., 1997; Pike et al., 1998) and human (Clark et al., 1999) brain injury, and in the chronic period following traumatic spinal cord injury (Emery et al., 1998; Springer et al., 1999). That caspase-mediated cell death may participate in the pathobiology of CNS injury was further substantiated by Moskowitz and co-workers, who used both caspase inhibitors and transgenic mice overexpressing mutant caspases to demonstrate that reduced caspase activity led to neuroprotection in models of stroke (Friedlander et al., 1997; Hara et al., 1997; Endres et al., 1998; Fink et al., 1998). Similarly, posttraumatic apoptotic death and neurological deficits were reduced by administration of the caspase inhibitor, z-DEVD-fmk following lateral fluid-percussion brain injury in the rat (Yakovlev et al., 1997).

Both JNK and ERK1/2 are known regulators of cell survival/death in a number of neural and nonneural systems in vitro, with phosphorylation (activation) of JNK signaling being associated with neuronal cell death and activation of ERK1/2 linked to cell survival (Xia et al., 1995; Jarvis et al., 1997; Lannuzel et al., 1997). In vivo, systemic administration of kainic acid led to an acute and sustained decreases in phospho-ERK1/2 levels, and a concomitant increase in phospho-JNK in apoptotic neurons within the cortex and hippocampus (Mielke et al., 1999). Delayed neuronal death following global cerebral ischemia was preceded by a sustained increase in activated JNK (Ozawa et al., 1999), while increased ERK1/2 signaling was associated with neuroprotection in a model of ischemic preconditioning (Shamloo et al., 1999). Activated JNK was evident both in apoptotic neurons and in apoptotic oligodendrocytes following compressive spinal cord injury (Nakahara et al., 1999). Inhibition of JNK directly or blocking of upstream activators of JNK have been reported to attenuate apoptotic cell death in vitro (Xia et al., 1995) and in vivo (Saporito et al., 1999). Gene-targeted disruption of JNK3, the brain isoform of JNK, resulted in mice that were resistant to kainic acid-mediated hippocampal cell death and exhibited reduced seizure activity and mortality (Yang et al., 1997a). Little to no information regarding the changes in JNK/ERK signaling following TBI is currently available.

CELLULAR MECHANISMS UNDERLYING APOPTOTIC CELL DEATH IN TBI: DNA DAMAGE

Although controlled DNA fragmentation (i.e., breakage of both DNA strands) is one biochemical hallmark associated with apoptosis (see above), it has also been reported that single and/or double DNA strand breaks may trigger apoptotic cell death (Vamvakas et al., 1997; Shaikh et al., 1998). Both ischemic and traumatic brain injuries in animals and man result in single- or double-stranded DNA breaks in neuronal and glial DNA (Chopp et al., 1996; Chen et al., 1997; Yakovlev et al., 1997; Conti et al., 1998; Love et al., 1998; Shaikh et al., 1998; Clark et al., 1999; Jin et al., 1999). While activation of endonucleases can result in double-stranded breaks in DNA, single-stranded breaks typically occur due to oxidative damage (Liu et al., 1996). Oxidative damage as a result of oxygen free radical generation has been suggested to contribute to the induction of neural apoptosis (Boobis et al., 1989; Greenlund et al., 1995). Oxygen-centered free radicals, or reactive oxygen species (ROS), such as superoxide anion, the hydroxyl radical, or singlet oxygen, are generated as a consequence of reduction of oxygen to water, or as a byproduct of certain enzymatic reactions. Neurologic insults such as stroke or TBI have been associated with an increase in ROS, suggesting that oxidative stress could be one pathway of secondary injury (Ikeda and Long, 1990; Chan, 1996). In addition to causing DNA strand breaks, ROS can mediate the formation of DNA–protein adducts and/or oxidative adducts of the nitrogen bases (Collins et al., 1996). While all nitrogen bases are susceptible to oxidation, the most abundant product is 7,8-dihydro-8-oxoguanine (8-OH-guanine), and can therefore be easily measured (Collins et al., 1996). Whereas an increase in multiple species of oxidized nitrogenous bases has been detected in cortical DNA following focal cerebral ischemia (Liu et al., 1996), it is unclear at the present time whether the increase in free radical production observed following TBI leads to oxidative DNA damage.

Damage to the DNA activates intracellular pathways that lead to either growth arrest, apoptosis, or repair and elimination of damaged DNA (Evan and Littlewood, 1998), a choice that is made based on the cell type, extent of damage, and/or environment. One major component of the DNA damage response is the induction and upregulation of the tumor suppresser gene, *p53*, also termed the "guardian of the genome" (Evan and Littlewood, 1998). Induction of *p53* mRNA has been associated with neuronal damage following excitotoxic, ischemic, and traumatic brain injuries (Chopp et al., 1992; Sakhi et al., 1994; Hughes et al., 1996; Kaya et al., 1999; Napieralski et al., 1999). Increased *p53* mRNA and *p53* protein were observed in regions that exhibit neuronal apoptosis and in neurons that were TUNEL(+) (Kaya et al., 1999; Napieralski et al., 1999). Wild-type *p53* is a transcription factor for genes such as wild-type *p53*-activated fragment (WAF1/p21) (Artuso et al., 1995), the proapoptotic factor Bax (Miyashita and Reed, 1995), and the growth-arrest and DNA damage-inducible gene, *GADD45* (Zhan et al., 1998). Therefore, the consequences of *p53* induction are many: while WAF1 and GADD45 can cause cell cycle arrest and facilitate DNA repair and eventual cell survival (Artuso et al., 1995), Bax can induce cell death (see above) (Fig. 11.3).

Base excision and nucleotide excision repair are two primary mechanisms that are responsible for repairing damaged DNA (Sancar, 1995). The base excision repair (BER) pathway is believed to repair oxidative DNA damage and involves the sequential and coordinated activities of repair enzymes such as glycosylases (to hydrolyze the glycosyl bond between the base and sugar and remove the oxidized base), endonucleases (to break the DNA strand), polymerase β (to replace the absent base), and ligases (which reform the phosphodiester bond and seal the nicked DNA strand) (Fig. 11.4). Nucleotide excision repair is mediated by a combination of exo- and endonuclease activities that remove a patch of the DNA strand (typically 27 to 29 nucleotides), which is subsequently filled in by DNA polymerases (Sancar, 1995).

Recent reports suggest that the DNA damage that occurs following ischemic brain injury may be subjected to repair processes (Chopp et al., 1996; Liu et al., 1996; Love et al., 1998; Shaikh et al., 1998; Kawase et al., 1999). Liu and co-

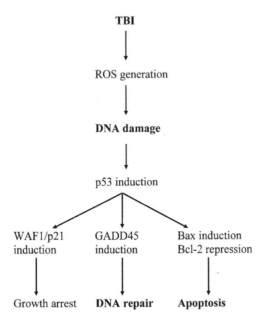

Figure 11.3 TBI may lead to DNA damage via the generation of reactive oxygen species (ROS). In turn, damaged DNA may induce *p53*, which could mediate the appropriate neuronal response (i.e., survival via DNA repair, or death via apoptosis).

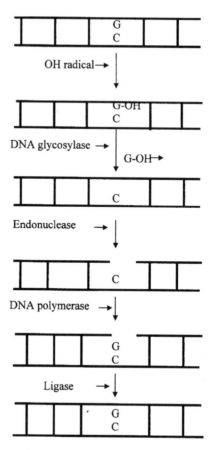

Figure 11.4   The base excision repair pathway to remove 8-OH guanine (G-OH) from DNA.

workers (1996) reported that, within 4 to 6 h following experimental ischemia, a reduction of glycosylase activity was observed, suggesting that BER processes have been activated. In contrast, a decrease in nuclear levels of the endonuclease associated with BER following global cerebral ischemia suggests that neuronal apoptosis occurs as a result of a failure of DNA repair processes (Kawase et al., 1999). Indirect evidence for the activation of DNA repair following ischemia arises from the observations of increased activity of poly(ADP-ribose) polymerase (PARP) (Endres et al., 1997; Shaikh et al., 1998). While the exact role of PARP activation in DNA repair has yet to be determined, the ability of PARP to bind to damaged DNA suggests that it may serve a role in targeting the repair enzymes to the lesioned area on the DNA molecule (Satoh and Lindahl, 1992). Similar to the observations following ischemia, LaPlaca and co-workers reported that TBI in rats induced PARP activation as early as 30 min post injury (LaPlaca et al., 1999). Because PARP uses nicotinamide–adenine dinucleotide as its substrate and thereby depletes cellular stores of energy, it has been suggested that PARP activation following CNS injury may be detrimental (Eliasson et al., 1997; Takahashi et al., 1997; Whalen et al., 1999).

THE APOPTOSIS–NECROSIS CONTINUUM DEBATE: IMPLICATIONS FOR THE PATHOLOGY OF TBI

Since the early 1990s, there has been a deluge in the number of studies reporting the presence of apoptosis in the CNS following excitotoxic, ischemic, or traumatic injuries, and in neurodegenerative diseases. More recently, it has been suggested that pathological (conventionally referred to as "necrotic") stimuli to the adult CNS may not necessarily result in classical apoptosis, such as that described during development of the nervous system (Roy and Sapolsky, 1999). Instead, based on the observations that morphological features of both necrosis and apoptosis appear in the same neural cell, and that apoptotic neural cells exhibit only some of the characteristics of developmental apoptosis, it has been argued that a continuum exists between apoptosis and necrosis (Cailliau et al., 1997; Nicotera et al., 1999). However, it is equally likely that the nature and/or intensity of the insult may regulate whether a complex cell such as a neuron undergoes apoptosis or necrosis. Whereas moderate–severe ischemia induces primarily necrotic cell death in the cortex (Charriaut-Marlangue et al., 1998), neuronal apoptosis is the predominant pattern of cell death following mild focal ischemia (Du et al., 1996). Alternatively, it has been reported that activation of the N-methyl-D-aspartate (NMDA) subtype of the glutamate receptor may lead to necrosis, while non-NMDA receptor activation may underlie apoptotic neuronal death (Cailliau et al., 1997). The presence of a continuum would suggest that intracellular pathways that lead to apoptosis and necrosis may also not be mutually exclusive. For example, although it has been proposed that the calcium-activated neutral proteases (calpains) may mediate necrosis, and that caspase-3 is activated only in apoptotic cells (Wang, 2000), calpain activation may also lead to apoptosis (Squier et al., 1994).

Based on the dependence of apoptosis on energy (in the form of ATP) (Tsujimoto, 1997; Green and Reed, 1998), it has been suggested that intracellular ATP concentrations may regulate whether a cell undergoes necrosis or apoptosis (Tsujimoto, 1997). Thus, as long as ATP is present within the injured cell, apoptotic pathways may be able to be initiated; once ATP is depleted (as a result of damage to the mitochondria), the injured cell may shift into a necrotic mode. This hypothesis may, in part, explain why neurons dying as a result of a pathological stimulus may exhibit features of both apoptosis and necrosis; that is, the apoptotic features may represent the temporal extent to which apoptotic pathways were active. Mitochondrial dysfunction with decreases in ATP levels has been documented following experimental TBI (Verweij et al., 1997; Xiong et al., 1997; Sullivan et al., 1998), although more recent data from the lateral fluid-percussion brain injury model suggest that TBI-induced decreases in ATP levels may not be sufficient to inhibit apoptosis (Lifshitz et al., 1999). Mitochondrial levels of ATP may decrease as a result of the formation of the mitochondrial permeability transition (MPT) pore

(Tsujimoto, 1997). The immunosuppressant cyclosporin A appears to inhibit the formation of the MPT, and it has been reported that reversal of trauma-induced mitochondrial damage by cyclosporin A treatment inhibits traumatic cortical cell loss (Scheff and Sullivan, 1999) and axonal injury (Buki et al., 1999; Okonkwo et al., 1999).

As more information regarding the pathological changes and the underlying cellular and molecular phenomena associated with TBI becomes available, it appears that TBI is a complex neurodegenerative disease. Thus, the strategies necessary to design a successful therapeutic regimen may need to be carefully planned and evaluated. Apoptotic pathways may provide reasonable targets for therapeutic interventions; however, it may be an understatement that an approach based on a single (or few) targets would be viewed as simplistic.

ACKNOWLEDGMENTS

The author thanks Drs. Tracy K. McIntosh and K. E. Saatman for many useful and timely discussions regarding the pathobiology of TBI. Studies described in this review were supported, in part, by NIH grants NS08803 and NS26818 (from NINDS), a VA Merit Review, and a Brain Injury Association grant to TKM.

ABBREVIATIONS

ATP	Adenosine triphosphate
BER	Base excision repair
$[Ca]_i$	Intracellular calcium concentration
CNS	Central nervous system
DNA	Deoxyribonucleic acid
ERK1/2	Extracellular signal-regulated kinase 1 and 2
GADD45	Growth associated and DNA damage inducible 45 kilodalton protein
8-OH-guanine	7,8-Dihydro-8-oxoguanine
JNK	c-Jun N-terminal kinase
MAPK	Mitogen-activated protein kinase
MPT	Mitochondrial permeability transition (pore)
NMDA	N-methyl-D-aspartate
PARP	Poly (ADP-ribose) polymerase
PCD	Programmed cell death
ROS	Reactive oxygen species
TBI	Traumatic brain injury

TUNEL   Terminal deoxynucleotidyl transferase-mediated dUTP nick end-labeling

WAF1   Wild-type *p53* activated fragment 1

REFERENCES

J. H. Adams, D. Doyle, D. I. Graham, A. E. Lawrence, D. R. McLellan, T. A. Gennarelli, M. Pastuszko, and T. Sakamoto, *Neuropathol. Appl. Neurobiol.*, 11, 299–308 (1985).

M. Artuso, A. Esteve, H. Bresil, M. Vuillaume, and J. Hall, *Oncogene*, 11, 1427–1435 (1995).

M. S. Beattie, S. L. Shuman, and J. C. Bresnahan, *Neuroscientist*, 4, 163–171 (1998).

A. R. Boobis, D. J. Fawthrop, and D. S. Davies, *Trends Pharmacol. Sci.*, 10, 275–280 (1989).

H. M. Bramlett, W. D. Dietrich, E. J. Green, and R. Busto, *Acta Neuropathol.*, 93, 190–199 (1997).

D. E. Bredesen, *Ann. Neurol.*, 38, 839–851 (1995).

A. Buki, D. O. Okonkwo, and J. T. Povlishock, *J. Neurotrauma*, 16, 511–521 (1999).

C. P. Cailliau, D. L. Price, and L. J. Martin, *J. Comp. Neurol.*, 378, 88–104 (1997).

J. Cervos-Navarro and J. V. Lafuente, *J. Neurol. Sci.*, 103, s3–s14 (1991).

P. H. Chan, *Stroke*, 27, 1124–1129 (1996).

C. Charriaut-Marlangue, S. Remolleau, D. Aggoun-Zouaoui, and Y. Ben-Ari, *Biomed. Pharmacol.*, 52, 264–269 (1998).

C. Charriaut-Marlangue and Y. Ben-Ari, *Neuroreport*, 7, 61–64 (1995).

J. Chen, S. H. Graham, P. H. Chan, P. Lan, R. L. Zhou, and R. P. Simon, *Neuroreport*, 6, 394–398 (1995).

J. Chen, K. Jin, M. Chen, W. Pei, P. Kawaguchi, D. A. Greenberg, and R. P. Simon, *J. Neurochem.*, 69, 232–245 (1997).

J. Chen, T. Nagayama, K. Jin, R. A. Steffler, R. L. Zhu, S. H. Graham, and R. P. Simon, *J. Neurosci.*, 18, 4914–4928 (1998).

M. Chopp, Y. Li, Z. G. Zhang, and S. O. Freytag, *Biochem. Biophys. Res. Commun.*, 482, 1201–1207 (1992).

M. Chopp, P. H. Chan, C. Y. Hsu, M. E. Cheung, and T. P. Jacobs, *Stroke*, 27, 363–369 (1996).

R. S. B. Clark, J. Chen, S. C. Watkins, P. M. Kochanek, M. Chen, R. A. Stetler, J. E. Loeffert, and S. H. Graham, *J. Neurosci.*, 17, 9172–9182 (1997).

R. S. B. Clark, P. M. Kochanek, M. Chen, S. C. Watkins, D. W. Marion, J. Chen, R. L. Hamilton, J. E. Loeffert, and S. H. Graham, *FASEB J.*, 13, 813–821 (1999).

M. A. Colicos and P. K. Dash, *Brain Res.*, 739, 120–131 (1996).

M. A. Colicos, C. E. Dixon, and P. K. Dash, *Brain Res.*, 739, 111–119 (1996).

A. R. Collins, M. Dusinska, C. M. Gedik, and R. Stetina, *Environ. Health Perspect.*, 104, 465–469 (1996).

A. C. Conti, R. Raghupathi, A. D. Rink, J. Q. Trojanowski, and T. K. McIntosh, *J. Neurosci.*, 18, 5663–5672 (1998).

M. J. Crowe, J. C. Bresnahan, S. L. Shuman, J. N. Masters, and M. S. Beattie, *Nat. Med.*, 3, 73–76 (1997).

W. D. Dietrich, O. Alonso, and M. Halley, *J. Neurotrauma*, 11, 289–301 (1994).

C. Du, R. Hu, C. A. Cseransky, C. Y. Hsu, and D. W. Choi, *J. Cereb. Blood Flow Metab.*, 16, 195–201 (1996).

M. J. L. Eliasson, K. Sampei, A. S. Mandir, P. D. Hurn, R. J. Traystman, J. Bao, A. Pieper, Z.-Q. Wang, T. M. Dawson, S. H. Snyder, and V. L. Dawson, *Nat. Med.*, 3, 1089–1095 (1997).

E. Emery, P. Aldana, M. B. Bunge, W. Puckett, A. Srinivasan, R. W. Keane, J. Bethea, and A. D. O. Levi, *J. Neurosurg.*, 89, 911–920 (1998).

M. Endres, Z.-Q. Wang, S. Namura, C. Waeber, and M. A. Moskowitz, *J. Cereb. Blood Flow Metab.*, 17, 143–151 (1997).

M. Endres, S. Namura, M. Shimizu-Sasamata, C. Waeber, L. Zhang, T. Gomez-Isla, B. T. Hyman, and M. A. Moskowitz, *J. Cereb. Blood Flow Metab.*, 18, 238–247 (1998).

G. Evan and T. D. Littlewood, *Science,* 281, 1317–1322 (1998).

I. Fineman, D. A. Hovda, M. Smith, A. Yoshino, and D. P. Becker, *Brain Res.*, 624, 94–102 (1993).

K. Fink, J. Zhu, S. Namura, M. Shimizu-Sasamata, M. Endres, J. Ma, T. Dalkara, J. Yuan, and M. A. Moskowitz, *J. Cereb. Blood Flow Metab.*, 18, 1071–1076 (1998).

G. B. Fox, L. Fan, R. A. Levasseur, and A. I. Faden, *J. Neurotrauma*, 15, 599–613 (1998).

R. M. Friedlander, V. Gagliardini, H. Hara, K. B. Fink, W. Li, G. MacDonald, M. C. Fishman, A. H. Greenberg, M. A. Moskowitz, and J. Yuan, *J. Exp. Med.*, 185, 933–940 (1997).

Y. Gavrieli, Y. Sherman, and S. A. Ben-Sasson, *J. Cell Biol.*, 119, 493–501 (1992).

T. A. Gennarelli, *J. Neurotrauma*, 11, 357–368 (1994).

T. A. Gennarelli, L. E. Thibault, and D. I. Graham, *Neuroscientist*, 4, 202–215 (1998).

F. Gillardon, H. Wickert, and M. Zimmermann, *Neurosci. Lett.*, 192, 85–88 (1995).

F. Gillardon, C. Lenz, K. F. Waschke, S. Krajewski, J. C. Reed, M. Zimmermann, and W. Kuschinsky. *Mol. Brain Res.*, 40, 254–260 (1996).

D. R. Green and J. C. Reed, *Science,* 281, 1309–1312 (1998).

L. J. S. Greenlund, T. L. Deckwerth, and E. M. Johnson, Jr, *Neuron*, 14, 303–315 (1995).

C. Gu, P. Casaccia-Bonnefil, A. Srinivasan, and M. V. Chao, *J. Neurosci.*, 19, 3043–3049 (1999).

B. J. Gwag, L. M. T. Canzoniero, S. L. Sensi, J. A. Demaro, J.-Y. Koh, M. P. Goldberg, M. Jacquin, and D. W. Choi, *Neuroscience*, 90, 1339–1348 (1999).

H. Hara, R. M. Friedlander, V. Gagliardini, C. Ayata, K. Fink, Z. Huang, M. Shimizu-Sasamata, J. Yuan, and M. A. Moskowitz, *Proc. Natl. Acad. Sci. USA*, 84, 2007–2012 (1997).

R. R. Hicks, H. D. Soares, D. H. Smith, and T. K. McIntosh, *Acta Neuropathol.*, 91, 236–246 (1996).

P. E. Hughes, T. Alexi, T. Yoshida, S. S. Schreiber, and B. Knusel, *Neuroscience*, 74, 1143–1160 (1996).

Y. Ikeda and D. M. Long. *Neurosurgery*, 27, 1–11 (1990).

W. D. Jarvis, F. A. Fornari, Jr., K. L. Auer, A. J. Freemerman, E. Szabo, M. J. Birrer, C. R. Johnson, S. E. Barbour, P. Dent, and S. Grant, *Mol. Pharmacol.*, 52, 935–947 (1997).

K. Jin, J. Chen, T. Nagayama, M. Chen, J. Sinclair, S. H. Graham, and R. P. Simon, *J. Neurochem.*, 72, 1204–1214 (1999).

J. M. Jurgensmeier, Z. Xie, Q. Deveraux, L. Ellerby, D. E. Bredesen, and J. C. Reed, *Proc. Natl. Acad. Sci. USA*, 95, 4997–5002 (1998).

M. Kawase, M. Fujimura, Y. Morita-Fujimura, and P. H. Chan, *Stroke*, 30, 441–448 (1999).

S. S. Kaya, A. Mahmood, Y. Li, E. Yavuz, M. Goksel, and M. Chopp, *Brain Res.*, 818, 23–33 (1999).

R. M. Kluck, E. Bossy-Wetzel, D. R. Green, and D. D. Newmeyer, *Science,* 275, 1132–1136 (1997).

M. J. Kotapka, D. I. Graham, J. H. Adams, and T. A. Gennarelli, *Acta Neuropathol.*, 83, 530–534 (1992).

S. Krajewski, J. K. Mai, M. Krajewska, M. Sikorska, M. J. Mossakowski, and J. C. Reed, *J. Neurosci.*, 15, 6364–6376 (1995).

A. Lannuzel, J. V. Barnier, C. Hery, H. Van Tan, B. Guibert, F. Gray, J. D. Vincent, and M. Tardiu, *Ann. Neurol.*, 42, 847–856 (1997).

M. C. LaPlaca, R. Raghupathi, A. Verma, A. Pieper, K. E. Saatman, S. H. Snyder, and T. K. McIntosh, *J. Neurochem.*, 73, 205–213 (1999).

A. LeBlanc, *Am. J. Pathol.*, 152, 329–332 (1998).

X. Li, H. Zou, C. Slaughter, and X. Wang, *Cell*, 89, 175–184 (1997).

J. Lifshitz, R. Raghupathi, F. A. Welsh, and T. K. McIntosh, *J. Neurotrauma*, 16, 990 (1999).

P. K. Liu, C. Y. Hsu, M. Dizdaroglu, R. A. Floyd, Y. W. Kow, A. Karakaya, L. E. Rabow, and J.-K. Cui, *J. Neurosci.*, 16, 6795–6806 (1996).

A. C. Lo, L. J. Houenou, and R. W. Oppenheim, *Arch. Histol. Cytol.*, 58, 139–149 (1995).

S. Love, R. Barber, and G. K. Wilcock, *Neuroreport*, 9, 955–959 (1998).

T. K. McIntosh, M. Juhler, and T. Wieloch, *J. Neurotrauma*, 15, 731–769 (1998).

D. F. Meaney, D. H. Smith, D. I. Shreiber, A. C. Bain, R. T. Miller, D. T. Ross, and T. A. Gennarelli, *J. Neurotrauma*, 12, 689–694 (1995).

D. E. Merry and S. J. Korsmeyer, *Annu. Rev. Neurosci.*, 20, 245–267 (1997).

K. Mielke, S. Brecht, A. Dorst, and T. Herdegen, *Neuroscience*, 91, 471–483 (1999).

M. Miyashita and J. C. Reed, *Cell*, 80, 293–299 (1995).

H. Mochizuki, K. Goto, H. Mori, and Y. Mizuno, *J. Neurol. Sci.*, 137, 120–123 (1996).

S. Nakahara, K. Yone, T. Sakou, S. Wada, T. Nagamine, T. Niiyama, and H. Ichijo, *J. Neuropathol. Exp. Neurol.*, 58, 442–450 (1999).

M. Nakamura, R. Raghupathi, D. E. Merry, U. Scherbel, K. E. Saatman, and T. K. McIntosh, *J. Comp. Neurol.*, 412, 681–692 (1999).

S. Namura, J. Zhu, K. Fink, M. Endres, A. Srinivasan, K. J. Tomaselli, J. Yuan, and M. A. Moskowitz, *J. Neurosci.*, 18, 3659–3668 (1998).

J. A. Napieralski, R. Raghupathi, and T. K. McIntosh. Mol, *Brain Res.*, 71, 78–86 (1999).

R. Nath, A. Probert, Jr., K. M. McGinnis, and K. K. W. Wang, *J. Neurochem.*, 71, 186–195 (1998).

J. K. Newcomb, X. Zhao, B. R. Pike, and R. L. Hayes, *Exp. Neurol.*, 158, 76–88 (1999).

P. Nicotera, M. Leist, and L. Manzo, *Trends Pharmacol. Sci.*, 20, 46–51 (1999).

P. Nilsson, H. Laursen, L. Hillered, and A. J. Hansen, *J. Cereb. Blood Flow Metab.*, 16, 262–270 (1996).

D. O. Okonkwo, A. Buki, R. Siman, and J. T. Povlishock, *Neuroreport*, 10, 353–358 (1999).

R. W. Oppenheim, *Annu. Rev. Neurosci.*, 14, 453–501 (1991).

H. Ozawa, S. Shioda, K. Dohi, H. Matsumoto, H. Mizushima, C. J. Zhou, H. Funahashi, Y. Nakai, S. Nakajo, and K. Matsumoto, *Neurosci. Lett.*, 262, 57–60 (1999).

D. S. Park, E. J. Morris, L. Stefanis, C. M. Troy, M. L. Shelanski, H. M. Geller, and L. A. Greene, *J. Neurosci.*, 18, 830–840 (1998).

B. Pettman and C. E. Henderson, *Neuron.*, 20, 633–647 (1998).

B. R. Pike, X. Zhao, J. K. Newcomb, R. M. Posmantur, K. K. W. Wang, and R. L. Hayes, *Neuroreport*, 9, 2437–2442 (1998).

C. P. Portera, J. C. Hedreen, D. L. Price, and V. E. Koliatsos, *J. Neurosci.*, 15, 3775–3787 (1995).

J. T. Povlishock, D. E. Erb, and J. Astruc, *J. Neurotrauma*, 9, S198–S200 (1992).

J. T. Povlishock, R. L. Hayes, M. E. Michel, and T. K. McIntosh, *J. Neurotrauma*, 11, 723–732 (1994).

R. Raghupathi, S. C. Fernandez, H. Murai, S. P. Trusko, R. W. Scott, W. K. Nishioka, and T. K. McIntosh, *J. Cereb. Blood Flow Metab.*, 18, 1259–1269 (1998).

A. D. Rink, K. M. Fung, J. Q. Trojanowski, V. M.-Y. Lee, E. Neugebauer, and T. K. McIntosh, *Am. J. Pathol.*, 147, 1575–1583 (1995).

D. T. Ross, D. I. Graham, and J. H. Adams, *J. Neurotrauma*, 10, 151–165 (1993).

M. Roy and R. M. Sapolsky, *Trends Neurosci.*, 22, 419–422 (1999).

S. Sakhi, A. Bruce, N. Sun, G. Tocco, M. Baudry, and S. S. Schreiber, *Proc. Natl. Acad. Sci. USA*, 91, 7525–7529 (1994).

A. Sancar, *J. Biol. Chem.*, 270, 15915–15918 (1995).

M. S. Saporito, E. M. Brown, M. S. Miller, and S. Carswell, *J. Pharmacol. Exp. Ther.*, 288, 421–427 (1999).

M. S. Satoh and T. Lindahl, *Nature*, 356, 356–358 (1992).

S. W. Scheff and P. G. Sullivan, *J. Neurotrauma*, 16, 783–792 (1999).

A. Y. Shaikh, U. R. Ezekiel, P. K. Liu, and C. Y. Hsu, *Neuroscientist*, 4, 88–95 (1998).

M. Shamloo, A. Rytter, and T. Wieloch, *Neuroscience*, 93, 81–88 (1999).

Y. Shapira, G. Yadid, S. Cotev, and E. Shohami, *Neurol. Res.*, 11, 169–172 (1989).

S. L. Shuman, J. C. Bresnahan, and M. S. Beattie, *J. Neurosci. Res.*, 50, 798–808 (1997).

G. Smale, N. C. Nichols, D. R. Brady, C. E. Finch, and W. E. Horton, Jr, *Exp. Neurol.*, 133, 225–230 (1995).

F. M. Smith, R. Raghupathi, M.-A. Mackinnon, T. K. McIntosh, K. E. Saatman, D. F. Meaney, and D. I. Graham, *Acta Neuropathol.*, 100, 337–545 (2000).

J. E. Springer, R. D. Azbill, and P. E. Knapp, *Nat. Med.*, 5, 943–946 (1999).

M. K. T. Squier, A. C. K. Miller, A. M. Malkinson, and J. J. Cohen. J, *Cell, Physiol.*, 159, 229–237 (1994).

P. G. Sullivan, J. N. Keller, M. P. Mattson, and S. W. Scheff, *J. Neurotrauma*, 15, 789–798 (1998).

S. A. Susin, N. Zamzami, and G. Kroemer, *Biochim. Biophys. Acta*, 1366, 151–165 (1998).

R. L. Sutton, L. Lescaudron, and D. G. Stein, *J. Neurotrauma*, 10, 135–149 (1993).

K. Takahashi, J. H. Greenberg, P. Jackson, K. Maclin, and J. Zhang, *J. Cereb. Blood Flow Metab.*, 17, 1137–1142 (1997).

N. A. Thornberry and Y. A. Lazebnik, *Science,* 281, 1312–1316 (1998).

Y. Tsujimoto, *Cell Death Differ.*, 4, 429–434 (1997).

S. Vamvakas, E. H. Vock, and W. K. Lutz, *Crit. Rev. Toxicol.*, 27, 155–174 (1997).

M. van Engeland, L. J. W. Nieland, F. C. S. Ramaekers, B. Schutte, and C. P. M. Reutlingsperger, *Cytometry*, 31, 1–9 (1998).

B. H. Verweij, J. P. Muizelaar, F. C. Vinas, P. L. Peterson, Y. Xiong, and C. P. Lee, *Neurol. Res.*, 19, 334–339 (1997).

K. K. W. Wang, *Trends Neurosci.*, 23, 20–26 (2000).

M. J. Whalen, R. S. B. Clark, C. E. Dixon, P. Robichaud, D. W. Marion, V. Vagni, S. H. Graham, L. Virag, G. Hasko, R. Stachlewitz, C. Szabo, and P. M. Kochanek, *J. Cereb. Blood Flow Metab.*, 19, 835–842 (1999).

Z. Xia, M. Dickens, J. Raingeaud, R. J. Davis, and M. E. Greenberg, *Science*, 270, 1326–1331 (1995).

Y. Xiong, Q. Gu, P. L. Peterson, J. P. Muizelaar, and C. P. Lee, *J. Neurotrauma*, 14, 23–34 (1997).

A. G. Yakovlev, S. M. Knoblach, L. Fan, G. B. Fox, R. Goodnight, and A. I. Faden, *J. Neurosci.*, 17, 7415–7424 (1997).

D. D. Yang, C.-Y. Kuan, A. J. Whitmarsh, M. Rincon, T. S. Zheng, R. J. Davis, P. Pakic, and R. Flavell, *Nature*, 389, 865–870 (1997a).

J. Yang, X. Liu, K. Bhalla, C. N. Kim, A. M. Ibrado, J. Cai, T.-I. Peng, D. P. Jones, and X. Wang, *Science*, 275, 1129–1132 (1997b).

Y. Yoshiyama, T. Yamada, K. Asanuma, and T. Asahi, *Acta Neuropathol.*, 88, 207–211 (1994).

W. Young, *J. Neurotrauma*, 9, s9–s25 (1992).

Z. F. Zakeri, D. Quaglino, T. Latham, and R. A. Lockshin, *FASEB J.*, 7, 470–478 (1993).

Q. Zhan, I. T. Chen, M. J. Antinore, and A. J. Fornace, *Mol. Cell. Biol.*, 18, 2768–2778 (1998).

CHAPTER 12

MITOCHONDRIAL DYSFUNCTION FOLLOWING TRAUMATIC BRAIN INJURY

Y. XIONG AND C. P. LEE

Departments of Biochemistry and Molecular Biology, School of Medicine, Wayne State University, Detroit, Michigan

P. L. PETERSON

Department of Neurology, School of Medicine, Wayne State University, Detroit, Michigan

INTRODUCTION

Isolated mitochondria have served as useful tools for identifying site(s) of impairment associated with respiratory chain-linked oxidative phosphorylation and related processes. Since the early 1970s, a large number of neuromuscular diseases associated with mitochondrial dysfunction have been identified from biochemical studies of skeletal muscles biopsies. Systematic biochemical studies of brain lesions induced by TBI (traumatic brain injury) were not initiated until recently. This was primarily due to lack of suitable techniques for isolation and characterization of tightly coupled brain mitochondria. This chapter provides a brief survey of the current state of knowledge concerning mitochondrial dysfunction induced by head trauma, and a brief review of the following topics: (1) the relationship between mitochondrial structure and function in energy transduction and the role of mitochondria in apoptosis; (2) the unique properties of brain tissue in energy metabolism; (3) biochemical studies of brain mitochondrial injury induced by head trauma, and the importance of isolation and assay conditions of brain mitochondria; and (4) efficacy of in vivo treatment of TBI-injured rats with neuroprotective agents, for example, calcium blockers and antioxidants. Evidence accumulated in the literature supports the idea that TBI induces increase in the generation of reactive oxygen species (ROS) and perturbation of cellular calcium homeostasis, which consequently impairs mitochondrial electron transfer and energy transduction.

Head Trauma: Basic, Preclinical, and Clinical Directions, Edited by Leonard P. Miller and Ronald L. Hayes, Co-edited by Jennifer K. Newcomb
ISBN 0-471-36015-5 © 2001 John Wiley & Sons, Inc.

BRAIN ENERGY METABOLISM AND BRAIN INJURY

Energy metabolism of the brain is unique, possessing high aerobic metabolism with no significant capacity for anaerobic glycolysis and limited tissue stores of glucose. The adult human brain represents ~2 percent of total body weight yet it receives ~14 percent of the cardiac output (McHenry, 1978) and consumes ~20 percent of total body oxygen (Erecinska and Silver, 1989). Normal brain function is critically dependent upon a constant supply of oxygen and glucose to provide energy production from glycolysis and oxidative phosphorylation. Neuronal survival and normal neurologic function are therefore dependent upon adequate cerebral blood flow that delivers oxygen, glucose, and other nutrients, and removes carbon dioxide and other metabolic by-products. The sensitivity of the brain to disturbances in cerebral blood flow and energy generation is obvious. Over half a century ago, it was discovered that consciousness was lost 5 to 6 s following application of a pressure cuff to the necks of humans (Rossen et al., 1943). The brain has virtually no energy stores, and only small reserves of high-energy phosphate compounds and carbohydrates. Complete cerebral ischemia has been found to cause energy depletion within a few minutes in several animal species (Lust et al., 1985).

Traumatic brain injury (TBI) is the leading cause of death among individuals under the age of 45 years in the United States and Europe. Two million brain injuries occur per year in the United States and about 70,000 patients suffer from life-long neurologic motor and cognitive dysfunction. Brain damage following TBI results from two processes, primary injury and secondary injury. Primary injury is the result of immediate biomechanical damage and is amenable only to injury prevention. Secondary injury is an evolving process that occurs over hours to days following injury, thus providing a window of opportunity for therapeutic intervention. It is not understood at present what molecular mechanisms are involved in secondary injury (see Chapter 1); however, a decrease in cerebral blood flow (Bryan et al., 1995), increase in excitatory amino acids (Faden et al., 1989; Hayes et al., 1992; Palmer et al., 1993; McIntosh et al., 1998), perturbation of intracellular calcium homeostasis (Hovda et al., 1994; Xiong et al., 1997a), increased generation of reactive oxygen species (Hall, 1993; Smith et al., 1994; Shohami et al., 1997), and apoptosis (Rink et al., 1995; Colicos and Dash, 1996; Yakovlev et al., 1997; Chen et al., 1998) are thought to be involved. All of these factors, either alone or in combination, have been shown to be detrimental to mitochondrial function. More recently, a number of studies have provided evidence to support the idea that mitochondrial dysfunction might play a vital role in secondary injury after TBI (Xiong et al., 1997a, 1998; Sullivan et al., 1998).

MITOCHONDRIAL STRUCTURE AND COMPOSITION

Mitochondria are organelles of eukaryotic cells. The basic structure of the mitochondrion consists of an outer membrane, an inner membrane, the intermembrane space, and the matrix. It is well established that the inner membrane is the site of the respiratory chain and its related energy-transducing processes, such as the ATP synthase, the nicotinamide–adenine nucleotide transhydrogenase, and cation and anion translocators. The enzymes and cofactors associated with the tricarboxylic acid cycle and the β-oxidation of fatty acids, enzymes for biosynthesis of urea, ketones, amino acids, pyrimidines, nucleotides and hemes, and additionally mito-chondrial DNA (mtDNA) are located in the matrix. Adenylate kinase and creatine kinase are located in the intermembrane space. The outer membrane contains monoamine oxidase, long-chain acyl-CoA synthetase, NADH cytochrome-b_5 reduc-tase, cytochrome b_5, kynurenine 3-monooxygenase, and lysophosphatidate acyl-transferase 1, as well as receptors and other key components of the mitochondrial inner membrane import machinery (Baker and Schatz, 1991).

The inner membrane is extensively invaginated into folds or cristae, possesses reversible osmotic properties (e.g., they reversibly swell and contract), and is impermeable to most hydrophilic and ionized metabolites. The mitochondrial inner membrane is relatively rich in protein and consists of approximately 75 percent proteins and 25 percent lipids (DePierre and Ernster, 1977). More than two-thirds of the proteins are intrinsic. The respiratory chain and the ATP synthase constitute more than one-third of the total protein of the inner membrane, while the remainder includes various other enzymes, cation and anion translocators, and structural proteins. The lipids of the inner membrane are predominantly phospho-lipids; the main species are phosphatidylcholine, phosphatidylethanolamine, and cardiolipin. Cardiolipin is unique among phospholipids in animal cells and is essential for a number of energy-transducing enzymes (Cheneval et al., 1985; Hoch, 1992; Hoffmann et al., 1994). Cardiolipin differs from other phospholipids in that it is strongly acidic and possesses a relatively large proportion of poly-unsaturated fatty acids. The latter feature has been thought to be responsible for the sensitivity of cardiolipin to agents causing lipid peroxidation (Soussi et al., 1990a, b). The outer membrane contains twice as much phospholipid on a protein basis as the inner membrane and also contains a significant amount of cholesterol. In contrast to the inner membrane, the outer membrane does not possess reversible osmotic properties. It is able to swell upon a decrease in osmolarity, but it cannot contract in response to an increase in osmolarity. The outer membrane is permeable to both charged and uncharged molecules with a molecular mass less than 1000.

Evidence accumulated in the literature indicates that contact exists between inner and outer membranes of mitochondria and sites of contact do not preexist; therefore, dynamic structures are formed according to the transfer process (Brdiczka, 1991). Protein-transfer contact sites and energy-transfer contact sites are similar in the sense that their components lead to contact between the two membranes as a prerequisite for the specific transfer process. However, protein–transfer contact and energy–transfer contact are not the same since they are created by interaction of different components. In general, the components of the contacts are proteins that, besides their specific function (receptor, enzyme, pore), have the ability to interact with phospholipids or other proteins to form large complexes that constitute the contact sites. The benefit of this assembly is to guide optional metabolite reactions in a specific direction.

Another dynamic multiprotein complex, mitochondrial permeability transition (MPT) pore is formed in the contact site between the inner and outer mitochondrial membranes. It has been postulated to play an essential role in cellular metabolic functions. The proteins constituting the MPT pore are not fully known. When reconstituted into liposomes or black lipid membranes, the hexokinase/porin/ adenine nucleotide translocase (ANT) complex confers to the system permeability and conductance properties that resemble those of the MPT pore (Beutner et al., 1996). Further studies obtained with purified and reconstituted ANT indicate that ANT forms a channel for small molecules comparably to the MPT pore (Ruck et al., 1998). The well-characterized inhibitors of MPT such as cyclosporin A (cyclophilin D inhibitor), bongkrekic acid, and atractyloside (specific ligands for ANT) are able to prevent the apoptotic decrease in mitrochondrial membrane potential, $\Delta\psi_m$ decrease.

MPT may act as a sensor for Ca^{2+}, voltage, thiols, oxidoreduction status of the nicotinamide–adenine nucleotide pool, matrix pH, divalent cations, and adenine nucleotides. Periodic reversible pore opening under physiological conditions allows for the release of Ca^{2+} from mitochondrial matrix in maintaining the cellular calcium homeostasis, and facilitates the $\Delta\psi_m$-driven import of proteins into the mitochondrial matrix. However, massive MPT pore opening will culminate in cell death.

Mitochondrial DNA is a circular duplex. The human mtDNA was sequenced (Anderson et al., 1981) and shown to be 16,569 bp in length; it encodes 37 genes essential for mitochondrial respiratory chain-linked energy transduction: 13 poly-peptides, which include seven subunits (ND1, 2, 3, 4L, 4, 5, 6) of complex I, one subunit (cytochrome b) of complex III, three subunits (COX-1, COX-2 and COX-3) of complex IV, and two subunits (ATP-6 and ATP-8) of the H^+-translocating ATP synthase; two (12S and 16S) rRNAs; and 22 tRNAs. It is apparent that most mitochondrial proteins are encoded by nuclear (n)DNA and synthesized by cyto-plasmic ribosomes and imported into mitochondria (Hartl et al., 1989). However, all four energy-transducing complexes (complexes I, III, and IV and ATP synthase) contain one or more mtDNA-encoded unit.

MITOCHONDRIAL FUNCTIONS

Besides the classical concept of mitochondria serving as the "powerhouse" of the cell (ATP generation) it is now evident that mitochondria play crucial roles in various biological functions including electrolyte balance, calcium homeostasis, cellular signal transduction, antioxidant and immunologic defense (Lee, 1994), and apoptosis (Gunter et al., 1994; Liu et al., 1996; Petit et al., 1997; Kroemer et al., 1998; Mignotte and Vayssiere, 1998).

Respiratory Chain-linked Oxidative Phosphorylation

Oxidative phosphorylation is the process in which energy is generated from electron transfer via oxidation of substrates and is coupled through a transmembrane proton gradient to synthesize ATP. The electron transfer chain (also called the respiratory chain) transfers reducing equivalents from oxidizable substrates (NAD-linked and succinate) to molecular oxygen. The electron transfer chain consists of four multi-subunit complexes (I, II, III, and IV) linked by two mobile electron carriers, ubiquinone and cytochrome c. It transfers electrons from NADH via complex I (NADH-ubiquinone oxidoreductase) or from succinate via complex II (succinate-ubiquinone oxidoreductase) to ubiquinone, then via complex III (ubiquinol-cyto-chrome-c oxidoreductase) to cytochrome c, and finally via complex IV (cytochrome-c oxidase) to molecular oxygen with the formation of two water molecules. Free energy derived from electron transfer can be utilized for the synthesis of ATP from ADP and inorganic phosphate (P_i). Maximal ATP/O ratios of 3 for the oxidation of NAD-linked substrates (via complexes I–II–IV electron transfer chain) and 2 for the oxidation of succinate (via complexes II–III–IV) are the generally accepted values for mitochondrial oxidative phosphorylation (Lee et al., 1996).

Complexes I, III, and IV are membrane-bound and conserve energy by active translocation of protons across the membrane (Fig. 12.1). Complex I is the largest of them and catalyzes the transfer of electrons from NADH to ubiquinone; the energy derived is sufficient to synthesize one molecule of ATP per two electrons transferred. The mammalian enzyme contains 42 or 43 different subunits, one FMN, seven or eight Fe-S centers, covalently bound lipid, and at least three bound quinols (Walker et al., 1992; Friedich et al., 1998; Skehel et al., 1998). The monomeric complex I is $> 900\,\text{kDa}$, and is an L-shaped structure. Its three-dimensional structure is under investigation by several laboratories (Guenebaut et al., 1997; Friedrich et al., 1998;

Cytosolic side

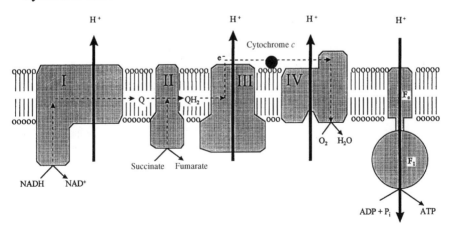

Matrix side

Figure 12.1 Schematic diagram of the respiratory chain and ATP synthase of the mitochondrial inner membrane. I, II, III, and IV represent complexes I, II, III and IV, respectively. Solid thick lines and arrows indicate proton translocation across the membrane. Dotted thin lines and arrows indicate the path of electron transfer.

Grigorieff, 1998). How the proton transport is coupled to electron transfer in complex I is not known and resolution of this awaits relevant structural information. Complex II is a component of the TCA cycle that transfers electrons from succinate to ubiquinone. It contains FAD and several Fe-S centers, and is anchored to the membrane by a b-type cytochrome. Complex II does not translocate H^+.

Complex III, or cytochrome $b-c_1$ complex, transfers electrons from ubiquinol to cytochrome c. This redox reaction is coupled to the generation of a proton gradient across the membrane via the Q cycle mechanism. The mammalian monomeric complex III contains 11 subunits ($\sim 240\,kDa$), but only three redox centers (cytochromes b, c_1 and Reskie Fe-S center). The existence of two active sites (Q_o and Q_i) in complex III and the bifurcation of the electron path are essential features of Mitchell's Q cycle mechanism (Mitchell, 1976). A quinol at the Q_o site can donate two electrons, one electron is transferred to the Fe-S center, then to cytochrome c_1; the second electron is transferred to the Q_i site via the hemes b_L and b_H of cytochrome b subunit, which is an electrogenic step (it creates part of the proton motive force) that is driven by the difference in redox potentials of the two hemes. Two electrons are transferred to the Q_i site after oxidation of two quinols at the Q_o site, to reduce one quinone. This mechanism leads to a net translocation of two protons for each electron transferred to cytochrome c. The structure of the bovine complex III has been deduced from X-ray crystallography (Iwata et al., 1998; Yu et al., 1999), indicating that complex III is in a stable dimeric form.

Complex IV, or cytochrome-c oxidase, generates a transmembrane proton gradient by a mechanism different from that of cytochrome $b–c_1$ complex. The bovine cytochrome-c oxidase contains 13 subunits. The three major subunits (COX-1, COX-2, COX-3) are encoded by mtDNA and form the functional core of complex IV. It has four redox centers, cytochromes a, a_3, Cu_A, and Cu_B. The active site (cytochrome a_3/Cu_B) resides in subunit I. Cytochrome c binds to the cytosolic side of the complex that donates electrons to the active site via Cu_A in subunit II and cytochrome a in subunit I, and is used to reduce O_2 to two water molecules. The protons needed for this reaction are taken from the mitochondrial matrix side through two channels, D- and K-channels; the same channels are used to pump one proton per electron across the membrane. Subunit III contains bound phospholipids but its functional role has yet to be established. A dimeric structure of bovine cytochrome-c oxidase was deduced from X-crystallography (Tsukihara et al., 1996). The mechanism of proton pumping in cytochrome-c oxidase remains to be elucidated.

The mitochondrial ATP synthase, or the $F_1F_0 - H^+$ translocating ATPase, or complex V, can synthesize ATP using a proton gradient across the membrane, and can also hydrolyze ATP to pump protons against an electrochemical gradient. Its essential structural features consist of three parts, a membrane sector (F_0), a catalytic component (F_1) and the stalk which links F_0 to F_1. F_1 is the catalytic unit and contains five different subunits (α, β, γ, δ, and ε) in a stoichiometry of $3:3:1:1:1$. The α and β subunits are homologous, both bind nucleotides but only β has catalytic activity. According to Boyer's binding exchange mechanism, each site would pass through three different states ("open," "loose," and "tight," corresponding to an empty state, a state with bound ADP and P_i, and a state with tightly bound ATP); at any given moment, the three sites would be in different states. Boyer and others have shown that energy is required for the binding of substrates and the release of ATP from the enzyme but not the formation of ATP from ADP and P_i. F_0 contains a number of hydrophobic subunits with the function of a proton channel and is linked to F_1 located on the matrix side of the membrane by a stalk consisting of two parallel structures referred to as a rotor and a stator (Boyer, 1997). The F_0 of the bacterial enzyme contains a tetramer of subunit a, a dimer of subunit b, and a dodecamer of subunit c. According to its crystal structure, a dodecamer of subunit c is connected to a complex of subunits γ and ε of F_1 forming the rotor; subunit a and a dimer of subunit b with subunit δ of F_1 form the stator arm, which has an interface with the oligomeric subunit c and links with F_1. The crystal structure of the bovine F_1-ATPase revealed the intrinsic asymmetry of the enzyme, which supports Boyer's mechanism that the enzyme operates by the rotational catalysis. The contact between the central γ subunit and the β subunits is a critical factor in the development of rotational model. The β and α subunits are three domain structures. Rotation of the γ subunit within the $\alpha_3\beta_3$ hexamer would facilitate the binding of the substrate and the release of product.

Mitochondrial Calcium Transport

Mitochondria actively participate in intracellular calcium regulation. Calcium is transported into mitochondria by means of an electrogenic carrier that is inhibited by ruthenium red and Mg^{2+}. Ca^{2+} can be pumped out primarily by means of the $2Na^+/Ca^{2+}$ antiport, which is inhibited by a wide variety of inhibitors including the Ca^{2+} antagonist diltiazem. There is a $2H^+/Ca^{2+}$ antiport, which is the most prominent mechanism of calcium efflux from mitochondria in tissues such as liver and kidney. The efflux of calcium is driven by the pH gradient, either directly or through the operation of the Na^+/H^+ antiport (Gunter and Pfeiffer, 1990; Gunter et al., 1994). Under physiological conditions, relatively low levels of mitochondrial Ca^{2+} stimulate the activity of matrix Ca^{2+}-sensitive dehydrogenase such as pyruvate dehydrogenase and isocitrate dehydrogenase (McCormack et al., 1990). This physiological response increases the supply of reducing equivalents to the electron transfer chain, enhancing ATP synthesis to meet the increased cellular energy requirements. This Ca^{2+} regulation is an important means of physically regulating mitochondrial metabolism by hormones and other stimuli. At higher intracellular Ca^{2+} concentration ($> 600\,\text{nM}$), the egress of Ca^{2+} becomes saturated while the entry pathway continues to allow electrogenic influx of Ca^{2+} (McCormack et al., 1990). This leads to mitochondrial Ca^{2+} overload (Gunter and Pfeiffer, 1990). Excessive Ca^{2+} cannot be retained by mitochondria and will be released again. This Ca^{2+} release leads to the opening/formation of mitochondrial permeability transition pore and substantial mitochondrial swelling, mitochondrial dysfunction, and eventually cell death.

Role of Mitochondria in Apoptosis

Evidence accumulated from intact cell apoptosis (Kroemer et al., 1998; Rosse et al., 1998) and cell-free (Newmeyer et al., 1994; Kluck et al., 1997) systems provides overwhelming support for the idea that mitochondria play a key role in apoptosis. In 1996, Liu et al. first reported that cytochrome c was involved in apoptosis. Cytochrome c is released from the intermembrane space into the cytosol at early steps of apoptosis, then combines with the cytosolic apoptotic activating factor (Apaf-1) and dATP activates conversion of the latent apoptosis-promoting protease pro-caspase-9 to its active form, caspase-9. Caspase-9 induces conversion of pro-caspase-3 to caspase-3, the key enzyme involved in apoptosis. Therefore, cytochrome c acts as a regulator of executive caspase activation (Zou et al., 1997; Skulachev, 1998; Hampton et al., 1998).

Yang and Cortopassi (1998) have reported that the release of cytochrome c in mouse liver mitochondria by canonical inducers of MPT is dependent on mitochondrial swelling. However, the mechanism remains controversial. By contrast, dATP induces a strong, dose-dependent release of cytochrome c that appears to be independent of mitochondrial swelling. Andreyev et al. (1998) have found that rat brain mitochondria do not undergo Ca^{2+}-induced permeability transition in the presence of ATP and Mg^{2+}, but do so in the absence of ATP and Mg^{2+}. Cytochrome c release from mitochondria occurs independently of the permeability transition.

Unlike liver mitochondria, Ca^{2+}-evoked swelling of brain mitochondria may be insufficient to disrupt the mitochondrial outer membrane. Additionally, brain mitochondria accumulate very little Ca^{2+} in the absence of adenine nucleotides (Rottenberg and Marbach, 1990) and are less prone to undergo permeability transition-mediated swelling than liver mitochondria (Kristal and Dubinsky, 1997). Bax is a proapoptotic member of the Bcl-2 protein family located in the outer mitochondrial membrane, endoplasmic reticulum, and nuclear membrane. Bax is able to induce cytochrome c release from isolated mitochondria in vitro, and release can be prevented by Bcl-x_L and CsA, although Bax does not induce mitochondrial swelling (Jurgensmeier et al., 1998). Bax may form a pore in the outer membrane of mitochondria that allows cytochrome c to leak out, as Bax has been shown to form channels in synthetic membranes and may even create very high-conductance channels under certain circumstances (Bernardi et al., 1994). The study of Eskes et al. (1998) suggests the existence of two distinct mechanisms leading to cytochrome c release: one stimulated by Ca^{2+} and inhibited by CsA; the other Bax-dependent, Mg^{2+}-sensitive, but CsA-insensitive. Apoptosis may occur independently of or dependently upon cytochrome c release in different cells and by different apoptosis inducers (Chauhan et al., 1997; Tang et al., 1998). Bcl-2 may attenuate apoptosis either by preventing opening of the permeability transition pore or by binding released cytochrome c (Skulachev, 1998).

It has been suggested that MPT is a central coordinating event of apoptosis (Marchetti et al., 1996). In a number of experiments, the early stage of apoptosis that precedes nuclear disintegration is characterized by disruption of the mitochondrial membrane potential ($\Delta\psi_m$). This $\Delta\psi_m$ disruption is mediated by the opening of permeability transition pores and appears to be critical for the apoptotic cascade, since it is directly regulated by Bcl-2, and mitochondria induced to undergo MPT in vitro become capable of inducing nuclear chromatinolysis in a cell-free system of apoptosis. The finding that Bcl-2 prevents the MPT-mediated $\Delta\psi_m$ decrease both in cells and in isolated mitochondria adds further support. Bongkrekic acid, a specific inhibitor of MPT and a ligand of the mitochondrial adenine nucleotide translocase, prevents apoptosis. The consequences of mitochondrial dysfunction, such as uncoupling of the respiratory chain, hyperproduction of superoxide anion, disruption of mitochondrial biogenesis, outflow of matrix Ca^{2+} and glutathione, and release of soluble intermembrane proteins, entails a bioenergetic catastrophe. Eventually, disruption of plasma membrane integrity (necrosis) and/or the activation of specific apoptogenic proteases (caspases) by mitochondrial proteins, such as cytochrome c and apoptosis-inducing factor, with secondary endonuclease activation (apoptosis) will occur. The relative rates of these two processes (bioenergetic catastrophe versus protease and endonuclease activation) determine whether a cell will undergo primary necrosis or apoptosis.

MITOCHONDRIAL DYSFUNCTION INDUCED BY TRAUMATIC BRAIN INJURY

Utilization of Isolated Mitochondria to Study Brain Injury

In contrast to the heart and liver, the isolation of mitochondria from the brain has been complicated by its high myelin and lipid content. The separation of mitochondria from other membraneous constituents has been facilitated by increasing the density of the medium. This was accomplished either by the introduction of Ficoll into the fractionation medium, as described by Basford (1967), or by subjecting the crude preparation to a Ficoll gradient, as described by Clark and associates (Clark and Nicklas, 1970; Lai and Clark 1979). However, the yields of mitochondria were low, with $\sim 2\,mg$ mitochondrial protein per gram wet weight in the Basford preparation (1967) and approximately 3 percent recovery of mitochondrial enzymes in the Clark and Nicklas preparation (1970). In addition, with most, if not all, procedures documented in the literature, at least four to six rats were used for each preparation owing to the multiple steps involved in the preparation and to the relatively low recovery of mitochondrial protein. These factors make studies of brain injury on mitochondrial function difficult to interpret accurately, due to interanimal variability and the high aerobic metabolism and low endogenous energy stores of the brain. Although a span of a few minutes between the handling of two rats may not have significant effects in the case of liver and heart, it is a critical factor with respect to the brain, particularly with brain derived from head-injured rats (Lee et al., 1993). In addition, it is not possible to control physiological factors that would impact on study outcome in four to six rats as compared to one rat.

In our laboratory, a simple and fast procedure has been established to isolate intact brain mitochondria from a single rat with high quality and good yield

(Sciamanna et al., 1992; Lee et al., 1993). This procedure is particularly valuable for preparations from the brain following head injury (ischemia and trauma) (Sciamanna et al., 1992; 1993; Xiong et al., 1997a, b, 1998, 1999). The entire procedure can be completed within one hour. The mitochondrial preparation is stable for at least three hours with virtually no loss of functional activities. Respiratory and phosphorylating properties of our preparation (derived from differential centrifugation) are comparable to those of nonsynaptic mitochondria isolated by the Percoll density gradient centrifugation (Dunkley et al., 1988; Davey et al., 1997). The yield of our mitochondrial preparation is more than three times that of the Percoll gradient method (Table 12.1). It should be mentioned that nonsynaptic mitochondria amount to more than 90 percent of the total mitochondria (both synaptic and nonsynaptic). More recently, our method for mitochondrial preparation from a single rat brain has been refined to isolate mitochondria in only 1 h from one hemisphere of a rat following traumatic brain injury, which enables us to make comparative studies of metabolic functions of mitochondria derived from ipsilateral (IH) and contralateral (CH) hemispheres of the rat brain (Xiong et al., 1997a).

Effect of TBI on Mitochondrial Functions

The controlled cortical impact injury (CCII) model reproduces many features of severe human TBI both histopathologically and neurologically, including cortical contusion, diffuse axonal injury, and impairment in memory. One of the most important features of this model is that the severity of injury can be precisely controlled by the velocity and deformation depth with consistent reproducibility (Xiong et al., 1997a). Figure 12.2 shows typical polarographic traces of brain mitochondria isolated from a sham-injured rat (A) and the IH of a TBI-rat (B, C) with glutamate and malate as substrates. The respiratory rates were clearly

TABLE 12.1   Comparison of Mitochondria Isolated with Percoll Gradient and Differential Centrifugation

	Percoll Gradient[a]		Differential Centrifugation[b]
	Nonsynaptic Mitochondria[c] ($n = 3$)	Synaptic Mitochondria ($n = 2$)	Total Mitochondria[d] ($n = 7$)
Respiratory rate[e]			
State 3	223.7 ± 73.0	58.9 ± 5.5	213.6 ± 7.1
State 4	37.6 ± 12.0	41.6 ± 0.7	36.8 ± 1.8
RCI	6.1 ± 0.3	1.4 ± 0.2	5.6 ± 0.4
P/O ratio	2.7 ± 0.1	2.7 ± 0.3	2.8 ± 0.1
Yield (mg protein/g brain)	2.8 ± 0.7	1.5 ± 0.5	9.7 ± 0.5

[a] Prepared according to Dunkley et al. (1988) and Davey et al. (1997); [b] Prepared according to Lee et al. (1993); [c] Assayed in the presence of 0.4 mM EGTA; [d] Citrate synthase/acetyl cholinesterase $= 18$; succinate dehydrogenase/lactate dehydrogenase $= 65$; [e] Expressed as natoms O/min/mg protein.

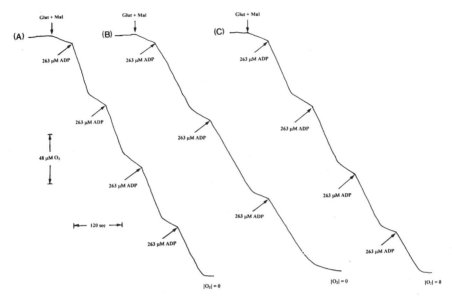

Figure 12.2 Polarographic traces of isolated forebrain mitochondria from sham (A) post TBI rats (B, C) at 12 h. The reaction mixture consisted of 150 mM sucrose, 25 mM Tris-HCl, 10 mM phosphate buffer, pH 7.4, and 0.80 mg protein (trace A) or 0.65 mg protein (traces B and C). The reaction was started upon the addition of 5 mM glutamate +2.5 mM malate. In (C) the reaction mixture was supplemented with 0.4 mM EGTA. Other additions were as indicated. Total volume 1.0 ml; temperature 30°C.

dependent on the presence (state 3) and absence (state 4) of added ADP. The state 3 and state 4 cycles were repeatable several times. The respiratory control indices (RCI) defined as the ratio of respiratory rate at state 3 and state 4 were >5 for sham mitochondria (Figure 12.2, trace A).

In contrast to sham animals, the state 3 respiratory rate of IH-mitochondria from rats subjected to TBI (trace B) was markedly impaired. The rate was decreased by nearly 50 percent, and both the P/O ratio and the RCI values were significantly decreased. Similar results were also obtained when glutamate and malate were replaced by pyruvate and malate as substrates. When the assay medium was supplemented with 0.4 mM EGTA (trace C), the respiratory activities exhibited by TBI-mitochondria were comparable to those of shams (trace A). Virtually identical results were obtained when EGTA was replaced by EDTA. The effects of added EGTA suggests that Ca^{2+} ions play an important role in TBI-induced mitochondrial dysfunction.

As compared with sham values, the state 3 respiratory rates of mitochondria from the hemisphere ipsilateral to impact were significantly impaired with an onset as early as 1 h post injury which persisted for 168 h with a nadir at 12 to 72 h (Xiong et al., 1997a). No significant change in the state 4 respiratory rates of IH mitochondria were seen up to 120 h post injury. With CH mitochondria, no significant change in the state 3 respiratory rates, but a marked increase in the state 4 respiratory rates, were observed. Consequently, a decline in RCI was observed in all cases tested. As expected, a decline in P/O ratios was also observed in most cases studied, though the extent of damage in the CH was much less than that in the IH. These findings do emphasize the diffuse nature of TBI induced by a focal impact. With succinate (+ rotenone) as substrate, the impairments induced by TBI to the respiratory rates at both state 3 and state 4 were much less severe than those observed with NAD-linked substrates; for example, the maximal decreases in state 3 respiratory rates were approximately 55 percent of sham for NAD-linked substrates and 75 percent of sham for succinate; the maximal increases in state 4 respiratory rates were about 155 percent of sham for NAD-linked substrates and 125 percent of sham for succinate. However, the energy-coupling capacities were significantly reduced, and comparable to those obtained with NAD-linked substrates. These results indicate that complex I is more susceptible to the effect of TBI, possibly due to its size and susceptibility to ROS-induced damage (Zhang et al., 1990; Xiong et al., 1997a).

Effect of In Vitro Treatment with EGTA on Mitochondrial Functions Following TBI

As shown in Figure 12.2, when the assay medium was supplemented with 0.4 mM EGTA (trace C), the state 3 respiratory rates, RCI, and P/O were restored to virtually sham level (trace A). Externally added EGTA is able to chelate Ca^{2+} and eliminates the Ca^{2+} transport across the mitochondrial inner membrane. Thus, added EGTA improves mitochondrial energy coupling by saving the energy for oxidative phosphorylation.

Using a unilateral controlled cortical impact model, Sullivan et al. (1998) demonstrated an immediate significant reduction in synaptosomal ATP levels in the injured half of the brain and specific regions of the injured half of the brain such as injured cortex and hippocampus. This reduction normalized by 6 h post injury. Following TBI, there is a significant increase in lipid peroxidation in the injured half of the brain and injured cortex at 30 min and 24 h post injury. The sharp decline in ATP levels during the first hour post injury in association with an increase in glucose uptake could indicate a decline in mitochondrial function. Reduction of ATP levels and mitochondrial dysfunction following TBI have been reported by several groups (Wagner et al., 1985; Yang et al., 1985; Proctor et al., 1988; Cadoux-Hudson et al., 1990; Xiong et al., 1997a).

On the other hand, no significant changes in ATP levels and impairment in mitochondrial function after TBI have been reported by others (Vink et al., 1988; Headrick et al., 1994; Prasad et al., 1994; Vink et al., 1994). These discrepancies may be related to the injury model and/or the species of animal employed, the severity of injury, and/or the conditions of procedures employed in different laboratories. There may be significant regional alterations in metabolism following TBI that are masked when analysis is carried out without specific dissection. In our study, the mitochondrial dysfunction after controlled cortical impact injury would have been masked if EGTA had been included in the assay medium (Xiong et al.,

1997a). For example, mitochondrial state 3 respiration and P/O ratios following TBI induced by fluid percussion injury (Vink et al., 1994) or CCII (Xiong et al., 1997a) were comparable to sham when the assay medium contained EGTA.

Mitochondrial Dysfunction After Human Head Injury

Mitochondria from human brain tissues have also been studied. The isolation and characterization of brain mitochondria are essentially the same as those for rat brain mitochondria according to the procedure of Lee et al. (1993), with minor modifications (Xiong et al., 1997a). State 3 respiratory rates of brain mitochondria derived from TBI patients were markedly impaired when compared to those of epilepsy and stroke patients. RCI and P/O ratios were also significantly decreased in TBI patients. When the assay medium was supplemented with the calcium chelator EGTA, in most, but not all, TBI patients state 3 rates, RCI, and P/O ratios were improved, suggesting that calcium ions partially play a role in mitochondrial dysfunction in human head injury (Verweij et al., 1997, 2000a). This strongly suggests that similar, if not identical pathological processes seen in the animal model also occur in humans.

Effect of In Vivo Treatment with Antioxidants and Calcium Channel Blockers on Mitochondrial Dysfunction Induced by TBI

With the CCII rat model, SNX-111, an N-type calcium channel blocker (Bowersox et al., 1997), was administered intravenously at various concentrations as a single bolus at 4 h post TBI, and the animals were sacrificed 12 h post injury (i.e., 8 h after injection). It was shown that SNX-111 produced a significant improvement of mitochondrial electron transfer and energy transfer activities with the optimal concentrations of 2 to 4 mg/kg (Verweij et al., 1997, 2000b). A time-course study of the effect of SNX-111 (4 mg/kg) administered after TBI on the mitochondrial electron transfer and energy coupling has also been carried out. A significant improvement was seen at 2 to 6 h after TBI, with an optimal effect at 4 h. SNX-111 exhibited beneficial effects on mitochondrial Ca^{2+} transport activity (data not shown) and mitochondrial respiratory and phosphorylating activities (Table 12.2). Unfortunately, the hypotensive effect of SNX-111 has confronted human head injury trials.

U-101033E is a new antioxidant of the pyrrolopyrimidine family that has been found to reduce infarct size when administered post injury in the mouse permanent middle cerebral artery occlusion model (Hall et al., 1996a) and to protect facial motor neurons following neonatal axotomy (Hall et al., 1996b). The advantage of this drug is that it can penetrate the blood–brain barrier to reach the brain. With the CCII rat model, U-101033E was given intravenously as two boluses at 5 min and 2 h post TBI (Xiong et al., 1997b). The effects on mitochondrial functions were evaluated in the dose range from 1 to 10 mg/kg. A bell-shaped dose–response profile was obtained on mitochondrial respiratory rates, RCI, and P/O ratio, with optimal doses of 2 to 3 mg/kg. Higher doses exhibited less beneficial effect, and in fact at 10 mg/kg some impairment was seen. The impairment at higher doses is not

TABLE 12.2 Mitochondrial Electron Transfer Activities and Energy-coupling Capacities from Each Hemisphere Following TBI with Glutamate and Malate as Substrates

Group	Electron Transfer Activities State 3 (natom O/min/mg protein)		Energy-coupling Capacities RCI		P/O	
	CH	IH	CH	IH	CH	IH
Sham	171.9±3.3	173.4±5.2	4.49±0.32	4.48±0.24	2.71±0.05	2.78±0.05
Injury	157.2±7.8	107.4±9.6*	3.40±0.24	3.17±0.34*	2.22±0.05*	1.90±0.06*
Vehicle[a]	146.7±3.7	114.3±5.0*	3.37±0.06	2.94±0.10*	2.52±0.14	2.01±0.05*
SNX-111 (mg/kg)						
0.5	229.2±25.6	203.3±22.8	3.05±0.31	3.11±0.11*†	2.64±0.04	2.58±0.11
1.0	222.5±12.2	197.4±11.6	3.05±0.05	3.11±0.06*†	2.60±0.03	2.30±0.03
4.0	251.1±35.5	225.3±8.6	4.20±0.28	4.23±0.42	2.71±0.06	2.69±0.02
U-101033E (mg/kg)						
1.0	170.8±15.4	91.5±11.4*†	3.94±0.43	2.40±0.12*†	2.46±0.10	1.96±0.07*†
3.0	166.2±12.6	192.0±17.8	3.96±0.26	3.68±0.17†	2.57±0.09	2.58±0.01
Combination (U + S) (mg/kg)						
0.5 U/0.5 S	170.5±9.9	163.5±12.3	4.70±0.72	4.42±0.54	2.61±0.09	2.43±0.10
1.0 U/1.0 S	193.0±19.8	228.6±6.5	3.71±0.26	4.33±0.11	2.44±0.10	2.43±0.06
3.0 U/4.0 S	221.9±13.9	236.4±6.2	4.45±0.58	4.96±0.21	2.43±0.19	2.50±0.11
NAC (163 mg/kg)						
30 min	197.4±35.6	206.5±27.0	4.62±0.49	4.51±0.76	2.53±0.04	2.46±0.05
1 h	190.0±12.8	202.4±12.4	4.25±0.14	4.45±0.03	2.65±0.05	2.50±0.06
2 h	128.6±4.8*	123.4±11.5*	2.83±0.26	2.92±0.29*	2.34±0.04	2.29±0.07*

Data are expressed as mean ±SEM ($n \geq 3$). CH, hemisphere contralateral to impact; IH, hemisphere ipsilateral to impact.

SNX-111 (S) was administered as a 0.5, 1.0, 4.0 mg/kg intravenous bolus 4 h post TBI. U-101033E (U) dissolved in 0.02 M citric acid was given intravenously over 30 s at 5 min and 2 h following TBI. N-Acetylcysteine (NAC) dissolved in saline was administered at 163 mg/kg intraperitoneally 30 min, 1 h or 2 h post TBI. The rats were sacrificed at 12 h post injury.

The reaction medium consisted of 150 mM sucrose, 25 mM Tris-HCl, 10 mM phosphate buffer, pH 7.4, and 0.4 to 0.9 mg of mitochondrial protein. The temperature was 30°C. The final concentrations of substrates were 5.0 mM/2.5 mM for glutamate/malate.

State 3 respiration was initiated by the addition of 263 μM ADP. Mitochondrial oxygen consumption in the presence of substrates and absence of ADP was defined as state 4 respiration (not shown). Respiratory control indices (RCI) were defined as the ratio of respiratory rates at state 3 and state 4. The P/O ratio was defined as the number of molecules of ADP phosphorylated per atom of oxygen consumed during state 3 respiration.

[a] Vehicle used in this table is normal saline; data for the vehicle citric acid are similar to those for normal saline shown in this table.

* $p < 0.05$ vs. sham; † $p < 0.05$ vs. combination.

surprising since antioxidants can also function as prooxidants under certain conditions. At the optimal doses, U-101033E significantly attenuated TBI-induced damage to brain mitochondrial respiratory chain-linked oxidative phosphorylation (Table 12.2). These data support our idea that oxidative stress plays an important role in TBI-induced mitochondrial dysfunction.

The combined therapy of SNX-111 and U-101033E on TBI-induced mitochondrial dysfunction is also shown in Table 12.2. The rationale for combined therapy is that secondary brain injury may originate through different biochemical mechanisms, such as ROS and Ca^{2+} overload. Ca^{2+} and ROS may act synergistically in the pathogenesis of brain mitochondrial and neuron damage (Braughler et al., 1985). SNX-111 has been shown to be effective in our TBI rat model (Verweij et al., 1997). Brain mitochondrial from injured and uninjured hemispheres were isolated and examined at 12 h post TBI. SNX-111 at 1.0 mg/kg significantly increased both state 3 and state 4 rates, and produced a slight increase in P/O ratios with virtually no change in RCI. U-101033E at 1.0 mg/kg did not show any beneficial effect. However, the combined treatment of SNX-111 at 1.0 mg/kg and U-101033E at 1.0 mg/kg restored not only state 3 rates and P/O ratios but also RCI to near sham values. These data demonstrate that the combination of these two drugs at reduced dosages suppresses secondary brain injury through different biochemical mechanisms and is more efficacious than either drug alone. One of the beneficial effects in using lower dosage is the elimination of undesirable side effects of high concentrations of drugs, such as hypotension with SNX-111. These data provide further evidence that both ROS and Ca^{2+} play major roles in the pathogenesis of TBI-induced mitochondrial dysfunction and support the idea of using combined therapy with lower dosages of drugs (Xiong et al., 1998).

N-Acetylcysteine (NAC) is a cysteine analogue (an antioxidant/GSH precursor) with multitherapeutic uses and is commonly used to treat the hepatotoxic consequences of acetaminophen overdose (Kelly, 1998). NAC can protect against ROS-induced injury, either by promoting glutathione (GSH) synthesis (Corcoran and Wong, 1986) or by direct scavenging action (Aruoma et al., 1989). NAC at 163 mg/kg has previously been shown to enhance hippocampal neuronal survival after transient forebrain ischemia in rats (Knuckey et al., 1995) and to restore cerebrovascular responsiveness following fluid percussion brain injury (Ellis et al., 1991). Recently we initiated a systematic study to evaluate the effects of NAC (administered intraperitoneally at 163 mg/kg either before or after TBI) on GSH levels in brain tissue and brain mitochondrial and the mitochondrial respiratory and energy-transducing functions following TBI.

Following TBI, GSH levels in brain tissues were decreased at all time points examined over a 14-day observation period, while mitochondrial GSH levels significantly decreased only at 3 days and 14 days. NAC treatment (163 mg/kg) given intraperitoneally within 1 h post TBI greatly restored brain GSH levels from 1 h to 14 days and mitochondrial GSH levels from 12 h to 14 days post TBI. NAC (administered intraperitoneally 5 min before injury, or 30 min or 1 h post injury) markedly restored mitochondrial electron transfer, energy-coupling capacity, and calcium uptake activity, and reduced calcium content absorbed to brain mitochondrial membranes when examined 12 h post TBI. NAC did not show protective effects when given 2 h post injury (Table 12.2). The result that delayed administration of the antioxidant NAC is not effective is consistent with the role of oxidative stress mechanisms in the acute pathophysiology of TBI. These data demonstrate that NAC administered at an early stage post injury can effectively reverse TBI-induced mitochondrial dysfunction. The protective effect of NAC may be related to its restoration of GSH levels in the brain (Xiong et al., 1999).

Possible Mechanisms of TBI-induced Mitochondrial Dysfunction

Evidence accumulated in the literature indicates that TBI induced increase in intracellular Ca^{2+}, ROS, and NO generation, extracellular glutamate, and cerebral ischemia. All of these factors either alone or in combination synergistically are detrimental to mitochondrial function.

The deleterious effects of cerebral ischemia on mitochondrial function have been reported. State 3 and state 4 respiration remained fairly stable until the cerebral blood flow was reduced to ~35 ml/100 g per min (Allen et al., 1995). At this rate and lower, there was a pronounced decrease in the rates of respiration in both state 3 and state 4 with both NAD- and FAD-linked substrates tested. Brain mitochondrial dysfunction after ischemia or followed by reperfusion has been demonstrated in many studies (Ginsberg et al., 1977; Hillered et al., 1984a,b; Sims, 1991; Sciamanna et al., 1992). Mitochondria isolated from ischemic brain (12 to 30 min ischemia) exhibited decreases in state 3 respiratory rates of 70 percent with NAD-linked substrates. RCI was decreased accordingly. A lesser effect was observed with FAD-linked substrates (Sciamanna et al., 1992). Calcium ions, reactive oxygen species, and glutamate have been considered mediators of ischemic brain damage regardless of whether it is due to global, forebrain ischemia or to focal ischemia (Sciamanna et al., 1992; Siesjo et al., 1995).

Mitochondrial Ca^{2+} uptake occurs when the extramitochondrial Ca^{2+} increases above the mitochondrial set point, the concentration at which the Ca^{2+} uniporter becomes more active than the Ca^{2+} efflux mechanism (Nicholls and Crompton, 1980). Ca^{2+} uptake utilizes proton motive force, diminishes the transmembrane potential, and stimulates electron transport until extramitochondrial Ca^{2+} is lowered below the set point. Ca^{2+} sequestration above a certain level can begin to compromise mitochondrial function, resulting in respiratory inhibition or uncoupling of oxidative phosphorylation, formation of nonspecific pores, or osmotic lysis. When presented with $Ca^{2+} \geq 10\,\mu M$, isolated mitochondria will divert their entire respiratory capacity from ATP synthesis to the accumulation of calcium ions (Nicholls and Akerman, 1982). Therefore, increased mitochondrial calcium content is a sensitive indicator of increased calcium fluxes from the extracellular into intracellular space. Hossmann et al. (1985) found that in animals with functional recovery after ischemia, neither tissue nor mitochondrial calcium content was significantly increased, but in animals without functional recovery both tissue and mitochondrial calcium content increased significantly. Sciamanna et al. (1992) demonstrated that the amounts of Ca^{2+} associated with the forebrain mitochondria were significantly increased by an ischemic insult of 15 min or longer. Using the controlled cortical impact model in rats, Xiong et al. (1997a) found that the first-order rate constant for mitochondrial Ca^{2+} uptake was significantly decreased 6 and 12 h post injury and calcium content absorbed to mitochondrial membranes was elevated significantly in the injured hemisphere 6 h to 14 days post injury. The increase in calcium content associated with mitochondrial membrane suggests that intracellular calcium concentration increases after TBI.

It is well established that the generation of ROS increases after TBI (Hall, 1993). Smith et al. (1994) demonstrated that there is an immediate, posttraumatic burst in hydroxyl radical formation (as early as 5 min), followed by a progressive increase in lipid peroxidation after cortical impact injury in the rat. In addition, Shohami et al. (1999) observed that the whole body appeared to be under oxidative stress within 24 h after brain injury. ROS include superoxide, nitric oxide, hydroxyl, peroxyl, and alkoxyl radicals, as well as nonradical oxygen metabolites such as hydrogen peroxide, lipid peroxide, singlet oxygen, and hypochlorous acid (Cadenas, 1989). While the brain uses 20 percent of the inspired oxygen, most of the oxygen molecules are utilized for the production of ATP molecules. However, a small proportion (about 2 to 5 percent) are used in alternative pathways leading to ROS production (Boveris and Chance, 1973; Chance et al., 1979). In the mitochondria, oxygen molecules are used in a series of reactions catalyzed by cytochrome-c oxidase that add four electrons to the dioxygen molecule and transform it into two water molecules without the release of any ROS. Mitochondria in cultured murine cortical neurons generate ROS following exposure to N-methyl-D-aspartate (NMDA) (Dugan et al., 1995). In addition, irreversible conversion of xanthine dehydrogenase into its ROS-producing oxidase form occurs through an uncharacterized protease released into the cytosol upon mitochondrial damage (Saksela et al., 1999). Substantial evidence has been accumulated that there is involvement of ROS and lipid peroxidation in the CNS injury (Kontos and Wei, 1986; Braughler and Hall, 1989, 1992; Ikeda and Long, 1990; Halliwell, 1992; Hall, 1993; Shohami et al., 1997). ROS inactivate mitochondrial electron transport chain-associated enzyme directly and/or indirectly through lipid peroxidation (Bindoli, 1988; Zhang et al., 1990). Hillered and Ernster (1983) demonstrated that ROS generated by hypoxanthine/xanthine oxidase in the presence of Fe^{2+} caused a severe inhibition of respiration with NAD-linked substrates. The damage could be prevented by catalase or mannitol but not superoxide dismutose (SOD), suggesting the hydroxyl radical is the damaging species. It has also been demonstrated that NO generation increases after TBI (Mesenge et al., 1996, 1998; Sakamoto et al., 1997; Wada et al., 1998). NO has been shown to inhibit and/or damage mitochondrial metabolic function (Bolanos et al., 1995, 1997, 1998; Lizasoain et al., 1996; Brown, 1997). The neuroprotective effect of antioxidants, U-101033E, and NAC further support the idea that ROS plays an important role in TBI-induced brain injury.

The amino acid neurotransmitters glutamate and aspartate, and many of their derivatives, are known as excitatory amino acids (EAAs). When present in excess,

EAAs can trigger a series of events leading to neuronal damage and death (see Chapter 4) (Choi, 1990). In the excitotoxic hypothesis, the implicated mechanisms of neuronal damage or death include an increase in intracellular Ca^{2+} followed by protein kinases and phospholipase activation, impaired mitochondrial metabolism, and generation of ROS (Choi, 1990; Beal, 1992; Hayes et al., 1992; Schulz et al., 1995). It has been demonstrated that TBI results in excessive increase of extracellular glutamate, which leads to activation of postsynaptic glutamate receptors, resulting in Ca^{2+} influx, oxygen radical production (Faden et al., 1989; Katayama et al., 1990; Muizelaar et al., 1993; Palmer et al., 1993; Smith et al., 1994). In vitro studies (Dugan et al., 1995) showed that mitochondria generate ROS in cortical neurons following exposure to NMDA and suggested that NMDA-mediated Ca^{2+}-dependent uncoupling of neuronal mitochondrial electron transfer may contribute to neuronal oxidative damage. Exposure of cultured cerebellar granule cells to $100\,\mu M$ glutamate plus glycine in the absence of Mg^{2+} causes Ca^{2+} loading of the in situ mitochondria and is excitotoxic, as demonstrated by a decline of the cellular ATP/ADP ratio, cytoplasmic Ca^{2+} deregulation, and extensive cell death (Budd and Nicholls, 1996). White and Reynolds (1996) demonstrated that mitochondria accumulate large amounts of Ca^{2+} during a toxic glutamate stimulus and further that Ca^{2+} efflux from mitochondria contributes to the prolonged $[Ca^{2+}]_i$ elevation after glutamate removal. Cyclosporin A prevents this effect, indicating that mitochondrial Ca^{2+} accumulation, and the subsequent MPT may be a critical early event specific to the NMDA receptor-mediated excitotoxic cascade. Ruthenium red, an inhibitor of mitochondrial Ca^{2+} uniporter, substantially lessens mitochondrial Ca^{2+} accumulation after glutamate exposure and protects against glutamate-induced neuronal death in the cerebellar cells (Dessi et al., 1995).

Acidosis has been demonstrated to occur in the ischemic brain (Marmarou, 1992; Hovda et al., 1992). Following experimental brain injury, injury-induced ionic flux is a result of both neuronal firing via direct mechanical force of the neurons as well as the activation of ligand-gated ion channels primarily associated with EAA (e.g., glutamate). This ionic destabilization places enormous energy demands on these cells in order to activate pumping mechanisms to reinstate normal ionic balance. The primary fuel used to acquire this energy is glucose, which results in a period of hyperglycolysis leading to the accumulation of lactate. This increased glucose metabolism lasts only during the acute period, after which these same cells exhibit a state of chronic metabolic depression for both glucose and oxygen (Hovda et al., 1992; Anderson and Marmarou, 1992). Hillered et al. (1984a,b) reported that acidosis inhibits ADP-stimulated respiration and that ATP production is virtually blocked at pH values of below 6. In vivo, acidosis may act in conjunction with other pathological events such as the activation of lysosomal enzymes, the release of ROS, and influx/release of Ca^{2+} and lead to cell injury and cell death.

Besides its effects on mitochondria, acidosis may also exaggerate brain damage by accelerating oxygen radical production via H^+-dependent reactions, some of which are catalyzed by iron released from protein binding by a lowering of pH; by perturbing the intracellular signal transduction pathway, leading to changes in gene expression or protein synthesis; and by activating endonucleases that cause DNA fragmentation.

CONCLUSIONS

Brain energy metabolism is unique and very vulnerable to disturbance of the supply of blood or oxygen. Even a relatively short period of ischemia would significantly impair the mitochondrial function to produce the ATP necessary for normal neuronal functioning. TBI induces many neurobiochemical changes that lead to secondary injury to neurons. Mitochondrial dysfunction may be either the result or the cause of some of these participating factors. Among them, the most important factors are ROS and calcium ions. They are the common pathways where many other detrimental mediators, EAA and acidosis, converge. They also interplay among each other. The fact that mitochondrial dysfunction induced by these mediators can be attenuated by therapeutic intervention is very encouraging. Additionally, the demonstration that similar, if not identical, changes take place in human TBI further supports efforts to pursue neuroprotective intervention. Although some promising progress has been made in the identification of injury mediators after TBI, further work must continue in order to understand the complex molecular cascades of secondary injury and prevent mitochondrial damage and overall neurologic deficits.

ACKNOWLEDGMENTS

Research done in our laboratory has been supported by funds from the Katz Foundation, the Tackett Foundation, and the Pharmacia/Upjohn Pharmaceutical Co.

ABBREVIATIONS

ANT	Adenine nucleotide translocase
CCII	Controlled cortical impact injury
CH	Contralateral hemisphere to impact
CNS	Central nervous system
CsA	Cyclosporin A
EAA	Excitatory amino acids
EDTA	Ethylenediaminetetraacetic acid
EGTA	Ethyleneglycol-bis-(β-aminoethyl ether)-N, N, N', N'-tetraacetate
FAD	Flavin–adenine dinucleotide
fura-2	2-(6-(Bis(carboxymethyl)amino)-5-(2-(2-(bis(carboxymethyl)amino)-5-methylephenoxy)ethoxy-2-benzofuranyl)
fura-2K$^+$	The potassium salt of fura-2
FMN	Flavin mononucleotide
GSH	Glutathione, reduced form
Hepes	4-(2-Hydroxyethyl)-1-piperazineethanesulfonic acid
IH	Ipsilateral hemisphere to impact
MPT	Mitochondrial permeability transition
mtDNA	Mitochondrial DNA

NAC   *N*-acetylcysteine
NAD   Nicotinamide–adenine dinucleotide
nDNA   Nuclear DNA
NMDA   *N*-Methyl-D-aspartate
NO   Nitric oxide
P_i Inorganic phosphate
RCI   Respiratory control indices
ROS   Reactive oxygen species
SOD   Superoxide dismutase
TBI   Traumatic brain injury
TCA   Tricarboxylic acid
$\Delta\psi_m$ Mitochondrial membrane potential

REFERENCES

K. L. Allen, A. Almeida, T. E. Bates, and J. B. Clark, *J. Neurochem.*, 64, 2222–2229 (1995).

B. J. Anderson and A. Marmarou, *Brain Res.*, 585, 184–189 (1992).

S. Anderson, A. T. Bankier, B. G. Barrell, M. H. de Bruijn, A. R. Coulson, J. Drouin, I. C. Eperon, D. P. Nierlich, B. A. Roe, F. Sanger, P. H. Schreier, A. J. Smith, R. Staden, and I. G. Young, *Nature*, 290, 457–5465 (1981).

A. Y. Andreyev, B. Fahy, and G. Fiskum, *FEBS Lett.*, 439, 373–376 (1998).

O. I. Aruoma, B. B. Halliwell, M. Hoey, and J. Butler, *Free Radic. Biol. Med.*, 6, 593–597 (1989).

K. P. Baker and G. Schatz, *Nature*, 349, 205–208 (1991).

R. H. Basford, *Methods Enzymol.*, 10, 96–101 (1967).

M. Beal, *Ann. Neurol.*, 31, 119–130 (1992).

P. Bernardi, K. M. Broekemeier, and D. R. Pfeiffer, *J. Bioenerg. Biomembr.*, 26, 509–517 (1994).

G. Beutner, A. Ruck, B. Riede, W. Welte, and D. Brdiczka, *FEBS Lett.*, 396, 189–195 (1996).

A. Bindoli, *Free Radic. Biol. Med.*, 5, 247–261 (1988).

J. P. Bolanos, S. J. Heales, J. M. Land, and J. B. Clark, *J. Neurochem.*, 64, 1965–1972 (1995).

J. P. Bolanos, A. Almeida, W. Stewart, S. Peuchen, J. M. Land, J. B. Clark, and S. J. Heales, *J. Neurochem.*, 68, 2227–2240 (1997).

J. P. Bolanos, A. Almeida, and J. M. Medina, *Brain Res.*, 787, 117–122 (1998).

A. Boveris and B. Chance, *Biochem. J.*, 134, 707–716 (1973).

S. Bowersox, J. Mandema, K. Tarczy-Hornoch, G. Miljanich, and R. R. Luther, *Drug Metab. Dispos.*, 25, 379–383 (1997).

P. D. Boyer, *Annu. Rev. Biochem.*, 66, 717–749 (1997).

J. M. Braughler and E. D. Hall, *Free Radic. Biol. Med.*, 6, 289–301 (1989).

J. M. Braughler and E. D. Hall, *J. Neurotrauma*, 9, S1–S7 (1992).

J. M. Braughler, L. A. Duncan, and T. Goodman, *J. Neurochem.*, 45, 1288–1293 (1985).

D. Brdiczka, *Biochim. Biophys. Acta*, 1071, 291–312 (1991).

G. C. Brown, *Mol. Cell. Biochem.*, 174, 189–192 (1997).

R. M. Bryan, L. Cherian, and C. Robert, *Anesth. Analg.*, 80, 687–695 (1995).

S. L. Budd and D. G. Nicholls, *J. Neurochem.*, 67, 2282–2291 (1996).

E. Cadenas, *Annu. Rev. Biochem.*, 58, 79–110 (1989).

T. A. Cadoux-Hudson, D. Wade, D. J. Taylor, B. Rajagopalan, J. G. Ledingham, M. Briggs, and G. K. Radda, *Acta Neurochir.*, 104, 1–7 (1990).

B. Chance, H. Sies, and A. Boveris, *Physiol. Rev.*, 59, 527–605 (1979).

D. Chauhan, P. Pandey, A. Ogata, G. Teoh, N. Krett, R. Halgren, S. Rosen, D. Kufe, S. Kharbanda, and K. Anderson, *J. Biol. Chem.*, 272, 29995–29997 (1997).

J. Chen, T. Nagayama, K. Jin, R. A. Stetler, R. L. Zhu, S. H. Graham, and R. P. Simon, *J. Neurosci.*, 18, 4914–4928 (1998).

D. Cheneval, M. Muller, R. Toni, S. Ruetz, and E. Carafoli, *J. Biol. Chem.*, 260, 13003–13007 (1995).

D. W. Choi, *Cerebrovasc. Brain Metab. Rev.*, 2, 105–147 (1990).

J. B. Clark and W. J. Nicklas, *J. Biol. Chem.*, 245, 4724–4731 (1970).

M. A. Colicos and P. K. Dash, *Brain Res.*, 739, 120–131 (1996).

G. B. Corcoran and B. K. Wong, *J. Pharmacol. Exp. Ther.*, 238, 54–61 (1986).

G. P. Davey, L. Canevari, and J. B. Clark, *J. Neurochem.*, 69, 2564–2570 (1997).

J. W. DePierre and L. Ernster, *Annu. Rev. Biochem.*, 46, 201–262 (1977).

F. Dessi, Y. Ben-Ari, and C. Charriaut-Marlangue, *Neurosci. Lett.*, 201, 53–56 (1995).

L. L. Dugan, S. L. Sensi, L. M. Canzoniero, S. D. Handran, S. M. Rothman, T. S. Lin, M. P. Goldberg, and D. W. Choi, *J. Neurosci.*, 15, 6377–6388 (1995).

P. R. Dunkley, J. W. Heath, S. M. Harrison, P. E. Jarvie, P. J. Glenfield, and J. A. Rostas, *Brain Res.*, 441, 59–71 (1988).

E. F. Ellis, L. Y. Dodson, and R. J. Police, *J. Neurosurg.*, 75, 774–779 (1991).

M. Erecinska and I. A. Silver, *J. Cereb. Blood Flow Metab.*, 9, 2–19 (1989).

R. Eskes, B. Antonsson, A. Osen-Sand, S. Montessuit, C. Richter, R. Sadoul, G. Mazzei, A. Nichols, and J.-C. Martinou, *J. Cell Biol.*, 143, 217–224 (1998).

A. Faden, I. P. Demediuk, S. S. Panter, and R. Rink, *Science*, 244, 798–800 (1989).

T. Friedrich, A. Abelmann, B. Brors, V. Guenebaut, L. Kintscher, T. Leonard, T. Rasmussen, D. Scheide, A. Schlitt, U. Schulte, and H. Weiss, *Biochim. Biophys. Acta*, 1365, 215–219 (1998).

M. D. Ginsberg, L. Mela, K. Wrobel-Kuhl, and M. Reivich, *Ann. Neurol.*, 1, 519–527 (1977).

N. Grigorieff, *J. Mol. Biol.*, 277, 1033–1046 (1998).

V. Guenebaut, R. Vincentelli, D. Mills, H. Weiss, and K. Leonard, *J. Mol. Biol.*, 265, 409–418 (1997).

T. E. Gunter and D. R. Pfeiffer, *Am. J. Physiol.*, 258, C755–C786 (1990).

T. E. Gunter, K. K. Gunter, S. S. Sheu, and C. E. Gavin, *Am. J. Physiol.*, 267, C313–C339 (1994).

E. D. Hall, *J. Emerg. Med.*, 11 (Suppl.), 31–36 (1993).

E. D. Hall, *J. Neurosci.*, 134 (Suppl.), 79–83 (1995).

E. D. Hall, P. K. Andrus, S. L. Smith, J. A. Oostveen, H. M. Scherch, B. S. Lutzke, T. J. Raub, G. A. Sawada, J. R. Palmer, L. S. Banitt, J. S. Tustin, K. L. Belonga, D. E. Ayer, and G. L. Bundy, *Acta Neurochir. Suppl.*, 66, 107–113 (1996a).

E. D. Hall, S. L. Smith, and J. A. Oostveen, *J. Neurosci. Res.*, 44, 293–299 (1996b).

B. Halliwell, *J. Neurochem.*, 69, 1609–1623 (1992).

M. B. Hampton, B. Zhivotovsky, A. F. Slater, D. H. Burgess, and S. Orrenius, *Biochem. J.*, 329 (Pt. 1), 95–99 (1998).

F. U. Hartl, N. Pfanner, D. W. Nicholson, and W. Neupert, *Biochim. Biophys. Acta*, 988, 1–45 (1989).

R. L. Hayes, L. W. Jenkins, and B. G. Lyeth, *J. Neurotrauma*, 9 (Suppl.), S173–S187 (1992).

J. P. Headrick, M. R. Bendall, A. I. Faden, and R. Vink, *J. Cereb. Blood Flow Metab.*, 14, 853–861 (1994).

L. Hillered and L. Ernster, *J. Cereb. Blood Flow Metab.*, 3, 207–214 (1983).

L. Hillered, L. Ernster, and B. K. Siesjo, *J. Cereb. Blood Flow Metab.*, 4, 430–437 (1984a).

L. Hillered, B. K. Siesjo, and K. E. Arfors, *J. Cereb. Blood Flow Metab.*, 4, 438–336 (1984b).

F. L. Hoch, *Biochim. Biophys. Acta*, 1113, 71–133 (1992).

B. Hoffman, A. Stockl, M. Schlame, K. Beryer, and M. Klingenberg, *J. Biol. Chem.*, 269, 1940–1944 (1994).

K. A. Hossmann, B. G. Ophoff, R. Schmidt-Kastner, and U. Oschlies, *Acta Neuropathol. (Berl.)*, 68, 230–238 (1985).

D. A. Hovda, D. P. Becker, and Y. Katayama, *J. Neurotrauma*, 9 (Suppl.), S47–S60 (1992).

D. A. Hovda, K. Fu, H. Badie, A. Samii, P. Pinanong, and D. P. Becker, *Acta Neurochir. Suppl. (Wein)*, 60, 521–523 (1994).

Y. Ikeda and D. M. Long, *Neurosurgery*, 27, 1–11 (1990).

S. Iwata, J. W. Lee, K. Okada, J. K. Lee, M. Iwata, B. Rasmussen, T. A. Link, S. Ramaswamy, and B. K. Jap, *Science*, 281, 64–71 (1998).

J. M. Jurgensmeier, Z. Xie, Q. Deveraux, L. Ellerby, D. Bredesen, and J. Reed, *Proc. Natl. Acad. Sci. USA*, 95, 4997–5002 (1998).

Y. Katayama, D. P. Becker, T. Tamura, and D. A. Hovda, *J. Neurosurg.*, 73, 889–900 (1990).

G. S. Kelly, *Alt. Med. Rev.*, 3, 114–127 (1998).

R. M. Kluck, S. J. Martin, B. M. Hoffman, J. S. Zhou, D. R. Green, and D. D. Newmeyer, *EMBO J.*, 16, 4639–4649 (1997).

N. W. Knuckey, D. Palm, M. Primiano, M. H. Epstein, and C. E. Johanson, *Stroke*, 26, 305–311 (1995).

H. A. Kontos and E. P. Wei, *J. Neurosurg.*, 64, 803–807 (1986).

B. S. Kristal and J. M. Dubinsky, *J. Neurochem.*, 69, 524–538 (1997).

G. Kroemer, B. Dallaporta, and M. Resche-Rigon, *Annu. Rev. Physiol.*, 60, 619–642 (1998).

J. C. Lai and J. B. Clark, *Methods Enzymol.*, 55, 51–60 (1979).

C. P. Lee, "Preface," in C. P. Lee, Ed., *Current Topics in Bioenergetics: Molecular Basis of Mitochondrial Pathology*, Vol. 17, Academic Press, San Diego, 1994, pp. xi–xxii.

C. P. Lee, M. Sciamanna, and P. L. Peterson, *Methods Toxicol.*, 2, 41–49 (1993).

C. P. Lee, Q. Gu, Y. Xiong, R. A. Mitchell, and L. Ernster, *FASEB J.*, 10, 345–350 (1996).

X. Liu, C. N. Kim, J. Yang, R. Jemmerson, and X. Wang, *Cell*, 86, 147–157 (1996).

I. Lizasoain, M. A. Moro, R. G. Knowles, V. Darley-Usmar, and S. Moncada, *Biochem. J.*, 314 (Pt. 3), 877–880 (1996).

W. D. Lust, H. Arai, Y. Yasumoto, T. S. Wittingham, B. Djuiricic, B. Mrsulja, and J. V. Passonneau, "Ischemic Encephalopathy," in D. W. McCandless, Ed., *Cerebral Energy Metabolism and Metabolic Encephalopathy*, Plenum Press, New York, 1985, pp. 79–112.

B. P. Marchetti, M. Castedo, S. A. Susin, N. Zamzami, T. Hirsch, A. Macho, A. Haeffner, F. Hirsch, M. Geuskens, and G. Kroemer, *J. Exp. Med.*, 184, 1155–1160 (1996).

A. Marmarou, *J. Neurotrauma*, 9, S551–S562 (1992).

J. G. McCormack, A. P. Halestrap, and R. M. Denton, *Physiol. Rev.*, 70, 391–425 (1990).

L. C. McHenry Jr., *Cerebral Circulation and Stroke*, Warren H. Green, St. Louis, MO, 1978.

T. K. McIntosh, M. Juhler, and T. Wieloch, *J. Neurotrauma*, 15, 731–771 (1998).

C. Mesenge, C. Verrecchia, M. Allix, R. R. Boulu, and M. Plotkine, *J. Neurotrauma*, 13, 11–16 (1996).

C. Mesenge, C. Charriaut-Marlangue, C. Verrecchia, M. Allix, R. R. Boulu, and M. Plotkine, *Eur. J. Pharmacol.*, 353, 53–57 (1998).

B. Mignotte and J.-L. Vayssiere, *Eur. J. Biochem.*, 252, 1–15 (1998).

P. Mitchell, *J. Theor. Biol.*, 62, 327–367 (1976).

J. P. Muizelaar, A. Marmarou, F. Young, S. C. Choi, A. Wolf, R. L. Schneider, and H. A. Kontos, *J. Neurosurg.*, 78, 375–382 (1993).

D. D. Newmeyer, D. M. Farschon, and J. C. Reed, *Cell*, 79, 353–364 (1994).

D. G. Nicholls and M. Crompton, *FEBS Lett.*, 111, 261–268 (1980).

D. G. Nicholls and K. Akerman, *Biochim. Biophys. Acta*, 683, 57–88 (1982).

A. M. Palmer, D. W. Marion, M. I. Botscheller, P. E. Swellow, S. D. Styren, and S. T. DeKosky, *J. Neurochem.*, 61, 2015–2024 (1993).

P. X. Petit, N. Zamzami, J. L. Vayssiere, B. Mignotte, G. Kroemer, and M. Castedo, *Mol. Cell. Biochem.*, 174, 185–188 (1997).

M. R. Prasad, H. S. Dhillon, T. Carbary, R. J. Dempsey, and S. W. Scheff, *J. Neurochem.*, 63, 773–776 (1994).

H. J. Proctor, G. W. Palladino, and D. Fillipo, *J. Trauma*, 28, 347–352 (1988).

K. Rink, M. Fung, J. Q. Trojanowski, V. M. Lee, E. Neugebauer, and T. K. McIntosh, *Am. J. Pathol.*, 147, 1575–1583 (1994).

T. Rosse, R. Olivier, L. Monney, M. Rager, S. Conus, I. Felay, B. Jansen, and C. Borner, *Nature*, 391, 496–499 (1998).

R. Rossen, H. Kabat, and J. P. Anderson, *Arch. Neurol. Psychiatry*, 50, 510–528 (1943).

H. Rottenberg and M. Marbach, *Biochim. Biophys. Acta*, 1016, 87–98 (1990).

A. Ruck, M. Dolder, T. Wallimann, and D. Brdiczka, *FEBS Lett.*, 426, 97–101 (1998).

K. I. Sakamoto, H. Fujisawa, H. Koizumi, E. Tsuchida, H. Ito, D. Sadamitsu, and T. Maekewa, *J. Neurotrauma*, 14, 349–353 (1997).

M. Saksela, R. Lapatto, and K. O. Raivio, *FEBS Lett.*, 443, 117–120 (1999).

A. F. Schinder, E. C. Olson, N. C. Spitzer, and M. Montal, *J. Neurosci.*, 16, 6125–6133 (1996).

J. B. Schulz, D. R. Henshaw, D. Siwek, B. G. Jenkins, R. J. Ferrante, P. B. Cipolloni, N. W. Kowall, B. R. Rosen, and M. F. Beal, *J. Neurochem.*, 64, 2239–2247 (1995).

M. A. Sciamanna and C. P. Lee, *Arch. Biochem. Biophys.*, 305, 215–224 (1993).

M. A. Sciamanna, J. Zinkel, A. Y. Fabi, and C. P. Lee, *Biochim. Biophys. Acta*, 1134, 223–232 (1992).

E. Shohami, E. Beti-Yannai, M. Horowitz, and R. Kohen, *J. Cereb. Blood Flow Metab.*, 17, 1007–1019 (1997).

E. Shohami, I. Gati, E. Beit-Yannai, V. Trembovler, and R. Kohen, *J. Neurotrauma*, 16, 365–376 (1999).

B. K. Siesjo, Q. Zhao, K. Pahlmark, P. Siesjo, K. Katsura, and J. Folbergrova, *Ann. Thorac. Surg.*, 59, 1316–1320 (1995).

N. R. Sims, *J. Neurochem.*, 56, 1836–1844 (1991).

J. M. Skehel, I. M. Fearley, and J. E. Walker, *FEBS Lett.*, 438, 301–305 (1998).

V. P. Skulachev, *FEBS Lett.*, 423, 275–280 (1998).

S. L. Smith, P. K. Andrus, J.-R. Zhang, and E. D. Hall, *J. Neurotrauma*, 11, 393–404 (1994).

B. Soussi, A. C. Bylund-Fellenius, T. Schersten, and J. Angstrom, *Biochem. J.*, 265, 227–232 (1990a).

B. Soussi, J. P. Idstrom, T. Schersten, and A. C. Bylund-Fellenius, *Acta Physiol. Scand.*, 138, 107–114 (1990b).

P. G. Sullivan, J. N. Keller, M. P. Mattson, and S. W. Scheff, *J. Neurochem.*, 15, 789–798 (1998).

D. G. Tang, L. L. Zhu, and B. Joshi, *Biochem. Biophys. Res. Commun.*, 242, 380–384 (1998).

B. F. Trump and I. K. Berezesky, *FASEB J.*, 9, 219–228 (1995).

T. Tsukihara, H. Aoyama, E. Yamashita, T. Tomizaki, H. Yamaguchi, K. Shinzawa-Itoh, R. Nakashima, R. Yaono, and S. Yoshikawa, *Science*, 272, 1136–1144 (1996).

B. H. Verweij, J. P. Muizelaar, F. C. Vinas, P. L. Peterson, Y. Xiong, and C. P. Lee, *Neurol. Res.*, 19, 334–339 (1997).

B. H. Verweij, J. P. Muizelaar, F. C. Vinas, P. L. Peterson, Y. Xiong, and C. P. Lee, *J. Neurosurg.*, 93, 815–820 (2000a).

B. H. Verweij, J. P. Muizelaar, F. C. Vinas, P. L. Peterson, Y. Xiong, and C. P. Lee, *J. Neurosurg.*, 93, 829–834 (2000b).

R. Vink, A. I. Faden, and T. K. McIntosh, *J. Neurotrauma*, 5, 315–330 (1988).

R. Vink, E. M. Golding, and J. P. Headrick, *J. Neurotrauma*, 11, 265–274 (1994).

K. Wada, K. Chatzipanteli, R. Busto, and W. D. Dietrich, *J. Neurosurg.*, 89, 807–818 (1998).

K. R. Wagner, P. A. Tornheim, and M. K. Eichhold, *J. Neurosurg.*, 63, 88–96 (1985).

J. E. Walker, J. M. Arizmendi, A. Dupuis, I. M. Fearnley, M. Finel, S. M. Medd, S. J. Pilkington, M. J. Runswick, and J. M. Skehel, *J. Mol. Biol.*, 226, 1051–1072 (1992).

R. J. White and I. J. Reynolds, *J. Neurosci.*, 16, 5688–5697 (1996).

Y. Xiong, Q. Gu, P. L. Peterson, J. P. Muizelaar, and C. P. Lee, *J. Neurotrauma*, 14, 23–34 (1997a).

Y. Xiong, P. L. Peterson, J. P. Muizelaar, and C. P. Lee, *J. Neurotrauma*, 14, 907–917 (1997b).

Y. Xiong, P. L. Peterson, B. H. Verweij, F. C. Vinas, J. P. Muizelaar, and C. P. Lee, *J. Neurotrauma*, 15, 531–544 (1998).

Y. Xiong, P. L. Peterson, and C. P. Lee, *J. Neurotrauma*, 16, 1067-1082 (1999).

A. G. Yakovlev, S. M. Knoblach, L. Fan, G. B. Fox, R. Goodnight, and A. I. Faden, *J. Neurosci.*, 17, 7415–7424 (1997).

J. C. Yang and G. A. Cortopassi, *Biochem. Biophys. Res. Commun.*, 250, 454–457 (1998).

M. S. Yang, D. S. Dewitt, D. P. Becker, and R. L. Hayes, *J. Neurosurg.*, 63, 617–621 (1985).

C.-A. Yu, H. Tian, L. Zhang, K.-P. Deng, S. K. Shenoy, L. Yu, D. Xia, H. Kim, and J. Deisenhofer, *J. Bioenerg. Biomembr.* 31, 191–199 (1999).

Y. Zhang, O. Marcillat, C. Giulivi, L. Ernster, and K. J. A. Davies, *J. Biol. Chem.*, 265, 16330–16336 (1990).

H. Zou, W. J. Henzel, X. Liu, and X. Wang, *Cell*, 90, 405–413 (1997).

CHAPTER 13

TRAUMATIC AXONAL INJURY

JOHN T. POVLISHOCK and JAMES R. STONE
Department of Anatomy, Medical College of Virginia, Campus of Virginia
Commonwealth University, Richmond, Virginia

INTRODUCTION

The goal of this chapter is to present an update on the pathobiology of traumatic axonal injury (TAI) in both animals and man. TAI has long been recognized as a component of traumatic brain injuries (TBI) of varying severity; our current understanding of the pathogenesis TAI suggests that with the exception of the most severe forms of traumatic brain injury, TAI does not involve direct renting of the axonal cylinder. Rather it involves subtle and varied intraaxonal perturbations that lead over time to progressive axonal failure, impaired axoplasmic transport, and disconnection of the axon. Currently, most agree that progressive or delayed axotomy contributes to most of the axonal injury found in experimentally injured animals and brain-injured humans, and emerging evidence suggests that the initiating factors involved in this pathogenesis may vary, not only as a function of fiber type but also of the severity of the injury. Thus, any treatment for blunting the progression of traumatically induced axonal injury must take into account these diverse initiating pathologies. This chapter will focus on what we currently understand regarding the initiating pathological factors involved in the genesis of TAI as well as what current therapies have been used in the laboratory with some degree of success.

THE CONCEPT OF TRAUMATIC AXONAL INJURY

The concept of diffuse axonal injury (DAI) has long been recognized in the literature. First described over 40 years ago by Strich and colleagues (Strich et al.,

Head Trauma: Basic, Preclinical, and Clinical Directions, Edited by Leonard P. Miller and Ronald L. Hayes, Co-edited by Jennifer K. Newcomb
ISBN 0-471-36015-5 © 2001 John Wiley & Sons, Inc.

1956, 1961), the presence of widespread or diffuse axonal damage was recognized as a consistent feature of traumatic brain injury.

In a pioneering study, Strich and colleagues (Strich et al., 1956) first advocated the role for white matter damage or axonal injury in a group of severely head-injured patients with significant morbidity who upon postmortem examination revealed little evidence of focal change and mass lesion formation, thereby prompting the question of the etiology of their morbidity. In those patients who survived 5 to 15 months post injury and who were unresponsive throughout their hospital course, Strich identified through multiple histopathological approaches widespread/diffuse white matter degeneration, accompanied by astrocytic invasion (Strich, 1956). These findings led her to posit that the morbidity seen with TBI was directly associated with axonal damage. In 1961, as a follow-up study, Strich examined another population of patients who survived from 2 days through 2 years. In these studies she confirmed diffuse white matter involvement and provided a comprehensive description of the progression of this white matter change (Strich, 1961). Specifically, she demonstrated that with shorter survival periods (days to weeks post injury) bulbous focal enlargements of the axons were detected in the same foci that with continued survival (several months) revealed Wallerian degenerative change reflected in the presence of axonal degeneration and myelin beading and breakdown. The inference here was that this axonal bulb formation and subsequent white matter degeneration were the continuation of one and the same process initially triggered by the traumatic episode (Strich, 1956).

Influenced by Cajal's work on central nervous system lesioning (Cajal, 1928), Strich assumed that the reactive bulbs seen in the early phases of traumatic injury represented the mechanical tearing of the axon, with its subsequent retraction and extrusion of its axoplasmic mass to form a bulb or spheroid termed a "retraction ball" based upon its assumed genesis. Since Strich's early work, numerous investigators have confirmed Strich and colleagues' observation that white matter/axonal damage is a consistent feature of traumatic brain injury in those patients whose traumatic course is uncomplicated by mass lesion or contusion formation, and thus may be a major player in their morbidity. In 1982, Adams and colleagues reexamined the occurrence of diffuse axonal injury in the postmortem examination of traumatically brain-injured humans in a rigorous effort to determine the precise foci anatomically involved and to correlate this information with the clinical course of the patients (Adams et al., 1982). Importantly, Adams and colleagues emphasized that TAI was a primary response to the traumatic event, rejecting the criticisms of others who had contended that it was a sequela of other insults such as edema, hypoxia, and hypotension (Graham, 1996). In addition to confirming the importance and primacy of traumatically induced axonal injury, Adams and colleagues made further important advancements by demonstrating that diffuse axonal injury occurred across the spectrum of traumatic brain injury, occurring in cases of mild, moderate, and severe insult (Adams et al., 1989). As one would anticipate, however, there were differences in the number of axons involved in these various injury states, with fewer numbers of axons and anatomical foci involved in mild versus moderate to severe injuries (Adams et al., 1989).

Based upon these early descriptive studies of the occurrence of axonal/white matter damage following traumatic brain injury, a relatively complete picture of the process of axonal damage began to emerge. Through the utilization of routine H&E and various silver stains, multiple investigators began to appreciate that the appearance of swollen reactive axons constituted a relatively early event, seen within the first days to weeks post injury, followed over time by the appearance of gliosis and then, over a course of several months, by Wallerian degeneration of the disconnected axonal segments. As noted above, all these changes were interpreted to be consistent with the mechanical tearing of the axon at the moment of the injury, with retraction of the axon into the proximal stump and the progressive degenerative change of the distal disconnected axonal segment. More recently, however, based upon evidence gleaned from the use of experimental laboratory animals, the correctness of this premise has been questioned. Specifically, as will be fully explicated in the subsequent passages, contemporary thought on the neuropathological sequelae of traumatic brain injury now holds that axons are not torn at the moment of injury. Rather, now most concur that the axons are more subtly perturbed, evoking changes within the focal axonal cytoskeleton that impair axoplasmic transport (Maxwell et al., 1997; Povlishock, 1992; Povlishock et al., 1983, 1992). This impaired transport is then recognized to progress, in many cases, to continued axonal swelling, lobulation, and ultimate detachment, resulting in the formation of the swollen, bulblike profile typically described in the early phases of human traumatic brain injury (Fig. 13.1) (Maxwell et al., 1997; Povlishock, 1992; Povlishock et al., 1983; Povlishock et al., 1992). The time involved from the initiation of axonal change to disconnection and maximal axonal swelling in traumatically brain-injured humans varies, typically occurring over a period of several hours or several days (Sherriff et al., 1994a,b,c; Wilkinson et al., 1999). To date, this progression of axonal change in man has been confirmed via multiple endpoints, including the use of antibodies targeting either cytoskeletal constituents or substances normally moved by anterograde axoplasmic transport. Using antibodies to the neurofilament subunits, Grady and colleagues confirmed progressive focal neurofilamentous change associated with impaired transport, swelling, and disconnection (Grady et al., 1993). Similarly, using a now universally accepted means of detecting traumatic induced axonal change, via antibodies targeting the amyloid precursor protein, which moves via anterograde axoplasmic transport, Sherriff and colleagues (Sherriff et al., 1994a,b,c) demonstrated a similar progression of events, noting that impaired transport could be seen within the first hours following traumatic insult. Further, based upon an analysis of 116 quadrants per brain-injured patient, Blumbergs and colleagues showed that this increase in axonal accumulation of amyloid precursor protein correlated with sites classically associated with diffuse axonal injury and, perhaps more importantly, confirmed that traumatically induced axonal damage occurred across the spectrum of traumatic brain injury ranging from mild through severe (Blumbergs et al., 1995).

INSIGHT INTO THE PATHOBIOLOGY UNDERLYING DAI

When TAI was first examined from the mechanistic perspective, experimental animals were used to model traumatic brain injury and therein assess the occurrence

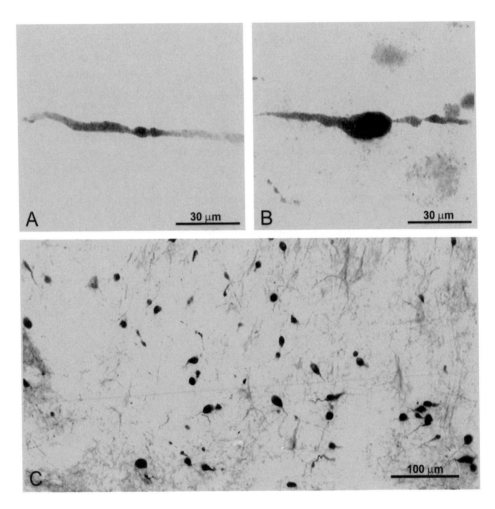

Figure 13.1 Parts (A) and (B), photographed from traumatically injured APP immunolabeled pig tissue, illustrate the progressive nature of TAI. In (A), at 4 h post injury, APP is seen accumulating at a focal site of traumatically impaired axoplasmic transport. At this relatively early time point post injury, the traumatically injured axon remains in continuity while showing some signs of axonal swelling due to the continued delivery of anterogradely transport organelles. In (B), at 6 h post injury, initial sites of focally impaired axoplasmic transport undergo continued APP immunoreactive organelle accumulation resulting in the formation of a swollen axonal bulb which, in this case, is in the process of disconnecting from its distal axonal segment. Part (C), photographed from traumatically injured, postmortem human hippocampal tissue illustrates the widespread nature of TAI at 12 h post injury. Immunostaining for the neurofilament light subunit 68 kDa reveals many traumatically injured axons scattered throughout the field. The majority of the injured axons in the field appear as grossly swollen, disconnected axonal bulbs and, as such, constitute the late stage of traumatically induced, delayed axotomy.

of TAI. As reviewed by Maxwell and colleagues (Maxwell et al., 1997), animal models do not replicate the full and diverse pathological spectrum of human traumatic brain injury, and thus do not fully replicate all the findings associated with human diffuse axonal injury. Yet these models do have utility for dissecting out specific features of TAI in a controlled fashion. In fact, animal models have helped provide insight into the nature of those events that lead to the intraaxonal perturbation, impaired axoplasmic transport, and disconnection alluded to in the previous passages. Specifically, in laboratory studies conducted in the 1980s, anterograde tracers were employed in animal models of TBI to assess the potential for impaired transport kinetics following traumatic brain injury (Povlishock et al., 1983, 1992). Using anterograde tracers, such as horseradish peroxidase, the anterograde axonal passage of this protein tracer was followed over time post injury to determine if mechanical severance with the random expulsion of the peroxidase, or focally impaired axoplasmic transport was the consequence of traumatically induced axonal injury. Through this approach, followed by light- and electron-microscopic analysis, it was found that traumatic brain injury typically triggered, in a diffuse fashion, focal impairments of axoplasmic transport, with some evidence of discrete multifocal change, particularly in the more severe forms of injury (Erb and Povlishock, 1988; Povlishock et al., 1983). Typically, these foci of impaired axoplasmic transport led to continued axonal swelling and lobulation, proceeding over a 3 to 12 h period to focal disconnection of the axon at the very site of swelling and lobulation. As the result of this focal disconnection, the proximal axonal segment, in continuity with its sustaining soma, continued to show modest axonal swelling at sites of disconnection, while the distal segment, separated from its sustaining soma, underwent the known sequelae of Wallerian degeneration (Erb and Povlishock, 1988; Povlishock et al., 1983). As part of this Wallerian degeneration, the nerve terminals associated with the disconnected axon degenerated and detached from the their neuronal target sites within the first 48 h of TBI, a process termed deafferentation (Erb and Povlishock, 1991). Following deafferentation, the remaining distal axonal shaft underwent the full progression of Wallerian degeneration, with the axon cylinder degenerating and its myelin sheath beading and breaking up over a lengthy posttraumatic time period (Erb and Povlishock, 1991).

Despite the fact that these laboratory findings emphasized an evolving focal intraaxonal change leading to disconnection/axotomy, once disconnected these axons showed a repertoire of change consistent with that described above in humans. Following upon these early observations using anterograde tracers in the cat motor system, these axonal changes were reevaluated in different motor and sensory fiber systems, animal models of injury, and various species, leading to confirmation by multiple investigators that these events were consistent features of TBI (Cheng and Povlishock, 1988; Erb and Povlishock, 1988; Gennarelli et al., 1989; Lewis et al., 1996; Maxwell et al., 1991; Ross et al., 1994; Smith et al., 1999a; Smith et al., 1997; Tomei et al., 1990). Because these experimental descriptions were all associated with focal, evolving change that ultimately led to disconnection/axotomy, Maxwell and colleagues coined the term delayed axotomy (Maxwell et al., 1997) to contrast this event from the immediate axotomy that had been posited in the original descriptions to TAI.

Based upon the sound foundation of these experimental studies, other studies of postmortem human tissue, using more indirect markers of impaired axoplasmic transport and axonal injury, confirmed, as noted above, this same progression of events in traumatically brain injured patients (Abou-Hamden et al., 1997; Blumbergs et al., 1994, 1995; Christman et al., 1994; Geddes et al., 1997; Gentleman et al., 1993, 1995; Gleckman et al., 1999; Grady et al., 1993; Oehmichen et al., 1999a,b; Sherriff et al., 1994a,b,c), leading to the universally accepted belief that the majority of axonal injury seen with traumatic injury occurs in a progressive fashion, with a delayed disconnection of the axon cylinder.

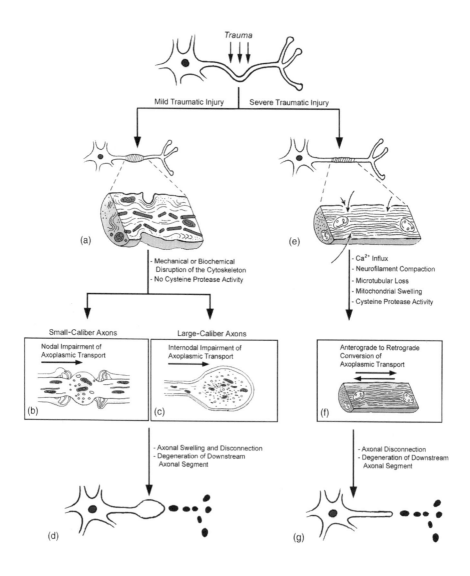

Despite this widespread recognition, however, the fact remained that, once injured, these axons ultimately did disconnect. Therefore, to successfully blunt this damaging progression, the initiating factors responsible for the events leading to delayed axotomy required detailed characterization. Identifying these changes, however, was not a trivial task and, as will be shown in the following passages, the description of these initiating changes was further complicated by the fact that axonal disconnection can be the final common pathway for multiple types of initiating traumatic axonal change. Simply stated, when first identified, it was assumed that the initiating mechanisms responsible for this delayed disconnection were the same across the spectrum of injury, in all fiber systems involved. However, on the basis of multiple studies, both from our laboratory as well as from others, it is now appreciated that this impression is too simplistic, in that multiple pathobiological processes appear to be involved in the initiation of the intraaxonal changes that lead to altered axoplasmic transport and disconnection (Fig. 13.2).

In the case of more severe forms of traumatic brain injury, it is now recognized that large-caliber axons demonstrate, in foci of injury, a disruption of their axolemmal integrity (Fig. 13.2e) (Pettus et al., 1994; Pettus and Povlishock, 1996; Povlishock and Pettus, 1996). This focally altered axolemmal permeability was first demonstrated at the locus of injury via the visualization of the intraaxonal passage of tracers normally confined to the extracellular environment (Pettus et al., 1994). Horseradish peroxidase as well as other large molecular-weight species were seen to cross the axolemma at the moment of impact, with the suggestion that the forces of injury caused a focal physical mechanoporation of the axolemma, allowing unrest-

Figure 13.2 This flowchart details how axons may differentially respond to TBI, based upon level of injury and fiber type involved. Mild TBI is seen to elicit local mechanical or biochemical disruption of the axonal cytoskeleton, focally impairing axoplasmic transport at sites of injury (a). This focal impairment of axoplasmic transport occurs primary at nodal and paranodal regions in small-caliber axons (b) and along internodal axonal segments in large-caliber axons (c). Both small- and large-caliber axons swell over time due to the continued delivery of organelles to focal sites of injury. This continued swelling ultimately results in the disconnection of a proximal axonal bulb from its distal axonal segment (d). Over time, this distal axonal segment undergoes Wallerian degeneration, with the downstream deafferentation of target sites (d). In contrast to these events associated with mild TBI, the forces associated with moderate to severe TBI overtly disrupt the axolemma, allowing for the entry of ions such as Ca^{2+} that are normally excluded by the intact axolemma (e). In attempt to buffer intraaxonal Ca^{2+}, mitochondria will actively sequester Ca^{2+}, resulting in the colloid-osmotic swelling of mitochondria and the uncoupling of oxidative phosphorylation (e). Additionally, Ca^{2+} triggers a number of intraaxonal enzymatic processes, resulting in neurofilament compaction and loss of the microtubular network (e). Ca^{2+} also activates cysteine proteases that trigger the anterograde to retrograde conversion of axoplasmic transport, effectively preventing axonal swelling at these sites of axonal damage (f). Distal axonal segments undergo Wallerian degeneration as local cytoskeletal damage and anterograde to retrograde conversion of transport disrupt its connection with the sustaining soma (g).

ricted passage of substances normally tightly regulated by the intact axolemma (Pettus et al., 1994). With mechanoporation, it was posited that an influx of damaging ions followed, with calcium figuring prominently (Pettus et al., 1994; Pettus and Povlishock, 1996). The potential involvement of calcium in this process has been demonstrated in experimental animal models where traumatic brain injury has been shown to induce altered axolemmal permeability, with a concomitant activation of calcium-dependent, calpain-mediated spectrin proteolysis, which most likely triggers continued axolemmal damage (Fig. 13.2e) (Buki et al., 1999a). With this altered axolemmal permeability and the influx of calcium ions, local intraaxonal cytoskeletal damage also has been observed (Pettus and Povlishock, 1996). Specifically, in these foci, neurofilaments undergo compaction with a toss of their highly phosphorylated sidearms, while the integrity of the microtubular network is lost (Fig. 13.2e) (Okonkwo et al., 1998; Pettus and Povlishock, 1996; Povlishock et al., 1997). Importantly, in concert with these cytoskeletal changes, the same increased intraaxonal calcium loads also apparently contribute to mitochondrial swelling, with a local release of cytochrome c and caspase-3 activation (Buki et al., 2000). This caspase activation, in turn, participates in the terminal degradation of the axonal cytoskeleton, leading to local intraaxonal failure (Buki et al., 2000).

To date, the above-described progression of intraaxonal events has been confirmed in multiple animal models and species. Some *in vitro* studies using mechanically loaded or electroporated giant squid axons have revealed similar changes, linking axolemmal failure to intraaxonal change and subsequent physiological and anatomical failure (Gallant and Galbraith, 1997). Other *in vitro* studies, focusing on rapidly stretched axons, have not confirmed altered axolemmal permeability, unless direct renting of the neurite was achieved (Smith et al., 1999b). Unfortunately, such differences *in vivo* versus *in vitro* speak to some of the shortcomings inherent in comparing small-caliber, unmyelinated and nontethered neurites assessed *in vitro* to large-caliber and myelinated axons anchored within the adult nervous system.

After identification of the above-described sequence of axolemmal disruption and calpain/caspase activation leading to cytoskeletal collapse, questions centered on how these intraaxonal abnormalities evoked impaired axoplasmic transport, axonal swelling, and subsequent disconnection. Initially, it was predicted that the neurofilament and microtubular damage described would directly impair axoplasmic transport, resulting in axonal swelling and disconnection (Povlishock, 1992). However, no study had demonstrated that such a relationship existed between these events. In fact, recent studies from our laboratory using double-label immunofluorescent approaches targeting both cytoskeletal damage associated with axolemmal disruption and impaired axoplasmic transport have shown that previous beliefs were an oversimplification of a highly complex process (Stone et al., 2000). Specifically, through double-labeling approaches it was recognized, in more severely injured axons, that the continued influx of calcium and the activation of various proteolytic processes triggered a conversion of anterograde to retrograde transport (Fig. 13.2f) comparable to that described in other experimental paradigms (Martz et al., 1989; Sahenk and Lasek, 1988). This effectively blunted the pooling of organelles within regions of cytoskeletal disruption and prevented the formation of axonal swelling (Stone et al., 2001). At present, there is not a full appreciation of the overall magnitude of this form of TAI, which does not evolve to axonal bulb formation. Yet its very description in experimental brain injury raises the question whether studies relying solely on the presence of axonal bulbs or clubs may underestimate the magnitude of traumatically induced axonal change occurring in either the experimentally injured animals or, more importantly, brain-injured humans.

While the above studies suggested that some axonal damage can occur without subsequent axonal swelling and formation of an axonal bulb, these double-label studies also confirmed that a separate population of axons did undergo organelle pooling, axonal swelling, and disconnection, similar to previous descriptions. Integrating previous studies focusing on TAI (Pettus et al., 1994; Pettus and Povlishock, 1996; Povlishock and Pettus, 1996; Yaghmai and Povlishock, 1992) with more recent work, we recognized that this class of swollen traumatically injured axons was not typically associated with an overt disruption of the axolemma or activation of cysteine proteases. In contrast, this class of axons, perhaps subjected to less tensile loading/stretching than those revealing overt axolemmal perturbation, manifested primary focal cytoskeletal change. This was reflected in neurofilament misalignment and/or disorganization, with the suggestion of parallel change in the local microtubular network (Fig. 13.2*a*) (Pettus et al., 1994; Pettus and Povlishock, 1996; Povlishock and Pettus, 1996; Stone et al., 1999; Yaghmai and Povlishock, 1992). As would be anticipated, these cytoskeletal changes led to local failure/blockage of axoplasmic transport with the subsequent accumulation of anterogradely transported substances (Figs. 13.2*b,c*). Further, in the absence of any massive axolemmal change and the activation of calcium-linked cysteine proteases, there was no conversion of axoplasmic transport from the anterograde to retrograde direction, which thereby permitted continued axonal swelling. Thus, the axons swelled, disconnected, and formed a bulb consistent with classical descriptions (Fig. 13.2*d*).

As noted, this progression was first demonstrated through multiple single-label immunocytochemical and ultrastructural approaches, with more recent double-label studies providing unequivocal evidence for a linkage between subtle intraaxonal cytoskeletal change and the genesis of impaired transport and intraaxonal swelling at the same anatomical site (Stone et al., 2001). Unfortunately, because immunofluorescent double-labeling approaches were employed, a comprehensive, quantitative assessment of the proportion of axons showing impaired axoplasmic transport versus anterograde to retrograde conversion has not been performed. Thus, it is difficult to speculate on the total percentage of the damaged axonal populations demonstrating each of these described pathologies. Further, as these changes were not studied across the full range of traumatic brain injury, from mild through severe, it is unknown whether one type of reactive change predominates in a specific injury. Perhaps, with mild injury, less tensile loading occurs, resulting in a lower proportion of axons experiencing axolemmal disruption, cysteine protease activation, and the anterograde to retrograde conversion of axoplasmic transport (Fig. 13.2*f*). Similarly, mild tensile loading could conceivably cause a greater number of focally injured axons to undergo cytoskeletal misalignment, resulting in impaired axoplasmic transport and swelling (Fig. 13.2a). Conversely, with more severe injury, it is conceivable that overt disruption of axolemmal integrity predominates, leading to catastrophic cytoskeletal change, anterograde to retrograde conversion, and the absence of impaired transport and axonal swelling (Fig. 13.2f).

Based upon the above, it is now clear that our understanding of the pathobiology of traumatic brain injury is becoming increasingly complex. This complexity is further illustrated by other findings from our laboratory demonstrating the occurrence of a new subclass of injured fibers within the class of axons undergoing focal cytoskeletal disruption, impaired axoplasmic transport, and axonal swelling in the absence of overt axolemmal disruption. Specifically, using a newly developed method of antigen retrieval compatible with electron-microscopic analysis (Stone et al., 1999), and antibodies to the amyloid precursor protein, known markers of traumatically induced axonal injury and impaired axoplasmic transport (Abou-Hamden et al., 1997; Ahlgren, 1996; Blumbergs et al., 1994, 1995; Bramlett et al., 1997; Gentleman et al., 1993; Koo et al., 1990; Li et al., 1995; McKenzie et al., 1996; Oehmichen et al., 1999a, 1999b; Sherriff et al., 1994a,b,c) our laboratories have confirmed many of the observations described above involving cytoskeletal misalignment and impaired axoplasmic transport. Moreover, they also identified a previously unrecognized subclass of axonal change involving fine-caliber thinly myelinated axons (Stone et al., 1999). In contrast to those axonal abnormalities described above, these axons revealed primary nodal blebbing, involving a pooling of organelles, and possible cytoskeletal disruption (Fig. 13.2f) (Stone et al., 1999). While not fully characterized, it appears that in these axons the nodal region is perturbed, perhaps allowing for transient ionic influx that disturbs the cytoskeleton, impairs transport kinetics, and results in local axonal swelling. In some cases, these axons continue to swell over time and go on to disconnect. In other cases, however, no evidence of disconnection is found, suggesting the potential for recovery. To date, these observations have been made only in small-caliber axons, bearing similarity to a series of changes described by Maxwell and colleagues in the guinea pig optic nerve fiber system, which is also populated by fine-caliber, thinly myelinated axons (Gennarelli et al., 1993; Maxwell, 1996; Maxwell and Graham, 1997; Maxwell et al., 1991). This linkage to a distinct change within a specific fiber type introduces the concept that the pathobiology of traumatically induced axonal injury may not only depend upon tensile loading forces associated with injury, but also may be related to the fiber type subjected to such loading. Such an observation is not without a biological basis, as it is well recognized that axons of varying caliber contain differing cytoskeletal composition. Large-caliber, heavily myelinated axons are neurofilament rich, with a relatively a sparse content of microtubules. Conversely, fine-caliber axons have a sparse neurofilament content, being composed primarily of microtubules (Hirokawa, 1991; Szaro et al., 1990).

White the above descriptions of traumatic axonal pathobiology suggest the existence of multiple mechanisms in the genesis of delayed axonal disconnection, and emphasize the significance of overt axolemmal disruption as a pivotal factor in the subsequent pathological cascade, caution must be exercised in too rigorously interpreting these findings. As noted, laboratory studies have consistently demonstrated either the presence or absence of axolemmal change in TAI (Pettus et al., 1994; Pettus and Povlishock, 1996; Povlishock and Pettus, 1996), and have consistently correlated this axolemmal disruption with Ca^{2+}-linked calpain activation (Buki et al., 1999a,b,c). However, importantly, this description of altered axolemmal integrity has relied on the use of large-molecular-weight tracers (Pettus et al., 1994; Pettus and Povlishock, 1996) whose exclusive use could underestimate the occurrence of more subtle axolemmal permeability change to small-molecular-weight solutes and/or ions. While not obviating the importance of previous observations, this leads to the question whether less dramatic axolemmal disruption can occur and allow for lesser degrees of Ca^{2+} influx. If one considers this potential, the above-described diverse intraaxonal responses to trauma may also be explained on this basis. Conceivably, specific levels of intraaxonal free calcium within a traumatically injured axon may predicate the precise pathobiological cascade that the injured axon experiences.

As noted, anterograde to retrograde conversion of transport has been shown to be dependent upon the activation of cysteine proteases (Sahenk and Lasek, 1988). As cysteine proteases such as calpains require micromolar levels of intracellular free calcium for activation (Kampfl et al., 1997; Wang, 2000), it is possible that the described overt axolemmal disruption with Ca^{2+} influx capable of cysteine protease activation could trigger the conversion of anterograde to retrograde transport (Fig. 13.2f). It is also conceivable that a less dramatic axolemmal permeability change, not detected by the tracers used, may not trigger this superthreshold response. Rather it may elicit more subtle calcium-mediated intraaxonal abnormalities capable of impairing the axonal cytoskeleton and the associated axoplasmic transport (Fig. 13.2a). That differing calcium thresholds can contribute to the generation of differing reactive axonal change is indirectly supported by previous work on calcium-calmodulin binding as a function of intracellular free calcium. With calcium concentrations of 1 µM, a half-maximal concentration of 22.5 nM calcium-bound calmodulin is achieved (Persechini and Cronk, 1999). As the high-affinity targets of this calcium-calmodulin are activated at calcium-calmodulin concentrations of ≤10 nM, it is likely that nanomolar concentrations of intracellular free calcium may result in calcium-bound calmodulin concentrations >10 nM, and activation of high-affinity calcium-calmodulin targets (Persechini and Cronk, 1999). One such high affinity target is the phosphatase calcineurin (Persechini and Cronk, 1999; Sola et al., 1999; Stemmer and Klee, 1994; Tokoyoda et al., 2000), which could contribute to cytoskeletal change via the alteration of cytoskeletal phosphorylation (Eyer and Leterrier, 1988; Halpain et al., 1998; Leterrier and Eyer, 1987).

Based upon the above, two distinct scenarios may then exist, both centering on pivotal rote for calcium in the generation of delayed axonal change. In mild TAI, subtle disruption of the axolemma or associated ion channels may permit the influx of submicromolar levels of calcium. These may be adequate to trigger high-affinity calcium-calmodulin targets such as calcineurin, but insufficient to activate micromolar calpain activity. Thus, although cytoskeletal damage may ensue, anterograde to retrograde conversion will not occur, resulting in the pooling of organelles and swelling in the focus of damage (Fig. 13.2a). In those cases, however, where the axon undergoes overt disruption of the axolemma, calcium concentrations may reach micromolar levels, allowing for the conversion of the anterograde to retrograde transport system (Fig. 13.2f). While these high levels of calcium may cause profound local cytoskeletal damage, the anterograde to retrograde transport conversion may blunt the accumulation of transported organelles, thereby preventing the formation of axonal swellings.

THERAPEUTIC INTERVENTIONS TARGETING TAI

The pathobiology of traumatically induced axonal injury as described above is complex and superficially would not seem an ideal target for therapeutic intervention. Yet, despite these limitations, remarkable progress has being seen in this field over the last five years with clear evidence from the experimental setting that therapeutic intervention in the early phases of injury can attenuate many of these evolving processes described in the previous passages and thereby effectively blunt the genesis of traumatically induced axonal injury. The first paper suggesting that traumatic axonal injury could be targeted for therapeutic intervention stemmed from the work of Marion and colleagues, who used a combination of hypothermia and steroids in animal models of traumatic brain injury (Marion and White, 1996). Through this approach, they demonstrated that hypothermia and steroids exerted statistically significant protection, reducing the numbers of traumatically injured axons that were identified by the use of markers of cytoskeletal/neurofilament change (Marion and White, 1996). Following upon these seminal observations, our laboratory reevaluated the potential protective effects of hypothermia, using a rigorously controlled induction of hypothermia followed by carefully regulated rewarming. In this series of studies, we focused on contemporary markers of traumatically induced axonal injury employing antibodies to amyloid precursor proteins (APP), which denote sites of altered axoplasmic transport and subsequent axonal damage (Koizumi and Povlishock, 1998). Additionally in the same studies, we also used other markers of axonal injury, including markers of cytoskeletal perturbation and calcium-mediated change (Buki et al., 1999b). Through these approaches, it was demonstrated that hypothermia followed by gradual rewarming provided statistically significant axonal protection, not only in terms of the reduction of total numbers of APP-labeled axons found in the injured brain, but also in terms of a reduction in the overall neurofilamentous and calcium-mediated cascades found in these injured fibers (Buki et al., 1999b; Koizumi and Povlishock, 1998). It is important to note that this protection was noted when hypothermia was used both prior to injury as well as within the first hour post injury (Koizumi and Povlishock, 1998). While clearly confirming that the protective effects of pre- and posttraumatic hypothermia through multiple endpoints, these studies, in themselves, did not provide detailed information as to precisely how hypothermia provided this axonal protection.

Buoyed by the findings of axonal protection with the use of hypothermia, effort then turned to other potential therapeutic strategies for the treatment of traumatically induced change. As reviewed in the previous passages, there appeared to be multiple targets for potential therapeutic intervention, most of which involve calcium-mediated change. The reported alterations in axolemmal permeability with the activation of calpains and mitochondrial swelling due to calcium overloading appeared obvious choices for therapeutic intervention. Although the use of established calpain inhibitors appeared reasonable, concerns existed that the therapeutic window for their potential use post injury was short, and thus not practical in a clinical situation. Calcium-induced mitochondrial swelling, on the other hand, appeared a more appropriate target as its genesis was more delayed and the subsequent mitochondrial demise was perceived as a terminal event in the processes that led to axonal failure and disconnection. Appreciating that the observed mitochondrial swelling was consistent with an opening of the mitochondrial permeability transition (MPT) pore, which signaled the loss of the mitochondria's electrochemical potential (Ankarcrona et al., 1995; Petit et al., 1997), this pore seemed an appropriate target for therapeutic intervention. It was posited that any mitochondrial protection would provide not only the local high-energy phosphates needed to maintain membrane pumps, but also blunt the release of cytochrome *c*, and any subsequent activation of caspases that participate in the terminal degradation of the axon cylinder (Buki et al., 2000; Cai et al., 1998; Gorman et al., 1999; Krajewski et al., 1999; Martinou et al., 1999; Susin et al., 1998, 1999a,b; Uehara et al., 1999).

In view of these factors and the fact that some members of the immunophilin family such as cyclosporin A (CsA) are known to bind with the mitochondrial permeability transition pore and blunt its opening in situations of calcium-loading and other permissive factors (Halestrap et al., 1997; Zoratti and Szabo, 1995) CsA was used to attenuate traumatically induced axonal damage. To date, two members of the immunophilin family, cyclosporin A and FK506, have been widely studied for their immunosuppressive effects. So called because they are believed to exert their action through binding to small intracellular regulatory proteins, the cyclophilins are recognized to inhibit the phosphatase calcineurin. Additionally, CsA, but not FK506, prevents mitochondrial permeability transition by blocking translocation of the mitochondrial matrix-specific cyclophilin D to the inner mitochondrial membrane. Using well-controlled models of traumatic brain injury, the use preinjury and early postinjury CsA administration resulted in a statistically significant reduction of the number of damaged axons per unit area (Buki et al., 1999c; Okonkwo and Povlishock, 1999). In addition to demonstrating convincing neuroprotection in terms of the reduction of APP immunoreactive axons, well-recognized markers of altered axoplasmic transport and axonal damage, these studies also provided further mechanistic insight into the potential modes of action of the CsA administration. Specifically, through parallel ultrastructural analyses, these studies confirmed that the CsA provided mitochondrial protection in foci of traumatically induced axonal change (Okonkwo and Povlishock, 1999). Further, through the use of antibodies targeting calcium-mediated changes, such as calpain-mediated spectrin proteolysis and neurofilament compaction, it was shown that these markers were also significantly reduced by CsA administration (Buki et al., 1999c).

It is of note that since these initial reports of the utility of CsA in traumatically induced axonal change, other laboratories have reported the potential efficacy of this drug in reducing the contusional damage also associated with traumatic brain injury (Scheff and Sullivan, 1999; Sullivan et al., 2000). While there is considerable evidence that CsA is neuroprotective and most likely acts through its action on the mitochondrial permeability transition pore, with the subsequent maintenance of mitochondrial integrity, there are several other modes of action of CsA that require further investigation. As noted above, it is well known that CsA, in addition to its effect on the MPT, is also an inhibitor of calcineurin, which has potentially significant cytoskeletal modulatory actions (Dawson et al., 1993, 1994; Sabatini et al., 1997). Although initial studies emphasized the role of mitochondrial permeability transition as a target for the protective effects of CsA, recent use of another member of the immunophilin family, FK506, targeting calcineurin without any effect upon mitochondrial permeability transition, also provided significant axonal protection (Singleton et al., 2000). While these studies suggest that multiple neuroprotective mechanisms may be operant in the pathobiology of traumatic axonal injury, they do not exclude the importance of therapies targeting the mitochondrial permeability transition. Rather, they emphasize the complexity of the disease, confirming the widely held impression that the treatment of traumatic brain injury and its specific components will most likely involve the use of polypharmacia employed at multiple time points to achieve maximum efficacy.

THE SIGNIFICANCE OF TRAUMATIC AXONAL INJURY IN RELATION TO OTHER PATHOLOGICAL CHANGES ASSOCIATED WITH TBI

Despite the remarkable progress made in characterizing those pathobiological events that lead to traumatically induced axonal injury, the question remains what is the overall neurological significance of axonal injury when it occurs in traumatically brain-injured animals and humans. As noted throughout this book, traumatic brain injury is a complex disease involving combinations of focal and diffuse change as well as an increased risk for exacerbated damage in the presence of secondary insults such as hypotension and/or hypoxia (Graham, 1996). On this basis, it is unlikely that traumatically induced axonal injury/diffuse axonal injury is the only player in the morbidity associated with human traumatic injury. TAI, however can be a major contributor to morbidity, at least in a specific population of traumatically brain-injured humans.

As noted on several occasions in this text, the specific pathobiological responses seen following traumatic brain injury are obviously a function of the initial traumatic insult. Falls and blows to the head result in more focal lesions, such as contusion and hematoma formation (Graham, 1996). Their damaging consequences are a direct function of the anatomical areas of the brain involved and/or the secondary pathologies evoked by related damage such as formation of edema and/or increased intracranial pressure. In contrast to injuries that involve focal lesions, other injuries, such as those involved in motor vehicle or auto–pedestrian accidents, can cause more diffuse/widespread insult to the brain, wherein diffuse axonal injury becomes a common occurrence together with other neuropathological changes involving widespread neuroexcitation and/or changes in blood flow and metabolism (Graham, 1996; Povlishock and Christman, 1995). In this population of traumatically brain-injured humans, it is recognized that traumatically induced axonal damage, diffuse axonal injury, is a consistent feature.

As detailed earlier in this chapter, postmortem studies of traumatically brain-injured humans have consistently found evidence of traumatically induced axonal injury across the spectrum of mild, moderate, through severe injury (Adams et al., 1989; Blumbergs et al., 1995). Further detailed topographic or sector analysis focusing on the occurrence of axonal injury in traumatically brain-injured humans reveals that axonal damage can be found in virtually every area of the brain, ranging from cortical and subcortical sites to diencephalic and brain stem involvement (Blumbergs et al., 1995). This was elegantly shown by the work of Blumbergs and colleagues (Blumbergs et al., 1995), who divided the brain into 116 sectors and performed routine histopathological analysis while also using antibodies to amyloid precursor protein to detect traumatically induced change. Through this approach, they confirmed that with increasing severity more sectors of the brain were involved (Blumbergs et al., 1995). The only shortcoming in these studies, as well as all others associated with human traumatic brain injury, was that, while they provided information on those brain regions consistently showing traumatically induced axonal change, they provided no information on the overall numbers of axons involved, particularly in relation to the uninjured axonal population. Thus, without quantitative assessments of the proportion of damaged fibers involved, it is difficult to speculate on the overall significance of this pathological change.

Although we know that TAI occurs and that there is some association with the patient's morbidity (Adams et al., 1989; Blumbergs et al., 1995), the precise interrelation of these factors remains unclear. In fact, despite its widespread occurrence in traumatically brain injured humans, there is a general impression that the overall numbers of fibers involved assessed through routine histological or immunocytochemical approaches still constitutes a relatively small proportion of the total fibers found in the sampled region or field. This impression is clearly borne out in the experimental setting where severely traumatically brain-injured animals followed by quantitative analysis to detect the number of damaged axons via APP immunocytochemistry revealed only 800 to 1000 damaged profiles per square millimeter of injured brain (Koizumi and Povlishock, 1998), a relatively modest number of damaged fibers given the overall mass of white matter found within an square millimeter. This presents a quandary as to what can be the overall clinical/neurological significance of this relatively modest degree of axonal injury. Traumatic brain injury can evoke widespread axonal injury; yet, are the numbers significant enough to translate into specific morbidity? Obviously this issue will require continued evaluation; however, as we have noted in this chapter, our overall impressions of the magnitude of traumatically induced axonal damage has been biased by the use of various methodologies focusing on axonal swelling or bulb formation alone. As noted, these approaches may target only a subpopulation of traumatically injured axons and thereby significantly underestimate the overall magnitude of traumatically induced axonal change. Preliminary studies conducted in our laboratory to address this issue suggest that this is the case (Stone et al., 2001). Moreover, in accepting the likely scenario that we have typically underestimated the overall number of damaged axons based upon routine morphological approaches, there is also the potential that these estimations of axonal damage may also underestimate the number of injured axons that maintain structural integrity while manifesting functional failure. Perhaps, the above-described traumatically induced axonal changes constitute the tip of the iceberg of those changes ongoing in the white matter and provide an underestimation of the actual change sustained by the brain.

These issues require further detailed investigation in animals and humans, but, based upon the above, we believe that these arguments are credible and, in this context, that traumatically induced axonal injury must be considered a contributor to the morbidity associated with traumatic brain injury.

FUTURE DIRECTIONS

As discussed in previous sections of this chapter, TAI is a complex pathobiological process involving multiple intraaxonal events within distinct axonal populations, ultimately leading to delayed axotomy and downstream deafferentation over time. While the complexity of TAI may appear to preclude complete therapeutic efficacy, recent investigations in laboratory animals have identified two promising therapeutic strategies. Using multiple markers of traumatic axonal damage, the administration of CsA and the induction of hypothermia both afford significant axonal protection following TBI (Buki et al., 1999c; Koizumi and Povlishock, 1998; Okonkwo et al., 1999; Okonkwo and Povlishock, 1999). These strategies have been shown to be effective when administered prior to injury as well as up to 1 h post injury in the rat. Despite this remarkable success in blunting axonal damage following TBI, additional studies are necessary to provide a more comprehensive understanding on the efficacy of CsA or hypothermia prior to the onset of clinical trials. Specifically, much of the work on CsA and hypothermia-mediated traumatic axonal protection has been performed using the impact acceleration model of TBI in rats (Foda and Marmarou, 1994; Marmarou et al., 1994). While this approach provides an excellent model for studying traumatic axonal damage, it does not represent the full repertoire of axonal change occurring in human TAI. Therefore, it would seem rational to study CsA administration or the induction of hypothermia across multiple models of TBI such as fluid percussion (Dixon et al., 1987; McIntosh et al., 1987; Sullivan et al., 1976), or nonimpact rotational acceleration (Smith et al., 1997, 1999a), in order to rule out any model-related specificity, while further appreciating the full spectrum of their neuroprotective properties. In addition to studying CsA administration or hypothermia induction in multiple animal models, future studies in these areas must also be directed toward the study of these approaches in multiple animal species. Previous studies have suggested that the progression of TAI is different in lisencephalic versus gyrencephalic animals, with gyrencephalic animals, including man, undergoing a more delayed postinjury progressive pathobiological time course than lisencephalic animals (Povlishock, 1992; Povlishock and Jenkins, 1995). Accordingly, it would seem important to explore the efficacy of CsA or hypothermia in gyrencephalic animals and determine its therapeutic window, issues that may be of immediate relevance to humans in view of their more comparable brain structure. As noted, studies in gyrencephalic animal models must define the therapeutic window for CsA administration or hypothermia induction. Although CsA administration and hypothermia induction have been shown to be effective in the rat up to 1 h post injury, the delayed progression of axonal pathobiology in higher-order gyrencephalic animals may afford a more prolonged window of opportunity for the blunting of axonal damage.

Future studies on TAI may also wish to explore the potential combined benefits of CsA and hypothermia in the same animal population. Although hypothermia has remained controversial in the clinical setting, laboratory studies have clearly shown its efficacy on multiple neuronal fronts (Farooque et al., 1997; Globus et al., 1995; Mitani et al., 1991; Smith and Hall, 1996). Thus, it would seem reasonable to explore whether the combination of hypothermia induction and CsA administration may enhance efficacy, and/or prolong the therapeutic window for treatment. In the clinical setting, it is reasonable to speculate that a patient could be cooled by emergency medical teams prior to arrival in a hospital setting, where the patient may then receive a postinjury treatment of CsA. Future studies may also focus upon determining whether the therapeutic window for CsA administration may be lengthened through the prior induction of hypothermia.

In addition to studies on CsA administration using multiple animal models and higher-order animals, it will also be important to conduct more critical evaluations of the precise mechanisms through which CsA elicits axonal protection. While emphasis has been placed upon the ability of CsA to block the MPT pore (Halestrap et al., 1997; Zoratti and Szabo, 1995), little consideration has been given to the fact that CsA acts as an inhibitor of the phosphatase calcineurin as well (Dawson et al., 1993, 1994; Sabatini et al., 1997). As mentioned previously in this chapter, MPT-related mitochondrial pathology has been linked to the overt permeabilization of the axolemma and subsequent flooding of Ca^{2+} within damaged axons (Buki et al., 1999c; Okonkwo et al., 1999; Okonkwo and Povlishock, 1999). Interestingly, studies on intracellular free Ca^{2+} concentrations have shown that calcium-calmodulin may activate the phosphatase calcineurin at nanomolar intracellular free Ca^{2+} concentrations (Persechini and Cronk, 1999), white MPT will not take place until micromolar levels of intracellular free Ca^{2+} occur (Zoratti and Szabo, 1995). As it is known that the phosphorylation state is critically important to maintain integrity of the cytoskeleton (Eyer and Leterrier, 1988; Halpain et al., 1998; Leterrier and Eyer, 1987), it is possible that the calcineurin inhibitor properties of CsA (Dawson et al., 1993, 1994; Sabatini et al., 1997) may elicit axonal protection at lower intracellular free Ca^{2+} concentrations than its MPT-blocking properties and, as such, may provide protection to a wider range of traumatically injured fibers. Determination of the precise mechanisms of CsA neuroprotection may therefore allow for the use of agents that are highly specific for either MPT blockade or calcineurin inhibition, depending upon which site provides for more complete axonal protection following TBI.

While the above passages address some of the extensively evaluated TAI therapies, it is important to also consider other therapeutic approaches such as those targeting calpain-mediated proteolysis. As noted in previous sections of this chapter, calpain activity has been demonstrated within sites of TAI, and is thought to contribute to the cytosketetal and membrane damage associated with traumatically induced delayed axotomy. It is reasonable to believe that the use of calpain inhibitors following TBI may blunt the pathobiological cascade associated with TAI, and may potentially afford axonal protection. While previous studies using the calpain inhibitor AK295 (Saatman et al., 1996) in fluid percussion and calpain inhibitor 2 (Posmantur et al., 1997) following cortical impact in animals have provided promising data, TAI was not studied in either of these studies. Thus, future studies using calpain inhibitors in TBI should assess their efficacy in blunting the pathobiological cascade associated with traumatically induced axotomy.

ABBREVIATIONS

APP   Amyloid precursor protein
CsA   Cyclosporin A
MPT   Mitochondrial permeability transition
TAI   Traumatic axonal injury
TBI   Traumatic brain injury
DAI   Diffuse axonal injury
CNS   Central nervous system
H&E   Hematoxylin and eosin

REFERENCES

A. Abou-Hamden, P. C. Blumbergs, G. Scott, J. Manavis, H. Wainwright, N. Jones, and J. McLean, *J. Neurotrauma*, 14(10), 699–713 (1997).

J. H. Adams, D. I. Graham, L. S. Murray, and G. Scott, *Ann. Neurol.*, 12(6), 557–563 (1982).

J. H. Adams, D. Doyle, I. Ford, T. A. Gennarelli, D. I. Graham, and D. R. McLellan, *Histopathology*, 15(1), 135–150 (1989).

S. Ahlgren, G. L. Li, and Y. Olsson, *Acta Neuropathol. (Berl.)*, 92(1), 49–55 (1996).

M. Ankarcrona, J. M. Dypbukt, E. Bonfoco, B. Zhivotovsky, S. Orrenius, S. A. Lipton, and P. Nicotera, *Neuron*, 15(4), 961–973 (1995).

P. C. Blumbergs, G. Scott, J. Manavis, H. Wainwright, D. A. Simpson, and A. J. McLean, *Lancet*, 344(8929), 1055–1056 (1994).

P. C. Blumbergs, G. Scott, J. Manavis, H. Wainwright, D. A. Simpson, and A. J. McLean, *J. Neurotrauma*, 12(4), 565–622 (1995).

H. M. Bramlett, S. Kraydieh, E. J. Green, and W. D. Dietrich, *J. Neuropathol. Exp. Neurol.*, 56(10), 1132–1141 (1997).

A. Buki, R. Siman, J. Q. Trojanowski, and J. T. Povlishock, *J. Neuropathol. Exp. Neurol.*, 58(4), 365–375 (1999a).

A. Buki, H. Koizumi, and J. T. Povlishock, *Exp. Neurol.*, 159(1), 319–328 (1999b).

A. Buki, D. O. Okonkwo, and J. T. Povlishock, *J. Neurotrauma*, 16(6), 511–521 (1999c).

A. Buki, D. O. Okonkwo, K. K. Wang, and J. Povlishock, *J. Neurosci.*, 20(8), 2825–2834 (2000).

J. Cai, J. Yang, and D. P. Jones, *Biochim. Biophys. Acta*, 1366(1–2), 139–149 (1998).

R. Cajal, "Degeneration and Regeneration of the White Matter," in R. M. May, Eds., *Degeneration and Regeneration of the Nervous System*, Hafner Publishing, New York, 1928.

C. L. Cheng and J. T. Povlishock, *J. Neurotrauma*, 5(1), 47–60 (1988).

C. W. Christman, M. S. Grady, S. A. Walker, K. L. Holloway, and J. T. Povlishock, *J. Neurotrauma*, 11(2), 173–186 (1994).

T. M. Dawson, J. P. Steiner, V. L. Dawson, J. L. Dinerman, G. R. Uhl, and S. H. Snyder, *Proc. Natl. Acad. Sci. U.S.A.*, 90(21), 9808–9812 (1993).

T. M. Dawson, J. P. Steiner, W. E. Lyons, M. Fotuhi, M. Blue, and S. H. Snyder, *Neuroscience*, 62(2), 569–580 (1994).

C. E. Dixon, B. G. Lyeth, J. T. Povlishock, R. L. Findling, R. J. Hamm, A. Marmarou, H. F. Young, and R. L. Hayes, *J. Neurosurg.*, 67(1), 110–119 (1987).

D. E. Erb and J. T. Povlishock, *Acta Neuropathol. (Berl.)*, 76(4), 347–358 (1988).

D. E. Erb and J. T. Povlishock, *Exp. Brain Res.*, 83(2), 253–267 (1991).

J. Eyer and J. F. Leterrier, *Biochem. J.*, 252(3), 655–660 (1988).

M. Farooque, L. Hillered, A. Holtz, and Y. Olsson, *J. Neurotrauma*, 14(1), 320–335 (1997).

M. A. Foda and A. Marmarou, *J. Neurosurg.*, 80(2), 301–313 (1994).

P. E. Gallant and J. A. Galbraith, *J. Neurotrauma*, 14(11), 811–822 (1997).

J. F. Geddes, G. H. Vowles, T. W. Beer, and D. W. Ellison, *Neuropathol. Appl. Neurobiol.*, 23(4), 339–347 (1997).

T. A. Gennarelli, L. E. Thibault, R. Tipperman, G. Tomei, R. Sergot, M. Brown, W. L. Maxwell, D. I. Graham, J. H. Adams, and A. Irvine, *J. Neurosurg.*, 71(2), 244–253 (1989).

T. A. Gennarelli, R. Tipperman, W. L. Maxwell, D. I. Graham, J. H. Adams, and A. Irvine, *Acta Neurochir. Suppl. (Wien)*, 57, 49–52 (1993).

S. M. Gentleman, M. J. Nash, C. J. Sweeting, D. I. Graham, and G. W. Roberts, *Neurosci. Lett.*, 160(2), 139–144 (1993).

S. M. Gentleman, G. W. Roberts, T. A. Gennarelli, W. L. Maxwell, J. H. Adams, S. Kerr, and D. I. Graham, *Acta Neuropathol. (Berl.)*, 89(6), 537–543 (1995).

A. M. Gleckman, M. D. Bell, R. J. Evans, and T. W. Smith, *Arch. Pathol. Lab Med.*, 123(2), 146–151 (1999).

M. Y. Globus, O. Alonso, W. D. Dietrich, R. Busto, and M. D. Ginsberg, *J. Neurochem.*, 65(4), 125–134 (1995).

A. M. Gorman, E. Bonfoco, B. Zhivotovsky, S. Orrenius, and S. Ceccatelli, *Eur. J. Neurosci.*, 11(3), 1067–1072 (1999).

M. S. Grady, M. R. McLaughlin, C. W. Christman, A. B. Valadka, C. L. Fligner, and J. T. Povlishock, *J. Neuropathol. Exp. Neurol.*, 52(2), 143–152 (1993).

D. I. Graham, "Neuropathology of Head Injury," in R. K. Narayan, J. E. Wilberger, and J. T. Povlishock, Eds., *Neurotrauma*, McGraw-Hill, New York, 1996.

A. P. Halestrap, C. P. Connern, E. J. Griffiths, and P. M. Kerr, *Mol. Cell Biochem.*, 174(1–2), 167–172 (1997).

S. Halpain, A. Hipolito, and L. Saffer, *J. Neurosci.*, 18(23), 9835–9844 (1998).

N. Hirokawa, "Molecular Architecture and Dynamics of the Neuronal Cytoskeleton," in R. D. Burgoyne, Ed., *The Neuronal Cytoskeleton*, Wiley-Liss, New York, 1991.

A. Kampfl, R. M. Posmantur, X. Zhao, E. Schmutzhard, C. L. Clifton, and R. L. Hayes, *J. Neurotrauma*, 14(3), 121–134 (1997).

H. Koizumi and J. T. Povlishock, *J. Neurosurg.*, 89(2), 303–309 (1998).

E. H. Koo, S. S. Sisodia, D. R. Archer, L. J. Martin, A. Weidemann, K. Beyreuther, P. Fischer, C. L. Masters, and D. L. Price, *Proc. Natl. Acad. Sci. U.S.A.*, 87(4), 1561–1565 (1990).

S. Krajewski, M. Krajewska, L. M. Ellerby, K. Welsh, Z. Xie, Q. L. Deveraux, G. S. Salvesen, D. E. Bredesen, R. E. Rosenthal, G. Fiskum, and J. C. Reed, *Proc. Natl. Acad, Sci. U.S.A.*, 96(10), 5752–5757 (1999).

J. F. Leterrier and J. Eyer, *Biochem. J.*, 245(1), 93–101 (1987).

S. B. Lewis, J. W. Finnie, P. C. Blumbergs, G. Scott, J. Manavis, C. Brown, P. L. Reilly, N. R. Jones, and A. J. McLean, *J. Neurotrauma*, 13(9), 505–514 (1996).

G. L. Li, M. Farooque, A. Holtz, and Y. Olsson, *Neurotrauma*, 12(3), 269–277 (1995).

D. W. Marion and M. J. White, *J. Neurotrauma*, 13(3), 139–147 (1996).

A. Marmarou, M. A. Foda, W. van den Brink, J. Campbell, H. Kita, and K. Demetriadou, *J. Neurosurg.*, 80(2), 291–301 (1994).

I. Martinou, S. Desagher, R. Eskes, B. Antonsson, E. Andre, S. Fakan, and J. C. Martinou, *J. Cell Biol.*, 144(5), 883–889 (1999).

D. Martz, J. Garner, and R. J. Lasek, *Brain Res.*, 476(1), 199–203 (1989).

W. L. Maxwell, *Microsc. Res. Tech.*, 34(6), 522–535 (1996).

W. L. Maxwell and D. I. Graham, *J. Neurotrauma*, 14(9), 603–614 (1997).

W. L. Maxwell, A. Irvine, D. I. Graham, J. H. Adams, T. A. Gennarelli, R. Tipperman, and M. Sturatis, *J. Neurocytol.*, 20(3), 157–164 (1991).

W. L. Maxwell, J. T. Povlishock, and D. L. Graham, *J. Neurotrauma*, 14(7), 419–440 (1997).

T. K. McIntosh, L. Noble, B. Andrews, and A. I. Faden, *Cent. Nerv. Syst. Trauma*, 4(2), 119–134 (1987).

K. J. McKenzie, D. R. McLellan, S. M. Gentleman, W. L. Maxwell, T. A. Gennarelli, and D. I. Graham, *Acta Neuropathol. (Berl.)*, 92(6), 608–613 (1996).

A. Mitani, F. Kadoya, and K. Kataoka, *Brain Res.*, 562(1), 465–481 (1991).

M. Oehmichen, C. Meissner, V. Schmidt, I. Pedal, and H. G. Konig, *Int. J. Legal Med.*, 112(4), 261–267 (1999a).

M. Oehmichen, I. Theuerkauf, and C. Meissner, *Acta Neuropathol. (Berl.)*, 97(5), 491–494 (1999b).

D. O. Okonkwo and J. T. Povlishock, *J. Cereb. Blood Flow Metab*, 19(4), 443–451 (1999).

D. O. Okonkwo, E. H. Pettus, J. Moroi, and J. T. Povlishock, *Brain Res.*, 784(1–2), 1–6 (1998).

D. O. Okonkwo, A. Buki, R. Siman, and J. T. Povlishock, *Neuroreport*, 10(2), 353–358 (1999).

A. Persechini and B. Cronk, *J. Biol. Chem.*, 274(11), 6827–6830 (1999).

P. X. Petit, N. Zamzami, J. L. Vayssiere, B. Mignotte, G. Kroemer, and M. Castedo, *Mol. Cell Biochem.*, 174(1–2), 185–188 (1997).

E. H. Pettus and J. T. Povlishock, *Brain Res.*, 722(1–2), 1–11 (1996).

E. H. Pettus, C. W. Christman, M. L. Giebel, and J. T. Povlishock, *J. Neurotrauma*, 11(5), 507–522 (1994).

R. Posmantur, A. Kampfl, R. Siman, J. Liu, X. Zhao, G. L. Clifton, and R. L. Hayes, *Neuroscience*, 77(3), 875–888 (1997).

J. T. Povlishock, *Brain Pathol.*, 2(1), 1–12 (1992).

J. T. Povlishock and C. W. Christman, "Diffuse Axonal Injury," in S. G. Waxman, J. D. Kocsis, and P. K. Stys, Eds., *The Axon*, Oxford University Press, New York, 1995.

J. T. Povlishock and L. W. Jenkins, *Brain Pathol.*, 5(4), 415–426 (1995).

J. T. Povlishock and E. H. Pettus, *Acta Neurochir. Suppl. (Wien)*, 66, 81–86 (1996).

J. T. Povlishock, D. P. Becker, C. L. Cheng, and G. W. Vaughan, *J. Neuropathol. Exp. Neurol.*, 42(3), 225–242 (1983).

J. T. Povlishock, D. E. Erb, and J. Astruc, *J. Neurotrauma*, 9(Suppl. 1), 189–200 (1992).

J. T. Povlishock, A. Marmarou, T. McIntosh, J. Q. Trojanowski, and J. Moroi, *J. Neuropathol. Exp. Neurol.*, 56(4), 347–359 (1997).

D. T. Ross, D. F. Meaney, M. K. Sabol, D. H. Smith, and T. A. Gennarelli, *Exp. Neurol.*, 126(2), 291–299 (1994).

K. E. Saatman, H. Murai, R. T. Bartus, D. H. Smith, N. J. Hayward, B. R. Perri, and T. K. McIntosh, *Proc. Natl. Acad. Sci. U.S.A.*, 93(8), 3428–3433 (1996).

D. M. Sabatini, M. M. Lai, and S. H. Snyder, *Mol. Neurobiol.*, 15(2), 223–239 (1997).

Z. Sahenk and R. Lasek, *Brain Res.*, 460(1), 199–203 (1988).

S. W. Scheff and P. G. Sullivan, *J. Neurotrauma*, 16(9), 783–792 (1999).

F. E. Sherriff, L. R. Bridges, and S. Sivaloganathan, *Acta Neuropathol. (Berl.)*, 87(1), 55–62 (1994a).

F. E. Sherriff, L. R. Bridges, and P. Jackson, *Neuroreport*, 5(9), 1085–1088 (1994b).

F. E. Sherriff, L. R. Bridges, S. M. Gentleman, S. Sivaloganathan, and S. Wilson, *Acta Neuropathol. (Berl.)*, 88(5), 433–439 (1994c).

R. H. Singleton, J. R. Stone, D. O. Okonkwo, and J. Povlishock, *J. Neurotrauma*, in press (2001).

D. H. Smith, X. H. Chen, B. N. Xu, T. K. McIntosh, T. A. Gennarelli, and D. F. Meaney, *J. Neuropathol. Exp. Neurol.*, 56(7), 822–834 (1997).

D. H. Smith, X. H. Chen, M. Nonaka, J. Q. Trojanowski, V. M. Lee, K. E. Saatman, M. J. Leoni, B. N. Xu, J. A. Wolf, and D. F. Meaney, *J. Neuropathol. Exp. Neurol.*, 58(9), 982–992 (1999a).

D. H. Smith, J. A. Wolf, T. A. Lusardi, V. M. Lee, and D. F. Meaney, *J. Neurosci.*, 19(11), 4263–4269 (1999b).

S. L. Smith and E. D. Hall, *J. Neurotrauma*, 13(1), 123–136 (1996).

C. Sola, S. Barron, J. M. Tusell, and J. Serratosa, *Prog. Neurobiol.*, 58(3), 207–232 (1999).

P. M. Stemmer and C. B. Klee, *Biochemistry*, 33(22), 6859–6866 (1994).

J. R. Stone, S. A. Walker, and J. T. Povlishock, *Acta Neuropathol. (Berl.)*, 97(4), 335–345 (1999).

J. R. Stone, R. H. Singleton, and J. Povlishock, *J. Neuropathol. Exp. Neurol.*, in review (2001).

S. Strich, *J. Neurol. Neurosurg. Psychiatry*, 163–185 (1956).

S. J. Strich, *Lancet*, (2), 443–448 (1961).

H. G. Sullivan, J. Martinez, D. P. Becker, J. D. Miller, R. Griffith, and A. O. Wist, *J. Neurosurg.*, 45(5), 521–534 (1976).

P. G. Sullivan, M. Thompson, and S. W. Scheff, *Exp. Neurol.*, 161(2), 631–637 (2000).

S. A. Susin, N. Zamzami, and G. Kroemer, *Biochim. Biophys. Acta*, 1366(1–2), 157–165 (1998).

S. A. Susin, H. K. Lorenzo, N. Zamzami, I. Marzo, C. Brenner, N. Larochette, M. C. Provost, P. M. Alzari, and G. Kroemer, *J. Exp. Med.*, 189(2), 381–394 (1999a).

S. A. Susin, H. K. Lorenzo, N. Zamzami, I. Marzo, B. E. Snow, G. M. Brothers, J. Mangion, E. Jacotot, P. Costantini, M. Loeffler, N. Larochette, D. R. Goodlett, R. Aebersold, D. P. Siderovski, J. M. Penninger, and G. Kroemer, *Nature*, 397(6718), 441–446 (1999b).

B. G. Szaro, M. H. Whitnall, and H. Gainer, *J. Comp. Neurol.*, 302(2), 220–235 (1990).

K. Tokoyoda, Y. Takemoto, T. Nakayama, T. Arai, and M. Kubo, *J. Biol. Chem.*, 275(16), 11728–11734 (2000).

G. Tomei, D. Spagnoli, A. Ducati, A. Landi, R. Villani, G. Fumagalli, C. Sala, and T. Gennarelli, *Acta Neuropathol (Berl.)*, 80(5), 506–513 (1990).

T. Uehara, Y. Kikuchi, and Y. Nomura, *J. Neurochem.*, 72(1), 196–205 (1999).

K. K. Wang, *Trends Neurosci.*, 23(1), 20–26 (2000).

A. E. Wilkinson, L. R. Bridges, and S. Sivaloganathan, *Acta Neuropathol. (Berl.)*, 98(2), 197–202 (1999).

A. Yaghmai and J. Povlishock, *J. Neuropathol. Exp. Neurol.*, 51(2), 158–176 (1992).

M. Zoratti and I. Szabo, *Biochim. Biophys. Acta*, 1241(2), 139–176 (1995).

CHAPTER 14

VASCULAR ASPECTS OF SEVERE HEAD INJURY

MARIKE ZWIENENBERG and J. PAUL MUIZELAAR
Department of Neurological Surgery, University of California Davis, Sacramento, California

INTRODUCTION

During the 1990s a large body of evidence has become available indicating the importance of events at the level of the cerebrovasculature as factors contributing to the pathophysiology of severe head injury. These factors include ischemia, raised intracranial pressure (ICP), and posttraumatic vasospasm. Moreover, all are important mechanisms of secondary injury that may contribute substantially to the morbidity and mortality of severe head injury. In this chapter the role of these various vascular factors in the pathogenesis of severe head injury and their implications for head injury management are discussed.

Mortality from severe head injury has decreased slightly between 1980 and the present (Fig. 14.1) (Schroder, 1994). It is generally thought that this decrease is mainly due to increased recognition of the mechanisms of secondary brain injury and avoidance of secondary insults to the brain by optimizing cerebral perfusion and oxygenation. Improved prehospital care, resuscitation, and radiological diagnosis (i.e., rapid diagnosis of intracranial mass lesions) are also major contributors (Klauber et al., 1985). In addition, data indicate that early aggressive surgical and medical treatment of intracranial mass lesions and raised ICP, and cerebral perfusion pressure (CPP) therapy improve outcome, although no such treatment has been put to test in a randomized controlled clinical trail (McGraw, 1989; Cortbus et al., 1994; Rosner 1995, 1996).

Head Trauma: Basic, Preclinical, and Clinical Directions, Edited by Leonard P. Miller and Ronald L. Hayes, Co-edited by Jennifer K. Newcomb
ISBN 0-471-36015-5 © 2001 John Wiley & Sons, Inc.

303

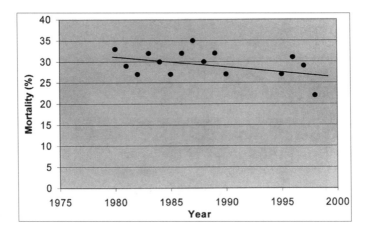

Figure 14.1   Mortality from severe head injury after 6 months at the Medical College of Virginia.

CEREBRAL METABOLISM AND CIRCULATION

Cerebral Metabolism

Cell metabolism involves the consumption of adenosine triphosphate (ATP) and the ensuing consumption of metabolic substrates to resynthesize ATP from adenosine diphosphate (ADP). ATP is generated both in the cytosol (via glycolysis) and in the mitochondria (via oxidative phosphorylation).

Glucose is the sole energy substrate of the brain, unless there is ketosis. The presence of oxygen determines whether glucose is metabolized aerobically or anaerobically. Under normal circumstances 95 percent of the energy requirements of the brain comes from the aerobic conversion of glucose to water and CO_2. ATP generation by this pathway is highly efficient. Glycolysis and subsequent oxidative phosphorylation result in the generation of 38 molecules of ATP for each molecule of glucose. In the absence of oxygen, conversion of glucose takes place by anaerobic glycolysis, but energy production is much less efficient. Only two molecules of ATP and two molecules of lactate are generated for each molecule of glucose.

Of the total energy generated, 50 percent is used for interneuronal communication and generation, release, and uptake of neurotransmitters (synaptic activity); 25 percent is used for maintenance and restoration of ion gradients across the cell membrane; and the remaining 25 percent is used for molecular transport, biosynthesis, and other, as yet unidentified, processes (Astrup, 1982; Siesjo, 1984). Most of the energy generated is consumed by neurons. Glial cells that make up almost 50 percent of the brain have a much lower metabolic rate than neurons and account for less than 10 percent of total cerebral energy expenditure (Siesjo, 1984). Compared to that of other organs, the metabolic demand of the brain is high in that it accounts for only 2 to 3 percent of the total body weight, does not do any mechanical work, and yet it receives 20 percent of all cardiac output.

Regulation of Cerebral Blood Flow

The reserves of glucose and glycogen within astrocytes are limited and there is no significant storage capacity for oxygen. Therefore, the brain depends on a continuous blood flow to supply the glucose and oxygen it requires. The brain possesses several mechanisms (autoregulation) to ensure substrate availability, both under normal circumstances and under circumstances of physiological stress.

Usually the brain is able to maintain an adequate supply of substrates by regulation of cerebral blood flow (CBF). CBF increases with vasodilatation and decreases with vasoconstriction (Fig. 14.2). Caliber changes mainly take place in the so-called "cerebral resistance vessels" (i.e., arterioles with a diameter of 30 to 300 μm) (Kontos et al., 1978). Control of CBF by adjustments in vessel caliber is commonly referred to as autoregulation of blood flow (Lassen, 1959). In humans several mechanisms, active under different circumstances, have been described.

Metabolic Autoregulation. CBF is functionally coupled to cerebral metabolism, changing proportionally with increasing or decreasing regional or global metabolic demand. Thus, the brain is able to precisely match local CBF to local metabolic needs. The relation between CBF and metabolism is expressed in the Fick equation: $CMRO_2 = CBF \times AVDO_2$, in which $CMRO_2$ is the cerebral metabolic rate of oxygen and $AVDO_2$ is the arterio-venous difference of oxygen. Global $CMRO_2$ is

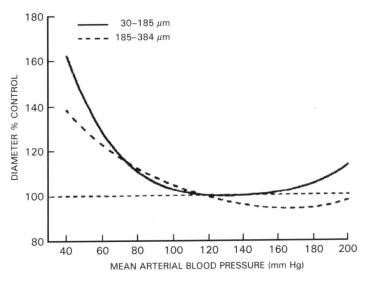

Figure 14.2 Relation between blood pressure and diameter of cerebral surface arteries and arterioles. The solid line represents diameter change of arterioles; the dashed line represents diameter change of the cerebral surface arteries. Adapted from Kontos et al. (1978).

thus obtained by multiplying global CBF with the global arterio-venous difference of oxygen. In general the brain responds to alterations of metabolism with changes in flow and thus has a tendency to keep $AVDO_2$ relatively constant. Examples of increasing metabolic demand are seizures and fever, in which a proportional increase in CBF are observed. Decreased metabolic demand and consequently diminished CBF is observed in case of anesthesia or deep coma (Nilsson et al., 1978). In comatose patients with severe head injury, $CMRO_2$ is typically reduced from a normal value of 3.3 mL/100 g per min to approximately 2.1 mL/100 g per min (Robertson, 1996). Normal metabolic coupling (proportional decrease in CBF) is maintained in approximately 45 percent of those suffering from severe head injury (Obrist et al., 1984).

Several investigators have reported CBF in excess of metabolism (luxury perfusion or hyperemia), in particular in the first 24 h after injury (Lassen, 1966; Obrist et al., 1984; Muizelaar et al., 1989a,b). The underlying mechanism uncoupling CBF from metabolism is poorly understood. Recent studies on mitochondrial function performed by our group have revealed that severe head injury may result in significant damage and dysfunction (Verweij et al., 1997; Xiong et al., 1997a,b; 1998), which may explain the low $CMRO_2$ values in the presence of normal CBF. Moreover, CBF may be preserved under these circumstances to support anaerobic glucose turnover and thus ensure ATP generation. Earlier work of Cox and Gonzalez revealed that CBF is in fact functionally coupled to the cerebral metabolic rate of glucose (CMRG) (Cox et al., 1993; Gonzalez and Sharp, 1985). In experimental and human brain injury, CMRG in excess of $CMRO_2$ has been reported (Hovda et al., 1995; Bergsneider et al., 1997).

Pressure Autoregulation. Pressure autoregulation is one of the mechanisms through which the brain is able to maintain a constant supply of substrates at the level set by metabolism. Factors governing CBF are expressed in the Poiseuille equation, $CBF = k \, (CPP \times d^4)/(8 \times l \times v)$. CPP represents cerebral perfusion pressure, d vessel diameter, l vessel length, and v blood viscosity. According to this equation, changes in CPP (i.e., arterial hypotension or increases in ICP) will be followed by changes in CBF unless diameter regulation ("pressure autoregulation") takes place. In humans, the limits of pressure autoregulation range from 40 to 150 mm Hg of perfusion pressure. Beyond these limits, vessel caliber follows flow passively, leading to collapse of the vessels at low pressure and forced dilation or "pressure breakthrough" at high pressures (Fig. 14.3).

Under normal circumstances small changes in CBF occur during CPP changes, even within the limits of autoregulation. Therefore it may be more appropriate to define autoregulation in terms of cerebrovascular resistance (CVR), that is, the change in CVR (Heistad and Kontos, 1983) (calculated as CPP/CBF) that occurs in response to a given change in CPP. Pressure autoregulation is considered intact if $0 \leq \Delta\%CPP/\Delta\%CVR \leq 2$ (Muizelaar et al., 1984, 1989a,b; Bouma and Muizelaar, 1990).

Several authors have investigated pressure autoregulation after severe head injury (Fieschi et al., 1974; Overgaard and Tweed, 1974; Enevoldsen and Jensen, 1978;

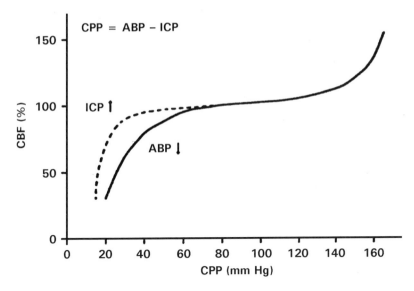

Figure 14.3 Pressure autoregulation in humans. The cerebral perfusion pressure (CPP) is defined as the mean arterial blood pressure (ABP) minus the intracranial pressure (ICP). Changes in cerebral blood flow (CBF) are expressed as percent change from baseline. At the lower limit of autoregulation, changes in ABP have a more profound effect on CBF than do changes in ICP.

Muizelaar et al., 1989a,b; Bouma and Muizelaar, 1992; Newell et al., 1996; Tiecks et al., 1996; Newell et al., 1997). Enevoldsen and colleagues found that autoregulation is usually intact during the first few days after head injury and subsequently only temporarily dysfunctional with no apparent effect on outcome (Enevoldsen and Jensen, 1978). In another study it was found that pressure autoregulation was always intact during the first 36 h and absent in 50 percent of the patients between 36 and 96 h post injury (Fieschi et al., 1974). Overgaard and Tweed related autoregulatory capacity to clinical outcome and found that patients had a better outcome when autoregulation was intact over the first week after injury. However, no such correlation could be found after the first week of injury (Overgaard and Tweed, 1974). We performed autoregulation tests in 117 severely head-injured patients using xenon-133 CBF measurements (Bouma and Muizelaar, 1992). Autoregulation was found intact in 51 percent of the patients, but no specific temporal pattern or a relation to clinical status could be determined.

The cause of defective pressure autoregulation is unknown. From a clinical study it has been suggested that brain stem lesions damaging an autoregulatory center within the brain stem (Enevoldsen and Jensen, 1978) may be responsible. We studied multimodality evoked potentials (MEP) in severely head-injured children but could not find a relation between the status of autoregulation and the site of the lesion as indicated by MEP abnormalities (Muizelaar et al., 1989). Autoregulation was defective in 15 of the 37 children studied. Endothelial damage may be responsible for the perturbation of "pressure autoregulation." In experimental brain injury, endothelial lesions are often present with severe ischemia or trauma (Wei et al., 1980). Oxygen radicals that are generated in the cerebral blood vessel walls, circulating leukocytes, and macrophages (Kontos and Wei, 1985) following injury may in part cause the endothelial damage (Ignarro et al., 1986; Beckman et al., 1990). Impairment of vascular reactivity can be prevented by administration of oxygen radical scavengers (Kontos and Wei, 1985; Ellis et al., 1991).

Viscosity Autoregulation. The second autoregulatory mechanism to maintain CBF at the set metabolic demand is viscosity autoregulation (Muizelaar et al., 1984, 1986; Hudak et al., 1989). According to Poiseulle's equation, CBF can vary with changes in the viscosity of blood. Blood viscosity changes with variations in hematocrit, gammaglobulin, and fibrinogen components of plasma protein. Increased viscosity would increase cerebrovascular resistance $(8 \times l \times v/d^4)$. By means of diameter adjustment ("viscosity autoregulation"), cerebrovascular resistance is decreased and CBF can be kept constant.

There are few studies available that have specifically evaluated the status of viscosity autoregulation after severe head injury. We evaluated the response of CBF to bolus administration of mannitol in patients with severe head injury (Muizelaar et al., 1984). In the group with intact pressure autoregulation only 5 out of 28 cases showed a more than 10 percent increase in CBF following mannitol administration. In the group with defective pressure autoregulation 11 out of 14 cases showed an increase in CBF by more than 10 percent of baseline in response to mannitol injection, accounting for a total of 16 out of 42 cases in which viscosity autoregulation appeared defective (38 percent). In the first group ICP decreased by more than 10 percent in 24 out of 28 cases (86 percent) and only in 5 out of 14 cases in the second group (36 percent).

Theories on Autoregulation. It is not clear what mechanism couples regional CBF to regional metabolism, nor are the exact mechanisms underlying pressure and viscosity autoregulation known. It is likely that a similar mechanism is involved in all three types of autoregulation, but this has not been unraveled yet. Recently, the vascular endothelium has received much attention in both pressure and metabolic autoregulation, and investigators were able to elucidate some of the underlying mechanisms.

Vasoactive metabolites that are released from the active nerve cell are thought to be responsible for metabolic coupling. This concept is more than a century old. As early as 1890, Roy and Sherrington stated

> The chemical products of cerebral metabolism contained in the lymph, which bathes the walls of the arterioles of the brain, can cause variations in the caliber of the cerebral vessels. In the reaction the brain possesses an intrinsic mechanism by which its vascular supply can be varied locally in correspondence with local variations of functional activity

(Denny-Brown, 1979; Eccles and Gibson, 1979). The identity of these vasoactive agents is not known. Agents that are directly influenced by local energy metabolism, such as CO_2, H^+, O_2, adenosine, and ions like K^+ and Ca^{2+} have been proposed (Kontos et al., 1978; Kuschinsky and Wahl, 1978; Bouma, 1993), but most were rejected on various theoretical grounds (Siesjo, 1984).

The vascular endothelium plays an important role in maintaining the normal physiological function of the blood vessel wall by releasing relaxing and contracting factors and is therefore an interesting site mediating autoregulation. Substances released by endothelial cells and involved in vessel wall response include release of relaxing factors such as endothelium-derived relaxing factor/nitric oxide (EDRF/NO), endothelium-derived hyperpolarization factor (EDHF), and prostacyclin. Contracting factors released by the endothelium are respectively thromboxane A_2 and endothelins. These factors are illustrated in Fig. 14.4.

Nitric oxide (NO)/endothelium-derived relaxing factor (EDRF) is the primary mediator of endothelin-dependent relaxation (Furchgott and Zawadzki, 1980). EDRF is synthesized from L-arginine by the enzyme NO-synthase in the endothelial cell and, when released, diffuses into the smooth muscle cell. NO causes relaxation by augmenting cyclic GMP. Cyclic GMP in turn decreases the level of intracellular calcium, resulting in relaxation of the myofibrils (Rapoport and Murad, 1983).

The role of EDRF/NO in autoregulation is controversial (Tanaka, 1996). Most authors think that the main role of EDRF/NO is maintenance of basal cerebral blood flow. Garthwait and colleagues have shown, however, that EDRF/NO may mediate a functional coupling of metabolism and cerebral blood flow in certain types of neural activation (Garthwaite et al., 1988). They found that glutamate activation of the N-methyl-D-aspartate (NMDA) receptor causes a calcium-dependent release of a substance with properties similar to that of EDRF/NO. The observed vasodilation after glutamate activation was inhibited by administration of both an NMDA antagonist and a NO synthase inhibitor, suggesting coupling of neuronal activation and CBF through EDRF/NO release. It is thought that a mediator released from adjacent glutamate-responsive cells induces this EDRF/NO production by the endothelium, because endothelial cells do not possess functional ionotropic or metabotropic glutamate receptors (Morley et al., 1998).

Goadsby and colleagues, who simultaneously studied cerebral neuronal activity and local blood flow in cats, provided other evidence for EDRF/NO involvement in metabolic coupling (Goadsby et al., 1992). It was found that intravenous administration of N-nitro-L-arginine methyl ester (L-NAME), a potent nitric oxide synthase inhibitor, resulted in a complete blockade of the hyperemia associated with spreading depression but did not cause a change in resting cell firing or cause a change in spreading depression-evoked increases in firing rate.

Release of EDHF from the endothelium causes hyperpolarization (through potassium channels), a decrease in intracellular calcium in the smooth muscle cell, and relaxation. The identity, the pathway of synthesis, and the role of EDHF in autoregulation are presently unknown.

The third major endothelium-derived vasodilator is the arachidonic acid metabolite prostacyclin (PGI_2). Prostacyclin was the first endothelial vasoactive

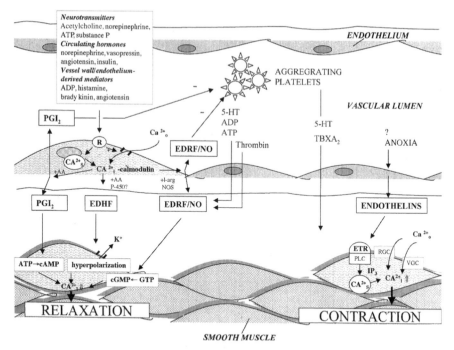

Figure 14.4 Mechnisms of vascular smooth muscle contraction and relaxation. Main factors involved in smooth muscle relaxation are the arachidonic acid cycle (AA) metabolite prostacyclin (PGI_2), endothelium-derived hyperpolarization factor (EDHF), and endothelium-derived relaxing factor (EDRF) or nitric oxide (NO). All three are synthesized in endothelial cells upon activation by various stimuli. The Ca_i^{2+}–calmodulin complex is a cofactor in the synthesis of all three factors. In the smooth muscle cell PGI_2 and EDRF stimulate respectively guanyl and adenyl cyclase, resulting in a decrease of intracellular calcium (Ca_i^{2+}) and smooth muscle relaxation. Decrease of Ca_i^{2+} by EDHF is mediated through opening of a potassium channel and hyperpolarization of the cell membrane. Aggregating platelets release a variety of vasoactive metabolites with both vasorelaxant and vasoconstrictor properties. PGI_2 and EDRF/NO are thought to inhibit platelet aggregation. Endothelin synthesis and release is thought to be stimulated by anoxia and other yet unknown factors. Binding of endothelin to the endothelin receptor (ETR) on the smooth muscle cell membrane and subsequent coupling to phospholipase C (PCL) results in generation of inositol 3-phosphate (IP_3) recruitment of calcium (Ca_s^{2+}) from intracellular stores and smooth muscle contraction. In addition, calcium (Ca_o^{2+}) enters the cell through activated receptor gated channels (RGC) and upon membrane depolarization through voltage-gated channels (VGC).

substance discovered in the late 1970s. PGI_2, generated through the cyclooxygenase pathway of the arachidonic acid metabolism, is synthesized by its specific enzyme prostacyclin-synthetase and exerts a strong vasodilating effect. Like EDRF, PGI_2 release is stimulated by increased shear stress on the vessel wall. However, its role in autoregulation is unknown.

The observation that removal of the endothelium in canine femoral arteries significantly reduced the contractions generated in response to various vasoconstrictors and hypoxia was the first indication that endothelium not mediates only relaxation of the underlying smooth muscle but also vasoconstriction. Evidence accumulated over the past years has established a main role for endothelium-dependent vasoconstriction in both peripheral and cerebral circulation. The observation that rapid elevation of transmural pressure triggers vasoconstriction (Bayliss effect) and that this response is prevented by removal of the endothelium has led to the idea that pressure autoregulation may be endothelium-mediated (Rubanyi, 1988; Rubanyi et al., 1990).

Two major endothelium-derived contracting factors are thromboxane A_2 and endothelin. Thromboxane A_2 is generated in small amounts from endothelial cells (Davies and Hagen, 1993) but mostly produced in platelets via the enzyme thromboxane-synthetase. Thromboxane A_2 is a powerful vasoconstrictor and enhances platelet aggregation. Endothelins are the most recently discovered endothelium-derived vasoactive agents and are extremely potent vasoconstrictors. Endothelins are formed in endothelial cells by the conversion of big-endothelin to endothelin by one or two endothelin-converting enzymes (ECE) (Davies and Hagen, 1993).

Martainez-Orgado and colleagues evaluated the influence of endothelial factors on pressure autoregulation in a recent study (Martainez-Orgado et al., 1998). Middle cerebral arteries from 3- to 4-day-old piglets were cannulated, and diameter changes after transmural pressure variation were measured. Segments with intact endothelium showed vasodilation during pressure decrease and vasoconstriction during pressure increase. Segments without endothelium responded passively to pressure change. Their results suggested an endothelium-dependent autoregulatory mechanism, involvement of NO and K^+/Ca^{2+} channels in vasodilation during transmural pressure decrease, and involvement of endothelin-1 and prostanoids in vasoconstriction during pressure increase.

CO$_2$ Reactivity. Vascular caliber and cerebral blood flow are also responsive to changes in arterial PCO_2, a mechanism commonly referred to as CO_2 reactivity. Cerebral blood flow changes 2 percent to 3 percent for each mm Hg in $PaCO_2$, within the range from 20 to 60 mm Hg. Hypercarbia (hypoventilation) results in vasodilatation and higher CBF, and hypocarbia (hyperventilation) results in vasoconstriction and lower CBF. CO_2 reactivity is fundamentally different from autoregulation: vessel caliber changes and CBF follow changes in CO_2 passively. Autoregulation is an active compensatory or adaptive response, adjusting cerebral blood flow to metabolism. The vessels respond not to changes in $PaCO_2$ but to the pH in the perivascular space. CO_2 can cross the blood–brain barrier freely, thus changing perivascular pH. However, over 20 to 24 h, with a constant new level of $PaCO_2$, the pH in blood and the perivascular space returns to baseline, and the diameter of cerebral blood vessels also returns to baseline (Muizelaar et al., 1988). With CO_2 reactivity, changes in CBF are compensated for by changes in AVDO$_2$, so that a constant supply of substrates is maintained at the level set by metabolism (CMRO$_2$). In contrast, a constant AVDO$_2$ is a common feature of metabolic, pressure and viscosity autoregulation; CBF is tuned to metabolism, and therefore AVDO$_2$ can be kept constant.

CO_2 reactivity is usually preserved after severe head injury. CO_2 reactivity may be low early after injury but return to a normal 3 percent change per mm Hg CO_2 is found 24 hours after injury in most circumstances (Fieschi et al., 1974; Overgaard and Tweed, 1974; Enevoldsen et al., 1976; Cold and Jensen, 1978; Enevoldsen and Jensen, 1978; Obrist et al., 1984; Messeter et al., 1986). In experimental studies, temporarily reduced CO_2 reactivity has also been observed but returns to normal within a few hours (Zimmerman et al., 1987). In some cases a considerable difference between global and regional CO_2 reactivity is observed. Marion and colleagues determined CO_2 vasoresponsivity in 17 patients with severe closed head injury using stable xenon-enhanced computed tomography (Marion et al., 1991). Hemispheric, lobar, basal ganglia, and midbrain CBF values before and after pCO_2 reduction were used to determine CO_2 reactivity. CO_2 reactivity was expressed as the percentage change of CBF per mm Hg pCO_2. They reported that regional CO_2 reactivity was different from global CO_2 reactivity in at least one area in all but one patient. In some cases the difference was as large as 50 percent, particularly in patients with subdural hematomas or diffuse cerebral contusions. Patients with severely impaired CO_2 reactivity usually die or are left with severe neurological deficits (Overgaard and Tweed, 1974; Obrist et al., 1984). The pathological mechanisms leading to disturbed CO_2 regulation are poorly understood. Free radicals may play a role since it was shown in a cat model that administration of free radical scavengers prevented loss of vasoresponsivity following injury (Zimmerman et al., 1987).

Induction of hypocapnia by means of hyperventilation has long been a popular treatment to reduce ICP. At the same time, however, it reduces CBF, which may already be at critical ischemic levels in certain parts of the brain (Skippen et al., 1997). Therefore hyperventilation ($PCO_2 < 30$) should not be instituted prophylactically. Moreover, we previously showed that prolonged hyperventilation becomes ineffective after 24 h and in a randomized clinical trial it was shown that hyperventilation retards recovery after severe head injury (Muizelaar et al, 1991). In cases where $PaCO_2$ must be reduced to extremely low levels, hyperventilation can be combined with mannitol as this will improve CBF by reducing blood viscosity (Muizelaar et al., 1983). $AVDO_2$ measurement by jugular venous oxymetry is useful in these situations as it will indicate when vasoconstriction results in ischemic levels of CBF (Gopinath et al., 1994).

CEREBRAL BLOOD FLOW, CEREBRAL BLOOD VOLUME, AND AUTOREGULATION

Cerebral Blood Flow and Cerebral Blood Volume

Alterations in vascular caliber not only affect the perfusion of the brain, but cause a change in the total intravascular blood volume or cerebral blood volume (CBV). CBV is considered a major determinant of ICP (see "intracranial pressure"). The relationship between CBF and CBV can be characterized by the equation

$CBV = CBF \times MTT$, in which MTT is the mean transit time of the blood through the cerebral vasculature.

CBV is determined by the diameter of the vascular bed; that is, increasing vascular diameter CBV increases and vice versa. Vessels with a diameter between 30 and 300 μm, due to their relatively large number and still fairly large size, probably contain most of the intracranial blood volume. Caliber alterations in these vessels mainly take place in the arterioles (200 μm) (Kontos et al., 1978). The diameter of the venules remains more or less constant.

CBF, CBV, and Autoregulation

The status of autoregulation will determine the effect of certain treatment modalities, in particular those used to control ICP or CPP. As discussed previously, CBF is influenced by vascular diameter, but also by blood viscosity and cerebral perfusion pressure (CPP), while CBV is determined by vascular diameter only. In earlier work we reported on alterations of CBF, CBV (ICP), and $AVDO_2$ in response to a variety of physiological and pathological conditions (Muizelaar et al., 1989). These findings are summarized in Table 14.1. For example, a decrease in cerebral perfusion pressure within the limits of autoregulation will lead to compensatory vasodilation. CBF and $AVDO_2$ will remain constant. ICP, however, will increase due to the increase in vascular diameter and CBV. When pressure autoregulation is defective, a decrease in CPP will lead to a decrease in CBF (Poiseuille equation). Due to the decrease of CBV ($CBV = CBF \times MIT$), ICP will also decrease. Finally, an increase of $AVDO_2$ compensates for the reduced CBF.

TABLE 14.1 Status of CBF, CBV, and $AVDO_2$ Under Various Clinical Conditions

Feature with primary reduction	CBF	CBV (ICP)	$AVDO_2$
$CMRO_2$ (within physiological limits)	⇓	⇓	=
CPP (autoregulation intact)	=	⇑	=
CPP (autoregulation defective)	⇓	⇓	⇑
Blood viscosity (autoregulation intact)	=	⇓	=
Blood viscosity (autoregulation defective)	⇑	=	⇓
$PaCO_2$ (hyperventilation)	⇓	⇓	⇑
Large cerebral artery diameter (cerebral vasospasm)	⇓	⇑	⇑

RAISED INTRACRANIAL PRESSURE

Raised intracranial pressure (ICP) is a common complication of severe head injury and continues to be one of the main problems in the treatment of severely head-injured patients (Becker et al., 1977; Marshall et al., 1979; Miller, 1982; Marmarou et al., 1989; Marshall and Gautille, 1990). ICP is governed by the volume of the intracranial contents. The Monro–Kellie doctrine states that the total volume of the intracranial contents (cerebral blood volume, CSF, and brain parenchyma) is constant (Monro, 1783; Kettle, 1824). Increase in one of the three compartments must be accompanied by an equal decrease in one of the two other compartments, otherwise ICP will increase (Monro, 1783; Kellie, 1824). As long as these volume compensations are sufficient, ICP remains relatively constant (compensated state) in the range of 8 to 10 mm Hg above atmospheric level (Ekstedt, 1978). At a certain volume, however, this volume-buffering capacity is exhausted, resulting in an exponential pressure rise with any further increase in volume (Fig. 14.5).

When this curve is plotted on a semilogarithmic scale, a straight line is the result (Fig. 14.6) (Marmarou et al., 1978). The slope of this line is defined as the pressure–volume index (PVI) and represents the amount of volume that must be added to or withdrawn from the craniospinal axis in order to raise or decrease ICP by tenfold:

$$PVI = \frac{\Delta V}{\log(ICP_i/ICP_o)}$$

Change in volume is represented by ΔV, ICP_o is the pressure before volume change, ICP_i the pressure after volume change. PVI is thus a measure for the compliance ($\Delta V/\Delta P$) or tightness of the brain. Brain compliance can be estimated by injecting small quantities of fluid into the CSF space with simultaneous recording of ICP. This involves repeated injections of 2 to 3 ml in the CSF space, usually through lumbar infusion.

The normal PVL is 26 ± 4 ml (Shapiro et al., 1980); that is, 26 ml of volume will raise ICP from 1 to 10 mm Hg, but the same volume will also raise ICP from 10 to 100 mm Hg. Conversely, a change in volume of only 6.4 mL is required to increase ICP from 10 mm g (normal) to the treatment threshold of 20 mm Hg, indicating the sensitivity of ICP to volume changes (Marmarou, 1992; Yoshihara et al., 1995).

Another measure of brain compliance is the volume–pressure ratio (VPR). VPR describes the slope of the pressure volume curve at a given level of ICP and is defined as the change in ICP achieved by a 1 mL bolus addition of CSF volume (Miller et al., 1973; Miller and Pickard, 1974). VPR will vary linearly with ICP if the pressure–volume curve is fixed. The relationship with PVI under steady-state circumstances is: $VPR = ICP_o/(0.434PVI)$ (Marmarou, 1996). The precise sequence of events leading to ICP elevation and the exact contribution of each of the components remain elusive. Marmarou distinguished five factors that influence intracranial volume increase: (1) CSF system; (2) cerebral blood volume (CBV); (3) vasogenic edema [blood–brain barrier damage-associated edema (BBB edema)]; (4) cytoxic (neurotoxic) edema; (5) cytotoxic (ischemic) edema.

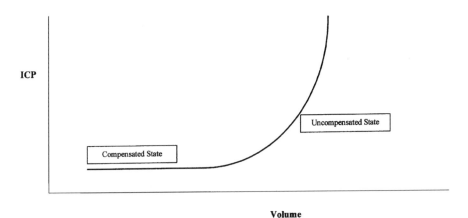

Figure 14.5   Response of intracranial pressure (ICP) to change of craniospinal volume.

CSF components (CSF resistance to outflow and absorption) account for approximately one-third of ICP elevation. This component can increase substantially in patients with subarachnoid hemorrhage due to increased outflow resistance as a result of blockage of the arachnoid villi. The remaining two-thirds are attributed to a "vascular component": increased blood volume and increased tissue water (vasogenic and cytotoxic edema) (Marmarou et al., 1987). Neurotoxic and ischemic edema are thought to be of cellular origin. Edema due to BBB damage is thought to be extracellular. Diffusion-weighted magnetic resonance imaging experiments in

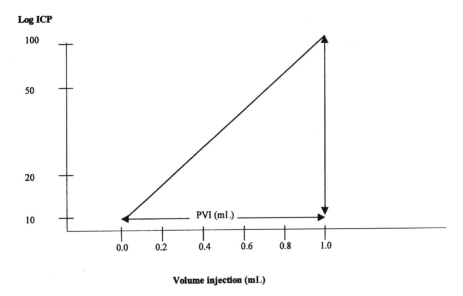

Figure 14.6   Relation between pressure and volume plotted on a semilogarithmic scale.

rodents indicate that there is a temporal pattern in the type of edema that develops. Immediately after injury the edema is thought to be predominantly vasogenic. Intracellular edema formation starts at 1 h post injury and is most dominant between 1 to 2 weeks post injury (Barzo et al., 1997).

Cerebral blood volume (CBV) is determined by the total diameter of the cerebrovascular bed. The cerebral veins contain most of the total blood volume, but their diameter and thus volume are relatively constant. In humans, approximately 20 mL of blood (i.e., one-third of total CBV) is located in the cerebral resistance vessels (300 to 15 μm). Since most autoregulatory and CO_2-dependent diameter variations take place in these vessels, CBV will mainly be determined by the diameter of these vessels. Typically, diameter varies between 80 percent and 160 percent of baseline, resulting in volume changes between 64 percent and 256 percent of baseline. With a baseline CBV of 20 mL in the resistance vessels, CBV will range from 13 mL (maximal vasoconstriction) to 51 mL (maximal vasodilatation). Given a PVI of 26, change from maximal vasoconstriction to maximal vasodilatation will be accompanied by an almost 29-fold change of ICP.

CEREBRAL ISCHEMIA

Ischemia, defined as CBF that is inadequate to meet the metabolic demands of the brain, is an important mechanism of secondary injury in patients with severe head injury. Ischemic brain damage is common, as evidenced by autopsy findings of patients who died after severe bead injury. Histological damage indicative of cerebral ischemia was seen in 90 percent of the cases (Graham et al., 1989). Bouma and colleages found ischemia (defined as CBF < 18 mL/dL with high $AVDO_2$ values) in 20 percent to 33 percent of the patients with severe head injury within 4 to 12 h of injury. Ischemia was associated with a poor prognosis. Of the intracranial lesions, acute subdural hematoma and diffuse cerebral swelling were most often associated with ischemia. Experimental data suggest that the brain becomes more vulnerable to ischemia after a head injury, while similar ischemic insults are well-tolerated under normal circumstances (Jenkins et al., 1989). Common metabolic and biochemical derangements or abnormal neurotransmitter–receptor interactions, which reach a lethal threshold when the insults are combined, may explain this increased vulner-ability (Bouma, 1993). Under circumstances of declining CBF (due to failure of pressure autoregulation or severe hypotension), the brain can initially protect itself from ischemia and maintain metabolic supply by increasing extraction of the required oxygen from the available blood flow. Clinically this results in an increased $AVDO_2$. Maximum oxygen extraction capacity is reached when $AVDO_2$ is approxi-mately double its normal value (±13 mL/100 mL), that is, when all the oxygen contained in the blood is extracted (Bouma et al., 1991). When CBF declines further, neuronal dysfunction will occur. Initially this will result in reduction of synaptic function (50 percent of the energy expenditure of the brain), but further lowering of CBF will cause membrane failure, sodium–potassium pump arrest, cell swelling and dysfunction, and finally cell death. The CBF threshold at which these changes occur

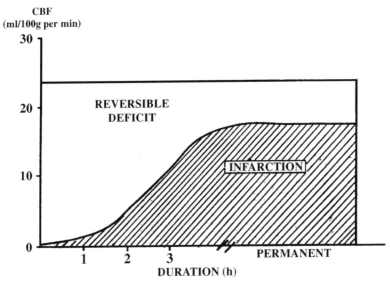

Figure 14.7   CBF and neuronal dysfunction.

has been found to be 18 mL/100 g per min (Jones 1981). The resultant cell damage depends on both the duration and depth of CBF depression (Fig. 14.7). Thus, at CBF of 10 mL/100 g per min the neurological deficit is reversible when the duration does not exceed 3 h. However, beyond 3 h irreversible damage occurs.

POSTTRAUMATIC VASOSPASM

Subarachnoid hemorrhage (SAH) is common after severe head injury. In a study from the NIH Traumatic Coma Databank, SAH was identified in 291 (39 percent) of 753 patients with severe head injury (Eisenberg et al., 1990). The occurrence of cerebral arterial spasm (vasospasm) after severe head injury has long been recognized (Macpherson and Graham, 1973). It is thought that intradural bleeding, which extends into the CSF spaces (subarachnoid, intraventricular, and subdural hemorrhage), plays a role in the pathogenesis of posttraumatic arterial spasm (Martin et al., 1995). The distribution of traumatic subarachnoid hemorrhage (TSAH), as visualized on CT scan, is different from the distribution seen after aneurysmal subarachnoid hemorrhage (ASAH). Unlike ASAH, TSAH is not limited to cisterns surrounding the circle of Willis but extends to supratentorial regions and interhemispheric fissures. In addition, computed tomography-detected subarachnoid hemorrhage disappears very early with TSAH and more gradually with ASAH (Fukuda et al., 1998).

Vasospasm can be demonstrated by either cerebral angiography or transcranial doppler ultrasonography (TCD) and occurs in approximately 25 percent to 40 percent of the patients with severe head injury (Martin et al., 1995). Like ASAH-associated vasospasm, the arteries typically affected by posttraumatic vasospasm are the large cerebral arteries, such as the supraclinoid internal carotid artery (ICA), the middle cerebral artery (MCA), the anterior cerebral artery (ACA), and the basilar artery (BA). The time course of TSAH associated vasospasm also resembles that of ASAH vasospasm, with onset occurring two or more days after injury, peak around two weeks after injury, and resolution after three weeks.

Pathophysiologically, vasospasm is an important posttraumatic secondary insult. MacPherson and Graham found a significant correlation between angiographic arterial narrowing and postmortem ipsitateral ischemic hemispheric damage (Macpherson and Graham, 1973). In addition, several studies of severely head-injured patients have shown low CBF values in combination with increased TCD velocities, indicating that vasospasm is associated with impaired cerebral perfusion (Lee et al., 1997; Martin et al., 1997). Fukuda and colleagues, however, reported that, unlike ASAH in which all low-density areas on the CT scans corresponded to vascular territories, low-density areas on the CT scans of patients with TSAH were rarely associated with vascular territories. Instead, the low-density areas contained deep-seated or gliding contusions (Fukuda et al., 1998). If pressure autoregulation is intact, vasospasm of the large intracranial arteries may be accompanied by an increase of cerebral blood volume (CBV), due to compensatory dilatation of the vessels in the microcirculation. A reduced CBF in the presence of increased CBV thus supports the diagnosis of large artery spasm. Schröder and colleages simultaneously evaluated early CBF and CBV in seven patients with severe head injury (Schröder et al., 1998). These patients were selected from a larger series of 51 patients because they exhibited both nonischemic and ischemic (CBF < 18 mL/100 g per min) areas on stable xenon-CT measurements. Both CBF and CBV were significantly lower in the ischemic zones, indicating that in the early phase after injury compromise of the microvasculature is the cause of ischemia, rather than vasospasm of the larger conductance vessels. No simultaneous studies have been performed at a later stage, when the highest incidence of vasospasm is expected. In an earlier study, Martin and colleagues, using CBF and TCD measurements, identified three different circulatory stages after severe head injury: phase I (hypoperfusion), phase II (hyperemia), and phase III (vasospasm) (Martin et al., 1997). The following parameters were evaluated (Table 14.2): CBF, TCD velocity in

TABLE 14.2   Circulatory Phases After Severe Head Injury

Phase	Days After injury	CBF (ml/100 g per min)	AVDO$_2$ (vol%)	CMRO$_2$ (mL/100 g per min)	$V_{(mca)}$ (cm/s)	HI
Hypoperfusion	0	Low	Normal	Depressed	Normal	Normal
		32.2 ± 2	5.4 ± 0.5	1.77 ± 0.18	56.7 ± 2.9	1.67 ± 0.11
Hyperemia	1–3	Relatively increased	Decreased	Depressed	Increased	Normal/ increased
		46.8 ± 3	3.8 ± 0.1	1.49 ± 0.82	86 ± 3.7	2.41 ± 0.1
Vasospasm	14–15	Decreased	Increased	Depressed	Increased	Increased
		35.7 ± 3.8	3.9 ± 0.1	1.46 ± 0.56	96.7 ± 6.3	2.87 ± 0.22

the middle cerebral artery, the hemispheric index (HI) calculated as the ratio of MCA and ICA velocity, the arterio-venous oxygen difference ($AVDO_2$, see "cerebral metabolism and circulation"), and the cerebral metabolic rate of oxygen ($CMRO_2$, see "cerebral metabolism and circulation"). Phase I occurs on the day of injury (day 0) and is defined by a low CBF (mean CBF $= 32.3 \pm 2$ ml/100 g per min), normal middle cerebral artery (MCA) velocity (mean $V_{(MCA)} = 56.7 \pm 2.9$ cm/s), normal hemispheric index (HI, mean HI $= 1.67 \pm 0.11$), and normal $AVDO_2$ (mean $AVDO_2 = 5.4 \pm 0.5$ vol%). The $CMRO_2$ is approximately 50 percent of normal (mean $CMRO_2 = 1.77 \pm 0.18$ mL/100 g per min) during this phase and remains depressed during the second and third phases. In phase II (relative hyperemia phase, days 1 to 3), CBF increases (46.8 ± 3 mL/100 g per min), $AVDO_2$ falls (3.8 ± 0.1 vol%), $V_{(MCA)}$ rises (86 ± 3.7 cm/s), and the HI remains less than 3 (2.41 ± 0.1). In phase III (vasospasm phase, days 4–15), there is a fall in CBF (35.7 ± 3.8 ml/100 g per min), a further increase in $V_{(MCA)}$ (96.7 ± 6.3 cm/s), and a pronounced rise in the HI (2.87 ± 0.22).

The etiology of posttraumatic vasospasm is unknown. Similar mechanisms to those in ASAH-associated vasospasm are thought to be involved. Recent research in ASAH-associated vasospasm has suggested an important role for endothelium and its mediators (Hirose et al., 1995; Roux et al., 1995; Seifert et al., 1995; Zuccarello et al., 1995; Caner et al., 1996; Zimmermann and Seifert, 1996, 1998; Zimmermann et al., 1996; Zimmermann, 1997; Sobey and Faraci, 1998; Pierre et al., 1999). Endothelium-mediated hyperreactivity of vascular smooth muscle due to release of endothelins or an imbalance between the production of endothelium-derived relaxing factor (EDRF) and prostacyclin (PGI_2) on one hand, and endothelium-derived contracting factors on the other hand (endothelins and thromboxane A_2) may play a pivotal role in TSAH associated vasospasm (Fig. 14.4).

CONCLUSION

Vascular factors appear to play an important role in the pathogenesis of severe head injury and contribute substantially to the morbidity and mortality of this affliction. However, the exact effects of severe head injury on the cerebral circulation and the consequences of therapeutic modulation of the vascular compartment are largely unknown. It has become clear how ICP is affected by changes in the cerebrovascular compartment and also that certain therapeutic modalities (such as hyperventilation) can have a profound effect on the cerebral circulation but with potentially severe side effects. Therefore, knowledge of the posttraumatic status of autoregulation and CO_2 reactivity is extremely important before therapy is instituted.

Cerebral vasospasm is a relatively new field in head injury research but requires in-depth exploration considering the large number of patients that might be affected. Mechanisms similar to those responsible for impairment of autoregulation may be at work. Once these mechanisms are elucidated there is a potential that new therapies can be developed. However, it should be kept in mind that therapies that influence one factor beneficially might effect another factor negatively. The net effect upon outcome can and should only be assessed in pragmatic randomized clinical trial.

ABBREVIATIONS

ACA	Anterior cerebral artery
ADP	Adenosine diphosphate
AMP	Adenosine monophosphate
ASAH	Aneurysmal subarachnoid hemorrhage
ATP	Adenosine triphosphate
$AVDO_2$	Arterio-venous difference of oxygen
BA	Basilar artery
CBF	Cerebral blood flow
CBV	Cerebral blood volume
CMRG	Cerebral metabolic rate of glucose
$CMRO_2$	Cerebral metabolic rate of oxygen
CPP	Cerebral perfusion pressure
CSF	Cerebrospinal fluid
CT	Computerized tomography
CVR	Cerebrovascular resistance
EDHF	Endothelium-derived hyperpolarization factor
EDRF	Endothelium-derived relaxing factor
GMP	Guanosine monophosphate
HI	Hemispheric index
ICA	Internal carotid artery
ICP	Intracranial pressure
MCA	Middle cerebral artery
MEP	Multimodality evoked potentials
MTT	Mean transit time
NMDA	N-methyl-D-aspartate
NO	Nitric oxide
PGI_2	Prostacyclin
PVI	Pressure-volume index
SAH	Subarachnoid hemorrhage
$TBXA_2$	Thromboxane A_2
TCD	Transcranial doppler
TSAH	Traumatic subarachnoid hemorrhage
ECE	Endothelin-converting enzyme
L-NAME	N-nitro-L-arginine methyl ether
UPR	Volume–pressure ratio

REFERENCES

J. Astrup, *J. Neurosurg.*, 56(4): 482–497 (1982).

P. Barzo, A. Marmarou, P. Fatouros, K. Hayasaki, and F. Corwin, *Acta Neurochir.*, 70, 119–122 (1997).

D. P. Becker, J. D. Miller, J. D. Ward, R. P. Greenberg, H. F. Young, and R. Sakalas, *J. Neurosurg.*, 47(4), 491–502 (1977).

J. Beckman, T. Beckman, J. Chen, P. Marshall, and B. Freeman, *Proc. Natl. Acad. Sci USA.*, 87, 1620–1624 (1990).

M. Bergsneider, D. A. Hovda, E. Shalmon, D. F. Kelly, P. M. Vespa, and N. A. Martin et al., *J. Neurosurg.*, 86(2), 241–251 (1997).

G. Bouma, "Cerebral Circulation After Severe Head Injury. A clinical study," Thesis. University of Amsterdam, 1993.

G. J. Bouma and J. P. Muizelaar, *J. Neurosurg.*, 73(3), 368–374 (1990).

G. J. Bouma and J. P. Muizelaar, *J. Neurotrauma*, 9 (Suppl. 1), S333–348 (1992).

G. J. Bouma, J. P. Muizelaar, S. C. Choi, P. G. Newlon, and H. F. Young, *J. Neurosurg.*, 75(5), 685–693 (1991).

H. H. Caner, A. L. Kwan, A. Arthur, A. Y. Jeng, R. W. Lappe, N. F. Kassell et al., *J. Neurosurg.*, 85(5), 917–922 (1996).

G. E. Cold and F. T. Jensen, *Acta Anaesthesiol. Scand.*, 22(3), 270–280 (1978).

F. Cortbus, P. A. Jones, J. D. Miller, I. R. Piper, and J. L. Tocher, *Acta Neurochir.*, 130(1–4), 117–124 (1994).

S. B. Cox, T. A. Woolsey, and C. M. Rovainen, *J. Cereb. Blood Flow Metab.*, 13(6), 899–913 (1993).

M. G. Davies and P. O. Hagen, *Ann. Surg.*, 218(5), 593–609 (1993).

D. Denny-Brown, *Selected Writings of Sir Charles Sherrington*. Oxford University Press, Oxford, 1979.

J. Eccles and W. Gibson, *Sherrington, His Life and Thought*. Springer International, Berlin, 1979.

H. M. Eisenberg, H. E. Gary, Jr., E. F. Aldrich, C. Saydjari, B. Turner, M. A. Foulkes et al., *J. Neurosurg.*, 73(5), 688–698 (1990).

J. Ekstedt, *J. Neurol., Neurosurg. Psychiatry*, 41(4), 345–353 (1978).

E. F. Ellis, L. Y. Dodson, and R. J. Police, *J. Neurosurg.*, 75(5), 774–779 (1991).

E. M. Enevoldsen, G. Cold, F. T. Jensen, and R. Malmros, *J. Neurosurg.*, 44(2), 191–214 (1976).

E. M. Enevoldsen and F. T. Jensen, *J. Neurosurg.*, 48(5), 689–703 (1978).

C. Fieschi, N. Battistini, A. Beduschi, L. Boselli, and M. Rossanda, *J. Neurol., Neurosurg. Psychiatry*, 37(12), 1378–1388 (1974).

T. Fukuda, M. Hasue, and H. Ito, *Neurosurgery*, 43(5), 1040–1049 (1998).

R. F. Furchgott and J. V. Zawadzki, *Nature*, 288(5789), 373–376 (1980).

J. Garthwaite, S. L. Charles, and R. Chess-Williams, *Nature*, 336(6197), 385–388 (1988).

P. J. Goadsby, H. Kaube, and H. L. Hoskin, *Brain Res.*, 595(1), 167–170 (1992).

M. F. Gonzalez and F. R. Sharp, *J. Comp. Neurol.*, 231(4), 457–472 (1985).

S. P. Gopinath, C. S. Robertson, C. F. Contant, C. Hayes, Z. Feldman, R. K. Narayan et al., *J. Neurol., Neurosurg. Psychiatry*, 57(6), 717–723 (1994).

D. I. Graham, I. Ford, J. H. Adams III, D. Doyle, G. M. Teasdale, A. E. Lawrence, et al., *J. Neurol., Neurosurg. Psychiatry*, 52(3), 346–350 (1989).

D. Heistad and H. Kontos, in Sheperd, J., and Abboud, F. Eds. *Handbook of Physiology, Section 2. The Cardiovascular System*, Vol. 3. American Physiologic Society, Bethesda: 1983, pp. 137–182.

H. Hirose, K. Ide, T. Sasaki, R. Takahashi, M. Kobayashi, F. Ikemoto et al., *Eur. J. Pharmacol.*, 277(1), 77–87 (1995).

D. A. Hovda, S. M. Lee, M. L. Smith, S. Von Stuck, M. Bergsneider, D. Kelly et al., *J. Neurotrauma*, 12(5), 903–906 (1995).

M. L. Hudak, M. D. Jones, Jr., A. S. Popel, R. C. Koehler, R. J. Traystman, and S. L. Zeger, *Am. J. Physiol.*, 257(3 Pt. 2), H912–H917 (1989).

L. Ignarro, R. Byrns, and K. Wood, *Circulation*, 74(4, Suppl. 2), 287 (1986).

L. W. Jenkins, K. Moszynski, B. G. Lyeth, W. Lewelt, D. S. DeWitt, A. Allen et al., *Brain Res.*, 477(1–2), 211–224 (1989).

T. Jones, *J. Neurosurg.*, 54, 773–782 (1981).

G. Kellie, *Trans. Med. Chir. Soc. Edinburgh*, 84–169 (1824).

M. R. Klauber, L. F. Marshall, B. M. Toole, S. L. Knowlton, and S. A. Bowers, *J. Neurosurg.*, 62(4), 528–531 (1985).

H. Kontos and E. Wei, *J. Neurosci.*, 64, 803–807 (1985).

H. A. Kontos and E. P. Wei, *Ann. Biomed. Eng.*, 13(3–4), 329–334 (1985b).

H. A. Kontos, E. P. Wei, R. M. Navari, J. E. Levasseur, W. I. Rosenblum, and J. L. Patterson, Jr., *Am. J. Physiol.*, 234(4), H371–H383 (1978).

W. Kuschinsky and M. Wahl, *Physiol. Rev.*, 58(3), 656–689 (1978).

N. Lassen, *Physiol. Rev.*, 39, 183–238 (1959).

N. A. Lassen, *Lancet*, 2(7473), 1113–1115 (1966).

J. H. Lee, N. A. Martin, G. Alsina, D. L. McArthur, K. Zaucha, D. A. Hovda et al., *J. Neurosurg.*, 87(2), 221–233 (1997).

P. Macpherson and D. I. Graham, *J. Neurol., Neurosurg. Psychiatry*, 36(6), 1069–1072 (1973).

D. W. Marion, J. Darby, and H. Yonas, *J. Neurosurg.*, 74(3), 407–414 (1991).

A. Marmarou, *J. Neurotrauma*, 9 (Suppl. 1), S327–S332 (1992).

A. Marmarou, in Narayan, R. Jr. and Povlishock, J. Eds. *Neurotrauma*. New York: McGraw-Hill, 1996, pp. 413–428.

A. Marmarou, K. Shulman, and R. M. Rosende, *J. Neurosurg.*, 48(3), 332–344 (1978).

A. Marmarou, A. L. Maset, J. D. Ward, S. Choi, D. Brooks, H. A. Lutz et al., *J. Neurosurg.*, 66(6), 883–890 (1987).

A. Marmarou, R. Anderson, and J. Ward, in Hoff, J. and Betz, A. Eds., *Intracranial Pressure VII*. Springer-Verlag: New York, 1989, pp. 549–551.

L. F. Marshall and I. Gautille, *Acta Neurochir. Suppl.*, 51, 300–301 (1990).

L. F. Marshall, R. W. Smith, and H. M. Shapiro, *J. Neurosurg.*, 50(1), 26–30 (1979).

J. Martainez-Orgado, R. Gonzaalez, M. J. Alonso, M. A. Rodraiguez-Martainez, C. F. Saanchez-Ferrer, and J. Marain, *Pediat. Res.*, 44(2), 161–167 (1998).

N. A. Martin, C. Doberstein, M. Alexander, R. Khanna, H. Benalcazar, G. Alsina et al., *J. Neurotrauma*, 12(5), 897–901 (1995).

N. A. Martin, R. V. Patwardhan, M. J. Alexander, C. Z. Africk, J. H. Lee, E. Shalmon et al., *J. Neurosurg.*, 87(1), 9–19 (1997).

C. McGraw, in Hof, I. and Betz, A. Eds. *Intracranial Pressure VII*. Springer-Verlag: Berlin, 1989, pp. 839–841.

K. Messeter, C. H. Nordstreom, G. Sundbearg, L. Algotsson, and E. Ryding, *J. Neurosurg.*, 64(2), 231–237 (1986).

J. D. Miller, *Clin. Neurosurg.*, 29, 103–130 (1982).

J. D. Miller and J. D. Pickard, *Injury*, 5(3), 265–268 (1974).

J. D. Miller, J. Garibi, and J. D. Pickard, *Arch. Neurol.*, 28(4), 265–269 (1973).

A. Monro, Edinburgh, 1783.

P. Morley, D. L. Small, C. L. Murray, G. A. Mealing, M. O. Poulter, J. P. Durkin et al., *J. Cereb. Blood Flow Metab.*, 18(4), 396–406 (1998).

J. P. Muizelaar, E. P. Wei, H. A. Kontos, and D. P. Becker, *J. Neurosurg.*, 59(5), 822–828 (1983).

J. P. Muizelaar, H. A. D. Lutz, and D. P. Becker, *J. Neurosurg.*, 61(4), 700–706 (1984).

J. P. Muizelaar, E. P. Wei, H. A. Kontos, and D. P. Becker, *Stroke*, 17(1), 44–48 (1986).

J. P. Muizelaar, H. G. van der Poel, Z. C. Li, H. A. Kontos, and J. E. Levasseur, *J. Neurosurg.*, 69(6), 923–927 (1988).

J. P. Muizelaar, A. Marmarou, A. A. DeSalles, J. D. Ward, R. S. Zimmerman, Z. Li et al., *J. Neurosurg.*, 71(1), 63–71 (1989a).

J. P. Muizelaar, J. D. Ward, A. Marmarou, P. G. Newlon, and A. Wachi, *J. Neurosurg.*, 71(1), 72–76 (1989b).

J. P. Muizelaar, A. Marmarou, J. D. Ward, H. A. Kontos, S. C. Choi, D. P. Becker et al., *J. Neurosurg.*, 75(5), 731–739 (1991).

D. W. Newell, J. P. Weber, R. Watson, R. Aaslid, and H. R. Winn, *Neurosurgery*, 39(1), 35–43; discussion 43–44 (1996).

D. W. Newell, R. Aaslid, R. Stooss, R. W. Seiler, and H. J. Reulen, *Acta Neurochir.*, 139(9), 804–817 (1997).

B. Nilsson, S. Rehncrona, and B. Siesjo, in Purves, M. Ed., *Cerebral Vascular Smooth Muscle and its Control*. Ciba Foundation Symposium. Elsevier, Amsterdam, 1978, pp. 119–218.

W. D. Obrist, T. W. Langfitt, J. L. Jaggi, J. Cruz, and T. A. Gennarelli, *J. Neurosurg.*, 61(2), 241–253 (1984).

J. Overgaard and W. A. Tweed, *J. Neurosurg.*, 41(5), 531–541 (1974).

L. N. Pierre, A. P. Davenport, and Z. S Katusic, *Stroke*, 30(3), 638–643 (1999).

R. M. Rapoport and F. Murad, *Circ. Res.*, 52(3), 352–357 (1983).

C. Robertson, in Narayan, R. Jr. and Povlishock, J. Eds., *Neurotrauma*. McGraw-Hill, New York, 1996, pp. 487–501.

M. J. Rosner, *Neurosurg. Clin. N. Am.*, 6(4), 761–773 (1995).

M. J. Rosner, *Crit. Care Med.*, 24(7), 1274; discussion 1275–1276 (1996).

M. J. Rosner, S. D. Rosner, and A. H. Johnson, *J. Neurosurg.*, 83(6), 949–962 (1995).

S. Roux, B. M. Leoffler, G. A. Gray, U. Sprecher, M. Clozel, and J. P. Clozel, *Neurosurgery*, 37(1), 78–85; discussion 85–86 (1995).

G. M. Rubanyi, *Am. J. Physiol.*, 255(4 Pt. 2), H783–H788 (1988).

G. M. Rubanyi, A. D. Freay, K. Kauser, A. Johns, and D. R. Harder, *Blood Vessels*, 27(2–5) 246–257 (1990).

M. Schroder, "Early Ischemia After Severe Head Injury in Humans," Clinical study, Vrije Universiteit Amsterdam, 1994.

M. L. Schroder, J. P. Muizelaar, P. P. Fatouros, A. J. Kuta, and S. C. Choi, *Neurosurgery*, 42(6), 1276–1280; discussion 1280–1281 (1998).

V. Seifert, B. M. Leoffler, M. Zimmermann, S. Roux, and D. Stolke, *J. Neurosurg.*, 82(1), 55–62 (1995).

K. Shapiro, A. Marmarou, and K. Shulman, *Ann. Neurol*, 7(6), 508–514 (1980).

B. K. Siesjo, *J. Neurosurg.*, 60(5), 883–908 (1984).

P. Skippen, M. Seear, K. Poskitt, J. Kestle, D. Cochrane, G. Annich et al., *Crit. Care Med.*, 25, 1402–1409 (1997).

C. G. Sobey and F. M. Faraci, *Clin. Exp. Pharmacol. Physiol.*, 25(11), 867–876 (1998).

K. Tanaka, *Keio J. Med.*, 45(1), 14–27 (1996).

F. P. Tiecks, C. Douville, S. Byrd, A. M. Lam, and D. W. Newell, *Stroke*, 27(7), 1177–1182 (1996).

B. H. Verweij, J. P. Muizelaar, F. C. Vinas, P. L. Peterson, Y. Xiong, and C. P. Lee, *Neurol. Res.*, 19(3), 334–339 (1997).

E. P. Wei, W. D. Dietrich, J. T. Povlishock, R. M. Navari, and H. A. Kontos, *Circ. Res.*, 46(1), 37–47 (1980).

Y. Xiong, Q. Gu, P. L. Peterson, J. P. Muizelaar, and C. P. Lee, *J. Neurotrauma*, 14(1), 23–34 (1997a).

Y. Xiong, P. L. Peterson, J. P. Muizelaar, and C. P. Lee, *J. Neurotrauma*, 14(12), 907–917 (1997b).

Y. Xiong, P. L. Peterson, B. H. Verweij, F. C. Vinas, J. P. Muizelaar, and C. P. Lee, *J. Neurotrauma*, 15(7), 531–544 (1998).

M. Yoshihara, K. Bandoh, and A. Marmarou, *J. Neurosurg.*, 82(3), 386–393 (1995).

R. Zimmerman, J. Muizelaar, E. Wei, and H. Kontos, in J. Cervos-Navarro and R. Ferszt, Eds. *Stroke and Microcirculation*. Raven Press: New York, 1987, pp. 303–309.

M. Zimmermann, *J. Neurosurg. Sci.*, 41(2), 139–151 (1997).

M. Zimmermann and V. Seifert, *Zentrabl. Neurochir.*, 57(3), 143–149 (1996).

M. Zimmermann and V. Seifert, *Neurosurgery*, 43(4), 863–875; discussion 875–876 (1998).

M. Zimmermann, V. Seifert, B. M. Leoffler, D. Stolke, and W. Stenzel, *Neurosurgery*, 38(1), 115–120 (1996).

M. Zuccarello, A. Romano, M. Passalacqua, and R. M. Rapoport, *Am. J. Physiol.*, 269(3 Pt. 2), H1009–H1015 (1995).

PART III

CLINICAL DIRECTIONS

CHAPTER 15

THE EPIDEMIOLOGY AND ECONOMICS OF HEAD TRAUMA

DAVID J. THURMAN

Rehabilitation Research and Disability Prevention, National Center for Injury Prevention and Control, Atlanta, Georgia

INTRODUCTION

Since the late 1970's, head trauma—or, more specifically, traumatic brain injury (TBI)—has been a focus of epidemiological research. In this time, studies of the incidence, causes, and consequences of TBI have established that it is a major public health problem, one that deserves ongoing surveillance and dedicated prevention efforts (Committee on Trauma Research, 1985; U.S. Department of Health and Human Services, 1989). The purpose of this chapter is to describe what is known of the epidemiology of head trauma: the number of people who are affected, the associated risk factors and external causes, and the distribution of severity and outcome of TBI in populations. Based on epidemiological data, this chapter will also include estimates of the economic impact of TBI in the United States.

Definitions

The primary epidemiological measure examined in this review is the *incidence rate*, that is, the number of people with onset of the condition in a defined population within a defined time interval, for example, 50 TBI-related deaths per 100,000 population per year. The incidence rate is a measure of risk. A related epidemiological measure is *prevalence*, a proportion reflecting the distribution of people in a defined population who are living with the condition or its effects at a given time, for example, 2 percent of the U.S. population living with TBI-related disability. *Population-based* research is necessary to measure incidence and prevalence, using methods to enumerate the occurrence or presence of the condition either in the entire population of interest or in a representative sample of the population.

Head Trauma: Basic, Preclinical, and Clinical Directions, Edited by Leonard P. Miller and Ronald L. Hayes, Co-edited by Jennifer K. Newcomb
ISBN 0-471-36015-5 © 2001 John Wiley & Sons, Inc.

Population-based epidemiological research should be distinguished clearly from descriptive studies based on hospital case series, which constitute most of the clinical literature on traumatic brain injuries. Such case series may not be representative of the entire population of persons with brain injury. While they may provide important information about causes and outcomes, they usually cannot accurately describe incidence rates and may not accurately describe the population distribution of risk factors, causes, severity, and other characteristics of interest. Hence, the extensive literature describing non-population-based case series is not reviewed in this chapter.

In both epidemiological studies and *surveillance*, which is the ongoing systematic collection and analysis of information to monitor health problems (Buehler, 1998), accurate measurements or estimates of incidence and prevalence require valid *case definitions* of the condition—practical and consistent criteria for including cases in the study—as well as valid and consistent methods for ascertaining cases. Similarly, the accurate measurement of risk factors, severity, and outcome requires the collection of data based on valid and reliable definitions of these characteristics. In published studies of traumatic brain injury during the last two decades, case definitions, case ascertainment methods, and data element definitions have varied substantially. In 1995, in response to such limitations of previous studies of TBI incidence, the U.S. Centers for Disease Control and Prevention (CDC) published *Guidelines for Surveillance of Central Nervous System Injury* (Thurman et al., 1995) to provide standard definitions of traumatic brain and spinal cord injuries. The clinical case definition of *traumatic brain injury* (craniocerebral trauma) can be summarized as an occurrence of injury to the head (arising from blunt or penetrating trauma or from acceleration–deceleration forces) that is associated with symptoms or signs attributable to the injury—decreased level of consciousness, amnesia, other neurological or neuropsychological abnormalities, skull fracture, diagnosed intracranial lesions—or death. The *Guidelines* also provide a standard TBI case definition for data systems. This definition includes *International Classification of Diseases, Ninth Revision* (ICD-9) (WHO, 1977) or *International Classification of Diseases, Ninth Revision, Clinical Modification* (ICD-9-CM) (U.S. Department of Health and Human Services, 1989) diagnostic codes in the ranges 800.0–801.9, 803.0–804.9, and 850.0–854.1 for cases regardless of survival status, and the additional diagnostic codes 873.0–873.9, 905.0, and 907.0 for cases resulting in death. In addition, the *Guidelines* define data elements necessary to describe the occurrence and severity of these injuries, their external causes, and associated risk factors. The core of these data elements can be obtained from hospital discharge reports, which are readily available to most state health departments. The most recently published epidemiological studies of TBI in the United States have used these standards.

OVERVIEW OF STUDIES OF TBI INCIDENCE

TBI-related Hospital Admissions and Deaths—United States

Table 15.1 summarizes the incidence rates reported in selected epidemiological studies of TBI-related hospitalizations or TBI-related hospitalizations and death in

TABLE 15.1   Selected U.S. Studies of TBI Incidence

Year(s) Studied	Locality	Incidence Rate	Reference
1935–1974	Olmsted Co., Minnesota	193[b]	Annegers et al. (1980)
1974	United States	200[a]	Kalsbeek et al. (1980)
1978	San Diego Co., California	294[b]	Klauber et al. (1981)
1978	North Central Virginia	175[a]	Jagger et al. (1984)
1979–1980	Inner-city Chicago, Illinois	403[b]	Whitman et al. (1984)
1979–1980	Rhode Island	152[a]	Fife et al. (1986)
1977–1981	United States	136[a]	Fife (1987)
1980–1981	Bronx, New York	249[b]	Cooper et al. (1983)
1981	San Diego Co., California	180[b]	Kraus et al. (1984)
1986	Maryland	132[b]	MacKenzie et al. (1989)
1990–1992	Utah	108[b]	Thurman et al. (1996)
1991–1992	Colorado	101[b]	Gabella et al. (1997)
1990–1993	Colorado, Missouri, Oklahoma and Utah	102[b]	Centers for Disease Control and Prevention (1997)
1991–1993	Alaska	130[a]	Warren et al. (1995)
1994	Seven States[c]	92[b]	Thurman et al. (1999)

[a] TBI-related hospitalizations per 100,000 population per year.
[b] TBI-related combined hospitalizations and deaths per 100,000 population per year.
[c] Arizona, Colorado, Minnesota, Missouri, New York (excluding New York City), Oklahoma, and South Carolina.

U.S. localities. Before 1990, different case definitions for TBI and varied methods of collecting data made it difficult to compare information from these studies, combine data across studies, and thus estimate the national incidence of TBI (Kraus and McArthur, 1996). In the case definition, for example, not all studies included skull fractures without other neurological symptoms, and, as noted, some excluded immediate deaths that did not involve hospitalization. Most studies focused on limited geographic areas that were not necessarily representative of the United States as a whole. Comparisons of incidence rates among studies have also been complicated by inconsistent age adjustment.

Despite these limitations, however, the studies together suggest some broad trends in TBI incidence. In studies published before 1990, the reported annual incidence of TBI in different localities ranged from 132 to 403 injuries per 100,000 population, with the best estimate of national incidence at about 200 per 100,000 population (Kraus, 1993). Based on studies published since 1990, the national incidence of TBI-related hospitalizations and deaths appears closer to 100 per 100,000 population per year. It can be noted that recent studies that have been supported by the CDC are more easily compared, since they rely on a standard case definition and somewhat more standard methods of case ascertainment and data collection.

TBI-related Hospitalizations and Deaths—International

Table 15.2 summarizes the incidence rates reported in selected epidemiological studies of TBI-related hospitalizations or TBI-related hospitalizations and death in localities other than the United States. Varied case definitions, varying quality of national or regional health data sources, and different methods of identifying cases and collecting data make comparisons between international studies difficult. These problems are compounded in developing countries (Chiu et al., 1996). At the present time, there are too few published studies for it to be possible to form confident conclusions about TBI incidence worldwide or to describe international trends. Clearly more data are needed. To improve the quality of international data, the World Health Organization Advisory Committee on Neurotrauma Prevention has recommended standards for TBI surveillance and epidemiological studies (WHO, 1996).

Trends in TBI Incidence—United States

The apparent decline in TBI incidence rates suggested by U.S. studies has been examined in detail in two recent studies using national data. From 1979 through 1992, the TBI-associated death rate in the United States decreased 22 percent from 24.6 per 100,000 population to 19.3 per 100,000 population (Sosin et al., 1995). Most of the decrease resulted from a 42 percent decline in motor vehicle-related deaths, from 11.4 per 100,000 population in 1979 to 6.6 per 100,000 in 1992. During the same period, firearm-related TBI deaths increased 9 percent, from 7.7 per 100,000 in 1979 to 8.5 per 100,000 in 1992. Firearms use surpassed transportation crashes as the leading cause of death from TBI in 1990. Rates of TBI-associated death due to falls and other causes decreased slightly during this period. The CDC conducted a further examination of these trends through 1994, which are illustrated in Figure 15.1 (Thurman et al., 1999).

TABLE 15.2. Selected International Studies of TBI Incidence

Year(s) Studied	Locality	Incidence Rate[a]	Reference
1974	Scotland	313	Jennet and MacMillan (1981)
1974	Akershus County, Norway	236	Nestvold et al. (1988)
1979–1980	Trøndelag, Norway	200	Edna and Cappelen (1984)
1986	Aquitaine, France	281	Tiret et al. (1990)
1986–1987	Johannesburg, South Africa	316	Brown and Nell (1991) Nell and Brown (1991)
1988	New South Wales, Australia	100	Tate et al. (1998)
1988	Cantabria, Spain	91	Vasquez-Barquero et al. (1992)
1991–1992	Bangalore, India	122	Gururaj (1995)
1988–1994	Taipei, Taiwan	220	Chiu et al. (1997)

[a] TBI-related hospitalizations or combined hospitalizations and deaths per 100,000 population per year.

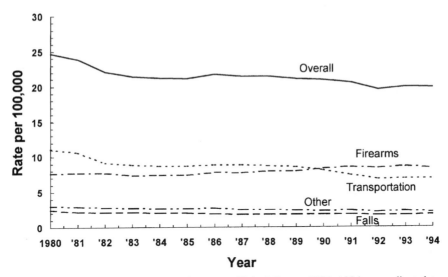

Figure 15.1   TBI-related death rates by cause, United States, 1980–1994, age-adjusted to 1990 U.S. population.

In contrast, an analysis of data from the National Hospital Discharge Surveys of 1980 through 1995 documented a steep decline of 51 percent in TBI-related hospitalization rates; they decreased from 199 to 98 per 100,000 per year over the period of this study (Thurman and Guerrero, 1999). The decline in rates of hospital admission occurred mainly among injuries classified as non-life-threatening. A comparison of findings in these two analyses indicates a disproportionately large reduction in rates of nonfatal TBI resulting in hospitalization. This decrease may reflect some success in injury prevention measures, but it appears also to be the result of recent changes in hospital admission policies that discourage inpatient care for less severe injuries. The apparent shift away from inpatient care underscores the need for surveillance of TBI patients treated in emergency departments and other outpatient settings.

RECENT EPIDEMIOLOGICAL FINDINGS FROM THE UNITED STATES

Mortality

Recent reports from the Centers for Disease Control and Prevention summarize information on TBI deaths, using data from the National Center for Health Statistics (NCHS) Multiple Cause of Death Public Use Data collected in 1994 (Thurman et al., 1999). In that year, 51,350 persons died from traumatic brain injury; most of these deaths were related to firearms, transportation (involving motor vehicle occupants, pedestrians, bicyclists, motorcyclists, and others), or falls.

In 1994, death rates among males were 3.3 times higher than among females (30.7 per 100,000 males compared with 9.3 per 100,000 females) (Fig. 15.2a). Rates were highest among persons aged 75 years and older, with a smaller peak among those aged 15–24 years.

The leading causes of TBI-associated death among males varied with age (Fig. 15.2b). Firearm-related injuries were the leading cause of TBI-associated death among males 15 to 84 years of age; transportation-related injuries among those under 15 years of age; and falls among those 85 years of age and older. For females, the leading causes of TBI-related deaths also varied with age (Fig. 15.2c). Transportation-related injuries were the leading cause of TBI among females from

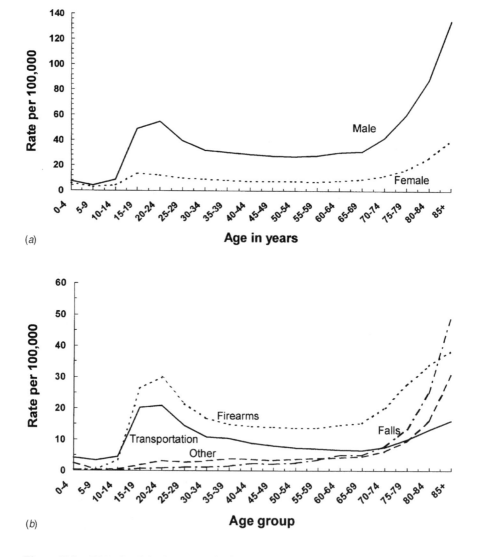

Figure 15.2   TBI-related death rates, United States, 1994, by age and sex (a) and by age and cause for males (b) and females (c). Note the different y-axis scales for males and females.

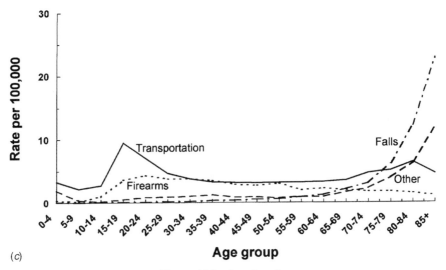

(c)

Age group

Figure 15.2   (*continued*).

birth to 74 years of age, although the death rates for firearms and transportation were almost identical among women aged 30 to 54 years. As in the older male population, falls were the leading cause of TBI-associated death among women 75 years of age and older.

TBI-associated death rates in 1994 differed by race as well (Fig. 15.3): 25.5 per 100,000 for African Americans; 19.0 per 100,000 for whites; and 15.3 per 100,000 for all other racial groups combined. Among African Americans, injury from firearm use was the leading cause of TBI-associated death, with a rate of 13.6 per 100,000. This rate was more than two times higher than the rate for injuries related to transportation, the next leading cause among African Americans. Firearm-related injuries were also the leading cause of TBI-associated death among whites, with a rate of 7.9 deaths per 100,000—just slightly higher than the transportation-related rate (7.3 per 100,000). Injury related to transportation was the leading cause of TBI-associated death among all other racial groups (6.1 per 100,000).

Morbidity and Mortality

Since 1990, CDC has supported statewide surveillance of TBI-related hospital-izations and deaths in several states, using standard case definitions and methods noted above. An epidemiological analysis of TBIs occurring in 1994 in Arizona, Colorado, Minnesota, Missouri, Oklahoma, New York State (excluding New York City), and South Carolina is included in the report cited above (Thurman et al., 1999).

The crude annual incidence rate of TBI for all seven states combined was 90.9 per 100,000 population (91.8 per 100,000, age-adjusted to the 1990 U.S. population).

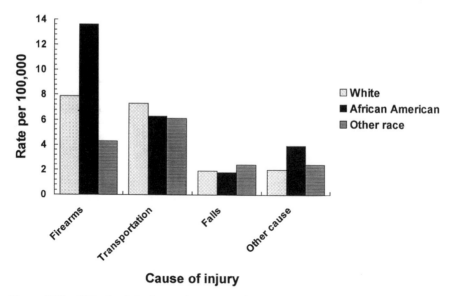

Figure 15.3   TBI-related death rates by cause and race, United States, 1994, age-adjusted to 1990 U.S. population.

The crude rate of hospitalizations for TBI in the seven states combined was 75.5 per 100,000. The overall TBI-related death rate was 20.5 per 100,000 (20.7 per 100,000, age-adjusted) (Fig. 15.4). The median age at the time of injury was 32 years. The incidence rate of TBI was highest among persons 75 years of age and older (191.1 per 100,000) and among persons 15 to 24 years (145.1 per 100,000) (Fig. 15.5). Most TBIs (66.7 percent) occurred among males, with the rate among males being about twice the rate among females (124.1 and 59.1 per 100,000, respectively).

Transportation-related crashes (involving motor vehicles, bicycles, pedestrians, and recreational vehicles) accounted for 49 percent of all TBIs; falls accounted for an additional 26 percent (Fig. 15.6). Firearm use accounted for 10 percent of all TBIs in the seven states, and assaults not involving firearms accounted for 8 percent of reported injuries. Nearly two-thirds of firearm-related TBIs (66.5 percent) were classified as suicidal in intent (Fig. 15.7). The leading causes of TBI varied by age in the seven states. Falls were by far the leading cause of TBI among persons aged 75 years and older (at a rate of 126.6 per 100,000), whereas transportation-related crashes led the list for persons aged 15 to 24 years (97.9 per 100,000) (Fig. 15.8).

The consistency of findings in these seven states, located in different regions of the United States, suggests that these data are fairly representative of the U.S. population. The incidence of TBI described in this report also resembles that from an analysis of National Hospital Discharge Survey (NHDS) data. The crude TBI-related hospitalization rate estimated from the NHDS data was 94 per 100,000 population (Thurman et al., 1999). The combined TBI-related hospitalization rate obtained from Arizona, Colorado, Minnesota, Missouri, New York State, Oklahoma, and South

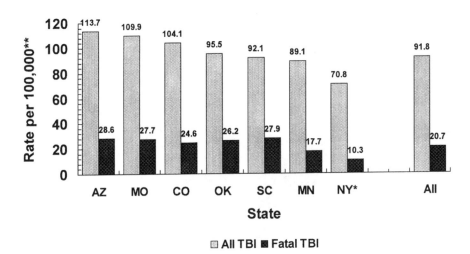

Figure 15.4   Rates of TBI-related hospitalization and death, seven states (Arizona, Colorado, Minnesota, Missouri, New York (excluding New York City), Oklahoma, and South Carolina), 1994.

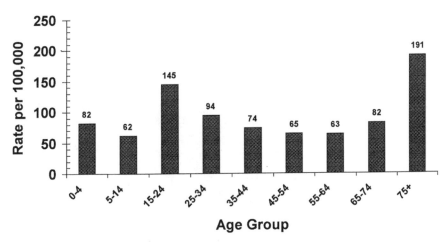

Figure 15.5   Rates of TBI-related hospitalization and death by age group, seven states (Arizona, Colorado, Minnesota, Missouri, New York (excluding New York City), Oklahoma, and South Carolina), 1994.

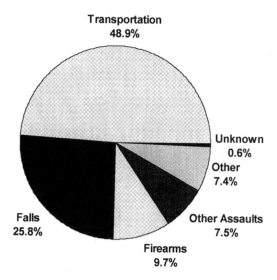

Figure 15.6   Rates of TBI-related hospitalization and death by external cause of injury, seven states [Arizona, Colorado, Minnesota, Missouri, New York (excluding New York City), Oklahoma, and South Carolina], 1994.

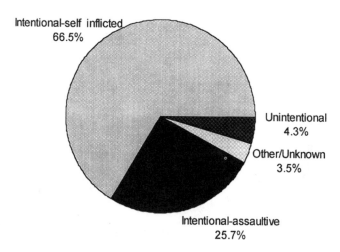

Figure 15.7   Proportion of firearm-related TBI by intent, seven states (Arizona, Colorado, Minnesota, Missouri, New York (excluding New York City), Oklahoma, and South Carolina), 1994.

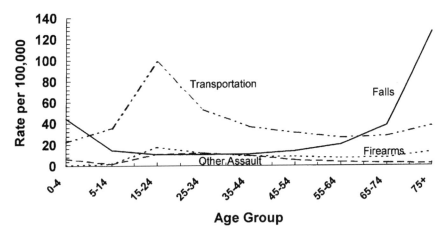

Figure 15.8 Rates of TBI-related hospitalization and death by age group and external cause of injury, seven states [Arizona, Colorado, Minnesota, Missouri, New York (excluding New York City), Oklahoma, and South Carolina], 1994.

Carolina is approximately 20 percent lower than the corresponding rate estimated from the NHDS. This moderate divergence in rates may be explained in part by (1) the lack of adjustment in the NHDS for repeated hospital admissions and inter-hospital transfers, (2) differences in sampling methods between the statewide enumerations of injuries in seven states and the NHDS sample of 478 hospitals across the United States (NCHS, 1997), and (3) perhaps other differences in methods that have not yet been elucidated.

Nonfatal TBIs Not Admitted to Hospitals

In the United States, the National Center for Health Statistics National Health Interview Survey (NHIS) has provided some information on the incidence of TBI treated on an outpatient basis (Sosin et al., 1996). In 1991, an estimated 1.54 million noninstitutionalized U.S. civilians sustained a brain injury that resulted in loss of consciousness but was not severe enough to cause death or long-term institutiona-lization, according to self-reported NHIS data collected with the 1991 Injury Supplement. Of these 1.54 million persons, 25 percent received no medical care for their TBI, 49 percent received care in an emergency department or other outpatient site, 9 percent received overnight hospital care, and 16 percent were admitted to a hospital for two or more days.

Limitations of the NHIS telephone survey methods—especially recall bias—may limit the accuracy of these estimates. A more recent study, using data from the National Hospital Ambulatory Medical Care Surveys of 1995–1996, may provide a more accurate estimate of the incidence of nonfatal TBIs that are treated and released from hospital emergency departments (EDS) (Guerrero et al., 2000) This analysis indicates an average annual incidence rate of such ED visits of 392 per 100,000

TABLE 15.3   Average Annual Incidence Rate of ED Visits Associated with TBI—United States, 1995–1996[a]

	Incidence Rate[b]	Estimated number[c] (%)[d]
Age (years)		
0–14	692	411 (40)
15–24	567	206 (20)
25–44	313	260 (25)
45+	180	149 (15)
Sex		
Female	306	412 (40)
Male	479	615 (60)
External cause		
Motor vehicle	86	225 (22)
Fall	123	322 (31)
Struck (unintentional)	80	209 (20)
Intentional	59	155 (15)
Other/unknown	44	116 (11)
Total	392	1027

[a] From Guerrero et al. (in preparation).
[b] Rate per 100,000 population per year.
[c] Numbers in thousands.
[d] Percent in categories of age, sex, or external cause.

population or about 1 million visits in the United States each year. Table 15.3 summarizes the incidence estimates of this study by age, sex, and external cause.

Severity and Outcome

Measures of severity made early in the clinical course of TBI have value in predicting longer-term outcomes. Several measures of TBI severity have been used in epidemiological studies. The simplest epidemiological measure of severity (and also outcome) is the proportion of cases that result in death, or the *case-fatality rate*. In the study of TBI-related hospitalizations and deaths in seven states during 1994, a total of 22.6 percent of all reported TBIs were fatal within the acute period of injury. Of all reported TBIs, 16.9 percent of cases died without being admitted to a hospital, while 5.6 percent died while receiving acute inpatient care. Further analysis revealed that this measure of severity varied greatly, depending on the cause. For example, 90.4 percent of firearm-related TBIs resulted in death, but only 10.2 percent of fall-related TBIs proved fatal (Fig. 15.9).

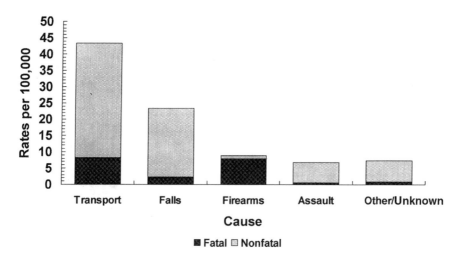

Figure 15.9   Rates of TBI-related hospitalization and death by external cause of injury and survival status, seven states (Arizona, Colorado, Minnesota, Missouri, New York (excluding New York City), Oklahoma, and South Carolina), 1994.

The case-fatality rate is of limited use for predicting long-term disability in populations. Thus, graded measures of severity have also been proposed for epidemiological studies of TBI. The Glasgow Coma Scale (GCS) is a widely used clinical measure of severity that assesses level of consciousness following TBI; valid GCS scores range from 3 (deep coma) to 15 (full alertness) (Teasdale and Jennett, 1974, 1976). The GCS, measured at the time of hospital admission, has been used in several epidemiological studies (Kraus, 1993). For example, in San Diego County in 1981, 82 percent of hospitalized cases were "mild" (GCS score 13–15), 9 percent were "moderate" (GCS score 9 to 12), and 9 percent were "severe" (GCS 3 to 8) (Kraus et al., 1984).

Some research indicates that the prediction of TBI outcome may be improved by supplementing GCS data with information about computed tomography (CT) brain scan findings (Williams et al., 1990). Currently, state surveillance programs in the United States collect both GCS and CT scan data, but population distributions of severity based on the combination of these data elements have not yet been published. Other research has found predictive value in the duration of posttraumatic amnesia (Levin et al., 1979). Nell and colleagues have recently proposed an enhancement of the GCS that incorporates a measure of duration of posttraumatic amnesia in persons with little or no depression of consciousness (Nell et al., 2000). Population-based studies that describe TBI severity with these measures have not yet been published.

Another severity classification used in recent epidemiological studies of TBI is ICDMAP-90© (Center for Injury Research and Policy, 1997), a computer algorithm that maps ICD-9-CM diagnostic codes to a six-level severity scale (ICD/AIS) that approximates the Abbreviated Injury Severity (AIS) Scale (Association for the

Advancement of Automotive Medicine, 1990). The analysis of recent trends of TBI incidence in the United States noted earlier used ICDMAP to estimate the severity distributions of hospitalized cases (Thurman and Guerrero, 1999). From the analysis of National Hospital Discharge Survey data collected in 1994–1995, 52 percent were "mild" (ICD/AIS score 1 or 2), 21 percent were "moderate" (ICD/AIS score 3), 19 percent were "severe" (ICD/AIS score 4 to 6), and 7 percent were unknown. The proportion of TBIs classified as "mild" among these 1994–1995 NHDS cases is considerably smaller than the proportion of TBIs classified as "mild" among 1980–1981 cases, described in the same report; it is also smaller than proportions reported in earlier studies (Kraus and McArthur, 1996). These findings indicate that a smaller proportion of less severe TBIs in the United States are now being admitted to hospitals.

Incidence of TBI-related Disability

There are few studies addressing the incidence of TBI-related disability. From the limited epidemiological data available, Kraus has estimated that about 83,000 or more U.S. residents were disabled by TBI in 1990 (Kraus and McArthur, 1996). The CDC has published a similar but more recent estimate based on 1994 data from the NHDS and 1996–1997 data from the Colorado TBI Registry and Follow-up System (Brooks et al., 1997). The latter system surveyed TBI survivors one year after injury and measured long-term disability by using the Functional Independence Measure (Research Foundation, 1995). NHDS data indicate that, during 1994, 230,000 persons hospitalized with TBI survived, and data from the Colorado TBI Registry and Follow-up System indicate that approximately 35 percent of hospitalized survivors of TBI are disabled one year after injury. This suggests that more than 80,000 persons in the United States experience the onset of long-term disability each year following hospitalization for TBI. This estimate may be conservative, since it does not include the unknown number persons with TBI who are not hospitalized but who may also experience long-term disability as a consequence of their injury.

Prevalence of TBI-related Disability

The prevalence of TBI-related disability is the proportion of persons in the population at a given time who have disability resulting from a traumatic brain injury. The lack of confident estimates of the incidence of TBI-related disability makes estimating prevalence even more difficult. In 1990, Willer and colleagues reviewed the subject and concluded that the best estimate then possible could be derived from the Health and Activity Limitation Survey in Canada, yielding a prevalence estimate of 74 per 100,000 (Willer et al., 1990). More recently, the CDC has estimated the prevalence of disability from TBI in the United States, using a model that incorporates data on the incidence of TBI, severity of injury, and likelihood of disability given a specific level of injury severity (Thurman et al., 1999; Guerrero et al., in preparation) Data for this model came from the following sources:

- National Hospital Discharge Survey data for 1970–1995. These data were used to estimate TBI incidence during these years, stratified by level of severity using ICDMAP-90$^{©}$.

- Preliminary follow-up data from the Colorado TBI Registry and Follow-up System. The probability of long-term disability within each severity stratum was estimated using Functional Independence Measure data. These probabilities were applied to TBI incidence estimates for 1980 or after; for injuries that occurred before 1980, the CDC used historical data reviewed by Kraus (Kraus and McArthur, 1996).

Based on this model, CDCs National Center for Injury Prevention and Control estimated that, in 1996, 5.3 million U.S. citizens (2 percent of the population) were living with disability as a result of a traumatic brain injury. This estimate is preliminary. It does not account for disability among people with TBI who visited emergency departments or outpatient clinics but were not admitted to the hospital. Limitations of existing data and methods may also compromise the accuracy of this estimate, leading to the expectation that substantial changes in future estimates of the prevalence of TBI-related disability are likely.

ESTIMATES OF ECONOMIC COSTS

Information about the economic costs of brain injury, when compared to estimates of costs of other health conditions, is important for making decisions about allocating resources for injury prevention, acute care, and rehabilitation. Knowledge of the current cost to society of TBI is limited. There are a few published studies of the cost of these injuries, mainly based on TBI incidence data and health care utilization and expenditure data collected in the 1980s. Max and colleagues analyzed U.S. incidence and cost data for 1985 TBIs that resulted in hospital admission or death (Max et al., 1991). They estimated that the total costs incurred over the lifetimes of those injured were approximately $37.8 billion. Their estimate included $4.5 billion in direct costs of medical care (hospital, extended, and other medical care and services); $20.6 billion in injury-related work loss and disability; and $12.7 billion in lost income resulting from premature death. A more recent study adjusted these estimates for inflation, yielding total costs of $48.3 billion in 1991 dollars (Lewin-ICF, 1992). To the extent that actual incidence rates of TBI remain relatively constant over time, and provided adjustments are made for inflation, such lifetime cost estimates may approximate annual costs of TBI to society.

Using different methods that analyze fatalities, hospital admissions, and emergency department visits, Miller and colleagues also estimated costs of TBI, based on national data collected in the United States between 1979 and 1989 (Miller, 1994). While their estimate of the annual direct costs of medical care for these injuries was similar—$5.8 billion in 1992 dollars—their estimate of total costs was much higher. In calculating total costs, they not only considered lost productivity, emergency service costs, funeral expenses, and legal and administrative costs, but also the cost of lost quality of life. By their report, lost quality of life accounts for more than two-thirds of the comprehensive costs of TBI. Taking all these factors into account, they estimated that TBIs in the United States each year result in total costs of $174 billion for nonfatal injuries and $100.8 billion for fatal injuries.

These studies are dated. A current study of TBI costs in the United States is needed to address recent changes in TBI incidence and health care practices. Until such a study is completed, the more conservative estimates provided by Max and co-workers may be updated by using incidence information from 1995 and adjusting for inflation as shown in Table 15.4, yielding a total cost estimate of $56 billion. There are limitations of this revised estimate. From available published data, it cannot separate direct costs of medical care from indirect morbidity and mortality costs, stratified by level of severity and, thus, does not take into account the additional inflation of medical care costs from 1985 to 1995. This estimate also does not take into account those TBIs treated only in hospital emergency departments, and it does not address the cost of lost quality of life. Thus, this estimate of $56.3 billion in total direct and indirect costs of TBI in the United States in 1995 may be conservative.

PREVENTION OF TBI

The frequency and severity of TBI in the population make it evident that the prevention of these injuries is of paramount importance to public health. The data reviewed consistently identify the following major causes of TBI toward which prevention efforts should be concentrated.

- *Motor Vehicle Crashes*. Transportation crashes are the leading cause of TBI-associated death among women and among persons under 15 years of age. Fortunately, the rate of TBI-associated death caused by transportation crashes in the United States has decreased approximately 40 percent since 1980. This drop is likely due to a combination of factors: an increase in seat belt and child safety seat use; an increase in the number of vehicles equipped with air bags; and a decrease in the incidence of impaired driving. Such positive changes deserve further support.
- *Firearms*. Violence is a leading cause of TBI in the United States—especially among males—and violence with firearms is the leading cause of TBI-associated death. Effective programs designed to decrease the occurrence of self-directed and interpersonal violence are critically needed.
- *Falls*. Falls are the third leading cause of TBI-associated death. Among women over 75 years of age and men over 85 years of age, falls are the leading cause of TBI-associated death. Falls are also a major cause of nonfatal TBI. Risk factors for falls among older persons may include the use of sedatives, antidepressants, or other psychotropic medications; and impairments of balance or lower extremity function. Although better data are needed to

TABLE 15.4 Estimated Lifetime Costs of TBI in the United States, 1995

TBI Severity	Estimated Cost per Injury		Estimated Incidence		Estimated Total Cost (millions of dollars) 1995[e]
	1985[a]	1995[b]	Rate, 1994–1995[c]	Number, 1995[d]	
Nonfatal					
Mild/unknown	$77,292	$109,473	58	152,476	$16,700
Moderate	$80,755	$114,378	21	55,207	$6,300
Severe	$141,377	$200,240	14[f]	36,805	$7,400
Fatal	$356,966	$505,591	19.5	51,263	$25,900
Total					$56,300

[a]From Max et al. (1991).
[b]Calculated by multiplying the 1985 estimated cost by the Consumer Price Index (CPI) ratio: (CPI 1995)/(CPI 1985) = 1.4164, obtained from the U.S. Bureau of Labor Statistics.
[c]Incidence rates per 100,000 population.
[d]Calculated by multiplying estimated rate (Thurman and Guerrero, 1999) by the estimate of the U.S. population in 1995 (262,889,634) from the U.S. Bureau of the Census.
[e]Calculated by multiplying 1995 estimated cost by 1995 estimated number, result rounded to nearest hundred million.
[f]Calculated by subtracting estimated incidence of fatal hospitalized TBI from estimated incidence of severe hospitalized TBI.

define the circumstances of fall injuries among older persons, effective interventions may involve modifying the environment to reduce fall hazards and the impacts of falls and, where possible, reducing the use of medications with side effects that increase the risk of falling.

To a large extent, the same measures that prevent traumatic brain injury also prevent other kinds of injury. Thus, broader strategies that effect general injury prevention and control, of which Rivara and colleagues have recently published a comprehensive review (Rivara et al., 1997a,b), have great relevance to brain injury prevention.

PUBLIC HEALTH AND THE PREVENTION OF TBI-RELATED DISABILITY

When the primary prevention of TBI occurrence fails, an effective public health response to TBI requires concerted programs to minimize adverse outcomes and disability. Basic and clinical research to improve the acute care and rehabilitation of persons with TBI is the subject of other chapters in this book, but the development of strategies to ensure that people with TBI have access to appropriate care and services and the development of policies to promote their independence and integration into the community are appropriate public health concerns.

To help persons living with the effects of TBI, we need better information on the nature and scope of these disabilities, including who experiences disability, which rehabilitation treatment methods are most effective, and what services are useful and readily available. Population-based follow-up surveillance is needed to provide more precise information on the longer-term impacts of these injuries. Standard measures for TBI outcomes need to be refined so that they will readily identify the adverse outcomes most amenable to prevention through rehabilitation and social support. A persons long-term outcome is related to the severity of the TBI. Better defining the relationship between the initial severity of an injury and a person's long-term outcome will help identify those persons who need ongoing medical care, rehabilitation, and other services. Such information will also help health practitioners and policy makers ensure that these services are available in the community.

To this end, with CDC support, the Colorado Department of Public Health and Environment, Craig Hospital in Denver, and the South Carolina Department of Disabilities and Special Needs are developing population-based follow-up registries of persons with TBI. Designed as models for other states, these registries will better define the proportion of persons with various outcomes associated with TBI, the services to which persons with TBI have been referred, and the services that have actually been delivered. Population-based state registries may also be useful in linking people with TBI to the services they need.

CONCLUSIONS

This chapter has reviewed epidemiological measures and estimates of traumatic brain injury incidence, severity, long-term outcomes, and cost. All of these findings indicate that TBI has a major impact on public health. Effective primary prevention programs are needed that are informed by accurate information regarding causes and populations at highest risk. More basic and clinical research is needed to improve the acute care and rehabilitation of TBI. Finally, more epidemiological research regarding TBI outcomes and disability is needed in order to develop policies that will ensure the availability of effective acute care, rehabilitation, and other services that will minimize disability among injured persons and promote their reintegration into the community.

ABBREVIATIONS

AIS	Abbreviated Injury Severity (Scale)
CDC	Centers for Disease Control and Prevention
CPI	Consumer Price Index
CT	Computed Tomography
ED	Hospital Emergency Department
GCS	Glasgow Coma Scale
GOS	Glasgow Outcome Scale
ICD-9	International Classification of Diseases, 9th Revision
ICD-9-CM	International Classification of Diseases, 9th Revision, Clinical Modification
ICD/AIS	Estimate of Abbreviated Injury Severity Scale score generated by ICDMAP software
NCHS	National Center for Health Statistics
NHDS	National Hospital Discharge Survey
NHIS	National Health Interview Survey
TBI	Traumatic Brain Injury
WHO	World Health Organization

REFERENCES

J. F. Annegers, H. D. Grabow, L. T. Kurland et al., *Neurology*, 30, 912–919 (1980).

Association for the Advancement of Automotive Medicine, *The Abbreviated Injury Scale*, 1990 Revision, Association for the Advancement of Automotive Medicine, Des Plains, IL, 1990.

C. A. Brooks, B. Gabella, R. Hoffman, D. Sosin, and G. Whiteneck, *Arch. Phys. Med. Rehabil.*, 78, S26–S30 (1997).

D. S. O. Brown and V. Nell, *Soc. Sci. Med.*, 13(3), 283–287 (1991).

J. W. Buehler, "Surveillance," in K. J. Rothman and S. Greenland, Eds., *Modern Epidemiology*, 2nd ed., Lippincott-Raven, Philadelphia, 1998, pp. 435–457.

Center for Injury Research and Policy of the Johns Hopkins University School of Public Health, *ICDMAP-90 Software*, The Johns Hopkins University and Tri-Analytics, Inc., Baltimore, 1997.

Centers for Disease Control and Prevention, *MMWR Morbidity and Mortality Weekly Report*, 46, 8–11 (1997).

W. T. Chiu, R. E. Laporte, G. Gururaj et al., "Head Injury in Developing Countries," in R. K. Narayan, J. E. Wilberger, Jr., and J. T. Povlishock, Eds., *Neurotrauma*, McGraw-Hill, New York, 1996, pp. 36–42.

W. T. Chiu, K. H. Yeh, Y. C. Li, Y. H. Gan, H. Y. Chen, and C. C. Hung, *Neurol. Res.*, 19, 261–264 (1997).

Committee on Trauma Research, National Research Council and Institute of Medicine, *Injury in America*, National Academy Press, Washington, D.C, 1985.

K. D. Cooper, K. Tabaddor, W. A. Hauser et al., *Neuroepidemiology*, 2, 70–88 (1983).

T.-H. Edna and J. Cappelen, *Scand. J. Soc. Med.*, 12, 7–14 (1984).

D. Fife, *Am. J. Public Health*, 77, 810–812 (1987).

D. Fife, G. Faich, W. Hollinshead, and B. Wentworth, *Am. J. Public Health*, 76, 773–778 (1986).

B. Gabella, R. E. Hoffman, W. W. Marine, and L. Stallones, *Ann. Epidemiol.*, 7, 207–212 (1997).

J. Guerrero, D. J. Thurman, and J. E. Sniezek, *Brain Injury*, 14, 181–186 (2000).

J. L. Guerrero, S. Leadbetter, D. J. Thurman, G. Whiteneck, and J. E. Sniezek, "A method for estimating the prevalence of disability from traumatic brain injury," manuscript in preparation.

G. Gururaj, *Neurol. India*, 43(Suppl.), 95–106 (1995).

J. Jagger, J. I. Levine, J. A. Jane, and R. W. Rimel, *J. Trauma*, 24, 40–44 (1984).

B. Jennett and R. MacMillan, *Br. Med. J.*, 282, 101–104 (1981).

W. D. Kalsbeek, R. L. McLaurin, B. S. Harris, and J. D. Miller, *J. Neurosurg.*, 53, S19–S24 (1980).

M.R. Klauber, E. Barrett-Connor, L. F. Marshall, and S. A. Bowers, *Am. J. Epidemiol.*, 113, 500–509 (1981).

J. F. Kraus, "Epidemiology of Head Injury," in P. R. Cooper, Ed., *Head Injury*, 3rd ed., Williams and Wilkins, Baltimore, 1993, pp. 1–25.

J. F. Kraus and D. L. McArthur, *Neurol. Clin.*, 14(2), 435–450 (1996).

J. F. Kraus, M. A. Black, N. Hessol et al., *Am. J. Epidemiol.*, 119, 186–201 (1984).

H. S. Levin, V. M. O'Donnell, and R. G. Grossman, *J. Nerv. Ment. Dis.*, 167, 675–687 (1979).

Lewin-ICF, "The Cost of Disorders of the Brain," *The National Foundation for Brain Research*, Washington, D.C., 1992.

E. J. MacKenzie, S. L. Edelstein, and J. P. Flynn, *MD Med. J.*, 38, 725–732 (1989).

W. Max, E. J. MacKenzie, and D. P. Rice, *J. Head Trauma Rehabil.*, 6, 76–91 (1991).

T. R. Miller, J. B. Douglass, M. S. Galbraith, D. C. Lestina, and N. M. Pindus, "Costs of Head and Neck Injury and a Benefit-cost Analysis of Bicycle Helmets," in *Head and Neck Injury*, Society of Automotive Engineers, Inc., Warrendale, PA, 1994, pp. 211–240.

NCHS, *Data File Documentation, National Hospital Discharge Survey, 1980–1995*, National Center for Health Statistics, Centers for Disease Control and Prevention, Rockville, MD, 1997.

V. Nell and D. S. O. Brown, *Soc. Sci. Med.*, 13, 289–296 (1991).

V. Nell, D. W. Yates, and J. Kruger, *Arch. Phys. Med. Rehabil.*, 81, 614–617 (2000).

K. Nestvold, T. Lundar, G. Blikra, and A. Lannum, *Neuroepidemiology*, 7, 134–144 (1988).

Research Foundation, State University of New York. *Guide for Use of the Uniform Data Set for Medical Rehabilitation Including the Functional Independence Measure (FIM) and Functional Assessment Measure (FAM)*, version 4.0, State University of New York, Buffalo, NY, 1995.

F. P. Rivara, D. C. Grossman, and P. Cummings, *N. Engl. J. Med.*, 337, 543–548 (1997a).

F. P. Rivara, D. C. Grossman, and P. Cummings, *N. Engl. J. Med.*, 337, 613–618 (1997b).

D. M. Sosin, J. E. Sniezek, and R. J. Waxweiler, *J. Am. Med. Assoc.*, 273, 1778–1780 (1995).

D. M. Sosin, J. E. Sniezek, and D. J. Thurman, *Brain Inj.*, 10, 47–54 (1996).

R. L. Tate, S. McDonald, and J. M. Lulham, *Austr. N.Z. J. Public Health*, 22, 419–423 (1998).

G. Teasdale and B. Jennett, *Lancet*, 2, 81–84 (1974).

G. Teasdale and B. Jennett, *Acta Neurochir.*, 34, 45–55 (1976).

D. J. Thurman, J. E. Sniezek, D. Johnson et al., *Guidelines for Surveillance of Central Nervous System Injury*, Centers for Disease Control and Prevention, Atlanta, GA, 1995.

D. J. Thurman, L. Jeppson, C. L. Burnett et al., *West. J. Med.*, 164, 192–196 (1996).

D. Thurman and J. Guerrero, *J. Am. Med. Assoc.*, 282, 954–957 (1999).

D. J. Thurman, C. Alverson, K. A. Dunn, J. Guerrero, and J. E. Sniezek, *J. Head Trauma Rehabil.*, 14, 602–615 (1999).

L. Tiret, E. Hausherr, M. Thicoipe et al., *Int. J. Epidemiol.*, 19, 133–140 (1990).

U.S. Department of Health and Human Services, *International Classification of Diseases, 9th Revision, Clinical Modification*, 3rd ed. (ICD-9-CM). U.S. Department of Health and Human Services, Washington D.C., 1989.

U.S. Department of Health and Human Services, *Federal Interagency Head Injury Task Force Report*, Department of Health and Human Services, Washington, D.C., 1989.

A. Vasquez-Barquero, J. L. Vasquez-Barquero, O. Austin, J. Pascual, L. Gaite, and S. Herrera, *Eur. J. Epidemiol.*, 8, 832–837 (1992).

S. Warren, M. Moore, and M. S. Johnson, *Alaska Med.*, 37, 11–18 (1995).

S. Whitman, R. Coonley-Hoganson, and B. T. Desai, *Am. J. Epidemiol.*, 4, 560–580 (1984).

WHO, Advisory Committee on Neurotrauma Prevention, *Standards for Surveillance of Neurotrauma*, World Health Organization, Geneva, Switzerland, 1996.

WHO, *International Classification of Diseases, 9th Revision* (ICD-9), World Health Organization, Geneva, Switzerland, 1977.

B. Willer, M. A. Abosh, and E. Dahmer, "Epidemiology of Disability from Traumatic Brain Injury," in R. Wood, Ed., *Neurobehavioral Sequelae of Traumatic Brain Injury*, Taylor and Francis, London, 1990, pp. 18–33.

D. H. Williams, H. S. Levin, and H. M. Eisenberg, *Neurosurgery*, 27, 422–428 (1990).

CHAPTER 16

CLINICAL PRESENTATION AND NEUROPSYCHOLOGICAL SEQUELAE OF TRAUMATIC BRAIN INJURY

SHARON A. BROWN and HARVEY S. LEVIN

Baylor College of Medicine, Department of Physical Medicine and Rehabilitation, Houston, Texas

INTRODUCTION

The neurobehavioral sequelae following traumatic brain injury (TBI) frequently include disturbances in cognitive, emotional, social, and behavioral functioning (Brooks et al., 1986; Giacino et al., 1991; Livingston and Livingston, 1985). The behavioral and psychosocial difficulties experienced by some patients are reported as being devastating not only to the patient but to the family and society as well, and are a frequent source of the residual disability (Levin et al., 1990). The Department of Health and Human Services: Interagency Head Injury Task Force Report (1989) noted the residual disabilities (physical and neurobehavioral) of a TBI are estimated to cost the public $25 billion yearly, in terms of hospitalization, rehabilitation, and lost wages or earning potential (Hamill et al., 1986).

This chapter will provide an overview of the neuropsychological sequelae of a TBI, including cognitive, behavioral, and psychosocial functioning. The cognitive domains to be addressed include learning and memory, attention and information processing, language and intellectual functioning, executive functioning, and behavioral-psychosocial functioning.

Head Trauma: Basic Clinical, and Preclinical Directions, Edited by Leonard P. Miller and Ronald L. Hayes, Co-edited by Jennifer K. Newcomb
ISBN 0-471-36015-5 © 2001 John Wiley & Sons, Inc.

CLINICAL PRESENTATION

Of the residual deficits after severe TBI, Jennett and co-workers (1981) found cognitive and behavioral disturbances to be the primary contributors to disability in about two-thirds of patients evaluated at six months. In the other one-third of patients, focal motor deficit and other neurophysical sequelae contributed equally or predominated as compared to neurobehavioral sequelae. The degree of impaired cognitive or behavioral functioning is related to the severity of the injury.

Deficits in neuropsychological functioning after TBI is related to the region of cerebral damage. Diffuse cerebral damage and injury to orbital, frontal, and temporal regions may lead to cognitive impairment across various domains, including verbal and nonverbal memory, attention and information processing speed, intellectual functioning, language, executive functions, motor speed and coordination, and visuospatial ability. Behavioral disturbances are often present, affecting psychosocial adaptation and mood (Bendixen and Benton, 1996; Brooks et al., 1986; Girard et al., 1996; Levin, 1993).

Memory

Of all the cognitive domains that may be disrupted by the effects of a TBI, memory is the most severely affected and the most frequently reported symptom by patients and relatives (Capruso and Levin, 1996; Levin, 1995). Memory deficits in patients sustaining a severe TBI frequently produce deficits in acquisition of new information, presented verbally or visually, with selective difficulty seen in encoding (Brooks, 1974, 1975) or retrieval (Goldstein and Levin, 1986). Deficits in other cognitive domains, such as attention or executive functioning, may also have an adverse impact on learning and memory. Memory disorders after TBI are often described according to the stage of recovery and by the specific memory paradigm (e.g., declarative versus procedural). Table 16.1 lists several tests that are often used in the assessment of memory functioning by memory paradigm.

Posttraumatic Amnesia. Anterograde amnesia (impairment in ability to recall newly acquired information) characterizes the memory disorder seen in the early stages of recovery, which is frequently referred to as posttraumatic amnesia (PTA). Russell and Nathan (1946) described PTA as the interval from the time of injury to the point of remembrance of waking up. This definition was later redefined as the interval during which current events have not been stored (Russell and Smith, 1961). Recently, Stuss et al. (1999) suggested using the term posttraumatic confusional state, as it is descriptive of the confusion experienced by the patient, in whom recovery of attentional skills precedes that of the more complex task of free recall.

The duration of PTA is primarily affected by the severity of the TBI, but age and drugs administered to the patient are also contributory. Ellenberg et al. (1996) noted other factors that influence PTA duration, including older age, lower first GCS (Glasgow Coma Scale) score, nonreactive pupils, longer time in coma, and extended use of phenytoin or steroids. However, PTA can be marked by intermittent periods of

TABLE 16.1   Tests Assessing Verbal and Nonverbal Memory

Memory	Test
PTA	Galveston Orientation and Amnesia Test
	Rivermead Behavioral Memory Test
STM	Wechsler Adult Intelligence Scale Digit Span
	Wechsler Memory Scale Digit Span
	Wechsler Memory Scale Visual Memory Span
Procedural memory	Maze Learning—Porteus Mazes
	Wechsler Intelligence Scale Children-III
	Mirror Reading Test[a]
	Pursuit Rotor Test[a]
Semantic memory	Mill-Hill Vocabulary Test
	Wechsler Adult Intelligence Scale Vocabulary Test
Episodic memory	Verbal Selective Reminding Test
	Wechsler Memory Scale-Revised
	Rey Adult Verbal Learning Test
	California Verbal Learning Test
	Benton Visual Retention Test
	Rey–Osterrieth Complex Figure Test

[a] Nonstandardized tests that are used in experimental paradigms or for research purposes.

lucidity. The Galveston Orientation and Amnesia Test (GOAT) is often used to assess the duration of PTA (Levin et al., 1979). A score of 66 or less (maximum of 100) indicates that the patient is not encoding new memory for daily events, hence a persisting PTA, while a score above 75 typically correlates with return of consistent day-to-day memories and an end of PTA. Ellenberg et al. (1996) found prospective measurement of PTA duration to be an important predictor of outcome; that is, PTA was shown to be related to global outcome and/or neurobehavioral sequelae of severe TBI, and that PTA provided incremental information, apart from coma duration, in outcome prediction at discharge and at six months post injury.

Residual memory deficits after resolution of PTA have been shown to be differentially impacted by the effects of TBI. Short-term memory or immediate memory appear to be least impacted by brain injury, with performance by TBI patients comparable to or approaching the performance by control groups (Brooks, 1972; Fodor, 1972; Lezak, 1979). Levin and colleagues (1982), however, found disparate findings for sparing of short-term memory. Based on the findings from the literature, they concluded that immediate memory span, as reflected by forward digit span (repeating sequences of three to nine digits) is comparatively resistant to the effects of head injury, although disturbed functioning may be noted in the early stages of recovery from severe injuries. On the other hand, persistent deficits of short-term memory appear to be confined to backward span (reversed order of presentation of sequences two to eight numbers long) and short-term visual memory. TBI patients may also experience a period of retrograde amnesia, the inability to recall experiences predating the brain injury (Russell, 1971), although it rarely extends beyond more than two days.

Procedural Versus Declarative Memory. The domains of long-term memory are differentially impacted by the effects of a severe brain injury. Procedural memory has been shown to be relatively spared, but not declarative memory. Procedural memory concerns "how to" knowledge; it is the acquisition of skills (Lachman et al., 1979; Squire, 1987), including perceptual, motor, and intellectual skills. Declarative memory, which concerns facts about the world or events that we can recount (Lachman et al., 1979), can be further subdivided into semantic and episodic memory (Tulving, 1972). Semantic memory represents one's knowledge of words and symbols, and the relations among them. Episodic memory is memory for personal events and recaptures the temporal and spatial context of one's past experiences.

Support for the relative preservation of procedural memory comes from the work of Ewert et al. (1989). Severely injured TBI patients were studied during PTA and again after resolution of PTA. Patient performance while in PTA evidenced a reduction in reading latencies across trials for mirror-image reading of words. Maze learning performance also improved, showing a reduction for time to completion and for number of entries into blind alleys. Accuracy for tracking a rotating target showed similar gains during learning while in PTA. Transfer of learning to the post-PTA phase was confirmed on the procedural tasks. The reading times declined after resolution of PTA as compared to the last session during PTA, despite an average interval of nearly three weeks between sessions. Gains in performance on the maze and pursuit rotor tasks were also noted. Timmerman and Brouwer (1999) found similar results for mirror-image reading. A reduction in reading latencies across sessions was found for severely injured TBI patients. Furthermore, response latency and error performance of the patients were not significantly different from those of control subjects; that is, the TBI patients learned the procedure as quickly as the control subjects.

Glisky (1992) used a data entry task to demonstrate procedural learning in a group of 10 amnesic patients, half of whom had sustained a closed head injury, while the remaining half sustained an aneurysm (3), encephalitis (1), or anoxia (1). Subjects were trained on the procedures for entering data into a computer and appeared to acquire the data-entry procedures in a relatively normal fashion. Compared to normal controls, the amnesic patients made only slightly more errors and improved their performance across trials at approximately the same rate as the controls. Mutter et al. (1994) used a serial pattern-learning paradigm with TBI patients. Subjects were asked to quickly respond to the appearance of an asterisk by pressing one of four response keys corresponding to its location. There were four learning trials, a trial of random placement of the asterisks, three additional learning trials, and a generation phase asking subjects to anticipate the location at which an asterisk would appear next. The authors found that persons sustaining a mild TBI performed identically to matched control subjects for normal learning and retention of a serial pattern. Patients who had a GCS score <13 performed at a significantly lower level than matched controls, but not significantly differently from patients with a GCS score ≥13. However, in the generation phase, both groups of TBI patients predicted the locations of the asterisks in the serial pattern as accurately as control subjects. The authors concluded that the effects of a TBI had a relatively minor impairment on the acquisition rate of the serial pattern knowledge, but the ability to recollect and use this knowledge, once acquired, seemed unaffected.

Although declarative memory has been demonstrated to be impacted by the effects of a TBI, the literature demonstrates that there is a disparity between the semantic and episodic domains. Semantic knowledge is relatively preserved after TBI, although it is impacted by poor subjective organization of the material, decreased speed of access, and passive learning strategies. Levin et al. (1986) found in their study investigating TBI patients' access to previously acquired semantic stores that the patients were able to appreciate the categorical relationship among the words, although they were inefficient at using the information to aid recall. Goldstein et al. (1989) found similar results in their study investigating effects of TBI on proactive interference. The TBI patients were sensitive to the semantic features present in the to-be-learned material, and demonstrated improvement in memory during the task shift. However, the TBI patients, as in Levin's study, were impaired in the ability to use this information to aid free recall. Baddeley (1987) found TBI patients performed similarly to control subjects on a vocabulary and verbal fluency test, measures that require access to semantic memory stores. The head-injured group's performance did not differ significantly from that of normal and elderly controls. Speed of access to semantic stores, however, was impaired in the TBI group.

Episodic memory is adversely affected by TBI and deficits are typically demonstrated on tests of word list learning, associating word pairs, and paragraph retention. The deficits are often manifested as impairments in acquisition, consolidation, and retrieval (Levin et al., 1979; Lezak, 1995). Crossen (1989) observed three distinct memory patterns in TBI and noted variation in the nature of the memory deficit sustained: (1) a selective encoding deficit that shows higher false recognitions and fewer correct recognitions; (2) a selective consolidation impairment that exhibits few false recognitions, but fewer than normal correct recognitions; and (3) a selective retrieval deficit that demonstrates few false recognitions and normal correct recognitions. On a selective reminding list learning task, Levin et al. (1979) found that patients who were severely disabled were impaired on consistent retrieval (recalling a correct word on a given trial and on all subsequent trials) and were inefficient for screening intrusive errors. Lezak (1979), using a serial learning task, found TBI patients to perform at a lower level of efficiency as indicated by the score on the fifth learning trial, relative to the performance on the first learning trial. She observed that few TBI patients improved their verbal learning ability within the first three years post trauma. Tabaddor et al. (1984) reported the performance of moderately and severely brain injured patients to be 6 and 5 standard deviations (SD) below the norm, respectively, on a selective reminding verbal list learning task.

Several authors have found nonverbal memory to be affected by the effects of a TBI in their investigations of learning and memory. Brooks (1972, 1974) found that

TBI patients performed significantly worse than patients with orthopedic injuries on reproduction of geometric designs (which were presented for 10 seconds). Similar findings were found by Brooks (1976) in a later study comparing severely injured TBI patients with control subjects on Visual Reproduction from the Wechsler Memory Scale. Tabaddor et al. (1984) found nonverbal learning, as measured by the Benton Test of Visual Retention, to be impaired for both moderately and severely brain-injured patients assessed at baseline. At six months post injury, impaired verbal and nonverbal memory functioning was noted, although a trend toward improvement for nonverbal memory was indicated. Overall, declarative memory deficits affect both verbal and nonverbal material and is not material-specific in the majority of patients.

Recognition memory may also be impaired after a brain injury and characterized primarily by excessive false-positive errors; that is, incorrectly identifying a new picture as one previously seen (Brooks, 1975; Hannay et al., 1979). Brooks (1974) noted impaired performance by TBI patients on Kimura's recurring figure recognition memory test consisting of both nonsense and geometric designs. In a prospective outcome study, Levin et al. (1988) found visual recognition memory to be impaired in a group of moderately and severely brain injured patients.

Another characteristic of memory functioning after TBI is the inclusion of extra-list words (intrusion errors). Levin et al. (1979) also found that the number of intrusions on a selective reminding test was markedly elevated in patients who were severely disabled, whereas the extra-list words were rare in patients who had achieved good recovery. Semantic errors tend to predominate among the types of intrusion errors made by TBI patients. Hannay et al. (1979) noted high false alarm errors (analogous to excessive intrusion on verbal recall) on a visual recognition memory task in moderately and severely brain-injured patients.

In summary, implicit learning, procedural learning and retention of visuomotor skills, and facilitation of performance through prior exposure to test materials (e.g., words) without conscious recall are relatively preserved following CHI. Preservation of semantic memory is demonstrated, although it is impacted by decreased subjective organization, decreased speed of access, and passive learning strategies. Episodic memory is more consistently impaired, as reflected in deficient learning, acquisition, consolidation, recall, and recognition of the material. Lesion location may somewhat impact the type of information to be recalled, with left and right hemisphere lesions affecting verbal and nonverbal material. Age at the time of injury and injury severity also affect memory performance. Older TBI patients (age 45+ years) have more severe memory deficits than younger patients after sustaining comparable injuries, perhaps reflecting their diminished reserve for recovery (Bendixen and Benton, 1996).

Attention and Information Processing

Attention has been defined as the ability to be aware of stimuli. This can refer to internal stimuli such as thoughts and memories, or external stimuli such as sights and sounds (Weber, 1990). Attention is not, however, a unitary concept and may comprise several components, including alertness, selectivity, effort, and information processing (Ponsford and Kinsella, 1987). Information processing refers to capacity and control (Ponsford and Kinsella, 1988). It is the amount of mental processing one can attend to within a given time and the ability to guide this process by directing and organizing whatever attentional capacity one has (Weber, 1990; Ponsford and Kinsella, 1987); or simply stated, it is the number of operations the brain can carry out at the same time (Gronwall, 1989). Attentional deficits may manifest as slowness of thought and response (McCaffrey and Gansler, 1992; Lezak, 1995). Diffuse cerebral damage, minute lesions and lacerations scattered throughout the brain substance, and damage to frontotemporal regions produced by TBI adversely affect the amount of and the speed with which one can process information (Gronwall, 1989; Lezak, 1995).

Attention and concentration difficulties are the second most frequently reported complaint of TBI patients (van Zomeren and Brouwer, 1994). Upon interview, brain-injured patients present with complaints of inability to concentrate or perform complex mental operations, confusion, and perplexity in thinking (Lezak, 1995). If the deficit is severe, the patient may appear highly distractible, or unable to maintain directed or focused attention (Lezak, 1995), particularly in the presence of distractors. The attentional deficit can be of a severity that limits the brain-injured patient's ability to perform well in stressful environments, such as driving in heavy traffic (Hinnant, 1999). The attentional problems may be manifested as difficulty concentrating on mental activities (such as reading) or performing two tasks simultaneously. Patients may misinterpret their slowed processing and attentional deficits as memory problems, even though performance on memory and attention tests typically reveals reduced auditory span, difficulty processing more than one thing at a time, and verbal retrieval problems (Lezak, 1995). Attentional deficits as a consequence of TBI have generally been described as those of sustained, selective, or divided attention, with information processing being the most impaired aspect of attentional deficits.

Sustained Attention. Sustained attention, or vigilance, requires that one maintain attentional activity over time. van Zomeren and Brouwer (1994) found that TBI patients showed an increase in response time for target detection when the patient was asked to complete sustained attention tasks of simulated driving and continuous choice reaction time. Accuracy of responses, on the other hand, was comparable for control and TBI groups. Brouwer and van Wolffelaar (1985) also found increased response latencies for TBI patients on sustained attention tasks. Using a signal detection task for discriminating small differences of loudness, the TBI patients showed less sensitivity than normal controls. Levin et al. (1988) found an interaction between severe head trauma and the ability to perform sustained attention tasks over time, noting worsening attentional performance over time. Spikman et al. (1996) also used a choice reaction time task and found no significant difference between severe TBI patients and control subjects. The investigators found that in the first blocks of the reaction time session, TBI patients performed more variably than the controls, but that, in the last part of the reaction time block, the difference in performance was no longer significant. Given that the task was not continuous, but consisted of a series of separate reaction time tasks that included short breaks, the investigators acknowledged that the task may not truly have been a sustained attention task.

Focused Attention. Selective or focused attention refers to the selection of specific stimuli to the exclusion of others as the focus of attention (Weber, 1990). For example, the subject may be asked to attend to only one of several inputs that are presented concurrently. Sohlberg and Mateer (1987) described a focused attention paradigm that required subjects to respond selectively to a sequence of stimuli presented one at a time while ignoring others. Focused attention is sensitive to the effects of diffuse brain damage. Reduced reaction times in situations that demand attentional focus and rapid response provide evidence of selective or focused attention deficits in patients sustaining a TBI (Hinnant, 1999). van Zomeren and Brouwer (1994) found that patients, at less than six months post injury, had focused attention impairments as evidenced by an increased sensitivity to interference from dominant response tendencies while performing modified Stroop tasks, visual reaction time tasks, and memory tasks. On a task that required suppression of an automatic response in the face of a conflicting response or unnecessary processing of redundant information, Stuss et al. (1988) found that TBI patients were less able than control subjects to ignore the redundant information. However, TBI patient performance was variable and detectable only after repeated assessments. The authors surmised that, although TBI patients could meet the demands of a focused attention task, they were inconsistent in maintaining an optimal level of performance. The ability to consistently maintain accurate performance appeared to erode over time. In a study by Spikman et al. (1996), the Stroop Color condition was used as a covariate for the Color-Word condition in order to study more closely the effect of TBI on distraction. The investigators found no difference between severe TBI patients and normal controls on the Stroop Color-Word condition adjusted for the Color condition. The authors concluded that TBI results in mental slowness but that the patients do not have specific difficulties in focused and divided attention. The TBI patients' performance, however, was disturbed compared to that of the controls, and the tasks were completed at a slower rate by the patients.

Divided Attention. Divided attention tasks ask the subject to attend to two or more inputs at the same time (Weber, 1990) and have been shown to be sensitive to the effects of diffuse injury. Divided attention deficits after TBI may be attributed to slow controlled processing, which results in a reduced capacity for controlled processing (Brouwer et al., 1989), that is, slowed or impaired information processing. Information processing is the most impaired aspect of attentional deficits in TBI patients. Slowed thinking and reaction times may result in significantly lowered scores on timed tests despite the capacity to perform the required task accurately. Additionally, as the complexity of the choice reaction time task increases and the time demands increase, brain-injured patients tend to show disproportionate slowing in mental processing speed (Levin, 1993; van Zomeren and Brouwer, 1994). This has also been demonstrated on visual reaction time tasks of rapid decision making and psychomotor speed (Levin, 1995). Tromp and Mulder (1991) noted that while motor complexity does not appear to affect response speed, task novelty can slow reaction time in TBI patients, which becomes interpreted as slowed information processing.

A significant relationship has been shown between injury severity and attentional impairments. Using the Paced Auditory Serial Addition Test (PASAT)—the addition of single digits presented at an increasingly rapid rate over trials—severely injured patients showed persistent slowing of performance (Levin, 1993). van Zomeren and Brouwer (1994) concluded that this nonspecific slowing was the most conspicuous phenomenon demonstrated in tasks showing slow information processing after severe brain injury. Stuss et al. (1988) also found TBI patients to be impaired on tasks of divided attention. Using a multiple choice reaction time paradigm, subjects responded to target items in three conditions: easy, complex, and redundant. For all three studies, the TBI patients were slower than the control subjects for all three choice reaction time tests, and both patient group and control subjects were slower for the complex choice than for either the easy or the redundant task. Stuss and colleagues defined the deficits in divided attention as slowness in consciously controlled information processing, an inability to process multiple bits of information rapidly and easily.

In summary, the diffuse effects of TBI may leave the patient having difficulty with mental speed, sustained attention (McCaffrey and Gansler, 1992), concentration, and performing mental operations (Gronwall and Wrightson, 1981). Lezak (1987) noted that deficits in attention are likely to underlie many other cognitive difficulties experienced by TBI survivors. Persons who have sustained a mild TBI (MTBI) usually recover from attention deficits within three months, in contrast to those with severe injuries, who may have more permanent deficits. MTBI patients, although they perform well on standard ability tests, might report that cognitive tasks demand more effort than prior to the injury. Table 16.2 provides a summary of several tests that are used in the assessment of attention, intelligence, language, and executive functioning.

Intellectual Functioning

In general, there appears to be an overall lowering of the intelligence quotient (IQ) following severe TBI, which has been interpreted by some to represent a relatively generalized impairment of cognitive functioning (Grafman and Salazar, 1995; Mayes et al., 1989). Diffuse cerebral swelling and the effects of a mass lesion sustained from a brain injury contribute to the intellectual impairment (Levin et al., 1982). This generalized impairment, however, frequently affects Performance IQ more than Verbal IQ, and is significantly impacted by injury severity. Verbal tests of intelligence provide a measure of premorbid, rote, overlearned information. Verbal intelligence may be least impacted by the effects of a brain injury, although focal damage to the language-specialized hemisphere, and cultural and educational limitations may lower the patient's performance. Mental speed and novel problem solving ability are inordinately affected by head trauma, possibly due to the

TABLE 16.2   Neuropsychological Tests

Domain	Test
Attention	Stroop Color Test
	Paced Auditory Serial Addition Test
	Symbol Digit Modalities Test
	Continuous Performance Test
	Visual Search and Attention Test
Intelligence	Wechsler Adult Intelligence Scale-Revised
	Wechsler Adult Intelligence Scale-III
Language	Multilingual Aphasia Exam
	Boston Naming Test
	Controlled Oral Word Association
	Token Test
	Discourse Analysis
Executive Functioning	Trail Making Test
	Wisconsin Card Sorting Test
	Halstead-Reitan Category Test
Personality	Minnesota Multiphasic Personality Inventory-2
	Neurobehavioral Rating Scale
	Beck Depression Inventory
	Personality Assessment Inventory

For a more comprehensive list of tests used in neuropsychological assessment, the reader is referred to Spreen and Strauss (1988).

relatively high concentration of contusion and diffuse axonal injury (DAI) in the frontal lobes, where these functions are localized. Greater demand is placed on mental and motor speed and novel problem solving skills for the Performance IQ subtests (Capruso and Levin, 1996), which are more sensitive to the residual effects of TBI than the Verbal Scale (VIQ) (Levin, 1993, 1995), and less closely related to educational background (Levin et al., 1982).

Using the Wechsler scales (i.e., The Wechsler Adult Intelligence Scales-WAIS, WAIS-Revised) as a measure of recovery of intellectual functioning, several researchers found a relation between severity of injury and intellectual functioning. In a study conducted by Levin et al. (1979), patients who had achieved a good recovery on the Glasgow Outcome Scale consistently scored within one standard deviation (SD), or above, of the population mean on the WAIS. Moderate to severe brain injury was shown to produce a more global impact than uniformly impaired intellectual functioning without regard to premorbid intellectual status (Levin et al., 1982; Mayes et al., 1989). Findings from Levin et al. (1979) showed that moderately disabled patients had Verbal and Performance IQ scores approximately one SD below normal (mean = 100, SD = 15) and that patients who were severely disabled had IQ scores greater than three SDs below normal, even after intervals as long as three years. They found that no patient had recovered to within two SDs of the population mean. Overall, outcome in patients without profound mental impairment was more clearly related to variations in PIQ as compared to VIQ. Mayes et al. (1989) also noted that patients with higher preinjury IQs may suffer more intellectual damage in relation to premorbid levels than individuals with lower IQs prior to injury. The greater the disparity between preinjury and postinjury IQs, the more profound the loss.

Aphasia and Other Communication Disorders

Classically defined linguistic disorders are atypical in patients sustaining TBI, with only about 2% of patients being aphasic. Heilman et al. (1971) found in his study of TBI patients that anomic aphasia was the most frequently identified language disturbance, followed by Wernicke's aphasia. However, these findings should be interpreted cautiously given that CT scans were not performed and patients who underwent surgery were excluded from the study. The anomic disturbance was found to be associated with damage sustained to the right orbitofrontal and left temporoparietal regions. Language deficits typically seen after head injury include impaired confrontation naming, deficits in comprehension of complex, multistage commands, writing praxis, and verbal fluency (Levin, 1993, 1995). Prose performance of TBI patients is characterized by a lack of organization and omission of portions of the essential information. Conversational speech tends to be tangential, poorly organized, and associated with difficulty in pragmatics and circumlocution, and has semantic paraphasias (Capruso and Levin, 1996; Levin, 1993). Studies examining discourse production further detail the disorganized nature of spontaneous speech produced by TBI patients. In comparison to normal controls, Coelho et al. (1995) found that TBI patients performed more poorly for intersentential cohesion (rule-based semantic organization) across sentences involving use of specific linguistic devices. Snow et al. (1997) found that TBI patients committed significantly more errors than normal and orthopedic controls on parameters such as sufficient information, accuracy, and informational redundancy. Similar findings were found by Hartley and Jensen (1992), who identified a confused discourse profile type that characterized patient performance, which included few accurate content, high inaccurate content, and a high number of clarity problems. This profile was reported as associated with impairment on indices of memory (Logical Memory from the Wechsler Memory Scale-R) and language (oral language portion of the Western Aphasia Battery).

The posttraumatic communication disorders typically seen after TBI were classified by Sarno (1980) as "subclinical" aphasic defects; the patient has adequate conversational language (albeit far from normal), yet shows clear language deficits on more challenging psychometric testing. Linguistic-based deficits may characterize the spontaneous speech, including impoverished cohesion and organization of meaning across sentences (Coelho et al., 1995). Dysarthria is the most common nonaphasic speech disturbance, and ranges in severity from minor articulation problems to nearly unintelligible, linguistically correct speech (Levin, 1993).

Executive Functioning

Executive functions (EF) are a type of supraordinate system that motivates self-initiated behavior and governs the efficiency and appropriateness of task performance (Capruso and Levin, 1996). Several components comprise executive functioning, including volition or the capacity for awareness of one's self, surroundings, and motivational state; planning or conceiving alternatives; and self-regulation or quality control (Stuss and Benson, 1986). Executive functions are concerned with self-regulation, flexibility in problem solving, planning, and decisions about allocating resources. EF impairment after TBI is seen despite having adequate performance on highly structured psychological and neuropsychological tests (Ylvisaker and Feeney, 1996). For example, Stuss et al. (1985) found impaired executive functioning despite intelligence within normal range and attainment of a good recovery in head-injured survivors. Impairment in EF after TBI has been attributed to frontal lobe damage (Burke et al., 1991).

Executive functioning deficits can occur in disparate neurobehavioral systems involving motor, verbal, or conceptual processes (Goldberg and Tucker, 1979). Disruption of function may be manifested in tasks of verbal fluency, hypothesis generation, use of feedback, and shift of conceptual strategies (Lezak, 1995). Verbal fluency tasks require the subject to generate as many words as possible from a single letter cue within a specified time. McDowell et al. (1997) found verbal fluency to be impaired in their group of TBI patients (GCS score <8 for six hours). This deficit was persistent even when effects of age and education were taken into consideration. Goldstein et al. (1994) found impaired verbal fluency performance in a group of older patients (≥50 years of age) who had sustained mild to moderate TBI. The patient group exhibited a significantly higher proportion of nonperseverative errors (illegal use of proper nouns) than normal controls, although the production of perseverative errors was similar for the two groups. Verbal fluency has been shown to be particularly impaired following injury to the dominant (left) prefrontal cortex, whereas design fluency (generating as many unique designs as possible in a specified time) was impaired following nondominant (usually right) prefrontal injury (Perret, 1974).

Executive function tasks that consist of formulating goals, effective planning, or carrying out plans are disrupted by the effects of a TBI. The Wisconsin Card Sorting Test (WCST), used to assess executive EF (Heaton et al., 1993), is a test of flexibility and adoption of new patterns. One must deduce the correct principle based on the examiners feedback of any given card placement as correct or incorrect. Stuss et al. (1985) found that TBI patients who had achieved a good recovery demonstrated significant deficits on the WCST. Goldstein et al. (1994) found that older (50 years of age or greater) TBI patients performed below control subjects for inferring conceptual relationships between items on a modified version of the WCST. Additionally, control subjects achieved a larger number of categories than did the TBI patients, although this difference missed significance ($p = 0.07$). The Halstead–Reitan Category Test (HCT) also assesses concept formation and shift of conceptual set as well as attention and visuospatial perception. Dikmen et al. (1983) found significantly impaired performance on this test among TBI patients throughout 18 months of follow-up.

The Trailmaking Test (TMT) provides a measure of flexibility as well as conceptual tracking, motor speed, and attention. Brouwer and co-workers (1989) reported that head-injured patients performed significantly slower than controls (van Zomeren and Brouwer, 1994). Stuss et al. (1985), on the other hand, did not find statistically significant impairment at a mean of 2.6 years after injury on the TMT. The above tasks (WCST, HCT, and TMT) share the common skill of flexibility. Lezak (1995) contended that TBI patients possess the capacity to perform tasks requiring flexibility, although it does not occur to them to use that available information or to anticipate future needs. Thus, the ability to plan, recognize, or choose alternatives may be impaired.

Difficulty with flexibility can be seen in the frequency with which perseverative errors are committed. Perseverative errors—the inability to terminate a sequence of behavior, be it a thought or a response (Lezak, 1995)—are common after injury to the prefrontal cortex or diffuse injury, which is evident when TBI patients are assessed using the Wisconsin Card Sorting Test (WCST) (Drewe, 1974). Severity of injury is also related to the perseverative error performance (Anderson et al., 1995). However, using a modified version of the WCST that required achievement of six categories or placement of 48 cards, McDowell et al. (1997) did not find their TBI patients' performance to be significantly worse than control subjects.

Goldstein and Levin (1991) also found impaired flexibility in their sample of TBI patients. Impaired performance was noted for ability to identify salient features and eliminate nonessential information on a task requiring question-asking strategies to identify undisclosed items. The investigators concluded that lack of mental flexibility and impaired self-initiated behavior were reflected in the patient's performance. McDowell et al. (1997) also found that TBI patients performed more poorly on dual-task reaction time paradigms compared to controls. The task required subjects to press the space bar as quickly as possible each time a dot appeared on the screen, which was set at random intervals. The task was presented three times and on the second administration subjects counted aloud from 1 to 10 repeatedly, placing minimal demands on the executive system. On the third administration, the subjects performed an oral digit span task, placing greater demand on the executive system. Speed of performance was significantly different between the groups in the single-task paradigm (patients at 390 ms and controls at 303 ms, $p < 0.001$). A consistent performance decrement was found on the visual reaction time task during dual-task performance for both counting and digit span, with digit span performance consistently worse for both groups. Analyses examining the impact of the TBI on the executive system revealed a significant effect for both subject groups and test conditions as well as an interaction between the two. That is, the dual-task measure was more difficult than the single task measure, and TBI patients, relative to the subject group, showed a larger impairment on the dual-task measure.

Executive function plays a significant role in discourse production and is generally typified as behaviors of goal setting, planning, and carrying out plans, which are disrupted by the effects of a TBI. Coelho et al. (1995) found impaired performance by TBI patients for "story structure" on a story generation task from a Norman Rockwell picture. Deficits were noted for producing an initiated event, an action, and a direct consequence. The authors found that "story structure" was the only parameter significantly correlated with the WCST perseverative response measure, a known measure of executive functioning. Tucker and Hanlon (1998) found similar results in their group of mild and moderate TBI patients. Subjects were asked to describe picture sequences depicting social interactions (items from the WAIS-R Picture Arrangement subtest). The patients differed significantly from controls for addressing the relevant details needed to produce a story congruent with the action depicted in the sequence. Accuracy, provision of essential information, and statement of implied meaning were deficient. The WCST perseverative response measure was also significantly related to the composite discourse score.

Shallice's supervisory attentional control system is a part of the executive functions of the frontal lobes and patients sustaining injury to this region, particularly focal left frontal lesions, do poorly on tests of supervisory attentional control (van Zomeren and Brouwer, 1994). The Tower of London Test (a test of supervisory attentional control) assesses the capacity to "look ahead" in planning moves of dowels from an initial position to match those of a sample provided. Ponsford and Kinsella (1992) found that head-injured patients, assessed one to seven months post injury, required more time than a control group to solve the problems, but committed the same number of errors (van Zomeren and Brouwer, 1994). Shallice (1982) and Shallice and Burgess (1991) found that brain-injured persons with predominantly left anterior lesions performed least well, while those with either left or right posterior lesions did as well as normal control subjects. Levin et al. (1991) found that TBI patients with anterior lesions performed at essentially the same level as control subjects and, on the most complex item (five moves), performed better than those with nonfrontal lesions.

Executive functioning affects all aspects of one's daily life and may be manifested as behaviors of disorganization, impulsivity, inflexibility, behavioral rigidity, and perseveration. Although possessing the required information, severely impaired TBI patients may fail to think to use this information unless externally cued. Self-correcting behaviors may follow the same pattern in that the patient knows there is an error but does nothing to correct it. Inflexibility, whether as perseveration or impaired conceptual shifting in response to changing circumstances, can compromise cognitive and social functioning alike. Lastly, although TBI patients may have attained a good recovery outcome, they may continue to exhibit executive functioning deficits that compromise their ability to maintain employment or return to a satisfactory psychosocial status (Lezak, 1987; McKinlay and Brooks, 1981).

Behavioral Disturbance

Behavioral disturbances are a common manifestation after severe brain injury, with personality change, slowness, irritability, bad temper, fatigue, depression, rapid mood change, tension and anxiety, and threats of violence as the most commonly reported sequelae (Brooks et al., 1986). Family members find these behavioral disturbances to be more burdensome than the residual cognitive or focal neurological deficits (Levin, 1993, 1995) and the emotional and personality disturbances are reported as more handicapping than are the residual cognitive and physical disabilities (Lezak, 1987). The behaviors may be manifested as a release of previously inhibited behaviors, giving rise to impulsivity or aggression, or inhibition of previously uncontrolled behaviors, yielding apathetic behavior. The patients' premorbid personality and the postinjury environment may also contribute to the long-term behavioral outcome.

The orbital-frontal regions have been implicated in behaviors of impulsivity, reduced anger control, aggressiveness, and sexual acting out (Ylvisaker and Feeney, 1996). Lezak (1988) reported impulsivity to be the most obvious manifestation of impaired control, and anger outbursts are the most commonly reported form of impulsivity. When frustrated, the TBI patient may engage in shouting, gestures, or diatribes that can be very distressing to the caregiver or a child. Elliott and Biever (1996) reported changes in sexual functioning to include impulsiveness, inappropriateness, changes in libido and sexual frequency, and global sexual difficulties. Sexually impulsive patients are a source of concern for the caregiver. For example, Lezak (1988) described a case depicting a teenage girl who could not bring her school friends home because her brother inevitably tried to kiss and fondle them, or of an elderly woman who complained that her husband felt for her breasts whenever she bent over to pour his coffee. To the contrary, Kreuter et al. (1998) found that many of the TBI patients in his study reported decreased ability for erection, orgasm, and desire, and a diminished frequency in intercourse. Sandel et al. (1996) found that sexuality was related to location of injury; that is, patients with frontal lobe lesions reported a higher level of satisfaction and functioning than those without frontal lesions. The orbital-frontal regions have been implicated in behaviors of impulsivity, lability, reduced anger control, aggressiveness, sexual acting out, and poor social judgment (Ylvisaker and Feeney, 1996). Also, right hemisphere injuries were correlated with higher scores on reports of sexual arousal and sexual experiences.

Irritability or aggressiveness is another frequently reported behavioral disturbance manifested after severe brain injury (Levin, 1995; Silver and Yudofsky, 1994). When these behaviors are present, family members may report them as a change in the patient's personality or as having significantly increased in those patients who have not had a change in personality (Brooks and McKinlay, 1983). Irritability may be seen along with agitation, restlessness, and lethargy during PTA; and in the later stages of recovery (Brooks and McKinlay, 1983; Silver and Yudofsky, 1994). The behaviors range in severity from irritability to outbursts that may possibly result in damage to property or assault on others. The patient may develop low frustration tolerance and explosive behavior that can be set off by minimal provocation or occur without warning (Silver and Yudofsky, 1994). In severe cases, affected individuals cannot remain in the community or with their families, and often are referred to long-term psychiatric or neurobehavioral facilities. Outbursts of rage and violent behavior occur after damage to the inferior orbital surface of the frontal lobe and anterior temporal lobes (Silver and Yudofsky, 1994). Lezak (1987) believed that the brain-injured patient's uncontrolled anger may help to account for relative lack of success in resuming normal social relationships and activities.

Impaired social interaction, awareness, and insight can be present after severe brain injury (Levin, 1995). Patients may display a childlike egocentricity (Lezak, 1988) or may have impaired ability to be aware of social signals or to interpret them accurately. They may misperceive or lack understanding of socially meaningful gestures, facial expressions, or metaphoric verbalizations. With the diminished awareness, severely injured patients may cease dressing or grooming themselves appropriately and may be unaware that their appearance is distressing to others (Lezak, 1988). Deficient planning with unrealistic goal setting may be exhibited along with diminished motivation (Levin, 1995). There is a lack of insight into how their behaviors are distressing to the caregiver or the level of burden on the caregiver (Lezak, 1988).

Major depressive disorders have been reported in patients with TBI. Fedoroff et al. (1992) found as many as 25 percent of their patient sample to have major depression. Jorge et al. (1993) found that in TBI patients assessed at hospital admission and 3, 6, and 12 months post injury, 28/66 (17 in the acute stage and 11 during the follow-up) met DSM-III-R diagnostic criteria for major depression at some time during the study duration. Disruption of mood and emotion occurs when damage is sustained to the left dorsolateral frontal and/or left basal ganglia lesions (Jorge et al., 1993). TBI patients who experience depression may also report worry, hopelessness, suicidal ideation, social withdrawal, and irritability (Levin, 1995; Grafman and Salazar, 1995). The depression may be transient, but frequently is chronic (Lezak, 1988). McKinlay et al. (1981) reported evidence, although indirectly, of depressed mood in about one-half of their patients at 3, 6, or 12 months following severe brain injury. Prevalence of depression in brain-injured patients varies, ranging from 6 percent to 77 percent (Robinson and Jorge, 1994), depending on the source of information. For example, Kinsella et al. (1988) reported that 33 percent of their 39 severely injured patients were depressed. The depressive symptomatology may feed on and exacerbate the patient's other emotional and social maladaptations (Lezak, 1988). Behaviors of emotional lability, apathy, and low energy may also be concomitant with the mood disorder (Robinson and Jorge, 1994). Jorge et al. (1993) and Fedoroff et al. (1992) found that major depression was strongly related to poor social functioning.

Behavioral disturbances after brain injury may be persistent over time. Brooks and McKinlay (1987) reported that changes in personality were evident 12 months post injury in their sample of TBI patients. Lezak (1987) found that over a five-year period, 70 percent or more of the patients assessed experienced some difficulty handling anger. Problems were also identified in areas of initiative, significant relationships, social contact, work/school, leisure, driving, and social appropriateness.

SUMMARY

Traumatic brain injury affects thousands of people in the United States each year and the economic costs are estimated to be billions of dollars in hospitalization, rehabilitation, and lost wages. Physical, cognitive, and emotional disturbances characterize the neurobehavioral sequelae of severe TBI, with the cognitive and behavioral deficits having the more devastating effects on the patient and family. As illustrated in Figure 16.1, the interaction between the pathophysiological changes resulting from a TBI and neuropsychological functioning significantly affect outcome, often adversely impacting social and environmental functioning. Diffuse cerebral damage and focal lesions sustained at the time of impact of the injury are responsible for the deficits in cognitive and behavioral functioning. Of the cognitive deficits, TBI patients complain most frequently about difficulties in memory, and impairment in other cognitive domains, such as attention and concentration and executive functioning, may exacerbate the patient's perception of his memory functioning. Executive functioning is also greatly affected by TBI. Deficits in executive functioning may impair the ability to plan, organize, problem solve, and sequence information. Impulsivity, inflexibility, and rigidity may characterize the TBI patient's behavior. Visual perceptual deficits may be more subtle and include acuity, visual fields, or diploplia (double vision). However, more severe impairment has been noted that included hemi-inattention and neglect. The behavioral manifestations exhibited by patients sustaining a TBI are reported by family members to be of a greater burden to the family than the cognitive or physical deficits. Impulsivity, irritability and aggression, disinhibition, and impaired awareness are common manifestations of the behavioral disturbances seen after TBI. The patients often have little insight into their deficits or behaviors. Additionally, from 33 percent to 77 percent of TBI patients experience a major depressive episode, which has been shown to be related to poor social functioning. As a result of the cognitive and

Conceptual Model of Neuropsychological Sequelae and Outcome of TBI

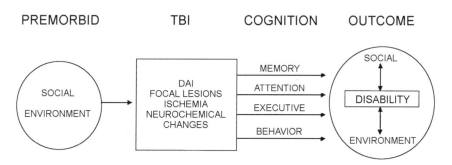

Figure 16.1   The neuropsychological sequelae resulting from a traumatic brain injury (TBI) can be devastating and have deleterious effects on psychosocial functioning. Impairments in cognitive and behavioral functioning adversely affects the ability to interact with the environment, including ability to work or attend school, or to have meaningful relationships. This impaired interaction often is the major source of disability for persons who have sustained a severe TBI.

behavioral deficits characteristic of a severe TBI, return to independent community living is impacted, which compromise the patient's ability to maintain employment or return to a satisfactory psychosocial status.

ACKNOWLEDGMENTS

This project was supported in part by NIH grants NS-21889 and NS-2188951, CDC-R49/CCR612707, TIRR-RRTC = H133B990014.

ABBREVIATIONS

CT	Computerized tomography
DAI	Diffuse axonal injury
DSM-III-R	Diagnostic and Statistical Manual, Third Edition—Revised
EF	Executive function
GCS	Glasgow Coma Scale
GOAT	Galveston Orientation and Amnesia Test
GOS	Glasgow Outcome Scale
HCT	Halstead–Reitan Category Test
IQ	Intelligence quotient
MTBI	Mild traumatic brain injury
PASAT	Paced Auditory Serial Addition Test
PIQ	Performance Intelligence Quotient
PTA	Posttraumatic Amnesia
SD	Standard deviation
STM	Short-term memory
TBI	Traumatic brain injury
TMT	Trailmaking Test
VIQ	Verbal Intelligence Quotient
WAIS-R	Wechsler Adult Intelligence Scale—Revised
WCST	Wisconsin Card Sort Test
WMS	Wechsler Memory Scale

REFERENCES

C. V. Anderson, E. D. Bigler, and D. D. Blatter, *J. Clin. Exp. Neuropsychol.*, 17(6), 900–908 (1995).

A. Baddeley, J. Harris, A. Sunderland, K. P. Watts, and B. Wilson, Closed head injury and memory, in H. S. Levin, J. Grafman, and H. M. Eisenberg, Eds., *Neurobehavioral Recovery from Head Injury*, Oxford University Press, New York, 1987, pp. 295–317.

B. Bendixen and A. L. Benton, Cognitive and Linguistic Outcome in H. S. Levin, A. L. Benton, J. P. Muizelaar, and H. M. Eisenberg, Eds., *Catastrophic Brain Injury*, Oxford University Press, New York, 1996, pp. 121–151.

D. F. Benson, D. T. Stuss, M. A. Naeser, W. S. Weir, E. F. Kaplan, and H. L. Levine, *Arch Neurol.*, 38(3), 65–69 (1981).

D. N. Brooks, *J. Nerv. Ment. Dis.*, 155(5), 350–355 (1972).

D. N. Brooks, *Cortex*, 10, 224–230 (1974).

D. N. Brooks, *Cortex*, 11, 329–340 (1975).

D. N. Brooks, *J. Neurol. Neurosurg. Psychiatry*, 39, 593–601 (1976).

D. N. Brooks, *Cortex*, 11, 329–340 (1979).

D. N. Brooks and D. N. Aughton, *Int. Rehab. Med.*, 1(4), (1979).

D. N. Brooks and W. McKinlay, *J. Neurol. Neurosurg. Psychiatry*, 46, 336–344 (1983).

N. Brooks, L. Campsie, C. Symington, A. Beattie, and W. Mckinlay, *J. Neurol. Neurosurg. Psychiatry*, 49, 764–770 (1986).

N. Brooks, W. McKinlay, C. Symington, A. Beattie, and L. Campsie, *Brain Inj.*, 1(1), 5–19 (1987)

W. H. Brouwer and P. C. Van Wolffelaar, *Cortex*, 21, 111–119 (1985).

W. H. Brouwer, R. W. H. M. Ponds, P. C. Van Wolffelaar, and A. H. van Zomeren, *Cortex*, 25, 219–230 (1989).

W. H. Burke, A. H. Zencius, M. D. Wesolowski, and F. Doubleday, *Brain Inj.*, 5(3), 241–252 (1991).

D. X. Capruso and H. S. Levin, in Neurobehavioral Outcome in Head Trauma, R. Evans, Ed., *Neurology and Trauma*, W. B. Sanders, Philadelphia, 1996, pp. 201–220.

C. A. Coelho, B. Z. Liles, and R. J. Duffy, *Brain Injury*, 9(5), 471–477 (1995).

J. R. Crossen and A. N. Wiens, *Clin. Neuropsychologist*, 2(4), 393–399 (1988).

Department of Health and Human Services, *Interagency Head Injury Task Force Report*, Department of Health and Human Services, Washington, D.C., 1989.

S. Dickerson-Mayes, L. E. Pelco, and C. J. Campbell, *Brain Inj.*, 3(3), 301–313 (1989).

S. Dikmen, R. M. Reitan, and N. R. Temkin, *Arch. Neurol.*, 40, 333–338 (1983).

E. A. Drewe, *Cortex*, 10, 159–170 (1974).

J. H. Ellenberg, H. S. Levin, and C. Saydjari, *Arch Neurol.*, 53, 782–791 (1996).

M. L. Elliott and L. S Biever, *Brain Inj.*, 10(10), 703–717 (1996).

E. Elovic and T. Antoinette, Epidemiology and Primary Prevention of Traumatic Brain Injury, in L. J. Horn, and N. D. Zalser, Eds., *Medical Rehabilitation of Traumatic Brain Injury*, Hanley & Belfus, Philadelphia, 1996, pp. 1–29.

J. Ewert, H. S. Levin, M. G. Watson, and Z. Kalisky, *Arch. Neurol.*, 46, 911–926 (1989).

J. P. Fedoroff, S. E. Starkstein, A. W. Forrester, F. H. Geisler, R. E. Jorge, S. V. Arndt, and R. G. Robinson, *Am. J. Psychiatry*, 149(7), 918–923 (1992).

I. E. Fodor, *J. Neurol. Neurosurg. Psychiatry*, 35, 818–824 (1972).

T. A. Gennarelli, H. R. Champion, and W. S. Copes, *International Research Council on Biokinetics of Impact*, 167–178 (1992).

T. A. Gennarelli, H. R. Champion, W. J. Saco, W. S. Copes, and W. M. Alves, *J. Trauma*, 29(9), 1193–1202 (1989).

J. T. Giacino, M. A. Kezmarsky, J. DeLuca, and K. D. Cicerone, *Arch. Phys. Med. Rehabil.*, 11, 897–901 (1991).

D. Girard, J. Brown, M. Burnett-Stolnack, N. Hashimoto, S. Hier-Wellmer, O. Z. Perlman, and C. Seigerman, *Brain Inj.*, 10(9), 663–676 (1996).

E. L. Glisky, *Neuropsychologia*, 30(10), 899–910 (1992).

E. Goldberg and L. D. Costa, *Brain Lang.*, 14, 144–173 (1981).

E. Goldberg and D. Tucker, *J. Clin. Neuropsychol.*, 4, 273–288 (1979).

F. C. Goldstein and H. S. Levin, *Brain Cogn.*, 17(1), 23–30 (1991).

F. C. Goldstein, H. S. Levin, and C. Boake, *Cortex*, 25, 541–554 (1989).

F. C. Goldstein, H. S. Levin, R. M. Presely, J. Searcy, A. R. T. Colohan, H. M. Eisenberg, B. Jann, and L. Betrolino-Kusnerik, *J. Neurol. Neurosurg. Psychiatry*, 57, 961–966 (1994).

Grafman and Salazar, Recovery of Function in Adults: Lessons for the Study of Pediatric Head Injury Outcome, in S. H. Brohman and M. E. Michel, Eds., *Traumatic Brain Injury in Children*, Oxford Press, New York, 1995.

D. Gronwall, Cumulative and Persisting Effects of Concussion on Attention and Cognition, in H. S. Levin, H. M. Eisenberg, and A. Benton, Eds., *Mild Brain Injury*, Oxford University Press, New York, 1989, pp. 153–162.

D. Gronwall and P. Wrightson, *J. Neurol. Neurosurg. Psychiatry*, 44, 889–895 (1981).

R. W. Hamil, P. D. Wolf, J. V. McDonald, L. A. Lee, and M. Kelly, *Ann. Neurol.*, 21, 438–443 (1986).

H. J. Hannay, H. S. Levin, and R. G. Grossman, *Cortex*, 15, 269–283 (1979).

L. L. Hartley and P. J. Jensen, *Brain Inj.*, 6(3), 271–282 (1992).

R. K. Heaton, G. J. Chelune, J. L. Talley, G. G Kay, and G. Curtis, *Wisconsin Card Sorting Test (WCST) Manual Revised and Expanded*, Psychological Assessment Resources, Odessa, FL, 1993.

K. M. Heilman, A. Safran, and N. Geschwind, *J. Neurol., Neurosurg. Psychiatry*, 34, 265–269 (1971).

D. W. Hinnant, Neurobehavioral Consequences—Assessment, Treatment, and Outcome, in D. W. Marion, Ed., *Traumatic Brain Injury*, Thieme, New York, 1999, pp. 187–197.

B. Jennet, J. Snoek, M. R. Bond, and N. Brooks, *J. Neurol. Neurosurg. Psychiatry*, 44, 285–293 (1981).

R. E. Jorge, R. G. Robinson, S. E. Starkstein, S. V. Arndt, A. W. Forrester, and F. H. Geisler, *Am. J. Psychiatry*, 150(6), 916–921 (1993a).

R. E. Jorge, R. G. Robinson, S. V. Arndt, S. E. Starkstein, S. V. Arndt, A. W. Forrester, and F. H. Geisler, *J. Affect. Disord.*, 27(4), 233–243 (1993b).

W. D. Kalsbeek, R. L. McLaurin, B. S. Harris and J. D. Miller, *J Neurosurg.*, Suppl. S19–31 (1980).

G. Kinsella, C. Moran, B. Ford, and J. Ponsford, *Psychol. Med.*, 18(1), 57–63 (1988).

M. R. Klauber, E. Barrett-Connor, L. F. Marshall, and S. A. Bowers, *Am. J. Epidemiol.*, 5, 500–509 (1981).

M. R. Klauber, B. Barrett-Connor, L. F. Marshall, and S. A. Bowers, *Am J. Epidemiol*, 113, 500 (1981).

M. Kreuter, A. G. Dahllof, G. Gudjonsson, M. Sullivan, and A. Siosteen, *Brain Inj.*, 12(5), 349–368 (1998).

R. Lachman, J. Lachman, and E. C. Butterfield, *Cognitive Psychology and Information Processing, An Introduction*, Lawrence Erlbaum Associates, Publishers, Hillsdale, New Jersey, 1979.

H. S. Levin, Neurobehavioral sequelae of closed head injury, in P. Cooper, Ed., *Head Injury*, 3rd Ed., Williams and Wilkins, Baltimore, MD, 1993, pp. 525–551.

H. S. Levin, *J. Neurotrauma*, 12(4), 601–610 (1995).

H. S. Levin, A. L. Benton, and R. G. Grossman, *Neurobehavioral Consequences of Closed Head Injury*, Oxford University Press, New York, 1982.

H. S. Levin and H. M. Eisenberg, *Neurosurg. Clin N. Am.*, 2(2), 457–472 (1991).

H. S. Levin, S. Mattis, R. M. Ruff, H. E. Eisenberg, L. F. Marshall, K. Tabaddor, W. M. High, Jr., and R. F. Frankowski, *J. Neurosurg.*, 66, 234–243 (1987).

H. S. Levin and F. C. Goldstein, *J. Clin. Exp. Neuropsychology*, 8(6), 643–656 (1986).

H. S. Levin, F. C. Goldstein, W. M. High, Jr., and H. M. Eisenberg, *J. Neurol., Neurosurg. Psychiatry*, 51, 1294–1301 (1988).

H. S. Levin. H. E. Gary, Jr., H. M. Eisenberg, R. M. Ruff, J. G. Barth, J. Kreutzer, W. M. High, Jr., et al., *J. Neurosurg.*, 73, 699–709 (1990).

M. Lezak, *J. Head Trauma Rehabil.*, 2(1), 57–69 (1987).

M. Lezak, *J. Clin. Exp. Neuropsychology*, 10(1), 111–123 (1988).

M. Lezak, *Neuropsychological Assessment*, 3rd Ed., Oxford University Press, New York, 1995.

M. G. Livingston and H. M. Livingston, *Int. Rehab. Med.*, 7, 145–149 (1985).

M. G. Livingston, D. N. Brooks, and M. R. Bond, *J. Neurol. Neurosurg. Psychiatry*, 48, 876–881 (1985)

J. L. Mathias and J. L. Coats, *J. Clin. Exp. Neuropsychol.*, 21(2), 200–215 (1999).

A. J. Mattson and H. S. Levin, *J. Nerv. Ment. Dis.*, 178(5), 282–291 (1990).

S. D. Mayes, L. E. Pelco, and C. J. Campbell, *Brain Inj.*, 3(3), 301–313 (1989).

S. McDowell, J. Whyte, and M. D'Esposito, *Neuropsychologia*, 35(10), 1341–1353 (1997).

W. W. McKinlay, D. N. Brooks, M. R. Bond, D. P., Martinage, and M. M. Marshall, *J. Neurol. Neurosurg. Psychiatry*, 44, 527–533 (1981).

S. A. Mutter, J. H. Howard, Jr., and D. V. Howard, *J. Clin. Exp. Neuropsychol.*, 16(2), 271–288 (1994).

E. Perret, *Neuropsychologia*, 12, 323–330 (1974).

J. L. Ponsford and G. Kinsella, *J. Clin. Exp. Neuropsychol.*, 10(6), 693–708 (1988).

J. Ponsford and G. Kinsella, *J. Clin. Exp. Neuropsychol.*, 14(5), 822–838 (1992).

R. G. Robinson and R. Jorge, Mood Disorders, in J. M. Silver, S. C. Yudofsky, and R. E. Hales, Eds., *Neuropsychiatry of Traumatic Brain Injury*, American Psychiatric Press, Inc., Washington, D.C., 1994, pp. 219–250.

W. R. Russell, *The Traumatic Amnesias*, Oxford University Press, New York, 1971.

M. E. Sandel, K. S. Williams, L. Dellapietra, and L. R. Derogatis, *Brain Inj.*, 10(10), 719–728 (1996).

T. Shallice, *Philos. Trans. R. Soc. Lond. B. Biol. Sci.*, 25; 298(1089), 199–209 (1982).

T. Shallice and P. W. Burgess, *Brain*, 114(Pt. 2), 727–741 (1991).

J. M. Silver and S. C. Yudofsky, Aggressive Disorders, in J. M. Silver, S. C. Yudofsky, and R. E. Hales, Eds., *Neuropsychiatry of Traumatic Brain Injury*, American Psychiatric Press, Inc., Washington, D.C., 1994, pp. 313–353.

E. Smith, *J. Neurol. Neurosurg. Psychiatry*, 37, 719–726 (1974).

P. Snow, J. Douglas, and J. Ponsford, *Brain Injury*, 11(6), 409–429 (1987).

M. M. Sohlberg and C. A. Mateer, *J. Clin. Exp. Neuropsychol.*, 9(2), 117–130 (1987).

J. M. Spikman, A. H. van Zomeren, and B. Deelman, *J. Clin. Exp. Neuropsychol.*, 18(5), 755–767 (1996).

O. Spreen and E. Strauss, *A Compendium of Neuropsychological Tests*, 2nd Ed., Oxford University Press, New York, 1998.

L. R. Squire, *Memory and Brain*, Oxford University Press, New York, 1987.

D. T. Stuss and D. F. Benson, *The Frontal Lobes*, Raven Press, New York, 1986.

D. T. Stuss, P. Elym, H. Hugenholtz, M. T. Richard, S. LaRochelle, C. A. Poirier, and I. Bell, *Neurosurgery*, 17, 41–47 (1985).

D. T. Stuss, L. L. Stethem, H. Hugenholtz, T. Picton, J. Pivik, and M. T. Richard, 1988.

D. T. Stuss, L. L. Stethem, T. W. Picton, E. E. Leech, and G. Pelchat, *Can. J. Neurol. Sci.*, 16, 161–167 (1989).

D. T. Stuss, J. P. Toth, D. Franchi, M. P. Alexander, S. Tipper, and F. I. Craik, *Neuropsychologia*, 37(9), 1005–1027 (1999).

K. Tabaddor, S. Mattis, and T. Zazula, *Neurosurgery*, 14(6), 701–708 (1984).

M. E. Timmerman and W. H. Brouwer, *Neuropsychologia*, 37, 467–478 (1999).

E. Tromp and T. Mulder, *J. Clin. Exp. Neuropsychol.*, 13, 821–830 (1991).

F. M. Tucker and R. E. Hanlon, *Brain Inj.*, 12(9), 783–792 (1998).

B. Tulving, Episodic and Semantic Memory, in E. Tulving and W. Donaldson, Eds., *Organization of Memory*, Academic Press, New York, 1972.

A. H. van Zomeren and W. H. Brouwer, *Clinical Neuropsychology of Attention*, Oxford University Press, New York, 1994.

A. M. Weber, *J. Head Trauma Rehabil.*, 5(1), 73–85 (1990).

M. Ylvisaker and T. Feeney, *Semin. Speech Lang.*, 17(3), 217–232 (1996).

CHAPTER 17

THE AMERICAN BRAIN INJURY CONSORTIUM

ANTHONY MARMAROU

Medical College of Virginia Commonwealth University, Richmond, Virginia

INTRODUCTION

Studies in 1995 and 1996 indicate that there are 280,000 traumatic brain injuries each year in the United States that require hospital admission. Of this group, 230,000 survive and an additional 50,000 die as a result of traumatic brain injury (Guerrero et al., 1996; Thurman and Guerrero, 1996; Sosin et al., 1995). Mortality associated with severe head trauma has decreased from 35 percent in the late 1980s to 25 percent in the late 1990s due to improved intensive care management and avoidance of secondary insult. Many consider this to be a plateau and that further improvement in outcome must come from pharmacological intervention. Heretofore, despite the development of many compounds exhibiting varying degrees of neuroprotection in the laboratory, no drugs have proven effective in the clinical setting. However, the reported success of the randomized prospective spinal cord injury trial utilizing high-dose steroid was the first indication that pharmacological treatment of the damaged central nervous system in man was possible (Bracken et al., 1990). The National Institutes of Health and the pharmaceutical industry jointly funded this trial, and it was common that investigators would seek funding from the federal government for the implementation of clinical trials. This was the case several years ago when most if not all head injury trials were funded exclusively by the NIH. For example, relatively small clinical trials conducted by the Medical College of Virginia in Richmond were funded by the NIH and included studies of barbiturate coma (Ward et al., 1985), hyperventilation (Muizelaar et al., 1991), and pegulated superoxide dismutase (Muizellar et al., 1993). However, the shrinking pool of research funds available from federal sources coupled with a shift in policy toward governmental funding of pharmaceutical product testing required that investigators move to the

Head Trauma: Basic, Preclinical, and Clinical Directions, Edited by Leonard P. Miller and Ronald L. Hayes, Co-edited by Jennifer K. Newcomb
ISBN 0-471-36015-5 © 2001 John Wiley & Sons, Inc.

private sector for conduct of clinical trials. Thus, a new approach was required to deal effectively with the many problems facing the clinical investigator in the industry–university relationship where primary differences in mission, policy differences in freedom of information, ownership of data, patent rights, and general reporting of scientific findings were problematic.

The American Brain Injury Consortium (ABIC) was formed in April 1993 by a small group of investigators with the mission of assisting in the design and implementation of clinical trials targeted toward improving outcome of the brain-injured patient. The administrative plan was kept as simple as possible, with participation voluntary by all hospitals and university centers. Participation as a center investigator required a pledge by the clinician to follow the scientific guidelines set forth by the consortium. Starting from a group of 20 centers in 1993, the ABIC has grown to 230 premier centers and 570 investigators throughout the United States and abroad.

ADMINISTRATIVE STRUCTURE

ABIC Chairman

The ABIC administrative structure was designed so that policy and scientific decisions could be made rapidly and effectively while at the same time involve all of its members. The structure consists of a chairman, technical director, and a 12 member executive board and center investigators (Fig. 17.1). The chairman represents the consortium in all matters and is the official to be contacted by groups interested in utilizing the expertise and services of the consortium. In addition, the chairman leads the executive board and general meetings and maintains responsibility for organizing and implementing the meeting agenda. The chairman is elected by the general membership and serves for a minimum term of two years.

Technical Director

The technical director's responsibilities are to assist the chairman, lead investigator, and consortium members in all financial and technical aspects of the study, including communication, data management, analysis, and quality control. The technical director also represents the consortium in all technical matters relating to trial design and implementation.

The Executive Board

The 12 members of the executive board are elected by the general membership and four members are elected each year. The responsibility of the executive board is to serve as an advisory group for the chairman, technical director, and lead investigator in all matters concerning the consortium. They also serve on subcommittees established by the ABIC chairman, which include legal, budget, research, and center qualification.

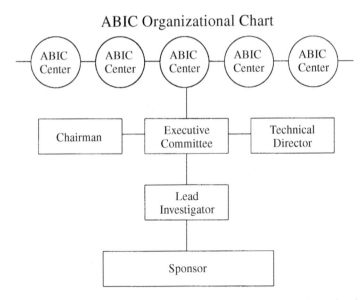

Figure 17.1 The administrative structure of the ABIC and its integration. The chairman of the consortium and the technical director have available the 12-member executive committee as advisors. The lead investigator is selected by the ABIC or appointed by the sponsor and coordinates the function of the consortium with the sponsor. The technical director is responsible for directing the ABIC technical center based in Virginia Commonwealth University, Richmond.

Lead Investigator

The lead investigator of a clinical trial implemented by the consortium must be a member of the consortium. Usually, one of the center investigators has been engaged in experimental or preliminary clinical studies and has developed a close liaison with the pharmaceutical company. It is the responsibility of the lead investigator to introduce the proposed study and together with the pharmaceutical company to present relevant preclinical and clinical data supporting the merits of the study. Upon endorsement of the study by the consortium, the lead investigator proposes scientific direction for the conduct of the study, coordinates scientific exchange between the consortium and the agency, and accepts responsibility for reporting the results of the study to the scientific community.

Center Investigators

The center investigator is entitled to one vote in all matters pertaining to the consortium. In the event there are several investigators from one center, all investigators may participate in ABIC meetings; however, only one vote is permitted from each center. The responsibilities of the center investigator are to decide which studies are to be implemented by the consortium based on the merits of the scientific data supporting the proposed clinical trial; to participate in all scientific and policy decisions of the consortium; to implement clinical trials at their respective center according to protocol; to manage head-injured patients according to American Association of Neurological Surgeons/ABIC guidelines adopted by the consortium; to propose or participate in substudies that may be warranted in conjunction with the main clinical trial; and to participate in special committees established by the consortium for management of centers, developing protocol guidelines consistent with standards of care, contractual matters, and publication.

Nurse Coordinators

The nurse coordinators from each center have primary responsibility for implementing the clinical trial and completing the clinical research forms in accordance with protocol. In addition, they are responsible for processing all IRB requirements; maintaining communication with the ABIC technical center and pharmaceutical company; reviewing proposed case report forms; surfacing patient management issues; completing forms necessary for the ABIC core data base; disseminating information from clinical reviews of patients entered into the trial; completing the monthly ABIC patient log; and participating in training of new coordinators.

Technical Center

The technical center of the ABIC resides at the Biotechnology Park of Virginia Commonwealth University in Richmond and is supervised by the technical director. The university has provided 5000 square feet of specialized facilities to house the technical center and its staff. The technical center works closely with the center investigators and the pharmaceutical company and provides expertise in the design, development, implementation and analysis of phases I through IV clinical trials. In addition, through the combined resources of the executive board and center investigations, the technical center coordinates preclinical animal studies, pretrial consultation, clinical operations, clinical data management, medical management, project management and statistical analysis essential to protocol design, safety monitoring board reporting, and final study reports. Funding of the technical center is derived from membership dues and services to pharmaceutical companies, which are necessary for conduct of a clinical trial by the ABIC.

The ABIC Core Database

The ABIC realized from its inception that it was essential that the vital data from traumatic brain-injured patients be archived and maintained. Prior to the formation of the ABIC, the only database information available on severe head injury was that of the NIH traumatic coma data bank (TCDB) (Foulkes and Eisenberg, 1991). This databank consisted of 1030 patients ranging from GCS (Glasgow Coma Score) 3 to 12, carefully monitored and documented during the period of 1987 to 1990. Unfortunately, the TCDB effort was not continued and thus there was no means of harvesting the wealth of clinical information derived from the survivors and nonsurvivors of severe brain trauma. At the outset, the ABIC adopted the principle that a "core" data set should be established that documents the pathophysiological course of all patients entered into clinical trials by the ABIC. At the same time, it was important to be highly selective so that the data collection process could be easily accomplished. It was decided to focus on that portion of data that is essential to publication. This generally includes the categories: patient demographics, parameters describing the severity of injury upon admission, experience of secondary insults of hypoxia and hypotension; CT descriptors; management and outcome. These elements, compacted into three pages of clinical research forms, comprise the ABIC core database and now serve as an extension of the traumatic coma databank experience.

The ABIC technical center archives and maintains the head injury database now totalling 3000 head-injured patients accrued from 1982 to present. In addition, demographic and injury severity information has been prospectively gathered on 15,000 patients as part of the monthly ABIC log instrument, which records data on all patients admitted to the ICU (Intensive Care Unit), and who form the selective cohort for clinical trials. The database includes patients from the TCDB and the major TBI trials. Initially, industry was reluctant to part with patient data; however, this has changed dramatically and companies are now offering their databases for research management and archiving by the ABIC. Thus, the history of emerging patterns of care and their influence on patient outcome are available from this master database. The databases are maintained in twin computer systems for maximum-security protection.

ABIC PATIENT CARE GUIDELINES

Management guidelines for the severely brain-injured patient were developed in 1995 as a joint initiative between the American Association of Neurological Surgeons (AANS), the Brain Trauma Foundation, and the AANS/Congress Joint Section on Neurotrauma and Critical Care (*J. Neurotrauma*, 1996). These evidence-based guidelines influence the treatment of head-injured patients throughout the world. The fact that only two treatments are considered "standards" point to the limited clinical prospective randomized studies. For example, monitoring of intracranial pressure (ICP) is considered an option due to the lack of a prospective randomized trial. As a trial of this nature would not be conducted in the United States today, the ABIC adopted several options as standards and members agree to treat patients within the boundaries of the ABIC patient care guidelines as an extension of the AANS guidelines.

Clinical Review of Patient Management

Clinical information documenting the intensive care of patients entered into clinical trials is transmitted to the Technical Center for review. The information includes ICU charts, medical notes and the ABIC core data set. The ICP component of the core data set documents ICP, CPP (cerebral perfusion pressure), temperature, and the therapy intensity level (TIL) (Maset et al., 1986) at hourly intervals for the first 5 days post injury. This information is entered into the technical center database, which provides graphical output summarizing the course of ICP, CPP, and TIL during the critical hours following injury (Fig. 17.2). Mean arterial blood pressure (MAP) is shown in the upper panel in combination with ICP. The solid line drawn at 20 mm Hg in the upper panel describes the ICP treatment threshold. The CPP is shown in the middle panel along with the ICP. The solid line drawn in the middle panel denotes the CPP threshold of 70 mm Hg, which is in accordance with ABIC/AANS guidelines. The bottom panel shows the temporal course of therapy intensity level, documenting the time during which sedation, drainage, mannitol, pressors, hyperventilation, and barbiturates were administered to the patient in an attempt to control brain swelling.

In the example shown, the graph depicts the clinical course of a 39-year-old male injured in a motor vehicle accident and admitted to the hospital with a subdural hematoma and a GCS of 7. Note that this required use of pressor therapy that was sustained for the duration of the monitoring period. Aggressive therapy was administered to maintain CPP within threshold and only brief excursions below a CPP of 70 mm Hg were experienced. This patient was managed appropriately and care was in compliance with recommended AANS/ABIC guidelines.

The first year's experience by the ABIC in determining compliance with AANS/ABIC guidelines is shown in Fig. 17.3. A total of 326 head-injured patients ranging in GCS from 3 to 8 treated by 84 level 1 trauma centers were classified as either compliant or noncompliant based on deviation from guidelines. The data elements available for review included (1) an initial screen form, which documented all demographics, prehospital status, presence of secondary insult and classification of CT used for randomization based on TCDB criteria (Marshall et al., 1991); (2) ICU charts for the first 5 days post injury documenting ICP and CPP variation at hourly intervals; and (3) therapy intensity levels documenting frequency of therapies for ICP and CPP management.

During the entire study period, 190 of 326 patients reviewed (58.6 percent) were classified as in compliance with AANS head injury guidelines. Deviations from guidelines were associated with the remaining 135 patients, representing 41.4 percent of the cohort. The highest percentage of deviations (52.7 percent) was attributed to use of sustained hyperventilation lowering $PaCO_2$ to less than 30 mm Hg. Periods of low CPP (<70 mm Hg) were attributed mainly to hypotension and accounted for 20.7 percent of deviations, while absence of ICP monitoring accounted for 14.6 percent of deviations.

The study showed that a significant number of deviations from recommended AANS guidelines occur and the greater percentage of deviations was attributed to sustained hyperventilation. The study supports the notion that publication of the guidelines in itself does not insure that the information filters down to the neurosurgical residents, intensivists, anesthesiologists, and trauma surgeons who are intimately involved in patient care. It is clear that a more aggressive campaign

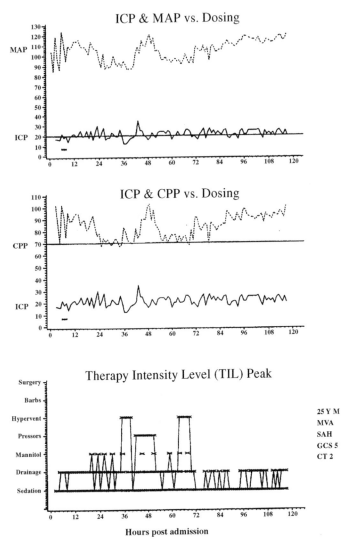

Figure 17.2   An example of a clinical review processed by the technical center and sent back to the investigator. Data are extracted from the ABIC core data forms, which require hourly measurement of ICP, BP, and the therapy intensity level (TIL) used in management for the first five days post injury. Solid lines indicate the treatment thresholds for ICP (<20 mm Hg) and CPP (>70 mm Hg) used by the ABIC. The flag (upper and middle panels) recorded at seven hours post injury indicates the time of drug dosing. Note that periods of aggressive hyperventilation were kept as brief as possible to avoid risk of ischemia. In the case presented, treatment thresholds were maintained and management of this patent was in accord with ABIC/AANS guidelines.

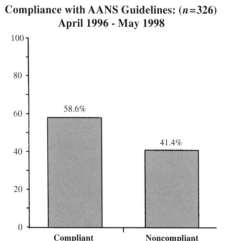

Figure 17.3 subtitle from chart:

Compliance with AANS Guidelines: ($n=326$)
April 1996 - May 1998

Figure 17.3 Assessment of compliance in 326 patients reviewed during the period immediately following the distribution of the AANS guidelines. Based on management guidelines by the ABIC and AANS, 41.4% of cases were considered noncompliant. Most of these deviations from guidelines were associated with the use of prolonged aggressive hyperventilation ($PaCO_2 < 30 \, mm \, Hg$).

must be launched to inform all disciplines as to the rationale and definition of AANS guidelines for traumatic brain injury. Moreover, it reinforces the concept that the clinical review process for monitoring the adherence to guidelines and eliminating management variation in clinical trials is essential.

OUTCOME MEASURES

One of the more complex issues in head injury research is the development of suitable outcome measures. At present, the Glasgow Outcome Scale (GOS) is the most widely used measure for grading outcome from severe brain injury (Jennet and Teasdale, 1981). Studies have shown that it is favored over other measures such as the disability rating scale (Gouvier et al., 1987). The GOS was devised to provide a coarse comparison in head injury outcome; however, the bimodal distribution of the GOS presents difficulties in trial design. For example, 70 percent of the patients will classify within two outcome categories, good recovery and death. The remaining 30 percent will be distributed among moderate disability, severe disability, and vegetative state. It is in this relatively small percentage of patients that an upscale movement can occur with successful pharmacological intervention and, as a result, the primary outcome parameter is usually dichotomized into Good/Mod and Sev/Veg/Dead. Clinical trials using the GOS, assessed at 6 months, are targeted to effect an upward movement of 15 percent to 20 percent of patients at a minimum of 85 percent power level.

GOS Reliability

The dichotomized GOS provides a degree of simplification in trial design. However, this may be confounded by interobserver reliability. The ABIC conducted a study to ascertain the reliability of the GOS among neurosurgeons, neuropsychologists, and nurse coordinators (Marmarou et al., 1999a). A total of 10 case reports describing outcome from 10 severely injured patients were placed on the internet and 34 ABIC members were asked to respond and rate the cases according to the GOS. Three months after receiving the responses, a GOS checklist was developed and distributed to the same group of investigators to repeat their ratings. To avoid bias, a second group of 46 ABIC investigators received the 10 case reports and the checklist at the same time and were asked to rate the case reports using the ABIC GOS checklist.

The mean accuracy of GOS rating of the 10 case reports without using the checklist equalled 68.84 percent $\pm$ 18.25 percent s.d. Using the checklist, the accuracy improved to 82.00 percent $\pm$ 11.57 percent. Interestingly, the percentage accuracy among nurse coordinators, neurosurgeons, and neuropsychologists with the checklist was not significantly different.

The effect of interobserver reliability of the GOS can be seen in Table 17.1, where the results of the analysis are shown for the correct GOS (vertical), as analyzed by a group of neuropsychologists, and the assessment by ABIC investigators (horizontal). Note that 31.91 percent of GOS Moderate were shifted to GOS Good. In addition, for patients with severe GOS, 56.99 percent were scored as Moderate and 2.15 percent were scored as Good outcome. Moreover, for vegetative patients, 18.18 percent were rated as Severe disability. Thus, in all categories there was a tendency for raters to shift upward to the better outcome category.

The GOS assessments using the structured check list are shown in Table 17.2. Patients in the Good category were rated most accurately. However, there still is a tendency to upgrade the outcome scoring. This is evident at 20.61 percent of Moderate patients shifted to GOS Good and 32.16 percent of Severe patients were rated as Moderately disabled. The comparison of GOS ratings using the checklist presented as dichotomized GOS is shown in Table 17.3. The reliability of Good and Moderate outcome assessment is excellent using the structured checklist. However, there still remains an upward shift of 17.4 percent of severe patients to the moderate

TABLE 17.1 Comparison of Correct GOS with Survey Answers—No Checklist (All Groups)

Rating	Correct GOS			
	G (%)	M (%)	S (%)	V (%)
G	**89.69**	10.39	0	0
M	31.91	**65.96**	2.13	0
S	2.15	56.99	**40.86**	0
V	0	0	18.18	**81.82**

TABLE 17.2 Comparison of Correct GOS with Survey Answers—With Checklist

Rating	Correct GOS			
	G (%)	M (%)	S (%)	V (%)
G	**99.12**	0.88	0	0
M	20.61	**79.39**	0	0
S	2.64	32.16	**65.20**	0
V 0	0	0	16.22	**83.78**

disability category. The differentiation of the lower end of moderate and upper end of severe disability categories is the most difficult to assess.

It is obvious from this analysis that interobserver reliability of GOS without use of the structured checklist is poor. Using the ABIC checklist, the accuracy was improved from 68.84 percent to 82.00 percent ($p < 0.002$). Presumably, if the same errors were made in each arm of a clinical trial, the effects would cancel. However, if the error was unbalanced, it could translate into a significant effect and jeopardize the outcome of a clinical trial.

The Expanded GOS

These problems cited above have been addressed by Teasdale et al. and a new approach to outcome assessment has resulted in the "expanded GOS" rating (GOSE) (Teasdale, 1999). Using this scale, assignments can be made to an extended 8-point scale as well as the original 5-point approach. Of great advantage is the use of a structured questionnaire (Wilson et al., 1998) for the GOSE, which facilitates the use for the scale and reduces interobserver variability as demonstrated in this

TABLE 17.3 Comparison of Correct GOS (Dichotomized)—with Checklist

	Correct GOS	
	G/M (%)	S/v (%)
G/M	100.0	0
S/V	17.4	82.6

In the dichotomized presentation of outcome, misclassifications of Good or Moderate are grouped and the G/M category appears as 100% correct. However, in poor outcome, 17.4% of patients which should have been scored as Severe or Vegetative were misclassified as Good/Moderate.

report. Another important aspect of the GOSE is that it can be reduced to the GOS in order to compare with historical outcome studies using the standard GOS rating.

Neuropsychological Measures

Neuropsychological testing has usually been applied to minor and moderately head-injured patients for assessment of motor skill and cognitive function during the recovery from TBI (Capruso and Levin, 1992; Levin et al., 1992; Williams et al., 1990). A broad battery of tests was applied to the TCDB population of severely and moderately injured patients. However, the time necessary to complete the battery was extensive and relatively limited data were derived from the severe patient cohort (Levin et al., 1990). The problem of test completion is a significant one in patients with less favourable outcome and as a result neuropsychometrics have seldom been applied to severe TBI. During the formation of the ABIC, it was proposed that a practical neuropsychological testing program be evolved to assess cognitive function and motor skill within the limitation of a 30-minute evaluation period. The result was the development of the ABIC neuropsychometric testing battery (Marmarou, 1996). The ABIC battery of tests evaluates five different dimensions, which include memory, attention, visual perception, motor functioning, and language. These were utilized in the Bradycor clinical trial in survivors of severe brain injury, which included patients with GCS 3 through 8 and one reactive pupil (Marmarou et al., 1999b). The completion rates at three months post injury for Good and Moderate outcome patients ranged from 80 percent to 90 percent and completion rates at six months were similar. As expected, since full completion of the test battery is an indicator of cognitive performance, rates for the severe disability group dropped to 27.5 percent and 38.5 percent at three and six months respectively. In the severe outcome group, 65 percent of patients were able to either partially or fully complete the battery at three months.

Perhaps the most striking feature of these data was that the average composite score of all dimensions among severe head injury survivors was only 19.9 percent of normal value. At six months, as the recovery process continued, the score increased from 19.9 percent to 31.5 percent. Patients classified as GOS Good scored only in the 40th percentile.

Thus, the impact of severe TBI even in GOS Good survivors is dramatic as they function at less than 50 percent normal level. It emphasizes that neuropsychometric testing should be coupled with GOS ratings in order to have a more complete assessment of outcome from severe TBI.

NIH Sponsorship of Clinical Trials

The NIH continues to play a pivotal role in the conduct of clinical trials in traumatic brain injury. New mechanisms are now available to fund studies. In 1996, $300 million was spent on clinical trials. More recently, a special clinical trial working group has been established by the NIH to facilitate support of trials with new mechanisms for investigators to apply for funding. This includes the NINDS pilot clinical trial grant and the NINDS clinical trial planning grant. This provides new impetus for evaluating products or therapies that are unlikely to be tested under the auspices of industry, for example, the recent hypothermia trial and the study of CPP versus ICP management.

The European Brain Injury Consortium (EBIC)

Following the formation of the ABIC, the administrative structure and core data forms were transmitted to Glasgow and, through the efforts of Graham Teasdale, Professor of Neurosurgery, the EBIC was organized. The EBIC mission is similar to the ABIC and both consortiums have worked together in trials that were designed for implementation in both continents. At present, all countries with major trauma centers in Europe are closely allied and follow the EBIC guidelines for management of severe head injury (Maas et al., 1997). The EBIC guidelines are based on pragmatic considerations, consensus, and expert opinion in addition to the considerations of the AANS evidence-based guidelines.

SUMMARY

The formation of brain injury consortiums in both the United States (ABIC) and Europe (EBIC) provides an effective mechanism for the design and conduct of head injury clinical trials. In the case of ABIC, seven centers have been established in Israel and they work closely with the ABIC. In addition, pilot centers have been organized in Japan, South Korea, Singapore, and South America. Collectively, the consortium concept has been extended worldwide and centers are prepared to evaluate new treatments and drugs as they become available for study.

ABBREVIATIONS

AANS   American Association of Neurological Surgeons
ABIC   American Brain Injury Consortium
CPP   Cerebral perfusion pressure
CRF   Case report form
EBIC   European Brain Injury Consortium
GCS   Glasgow Coma Scale
GOS   Glasgow Outcome Scale
GOSE   Expanded Glasgow Outcome Scale
ICP   Intracranial pressure
ICU   Intensive care unit
IRB   Internal review board
MAP   Mean arterial pressure

NINDS National Institute of Neurological Disorder and Stroke
SD   Standard deviation
TBI   Traumatic brain injury
TCDB   Traumatic coma data bank
TIL   Therapy intensity level

REFERENCES

M. B. Bracken, M. J. Shepard, W. F. Collins, T. R. Holford, W. Young, D. S. Baskin, H. M. Eisenberg, E. Flamm, L. Leo-Summers, J. Maroon, L. F. Marshall, P. L. Perot, J. Piepmeier, V. K. H. Sonntag, F. C. Wagner, J. E. Wilberger, and H. R. Winn, *N. Engl. J. Med.*, 332(20), 1405–1411 (1990).

D. X. Capruso and H. S. Levin, *Neurol. Clin.*, 10, 879–893 (1992).

M. A. Foulkes and H. Eisenberg, *J. Neurosurg.*, 75 (Suppl.), S1–S7 (1991).

W. D. Gouvier, P. D. Blanton, K. K. LaPonte, et al., *Arch. Phys. Med. Rehabil.*, 68, 94–97 (1987).

J. L. Guerrero, D. J. Thurman, and J. E. Sniezek, "National Hospital Ambulatory Medical Care Survey of the National Center for Health Statistics," United States, 1995–1996. Guidelines for the management of severe head injury. Introduction. *J. Neurotrauma*, 13(11), 643–645 (1996).

B. Jennett and Bond, *Lancet*, 79(5), 480–484 (1975).

J. S. Kreutzer, C. W. Devany, S. L. Myers, and J. H. Marwitz, "Neurobehavioral Outcome Following Traumatic Brain Injury. Review, Methodology, and implications for cognitive rehabilitation," in J. S. Kreutzer and P. H. Wehman, Eds., *Cognitive Rehabilitation for Persons with Traumatic Brain Injury*, Paul H. Brookes, Baltimore, MD, 1991.

H. S. Levin, H. E. Gary, Jr., H. M. Eisenberg, et al., *J. Neurosurg.*, 73, 699–709 (1990).

H. S. Levin, D. H. Williams, H. M. Eisenberg, W. M. High, Jr., and F. D. Guinto, Jr., *J. Neurol. Neurosurg. Psychiatry*, 55, 255–262 (1992).

A. I. Maas, M. Dearden, G. M. Teasdale, R. Braakman, F. Cohadon, F. Iannotti, A. Karimi, F. Lapierre, G. Murray, J. Ohman, L. Persson, F. Servadei, N. Stocchetti, and A. Unterberg, *Acta. Neurochir. (Wien)*, 139(4), 286–294 (1997).

A. Marmarou, *Acta Neurochir.*, Suppl. 66, 118–121 (1996).

A. Marmarou, A. Saunders, J. Kreutzer, and S. Choi, *"A Method to Increasing the Reliability of the GOS Assessment in Head Injury Patients"* presented at the American Association of Neurological Surgeons Congress, New Orleans, 1999a.

A. Marmarou, J. Nichols, J. Burgess, D. Newell, J. Troha, D. Burnham, L. Pitts, and the American Brain Injury Consortium Study Group, *J. Neurotrauma*, 16(6), 431 (1999b).

L. Marshall, S. Marshall, M. Klauber, et al., *J. Neurosurg.*, 75(Suppl.), S14–S20 (1991).

A. L. Mast, A. Marmarou, J. D. Ward, and H. F. Young, "Pressure-Volume Dynamics in Head-Injured Patients: A Preliminary Study," in J. D. Miller, G. M. Teasdale, J. O. Rowan, S. L. Galbraith, and A. D. Menedlow, Eds., *Intracranial Pressure VI*, Springer-Verlag, Berlin, 1986, pp. 647–651.

J. P. Muizelaar, A. Marmarou, J. D. Ward, H. A. Kontos, S. C. Choi, D. P. Becker, H. Gruemer, and H. F. Young, *J. Neurosurg.*, 75, 731–739 (1991).

J. P. Muizelaar, A. Marmarou, H. F. Young, S. C. Choi, A. Wolf, R. L. Schneider, and H. A. Kontos, *J. Neurosurg.*, 78, 375–382 (1993).

D. M. Sosin, J. E. Sniezek, and R. J. Waxweiler, *J. Am. Med. Assoc.*, 273(22), 1778–1780 (1995).

L. E. L. Teasdale, J. T. L. Pettigrew, G. Wilson, G. Murray, and B. Jennett, *J. Neurotrauma*, 15(8), 587 (1999).

D. J. Thurman and J. L. Guerrero, "National Hospital Discharge Survey," of the National Center for Health Statistics. Trends in hospitalization associated with traumatic brain injury—United States, 1980–1995, *JAMA*, 282(10), 954–957 (1999).

J. D. Ward, D. P. Becker, J. D. Miller, S. C. Choi, A. Marmarou, C. Wood, and P. G. Newlon, *J. Neurosurg.*, 62, 383–388 (1985).

D. H. Williams, H. S. Levin, and H. M. Eisenberg, *Neurosurgery*, 27, 422–428 (1990).

J. T. L. Wilson, L. E. L. Pettigrew, and G. M. Teasdale, *J. Neurotrauma*, 15(8), 573 (1998).

CHAPTER 18

GUIDELINES FOR MEDICAL AND SURGICAL MANAGEMENT IN HEAD TRAUMA PATIENTS IN THE UNITED STATES AND EUROPE

DOMENICO D'AVELLA, M. D., and GIUSTINO TOMEI*, M.D.

Department of Neurosciences, Neurosurgical Clinic, University of Messina Medical School and *Institute of Neurosurgery, Ospedale Maggiore Policlinico, IRCCS Milano, Italy.

M. Berardino, L. Beretta, G. L. Brambilla, G. Citerio, R. Delfini, F. Della Corte, F. Servadei, and N. Stocchetti
On behalf of the Neurotraumatology Study Group of the Italian Neurosurgery Society (SINch) and the Neurosurgical Anesthesia and Critical Care Study Group, Italian Society for Anesthesia, Analgesia, Reanimation and Intensive Care (SIAARTI)

BACKGROUND

The need for guidelines for severe head injury management arose in the United States following a survey showing that the quality of treatment in a substantial proportion of American trauma centers was far from optimal. A European survey (data collection in 1995) showed similar findings (Murray et al., 1999): the need for guidelines is worldwide. The Guidelines of the joint section on Neurotrauma and Critical care of the American Association of Neurological Surgeons and the Congress of Neurological Surgeon, supported by the Brain Trauma Foundation, were published in 1996 (Bullock et al., 1996). The Guidelines for the management of severe head injury in adults as evolved by the European Brain Injury Consortium (EBIC) were published in 1997 (Maas et al., 1997). Despite different methodological approaches adopted (evidence-based in the former and consensus and expert opinion in the latter), similar conclusions and recommendations are found and the U.S. and European Guidelines, reflecting the consensus already existing among major

Head Trauma: Basic, Preclinical, and Clinical Directions, Edited by Leonard P. Miller and Ronald L. Hayes, Co-edited by Jennifer K. Newcomb
ISBN 0-471-36015-5 © 2001 John Wiley & Sons, Inc.

neurotrauma centers throughout the world on basic management of patients with severe head injury. In Italy, since 1994 and independently of the United States, a group of neurosurgeons and intensivists have worked together to produce guidelines for minor head injury management, which were completed and published in 1996 (The Study Group on Head Injury of the Italian Society for Neurosurgery, 1996). Moving toward severe head injury was the next logical consequence. A group of 20 neurosurgeons and 20 neurointensivists was formed ("the experts"). The Brain Trauma Foundation permitted use of the American guidelines as a basis for literature review, discussion, and education. The Guidelines were divided into three parts: pre-hospital-admission care, and medical and surgical therapy. The last is not contained in the American guidelines. The step-by-step process was initiated in 1995 and completed in 1998. Meetings of the experts produced proposals that were discussed in general meetings involving a few hundred people all over the country. The Italian guidelines are a more detailed and educational version of the American guidelines. There are also several specific additions and changes, including the following.

- Practical suggestions for the referral policy from peripheral hospital to the regional hospital/university trauma centers added to the part of the American guidelines on prehospital care.
- A protocol detailing timing of computed tomography (CT) monitoring integrated into the guidelines using a modified Marshall classification.
- A chapter on surgical indications containing both general and specific criteria for surgery for acute epidural and subdural hematomas and brain contusions/intracerebral hematomas, detailing an algorithm containing clinical, CT, and monitoring-derived criteria for surgery in comatose patients.

INTRODUCTION

The prognosis for patients with traumatic brain injury (TBI) is drastically influenced by the quality of care in the first few hours after the trauma, and also particularly by the frequent concomitant clinical alterations, such as hypotension and hypoxia. Delayed recognition of lesions that can be dealt with surgically is another unfavorable prognostic factor.

Our understanding of the pathophysiology of trauma has improved markedly in recent decades (Teasdale and Graham, 1998; Maas et al., 1999). Experimental and clinical findings indicate that the brain damage does not cease with the impact (primary damage), but progresses over subsequent hours and days (secondary damage) (see Chapter 1). Surgical evacuation of intracranial masses has absolute therapeutic priority and there is no alternative approach. However, prevention and treatment of the extracerebral factors involved in secondary injury is the main aim of medical treatment. Scrupulous maintenance of systemic homeostasis not only prevents secondary brain ischemia or anoxia but also limits the development of intracranial hypertension in patients with no lesions likely to respond to surgery.

The idea of guidelines for the treatment of severe cranial trauma cases has proved ambitious elsewhere in the world and would have been inappropriate in our specific circumstances, given the methods underlying these recommendations. There is usually only scant scientific evidence of the efficacy of each component in the management of severe cranial trauma, as few studies employing correct methods have reached reliable conclusions. A critical review in terms of evidence of efficacy was made by the joint section on Neurotrauma and Critical care of the American Association of Neurological Surgeons and the Congress of Neurological Surgeons, supported by the Brain Trauma Foundation (Bullock et al., 1996). This, and the review based on expert opinions by the European Brain Injury Consortium (Maas et al., 1997), are landmarks from the methodological and clinical viewpoints, and have been used as the source and scientific basis for these Italian guidelines. However, some specific suggestions were needed for Italy, since the practical indications set out in the "Guidelines for the Management of Severe Brain Injury" (Bullock et al., 1996) do not cover all the clinical aspects and—above all—are not always easy to adapt to different regional organizations, where some of the concepts offered will not be clinically feasible. Many of the recommendations still have inadequate scientific backing and are under continuing review. The clinical and organizational indications must therefore be taken merely as suggestions on how to act.

It is important to stress that these are recommendations, not binding rules, because caution is always needed on account of the medicolegal implications and the need for safeguarding medical workers. If pragmatic recommendations could really be applied throughout Italy, they would probably have considerable impact in terms of reduction in mortality and disability. This was the conviction that in 1995 led a group of about 40 neurosurgeons, anesthesiologists, and intensivists, all belonging to the Neurotraumatology Study Groups of the Italian Society of Neurosurgery (SINCh) and the Italian Society of Analgesia, Anesthesia, Reanimation, and Intensive Therapy (SIAARTI), to draft Italian guidelines for the treatment of severe head injury. These guidelines were based on a mixture of scientific evidence, expert opinions and the current local clinical/organizational situation. The aim of the project is to provide a practical reference tool for all those dealing with severe cranial trauma, from the scene of traffic accidents to intensive care units. It sets out the minimal organizational and clinical goals to be reached throughout the country, in all emergency departments and hospitals with facilities for traumatic brain injury patients, even without neurosurgery and neurological intensive care units (ICU). This approach means that many of the guidelines will seem very modest compared to the advanced facilities available in many parts of Europe for emergency care and for neurotraumatology and intensive care. The guidelines will need continual critical review and updating. The approach is strictly clinical, and we have therefore kept it concise and schematic. These guidelines, which are grouped under several main headings (Table 18.1), were drafted by a combined group of neurosurgeons, intensivists, and anesthesiologists. Despite some methodological limitations, the recommendations therefore reflect a multidisciplinary consensus and provide a clear

TABLE 18.1 Guidelines of the Neurotraumatology Study Groups of SINCh and SIAARTI: List of Headings

1. Initial assessment and resuscitation of vital functions
2. Neurological evaluation
3. Hospital admission criteria
4. CT scanning
5. Monitoring systemic parameters in intensive care units
6. Monitoring intracranial pressure and jugular oxygen saturation
7. Medical treatment criteria
8. Surgical treatment criteria

example of the will to cooperate, which is what is needed more than anything else to improve the quality of organization and therapy.

INITIAL ASSESSMENT AND RESUSCITATION OF VITAL FUNCTIONS

The main goal of any treatment given before the patient is admitted to hospital must be to stabilize vital functions. This involves a series of assessments and steps. Absolute priority goes to prevention and treatment of hypotension and hypoxia, since these may have a dramatic impact on neurological outcome (Jones et al., 1994). The primary survey includes the following steps.

Airway Patency

Patients with altered level of consciousness [Glasgow Coma Scale (GCS) < 8] always require a definitive airway. This means tracheal intubation with the patient sedated or under analgesia (see Table 18.2 for protocol). The use of neuromuscular blocking drugs should be restricted to the intubation procedure. If necessary, short-acting neuromuscular blocking agents should be used to achieve positive-pressure breathing without a rise in intrathoracic pressure. Measures must be taken to protect the patient's cervical spine during the initial assessment and procedures to maintain airway patency. The orotracheal route is recommended for intubation. The naso-tracheal route is blind and is therefore not advisable. Airways must be protected to prevent gastric contents, blood, mucus, and so on, from entering. The risk of vomiting is high, so an aspirator must always be on hand. A nasogastric tube should be positioned through the mouth, on account of the risk of fractures of the skull base and ethmoid bone.

Breathing

All intubated patients must be ventilated, to obtain adequate oxygenation ($PaO_2 > 90$ mm Hg, $SaO_2 > 95$ percent) and to prevent hypercapnia ($PaCO_2 >$

TABLE 18.2   Sedation and Tracheal Intubation Protocols

Recommended sedation protocol for tracheal intubation of patients with severe brain injury
- Thiopental sodium 2–3 mg/kg i.v. or propofol 1–2 mg/kg i.v. or midazolam 0.2–0.3 mg/kg[a]
- If hypotensive or bleeding: ketamine 1 mg/kg + thiopental 1 mg/kg or midazolam 0.05–0.1 mg/kg
- Succinylcholine 1 mg/kg i.v. or vecuronium 0.1 mg/kg i.v.
- Lidocaine 1 mg/kg i.v.

Sequence of steps for intubation
1. Assessment of the airways
2. Manual stabilization of the spine
3. Preoxygenation of the patient
4. Removal of front of the cervical collar
5. Cricoid pressure
6. Induction of anesthesia and myorelaxation
7. Laryngoscopy and rapid intubation
8. Ventilation and auscultation
9. Replacing cervical collar

---

[a]Sedation/analgesia should be continued, using short-acting drugs so that neurological assessments can be made at regular intervals in the emergency department. Muscle relaxing drugs should be avoided if possible.

35 mm Hg) or hypocapnia ($PaCO_2$ < 30 mm Hg). Hypercapnia is avoidable as a factor aggravating brain injury and must absolutely be corrected if not prevented. Cerebral acidosis or vasodilatation can cause intracranial hypertension and secondary brain damage. Hyperventilation, which may lead to hypocapnia, is not advisable because cerebral vasoconstriction induced by the drop in blood CO_2 may cause cerebral hypoperfusion. This worsens the already critical situation of diminished cerebral blood flow or inadequate oxygen transport.

Circulation

Even a single episode of hypotension (systolic blood pressure (BP) < 90 mm Hg) in the early stages after trauma may increase mortality and disability. For safety's sake, therefore, it is advisable to keep systolic BP higher than 110 mm Hg in adults, throughout treatment, to ensure adequate cerebral perfusion pressure (CPP), calculated by subtracting mean intracranial pressure (ICP) from mean BP. The recommended measures to achieve these goals are shown in Table 18.3. If the patient presents clinical deterioration and clinical signs of uncal herniation (anisocoria, focal signs) before reaching a hospital, hyperventilation ($PaCO_2$ 25 to 30 mm Hg) and mannitol (e.g., 18 percent mannitol, 0.25 g/kg in 15 min) may be useful to limit the rise in ICP and compression of the brain stem, and gain time to reach neurosurgery, keeping BP high enough at all times. Mannitol may cause hypotension, and enlargement of a hematoma, and the hypocapnia may reduce brain blood flow to

TABLE 18.3 **Recommended Measures for Achieving Sustained High (> 110 mm Hg) Systolic Blood Pressure**

1. Identification of external bleeding and control by direct pressure (bear in mind that scalp lesions can cause copious bleeding, which is easily stopped once the cause has been identified and dealt with)
2. Initial restoration of blood volume using isotonic solutions (saline, Ringer lactate; hypotonic solutions such as 5 percent glucose should not be administered; osmotic diuretics (mannitol) are not recommended)

critical levels. To avoid iatrogenic damage, therefore, this aggressive approach must be duly weighed, and implemented only if all the above criteria are fulfilled. During primary transport, ECG, noninvasive BP, and arterial oxygen saturation, at least, should be monitored. Although there is always the risk of high BP due to traumatic stress facilitating cerebral edema in patients whose autoregulation is unbalanced, the danger that hypotensive drugs may cause hypoperfusion suggests that it is advisable to tolerate higher than normal BP—systolic up to BP 160 to 170 mm Hg—with adequate sedation and analgesia.

Disability: Neurological Examination

Neurological examination as described below (GCS, pupil diameter and pupillary light reflex) should be conducted following the procedures described.

Exposure: Thorough Examination and Assessment

Patients with head trauma should be fitted with a stiff collar to keep the cervical spine stable. All multiple-trauma patients must be checked for pneumothorax and hemoperitoneum. Multiple-trauma patients must receive prompt aggressive treatment to manage life-threatening injuries, as identified. Lesions such as pneumothorax or hemoperitoneum must be excluded. These are often overlooked in the early work-up, even once the patient has reached a hospital (Andrews et al., 1991). Prompt diagnosis and treatment for both these conditions can considerably reduce extra- and intrahospital mortality due to hypotension, hypoxia, and shock. A multidisciplinary clinical and organizational approach is required throughout the patient's early diagnostic stage, and subsequent stay in the ICU. Further recommendations that should be borne in mind are outlined in Table 18.4.

NEUROLOGICAL EVALUATION

Use the Glasgow Coma Scale (GCS) (Table 18.5) to describe the altered level of consciousness, on the basis of three components: eyes open, verbal responses, motor

TABLE 18.4   Anamnestic Work-up During Patient's Early Diagnostic Stage

1. Information can be collected from whoever provided first aid: How did the accident happen? Description of the scene, with an assessment of the damage to vehicles, for instance. Collect all possible details about what happened immediately after the accident. Was the patient conscious for even a short time before falling into a coma? Did she or he present convulsions, loss of fluid from the nose and/or mouth, cyanosis?
2. Age is an important prognostic factor. The prognosis may be worse for older people. Pathophysiological alterations caused by trauma differ in the young and old.
3. History: Obtain information on whether the patient had any previous pathology or allergic diathesis, was taking medicinal drugs, and had eaten, drunk alcohol, or used substances of abuse.

TABLE 18.5   Scale for Determination of Glasgow Coma Score

Definition of coma: A patient in coma cannot open his/her eyes, speak or obey simple commands (GCS < 8, or 8 if the patient utters incomprehensible sounds)

Glasgow Coma Scale

Eye opening (O)	Spontaneous	4
	In response to speech	3
	In response to pain	2
	No eye opening (also in cases with periorbital edema)	1
Verbal response (V)	Oriented	5
	Confused conversation	4
	Inappropriate speech	3
	Incomprehensible speech	2
	None (also for patients with tracheal tube)	1
Motor response (M)	Obeying command	6
	Localizing response to pain	5
	Flexor withdrawal	4
	Abnormal flexor response	3
	Extensor posturing to pain	2
	No response to pain	1

Overall GCS score = O + V + M (min 3–max 15)

responses (Marion and Carlier, 1994). A record must be made of the time when the evaluation was made and who made it. The patient should be examined as soon as vascular and respiratory homeostasis has been restored. For adequate interpretation, together with the scores for the three components, BP should be recorded, and whether the patient was under sedation. A standardized method (Table 18.6) should be employed to stimulate patients.

TABLE 18.6   Standardized Methodology for Obtaining GC Scores

1. Take the best motor response on the best side, and only of the arms.
2. The pain stimulus must always follow the verbal request. Stimuli should be of an adequate strength and duration, applied bilaterally, in the supraorbital area, to the trunk (knuckles on the breastbone) or to the nail bed, with a pencil, for example.
3. Always bear in mind the possibility of spinal cord or peripheral nerve injury and limb fractures.
4. The GCS should be documented and transmitted broken down into its three components and as the total. In comatose patients, whose eye opening score is obviously 1 and verbal response 1 or 2, the GCS differs only in the motor response to pain, which thus has considerable clinical and prognostic importance. We assume, when periorbital edema is such that the patient's eyes cannot be opened even passively, that GCS eye opening score (O) is indicated as 1 (E). For patients with a tracheal tube, the verbal response (V) is rated as 1 (T).
5. When the patient has been sedated, wait 10–20 min after the half-life of the drug employed.
6. Test localization by a stimulus to the thigh, so as to avoid confusion with flexor responses.
7. Abnormal flexion involves adduction of the arm, flexion of the wrist, and incarceration of the thumb (classical decortication).
8. Extension involves hypertonic arm adduction with pronation and flexion of the wrist (classic decerebration).
9. It is advisable to record the initial GCS after correcting hypotension, hypoxia, and so on, since the score may improve drastically after adequate reanimation.
10. A constant, homogeneous method must be used for neurological monitoring based on the GCS.

The state of the pupils must be clearly recorded so that the diameter and light reaction (photomotor reflex) can be established. Light in the examining room must be strong enough but not too bright. In patients with midriasis, assess and record the presence of drugs (epinephrine-like, atropine), stress and pain, and the possibility of peripheral lesions to cranial nerves II or III. Myosis may be due to anesthetics or opioids.

Neurological examination in the first 72 h comprises assessment of the GCS, pupil size, and reactions (see above) at admission, every hour or any time a neurological change occurs by the nursing staff, every 4 h or any time a neurological change occurs by the medical staff. In patients under sedation, leave a pharmacological "window" for assessment every 8 h during the first 72 h. Despite the highly sophisticated monitoring available in an ICU, clinical assessment of the patient is still essential. Records should be easy to read so that changes can be detected promptly; for example, nursing and medical staff may find an hour-by-hour daily chart useful. BP, ventilatory values, body temperature, and level of sedation at the time of neurological assessment must be entered on the chart. The use of drugs that are eliminated rapidly means that patients can be examined 15 to 20 min after discontinuing the drug during the first 72 h. New opioid analgesics offer this kind of prompt elimination.

HOSPITAL ADMISSION CRITERIA

The criteria offered here reflect the pragmatic approach taken by these guidelines and the wide variety of organizational settings throughout Italy. Clearly, a head trauma patient must be admitted to a certified trauma unit where the highest quality care and surveillance are available. Many deaths could be avoided if hospitals were better organized and more efficient. Emergency care may fail if hospital trauma centers are not able to offer full facilities around the clock and the quality of care in these centers depends largely on their having enough work to keep their procedures up-to-date and efficient. The national health emergency system is not organized at present to ensure this flow to trauma centers with specialized neurosurgery departments. This means that a large proportion of patients are admitted to hospitals closest to the scene without neurosurgical facilities. One aim of these recommendations is to indicate the best clinical approach in such nonspecialized settings. The intention is not to encourage admissions to nonspecialized units, but to help safeguard patients and provide prompt and appropriate attention in any logistic situation. Some likely scenarios depicting common situations are presented in Table 18.7. The main thing in any setting is that management of the severe cranial trauma patient has two equally important therapeutic priorities:

1. To identify and promptly treat any surgically removable lesions.
2. To prevent and treat any factors that might worsen the situation, and to maintain homeostasis.

CT SCANNING

The initial diagnosis may have to be modified during the acute phase on the basis of changes from the first CT scan. Some traumatic injuries—especially surgical cases—become evident only after a certain interval, so they are not detectable in the first CT scan (Servadei et al., 2000). The aim is to classify patients correctly on the basis of the initial lesions. For a uniform description, we refer here to Marshall's classification (Marshall et al., 1991), adding the type of lesion and whether it is single or multiple (Table 18.8). It is important to record whether there is intracranial air and whether the injury is closed or open. The criteria for follow-up CT are outlined in Table 18.9. Intracranial lesions may sometimes change considerably in size without causing any appreciable rise in ICP for a long time. The combination of clinical and instrumental monitoring with regular CT scans is the best way to follow space-occupying lesions. A CT scan must be done promptly to detect masses requiring surgery. However, even prompt investigation cannot detect lesions that are still forming. Negative findings at the first CT scan must therefore not induce a sense of false security, and subsequent checks and clinical observation remain indispensable, according to the procedures outlined above.

TABLE 18.7 Criteria for Admitting Comatose Trauma Patients to Hospital: Likely Scenarios

- Outside the hospital, a comatose patient has not been stabilized despite all primary reanimation efforts. Acute respiratory failure has not been solved by intubation and ventilation (e.g., chest trauma with hemopneumothorax), and severe cardiovascular insufficiency suggests internal hemorrhage. This patient must be taken to the nearest hospital with a 24-h general surgery unit, an ICU, and a radiology department offering full X-ray facilities and ultrasound. There is no need to rush specific tests for neurosurgical diagnosis before the patient is clinically stable. The hospital neurosurgical department should be advised so as to be ready to admit the stabilized patient for a CT scan and specialized assessment of intracranial lesions (and relative surgical interventions).
- Outside the hospital, a comatose patient has stable circulation and respiration and needs to be admitted to a hospital providing at least the following:

  - An Intensive Care Unit that can ensure ventilatory assistance, invasive arterial monitoring, serial blood gas analysis, hourly neurological checks (GCS and pupils), intensive care medical staff, and a ratio of at least one nurse to every two patients
  - 24-h CT scan service with staff to interpret the findings either on the spot or by telephone/computer.

At admission the following are indispensable:
1. Continuation and optimization of reanimation therapy
2. Diagnostic definition of brain injury (CT scan) and the cervical spine (including the cervicodorsal junction), within 3 h of trauma
3. Diagnosis of concomitant lesions (X-rays of the chest and pelvis and abdominal ultrasonography)
4. Neurosurgical consultation, either directly or using image and clinical information transmission systems, to establish whether transfer to a neurosurgical intensive care unit is urgent or can be planned.

The scarcity of intensive care beds for neurosurgery and the uniformity of medical reanimation therapies calls for cooperation between reanimation departments, so that surgical cases or those soon likely to need surgery can be sent preferably to hospitals with neurosurgical facilities, and patients whose conditions have been stabilized can continue reanimation treatment in nonneurosurgical units.

If the neurological consultant considers the patient can remain in a nonsurgical unit, therapy from that point on should be aimed at

- Maintaining cardiovascular and respiratory stability
- Clinical monitoring (GCS, pupils, focal signs) to detect any neurological deterioration suggesting progression, which would require the patient to be transferred immediately to a hospital with neurosurgical facilities
- CT scan at the 12th hour
- Complete spinal X-ray even if the patient presents no particular clinical signs
- Contact with the neurosurgeon for a second assessment.

Even in patients with no immediate intracranial masses, the risk period cannot be considered closed until at least a week has passed from the trauma.

- A hemodynamically stable patient in a hospital without neurosurgical facilities falls into a coma. The criteria for transfer to a neurosurgical department are neurological deterioration and instability with worsening of the GCS, particularly as regards the pupils (mydriasis, pinpoint pupils, anisocoria), and motor score. It is advisable to transfer the patient before doing any diagnostic investigations (CT scan).

TABLE 18.8   Modified Marshall's Classification of Traumatic Brain Injury

Class Definition	Features
Diffuse lesion I	No intracranial pathology detectable by CT scan
Diffuse lesion II	Cisterns visible with 0–5 mm shift, and/or high–medium density lesions $<25\,cm^3$ (bone or foreign body compression)
Diffuse lesion III (swelling)	Cisterns compressed or absent; 0–5 mm shift in the median line; high–medium density lesion $<25\,cm^3$
Diffuse lesions IV (shift)	>5 mm shift of the median line; high–medium density lesions $<25\,cm^3$
Mass evacuated	Any injury requiring surgical removal, specifying whether epidural, subdural, or intraparenchymal
Mass not evacuated	Subarachnoid hemorrhage; high–medium density lesions $>25\,cm^3$, not surgically evacuated, specifying whether single or multiple
Subarachnoid hemorrhage	Present/absent

TABLE 18.9   Criteria for CT Monitoring of Traumatic Brain Injury

If the admission CT scan was negative, repeat within 24 h.

If the patient was hypotensive, or had coagulation abnormalities, repeat within 12 h.

If the admission CT scan was not negative, repeat within 24 h if it was first done within 6 h of the trauma, and the patient presents no risk factors.

Repeat within 12 h if it was done in the first 3 to 6 h after the trauma.

Subsequent examinations should be scheduled 72 h and 5 to 7 days after the trauma.

In all cases of clinical deterioration (loss of two points on the GCS, pupillary or motor signs), rise in intracranial pressure (ICP) above 25 mm Hg, drop of CPP below 70 mm Hg or SjO_2 below 50 percent for more than 15 min, an unscheduled CT scan must be done.

MONITORING SYSTEMIC PARAMETERS IN INTENSIVE CARE UNITS

The main aim in preventing secondary brain damage is to maintain homeostasis while controlling intracranial pressure. This is the goal of all stages of treatment, but particularly reanimation. Continuous care and attention are needed to maintain BP (systolic BP > 110 mm Hg), to treat stress with sedation and analgesia as necessary to prevent movement, coughing, and neurovegetative responses, and help adapt to ventilation, to ensure adequate oxygen transport (keeping hemoglobin levels up and $SO_2 > 95$ percent), and to keep blood volume, carbon dioxide, sodium and glucose levels, and body temperature within normal limits. This alone is an effective therapeutic goal with considerable impact on outcome. Any shift from normal levels with a therapeutic aim—hypocapnia or hypothermia—must be carefully planned and executed in closely controlled conditions (see Medical Treatment Criteria later). Minimum standards of instrumental monitoring are indispensable to achieve these aims, and must obviously be available in a reanimation unit for severe cranial trauma patients. These standards are presented in Table 18.10.

Various measurements should be employed to ensure adequate oxygenation and the required level of blood CO_2. These include blood gas analysis every 8 h and any time there is neurological deterioration or change in cardiovascular conditions, jugular vein oxygen saturation (SjO_2), regulation of ventilatory support, SaO_2, and

TABLE 18.10   Minimum Standards of Instrumental Monitoring to be Available in Neuro-ICU

Invasive blood pressure: Continuous monitoring is mandatory with concomitant monitoring of ICP the CPP can be calculated.

Electrocardiograms

Central venous pressure (CVP): This gives a simple though rough indicator of blood volume. Restoring blood volume is extremely important for the control of BP. In patients with unstable hemodynamic conditions or under vasopressor treatment, a Swan–Ganz catheter should be placed.

Arterial oxygen saturation (SaO_2): This is important because even brief episodes of inadequate oxygen supply may have a negative prognostic impact. Saturation must always be at least 95 percent.

Hourly diuresis: This is another indirect indicator of perfusion. Hourly measurements are considered essential. In case of brain damage an oligouric or polyuric response may suggest hyper- or hyposecretion of ADH. A polyuric response to an osmotic load is quite common (hyperglycemia and administration of mannitol).

Body temperature: A rise in brain temperature increases the brain's oxygen needs and may aggravate an imbalance between demand and supply, contributing to cerebral ischemia. It is therefore essential to measure core temperature at least once an hour if it cannot be monitored continuously. It should be borne in mind that the brain temperature is normally higher than that usually measured in an ICU. Hyperthermia must be tackled promptly and aggressively.

---

end-expiratory CO_2, as change in temperature or sedation, end-expiratory CO_2 (ETCO$_2$), or airway pressures. A chest X-ray must be available round the clock, with a radiologist available for consultation. This X-ray must be done at admission, after positioning a CVP catheter, after urgent reintubation, for suspected pneumothorax, if indicated by auscultation and clinical objective findings, or if indicated by respiratory monitoring. Finally, a tracheobronchial endoscope must be available if needed.

With regard to laboratory tests, details of the principles of treating critical patients are beyond the scope of these guidelines. However, it is worth recalling the effect of blood sodium levels on water flow through the blood–brain barrier, and of blood glucose levels, which, if uncontrolled, may aggravate the damage caused by acid–base imbalance and the altered brain cell energy metabolism.

MONITORING INTRACRANIAL PRESSURE (ICP) AND JUGULAR OXYGEN SATURATION (SjO$_2$)

Monitoring Intracranial Pressure (ICP)

Monitoring ICP is fundamental. Intracranial hypertension is the main threat to survival in the acute phase of trauma, and cannot be detected by indirect methods. Even a CT scan cannot give acceptable qualitative and quantitative information. The indications for monitoring ICP are presented in Table 18.11. Monitoring should be started as soon as possible, once the patient is clinically stable and a diagnosis has been established (after instrumental examinations). Since the operating theatre is sterile, it is better to position equipment for monitoring there than at the patient's bedside in the reanimation unit. The first thing is to position a ventricular catheter. If the ventricle cannot be located after two attempts, a subdural or parenchymal catheter should be left. There are no fixed time limits with regard to duration of monitoring, and how long the catheter remains in place depends on the patient's clinical condition. To avoid complications, strictly aseptic techniques must be applied for cerebrospinal fluid (CSF) drainage and sampling. Closed drainage systems are best. Samples should be taken for cytochemical and bacteriological testing in all patients scheduled for CSF withdrawal, and in all cases after three days of monitoring. At the same time mean BP must be measured to permit continuous

TABLE 18.11   Indications for ICP Monitoring

---

1. All hemodynamically stable patients (systolic BP > 110 mm Hg and SO_2 > 95 percent) with a GCS < 8 and positive CT scan for brain damage (high-density lesions, i.e., hematoma or contusions, or low-density ones such as edema or compressed basal cisterns)
2. GCS < 8 but negative CT scan and at least two of the following:
   - Abnormal pupillary diameter and reflexes
   - Asymmetrical motor response
   - Hypotension
   - Age over 40 years

---

recording of CPP. The arterial pressure transducer can be kept at the level of the external acoustic meatus to give a good CPP reading (CPP = mean BP − ICP). When CSF is withdrawn for therapeutic purposes, the pressure recorded is not the ICP as the system is open. In case of bone decompression or CSF leakage, the monitor may give readings that underestimate the severity of brain swelling or are unreliable, depending on how the monitoring is done. In practice, especially in cases of bone decompression, even a small rise in ICP should be considered cause for alarm. In patients with subtentorial masses, cerebral herniation or brain stem compression may occur even when ICP, measured in the supratentorial compartment, is not high. It may be prudent to measure ICP in patients undergoing surgery for evacuation of intracranial hematomas, with a catheter placed at the end of the operation.

Monitoring Jugular Venous Oxygen Saturation (SjO_2)

The artery–jugular vein oxygen difference gives useful information on the ratio of cerebral blood flow to cerebral oxygen consumption. Instead of measuring the arteriovenous difference, which may be misleading in severely anemic patients, the difference in saturation, known as cerebral oxygen extraction (CEO_2), gives the difference between oxygen saturation in arterial blood and in the jugular vein (Dearden, 1991). Despite considerable limitations, this method does show up dangerous desaturation situations (Robertson, 1993), often caused by low CPP or excessive hyperventilation and hypocapnia. SjO_2 should be monitored round the clock, but the cost and reliability of the signal with optical fiber catheters remain problematic. Serial samples can be drawn from a normal venous catheter. A cooxymeter is needed to measure SjO_2. The indications, method, and serial sampling procedures are outlined in Table 18.12. The catheter should preferably be inserted on the side where the jugular is largest, as shown on the CT scan—usually the right. The value is "global," but considerable differences may be seen between the two sides. SjO_2 monitoring does not take the place of other cerebral monitoring, particularly ICP. Except as part of multiparametric monitoring, including ICP, its interpretation—especially if values are high—and utility as a guide to treatment are limited.

Since these guidelines are intended to provide only minimal requisites, no other brain monitoring systems have been considered. However, continuous or serial EEG (in simplified form and processed if necessary), multimodal evoked potentials, and transcranial doppler all have their indications. They provide additional information on the pathophysiological dynamics, to guide treatment and formulate a prognosis. In Italy, as many other countries, the EEG is indispensable to confirm death when the heart is still beating.

MEDICAL TREATMENT CRITERIA

The purpose of medical therapy in acute head injury patients is to prevent secondary brain damage. The secondary damage may be due to intra- or extracranial causes.

TABLE 18.12   Indications and Methodology for Monitoring Jugular Venous Oxygen Saturation

Indications
- Patients undergoing therapeutic hyperventilation
- Patients with GCS < 8 and multiparametric monitoring (advisable).

SjO_2 monitoring should be started as soon as possible. The normal range for CEO_2 is 25–45 percent

Method
- X-ray to check correct positioning with the tip of the catheter in the jugular bulb, which normally projects at the atlooccipital junction
- Frequent calibration (at least every 12 h) for optical fiber catheters
- Measurements of CEO_2 using a cooxymeter

Serial samples
- Every 12 h
- In case of clinical deterioration (reduction of two points on the GCS)
- ICP > 25 mm Hg or CPP < 70 mm Hg
- Changes in $ETCO_2$ or $PaCO_2$
- Changes in sedation
- Acute anemia

Contraindications
Local neck injury

Complications
Carotid puncture
Cases of thrombosis of the jugular vein and infection have been reported

Most secondary injuries have ischemic neuropathological consequences (Graham et al., 1989). Intracranial causes include intracranial hypertension, expansive lesions, edema, hydrocephalus, infections, convulsions, changes in regional and global blood flow, and damage caused by free radicals or excitotoxic agents. Extracranial causes include arterial hypotension, hypoxia, anemia, hyperthermia, hyper- or hypocapnia, electrolytic abnormalities (mainly low blood sodium levels), hyper- or hypoglycemia, and acid–base imbalance. The most important cause of injury is delay in diagnosis and failure to evacuate intracranial hematomas. Medical therapy in patients with lesions likely to respond to surgery is only a means of gaining time on the way to the operating theater. Medical therapy is not a substitute for surgical evacuation which, when indicated, is the only approach likely to be effective.

Hemodynamics

Normal blood volume must be reestablished as fast as possible, and maintained. External and/or internal hemorrhages must be promptly diagnosed and treated with absolute priority, or excluded. Pneumothorax and pericardial tamponade must also be diagnosed, and drained immediately, or excluded. There is no indication for water restriction. CPP should be kept higher than 70 mm Hg, so as to maintain cerebral blood flow, which is reduced in the early hours after trauma, and to avoid the harmful effects of hypotension (Changaris et al., 1987). This implies simultaneous control of ICP and mean arterial pressure (MAP). Every effort must be made to avoid hypotension, which must always be corrected immediately. Hypotension is not generally a result of the cranial trauma itself, but reflects an extracranial cause, which must be sought and corrected. These extracranial causes include blood loss, both visible [scalp lesions (especially in children), maxillofacial lesions, exposed fractures] and occult (intra/retroperitoneal or pelvic hematomas, hemothorax, fractures of the long bones, rupture of large blood vessels).

Normal MAP should be maintained at >90 mm Hg and invasive BP monitoring is advisable. The best site for cannulation is the radial artery, with the pressure transducer at the level of the external acoustic meatus, so that CPP can be calculated correctly. Patients often need vasoconstrictors to raise the MAP. Inotropic and vasoconstrictor agents are routinely employed in intensive care to boost the heart's performance or maintain blood pressure, or both. Since trauma patients are particularly susceptible to reductions in renal plasma flow, vasoconstrictor drugs must always be used with an eye to safeguarding renal perfusion. Vasoconstrictor drugs are not an alternative or substitute for the treatment of intracranial hypertension. Control of ICP must have absolute priority for maintaining or improving CPP. These drugs (Table 18.13) are recommended in the following circumstances: to raise MAP to normal levels (> 90 mm Hg) if it still remains low after restoring blood volume; to achieve CPP of >70 mm Hg when treating intracranial hypertension has not had adequate effect.

Ventilation and Oxygenation

Make sure that airways are patent with tracheal intubation in comatose patients (GCS < 8). Avoid, or immediately correct, any episodes of hypoxemia (PaO_2 < 60 mm Hg). In trauma patients it is advisable to keep PaO_2 at 90 mm Hg

TABLE 18.13 Recommended Vasoconstrictor Drugs

Dopamine: Infusion of 2 to 5 μg/kg per min increases cardiac contractility and output. Larger doses (up to 10 μg/kg per min) further increase output with limited effect on BP. At doses higher than 10 μg/kg per min, peripheral vascular resistances are increased, so MAP rises accordingly.

Norepinephrine: Raises BP and systemic vascular resistance. The recommended starting dose to raise BP is 0.02–0.04 μg/kg per min, which is definitely safe. Higher doses can be used if necessary, but care must be taken not to cause renal damage. Renal function must always be closely monitored during infusion of vasoactive drugs. The risk of renal insufficiency is considerably greater when vasoactive drugs are used together with others such as mannitol, aminoglycosides, or vancomycin. There is less risk when volemia is maintained with adequate liquid infusion.

with arterial hemoglobin saturation higher than 97 percent. Take measures to keep blood carbon dioxide levels normal ($PaCO_2 = 35$ to $40\,mm\,Hg$).

Sedation

Sedation and analgesia must always be ensured, after respiratory assistance, even when the head trauma is not associated with other lesions (Aitkenhead, 1989). The aims are to control stress response, to control pain, to facilitate tracheal tube tolerance and adaptation to ventilation, and to limit intracranial pressure increases resulting from medical or nursing maneuvers. The ideal sedative should have rapid onset and swift metabolism. It must not accumulate. It must have no active metabolites. It must reduce ICP and cerebral metabolism without raising cardiovascular depression. Its effects must be rapidly reversible after withdrawal, to permit neurological evaluation. It should be inexpensive. Needless to say, no single drug available today offers all these features. In selecting the drug for sedation, certain features must be borne in mind. In the first few hours, neurological examinations must be repeated frequently, preferably within minutes of discontinuing the drug. Hemodynamic stability is essential, especially in hypovolemic patients. Infusion must not be too fast, and intravenous boluses should be injected slowly. Continuous infusion with a pump is the best way of giving these drugs, and priority should be assigned to drugs causing the least possible cardiovascular depression. Listed in Table 18.14 are some of the most widely used drugs, with indicative dosages. Naturally, dosages depend on numerous clinical factors, on what other drugs are also being given, and on the duration of administration. The lowest useful dose should be used in order to limit adverse reactions.

Other Therapeutic Aspects

In patients with severe head injury, medical treatment involves various other important aspects with potential impact on the outcome. We will not describe them all in detail here since they are not specific to head trauma patients, and call simply for a state-of-the-art approach as applied in good general intensive care. Briefly, they include gastroprotection; respiratory system management; maintenance of water–electrolyte balance; control of infection; nutritional therapy; and physiotherapy. Under the heading of nutritional therapy, it is worth underlining that nutrition is a cornerstone of clinical improvement. Enteral feeding should be started as soon as possible. Patients with gastric intolerance may benefit from jejunal enteral nutrition. This facilitates the management of patients in the subacute phase and during rehabilitation.

Prevention of Seizures

Seizures are a frequent complication of brain injury and are referred to as "early" if they arise in the first week, and "delayed" after that. The incidence is higher in children. The severity of the trauma, depressed fractures of the skull, contusions, and

TABLE 18.14   Recommended Drugs for Sedation and Analgesia

Benzodiazepines: Diazepam (bolus 0.03 to 0.1 mg/kg). Continuous infusion leads to drug accumulation.
Midazolam (bolus 0.02 to 0.3 mg/kg; maintenance doses 0.05 to 0.1 mg/kg per h).
Lorazepam (bolus 0.02 to 0.05 mg/kg; maintenance doses 0.05 to 0.5 mg/kg per h).

The benzodiazepines have no analgesic effect. They do not affect intracranial or systemic (hemo)dynamics if infused at low doses. Bolus injections and high doses may cause mild hypotension and respiratory arrest; they may also modify objective neurological findings, particularly brain stem reflexes. They have anticonvulsant activity. They have a moderate effect on metabolism ($CMRO_2$) and cerebral blood flow (CBF). In certain cases, particularly the elderly and alcohol abusers, they give rise to paradoxical reactions with psychomotor restlessness.

Propofol: Bolus 1–2 mg/kg, maintenance doses 1–3 mg/kg per h. This drug has a sleep-inducing effect. It reduces brain metabolism, CBF and ICP. It is rapid-acting, with brief kinetics or elimination. High doses or bolus injection may give rise to hypotension. Continuous infusion supplies a high lipid intake. Reversibility diminishes after 36 to 72 h of infusion. Seizures have been reported after low-dose infusion.

Opioids: Morphine (2 to 10 mg i.v.), meperidine (15 to 75 mg i.m.) which, however, has cardiodepressive activity and is less easy to handle, and fentanyl (bolus 0.25 to 1.5 μg/kg, maintenance doses 0.3 to 1.5 μg/kg per h). New potent molecules have recently been introduced, with short half-lives. These drugs can be recommended as part of a sedation program even for patients without algogenic extracranial lesions. The aim is to "defend" against stress and the external stimuli and nursing maneuvers that may raise ICP. Association with muscle relaxants such as the benzodiazepines can prevent or reduce some of the side effects arising when these drugs are used continuously, for example, muscle rigidity.

Neuromuscular blocking agents: There are no indications for routine use of neuromuscular blocking agents. Generally, deep pharmacological sedation achieves satisfactory clinical results. If necessary, in the conditions listed below under the heading "Criteria for Use", select nondepolarizing muscle relaxants, administered as a controlled continuous infusion.

Criteria for use: Always associated with adequate sedation. In cases with severe intracranial hypertension. To facilitate adaptation to ventilation in cases with respiratory failure. To avoid/overcome difficulties in adapting to ventilation during transport. Facilities must be available to monitor curare levels.

Complications: Neurological examination is not possible in patients being given curare. Curare can mask an epileptic attack. Prolonged use appears to be related to a higher incidence of infection.

hematomas all appear to be risk factors. Patients receiving curare may present subclinical or "electric" patterns. Phenytoin and carbamazepine are effective against early posttraumatic convulsions but do not prevent delayed ones. In patients in the acute phase sedated with nonspecific anticonvulsant agents, such as benzodiazepines or propofol, prophylaxis may well be unnecessary. Pharmacological prophylaxis is not advisable for delayed attacks.

Medical Therapy for the Control of Intracranial Pressure

ICP must be measured as soon as possible, to permit treatment of intracranial hypertension. Monitoring ICP is usually reliable and causes few complications. Medical therapy is only needed when ICP is high. In adults treatment should be started if ICP stably exceeds 20–25 mm Hg (15 mm Hg if decompressive craniotomy has been done), meaning for at least 5 min. Before starting any specific treatment, a check must be made to exclude factors that may directly raise ICP and corrective measures must be taken if they are present. These factors are presented in Table 18.15.

Hyperpyrexia is a frequent cause of worsening in patients with severe head injury, and the resulting metabolic and dynamic changes increase the risk of secondary ischemic events. Fever must be tackled vigorously, without overlooking the fact that some antipyretic drugs have negative hemodynamic repercussions (lowering BP). Maintaining normal body temperature, using physical and pharmacological means, is an important goal of treatment, on a par with preventing infection. Moderate hypothermia (32 to 33°C) can perhaps now be considered a therapeutic option, though confirmation is still needed (see Other Options below). It is not free of sometimes serious complications.

Urgent Treatment of Suspected Intracranial Hypertension

Before monitoring is started, there is obviously no way of knowing whether ICP is high or not, and there would be no reason for therapy. However, in some conditions it is reasonable to suspect high ICP, especially when there are clinical signs of tentorial herniation. ICP tracings must always be assessed in parallel with frequent clinical examination, serial CT scans, and calculation of CPP. ICP should be kept below the threshold value, but CPP must be kept above 70 mm Hg. Some therapies lower ICP but at the same time reduce arterial BP. The resulting "apparently" lower ICP does not correspond to any improvement in CPP, which, however, is essential to improve CBF. Therapeutic choices must take into account all available clinical and instrumental findings. The literature suggests two therapeutic approaches:

- Targeted treatment, which assumes the cause of high ICP is known, by analyzing the data from multiparametric monitoring

TABLE 18.15   Extracerebral Factors That May Directly Raise ICP

- Obstruction to venous outflow (positioning of the head and neck, poor adaptation to ventilation, pneumothorax)
- Causes of cerebral vasodilatation (fever, hypercapnia, hypotension, seizures)
- Causes of arterial hypertension (pain, visceral stimuli, inadequate sedation)
- Shivering
- Low blood sodium
- Instrumental malfunction

- Stepwise treatment using less aggressive measures, with less risk of complications, before proceeding to more aggressive approaches if this does not give the desired result.

There is no proof that either approach is superior to the other, and it is not always possible, even with multiparametric monitoring, to identify the cause(s) of high ICP. Stepwise therapy can be recommended for its simplicity and the fact that it can be applied in centers without multiparametric monitoring facilities. Stepwise therapy starts with baseline sedation and analgesia, and employs CSF withdrawal, mannitol, and moderate hypocapnia, in that order. Mannitol is infused only after withdrawal of CSF has proved ineffective, and hyperventilation is kept as the last therapeutic option, when ICP remains higher than the threshold even after sedation, CSF withdrawal, and mannitol.

CSF withdrawal rapidly lowers the intracranial volume, reducing ICP, although often only for a short time. It can only be done if a ventricular catheter is already in place, and the CSF must be withdrawn slowly. The gradient between the catheter tip and the CSF drip should be about 10 cm H_2O, to avoid some of the problems listed below. Too fast withdrawal may cause collapse of the ventricular wall, which could worsen the shift in patients with a contralateral expansive process, or have a "suction" effect on the ventricular ependyma, with the risk of bleeding. The catheter should be handled as little as possible to limit the risk of infection. CSF withdrawal means that ICP cannot be measured at the same time, as the system is open. It must therefore be done intermittently.

In clinical practice mannitol has replaced other osmotic diuretics. It presumably has multiple mechanisms of action, the best known being its systemic and cerebral hemodynamic effects and the osmotic effect. The systemic and cerebral hemodynamic effects include expansion of blood volume, reduction of the hematocrit and of blood viscosity, increased cardiac output and BP, increased CPP, increased cerebral blood flow (CBF), particularly the microcirculation, and reduced ICP. The effects on CBF seem most obvious in patients with low CPP (<70 mm Hg). Mannitol reduces intracranial volume by inducing an osmotic pressure gradient in regions where the blood–brain barrier is intact, drawing fluid out of the extracellular space to the vessels (Kaufmann and Cardoso, 1992). Inject as repeated boluses (0.25 to 1.0 g/kg in 15 to 20 min). Mannitol passes across the damaged blood–brain barrier, so repeated doses may worsen ICP by inverting the osmotic gradient. This is more likely when the drug is given by continuous infusion. The effect is seen within 15 to 30 min of infusion, and lasts from 90 min to 6 h. Serum osmolarity must be monitored and kept lower than 320 mOsm. Replace water/electrolyte losses to avoid hypovolemia. At high doses mannitol can cause acute renal failure. This risk is higher if nephrotoxic drugs are used at the same time—antibiotics, vasoconstrictors—or in cases of sepsis. Combination with other diuretics such as furosemide does not seem useful, and the additive effect increases the risk of hypovolemia.

Hyperventilation ensures a rapid drop in ICP, resulting in cerebral vasoconstriction when cerebral vessels still react to changes in CO_2. Studies in healthy volunteers have shown that CBF drops 40 percent when $PaCO_2$ is reduced by 10 mm Hg. CBF is reduced by about 3 percent for each mm Hg reduction in $PaCO_2$. Hyperventilation has never been proved effective as a preventive measure and cannot be recommended, especially in the first 24 h (Muizelaar et al., 1991). Measurements of CBF in head trauma patients indicate that in most cases it is low in the early stages and comes close to the ischemic threshold in the first hours after trauma. Concomitant measurements of jugular vein oxygen saturation have shown that the reduction of saturation is correlated to ischemia and EEG slowing. Cerebral hypoperfusion raises the risk of ischemia, induced or aggravated by hypocapnia. The only prospective trial using preventive hyperventilation found the outcome was worse in patients kept hypocapnic.

In the prehospital phase, hyperventilation is indicated in patients with clinical signs of tentorial herniation (anisocoria and focal motor signals). In these extreme cases, hyperventilation is a means, with mannitol, of "gaining time" until a CT scan and surgery can be done. Moderate hypocapnia ($PaCO_2 = 30$ to 35 mm Hg) is unlikely to cause serious complications, and is frequently effective in controlling high ICP. Its "target" indication is absolute or relative cerebral hyperemia, but this is hard to diagnose and monitor in clinical settings. The best approach is caution, aimed at keeping hypocapnia within moderate limits only as long as necessary, depending on ICP, monitoring $ETCO_2$, and frequently measuring blood gases, including SjO_2 if possible.

Severe hypocapnia ($PaCO_2 = 25$ to 30 mm Hg) is a therapeutic option when intracranial hypertension fails to respond to standard therapy. It is advisable to check for cerebral ischemia by measuring SjO_2 and, when possible, CBF. This is not a standard therapeutic option, as there is no actual proof of its effectiveness, but it can be recommended in selected patients, in the light of today's knowledge.

Sodium Thiopental

Barbiturates appear to have some cerebral protective effect (Eisenberg et al., 1988), reducing intracranial pressure through two mechanisms: reduction of CBF and cerebral metabolism, and inhibition of free radical-mediated lipid peroxidation.

The main side effects of sodium thiopental are cardiovascular depression and hypertension, a higher incidence of sepsis, induction of hepatic enzymes and facilitation of pressure sores. Barbiturates are not indicated for sedation. Their prompt use for "cerebral protection" or prevention of intracranial hypertension has never been proved to give clinical benefit. High-dose thiopental is a therapeutic option in patients with intracranial hypertension refractory to standard therapies. This must, however, be considered an extreme approach—not a routine option—as there is no real evidence of its efficacy. It needs to be properly evaluated in a selected cohort of patients with intracranial hypertension refractory to therapy. The conditions in which treatment with barbiturates can be used include normovolemia and stable hemodynamic conditions, complete cardiovascular monitoring, preferably with Swan–Ganz catheter, possibility of EEG monitoring, adequate nursing resources available,. If necessary, inotropic and vasopressor drugs should be employed. The hemodynamic situation must be monitored, preferably with a

TABLE 18.16   Dosing Regimen for Sodium Thiopental

- Administer sodium thiopental 30 mg/kg by slow bolus injection. Maintenance doses vary widely, from 5 to 10 kg/h, but higher doses may be needed if EEG burst suppression is needed constantly for periods of 10 to 20 s. Doses should be tapered or raised gradually, and the lowest dose that suppresses EEG bursts as required should be used. This may vary widely from one patient to another, depending on the duration of their fusion and type of brain lesion. Since the correlation with cerebral metabolic depression is not linear, blood levels are of little help as a guide to treatment. Only the EEG burst suppression, monitored continuously, is correlated with a useful reduction in metabolism and blood flow (about 50 percent).
- English-language protocols suggest using pentobarbital in these regimens (loading dose 10 mg/kg in 30 min, then 5 mg/h for 3 h, and maintenance 1 mg/kg per h) (Eisenberg et al., 1988). Unfortunately, this drug is not available in Italy. Thiopental is more lipophilic and therefore presents more accumulation problems.

Swan–Ganz catheter as well as by standard monitoring methods (invasive and central venous pressure). The dosing regimen for sodium thiopental administration is given in Table 18.16.

Other Options

There are numerous therapeutic proposals in the literature for controlling ICP and of the medical treatment of head trauma. However, evidence of efficacy has never been obtained for any of them in controlled conditions. These proposals include the following.

- Hyperbaric oxygen.
- Vasoconstrictor drugs such as indomethacin and ergotamine (which, together with other measures, are part of "Lund's" therapy) (Eker et al., 1998).
- Moderate hypothermia was studied prospectively in a clinical trial and appeared to offer advantages compared to the conventionally treated group (see Chapter 19). However, another multicenter trial, from the United States, was discontinued on account of safety reasons. Further proof is needed before any recommendations can be formulated (Marion et al., 1997). First of all, however, the ratio of uncertain benefits to known risks must be borne in mind, in view of the risk of vascular instability and serious complications induced by keeping patients' temperature below 34°C.

Drugs for "Cerebral Protection"

Today's evidence is not in favor of the use of steroids (Dearden et al., 1986). A recent metaanalysis, however, laid the grounds for new prospective trials. Other molecules that had shown promising "brain protective" activity in laboratory investigations have been or are now being tested in clinical trials. For the time being, there is no molecule that has proved capable of significantly changing the long-term neurological outcome. These treatments have not only shown no convincing efficacy: some have extremely serious side effects, or involve high organizational and economic costs. New studies are needed to demonstrate their efficacy and safety before they can be proposed for use in clinical practice.

SURGICAL TREATMENT CRITERIA

Rapid diagnosis of intracranial space-occupying lesions and their prompt removal have absolute priority in the management of the severe head injury patient. Much of the improvement in prognosis achieved in the last twenty years can be attributed to the systematic adoption of an aggressive surgical approach. Nevertheless, some basic questions are still debated, such as the timing of surgery, the importance of removing necrotic/hemorrhagic tissue, and the possibility of conservative treatment.

The indication for surgery and the most appropriate strategy are dictated by the patient's clinical condition, neuroradiological findings, and the specific pathophysiological features of the lesion. Any attempt to present such a complex problem schematically must have limits. Here, therefore, we have simply tried to establish the main criteria for surgery in adults with severe cranial trauma. It must be borne in mind that only some of the recommendations offered are backed by rigorous scientific evidence. Most have never been proved in controlled randomized clinical trials but, from a review of the literature and our own clinical experience, they appear reasonable and useful in clinical practice, as it is usually organized today. We have grouped these guidelines for surgical treatment under the following three main headings.

Surgical Indications Based on Clinical and Neuroradiological Criteria, ICP and CPP

Clinical Criteria. A patient with severe head trauma is in coma (GCS < 8, or 8 if the patient cannot open his or her eyes and utters incomprehensible sounds). Neurological examination can be done once patient stabilization has been achieved, when all sedatives, or muscle relaxants, have been withdrawn, and time has been allowed for their elimination. When possible, a history must be taken, with details of any existing pathologies, and of the onset of the coma (immediate, after gradual loss of consciousness, after an interval of lucidity). The total GCS must be assessed, with particular reference to the motor response, and pupil diameter and pupillary light reflex must be recorded.

Neuroradiological Criteria, ICP and CPP. Absolute indications for surgery include focal lesions causing a shift of the median line more than 5 mm, and space-occupying lesions larger than 25 cm^3 (Marshall et al., 1991). The shift of the median line refers to the real, absolute value, obtained by measuring the shift on a CT scan and calculating the real value using a reference scale. As discussed in relation to the specific indications for each surgical pathology, the indication for surgery must be based on information from recent, preferably serial, CT scans. Nowadays many more hospitals are equipped to perform a CT scan within a short time of the trauma, and a new problem thus arises: From the early images obtained while the intracranial lesion is still evolving it is easy to underestimate its severity. This is why serial CT scans are recommended during the first days of observation (Servadei et al., 2000). The CT monitoring criteria are outlined in Table 18.9.

Relative indications are based on ICP and CPP. Surgery may be indicated for focal lesions not shifting the median line by more than 5 mm, or masses smaller than 25 cm^3 (types II, III, and IV diffuse lesions) (Marshall et al., 1991), if they cause a stable rise in ICP above 20 mm Hg, with a stable reduction in CPP—below 70 mm Hg—despite maximal medical therapy.

Brain Swelling. Brain swelling is the term used to describe an overall increase in the size of the brain mass, usually associated, regardless of its causes and characteristics, with increased ICP (Tomei et al., 1991). Brain swelling is normally explained by an increase in blood volume in the brain (hyperemia) rather than increased water, secondary to breakdown of the blood–brain barrier. However, recent data suggest that both components are involved, in varying proportions. The hemodynamic alteration arises rapidly after the trauma, and causes expansion of the cerebral vascular bed, mainly on the venous side. This is the vascular response to brusque acceleration and deceleration, and to stimulation of brain stem structures, or release of vasoactive substances. The increased venous blood volume leads to increased capillary pressure, and reduced cerebral compliance. Hyperemia can be induced or aggravated by disorders of pressure autoregulation, hypoxia, hypercapnia, hyperthermia, arterial hypertensive episodes, and venous obstruction.

Increased intracranial volume causes a reduction or disappearance of the basal cisterns, of the cerebral sulci, and the ventricular system, particularly the third ventricle, in patients with no expansive lesions calling for surgical treatment (Marshall et al., 1991). In all cases neuroradiological diagnosis must be confirmed after 12 h. Neuroradiological classification includes brain swelling in diffuse type III lesions or diffuse type IV lesions. Brain swelling is diagnosed in a patient with severe brain trauma (GCS < 8 after reanimation and cardiovascular, respiratory, and metabolic stabilization) presenting persistent intracranial hypertension (ICP > 20 mm Hg). For medical treatment protocol, see the previous section.

Surgical treatment of brain swelling is a "second-level therapy." There is a lack of controlled clinical studies confirming its utility, so it remains optional (Gower et al., 1988; Polin et al., 1997; Guerra et al., 1999). Indications for surgical treatment of brain swelling refer only to diffuse type III or IV lesions and do not include patients with diffuse lesions larger than 25 cm^3, whose treatment is dealt with in the specific sections on this point. In any event, surgery should be reserved for patients with persistent ICP > 20 mm Hg or CPP < 70 mm Hg, refractory to maximal medical therapy. Surgery for brain swelling involves unilateral or bilateral bone decompression (hemicraniectomy, frontal craniectomy, ample frontal–temporal–parietal craniectomy, bitemporal craniectomy), with an ample dural opening, with or without "internal" decompression (lobectomy). Mortality for diffuse type III lesions is over 30 percent, and only 16.4 percent have a chance of a good outcome, or moderate disability (Marshall et al., 1991). Ample decompressive craniectomy significantly relieves intracranial hypertension (Gower et al., 1988; Polin et al., 1997; Guerra et al., 1999). Generally speaking, decompressive craniectomy for treatment-resistant intracranial hypertension lowers mortality, although this has not always been confirmed. The resulting survival, however, is related to a high percentage of morbidity, so that some survivors remain in a permanent vegetative state.

In series of patients selected for age and GCS score, unilateral or bilateral decompressive craniectomy reduced mortality and improved overall outcome, with 58 percent of patients attaining social rehabilitation (Guerra et al., 1999). In a recent study in which patients with severe posttraumatic edema refractory to treatment underwent bilateral frontal craniectomy, the percentage of favorable outcomes was significantly higher than in nonoperated controls (Polin et al., 1997). In patients with "potentially salvageable brains," decompressive craniectomy can be considered as an alternative to other "second-level" therapies.

Acute Epidural and Subdural Hematomas

Acute Epidural Hematoma. For all focal lesions, the general criteria for surgical treatment are the same: $>25 \, cm^3$ volume, $>5 \, mm$ shift. Theoretically, isolated acute epidural hematoma in a patient without neurological deficits causes no mortality, and morbidity reflects only the inherent risks of surgery (Bricolo and Pasut, 1984). Overall mortality among patients with epidural hematomas is around 10 percent (Chesnut and Servadei, 1999). As a general rule, morbidity and mortality are directly related to the patient's level of consciousness at the time of surgery. Therefore any improvement in overall outcome in patients with these lesions depends on prompt diagnosis, and immediate intervention before neurological deterioration occurs. Most well-organized neurotrauma centers are well aware of this picture, but it is nevertheless worth underlining that a wrong or delayed diagnosis of epidural hematoma is often the explanation of a patient who "talks and dies" (Marshall et al., 1983; Lobato et al., 1991). The main way to avoid catastrophe is to remain suspicious and take a prompt CT scan for patients with no symptoms but who have reported loss of consciousness or have a cranial fracture (The Study Group on Head Injury of the Italian Society for Neurosurgery, 1996). Between 10 percent and 50 percent of patients with epidural hematomas have other intracranial lesions (Chesnut and Servadei, 1999). Since isolated epidural hematoma has a low mortality rate, it is these associated lesions that are primarily responsible for morbidity and mortality.

Specific criteria for surgical treatment of acute epidural hematomas are related to factors such as their site, association with other intracranial lesions, and hyperacute nature. Critical locations are the posterior or the temporobasal fossae. The standard treatment of an epidural hematoma in the posterior cranial fossa is to have it evacuated surgically and promptly (d'Avella, 2000). Although a recent literature review found no correlation between hematoma localization and outcome (Servadei,

1997a), temporobasal hematomas are widely considered to involve a high risk of neurological deterioration, and call for an aggressive approach. Epidural hematomas are associated with one or more other lesions in 10 to 50 percent of cases (Chesnut and Servadei, 1999). Intracranial compliance is reduced and an aggressive approach is called for, especially in patients with cerebral contusions. Extradural blood may collect as lesions presenting a mixed image of high and low density. This indicates the unstable, hyperacute nature of the hemorrhage, which generally also involves some coagulation abnormality (Zimmerman and Bilaniuk, 1982). Hyperacute hematomas must immediately be surgically evacuated (Servadei, 1997a) and the coagulation problem tackled (Olson et al., 1989; Hoots, 1996).

There is still controversy about conservative approaches for epidural hematomas. The criteria for conservative treatment in these patients is delineated in Table 18.17. Conservative treatment of epidural hematomas must always be conducted under strict medical control in a neurosurgical or intensive care ward with neurosurgical staff on call round the clock should urgent evacuation of the lesion become necessary.

Acute Subdural Hematoma. As for all focal lesions, the absolute criteria for surgical treatment are hematoma volume $>25\,cm^3$, midline shift $>5\,mm$. Subdural hematomas may be isolated or associated with other intracranial lesions. They are found with parenchymal lesions such as contusion and lacerations or hematomas (Servadei, 1997b), about 25 percent of these cases require surgery. A typical example is a satellite subdural hematoma in a patient with laceration of the temporal lobe where the hematoma must be evacuated and necrotic-hemorrhagic tissue must be vigorously debrided. Subdural hematoma is also frequently combined with diffuse axonal injury (Sahuquillo et al., 1988). In such cases the hematoma may not be the main cause of the neurological damage dictating the outcome. Acute subdural hematoma itself gives a clinical picture reflecting the mass effect and the intracranial hypertension it causes, the severity depending on the hematoma's size and speed of formation, and the combined effect of underlying parenchymal lesions. However, the pathophysiological mechanisms of acute subdural hematoma go

TABLE 18.17   Criteria for Conservative Treatment of Acute Epidural Hematomas

- The volume is $<25\,cm^3$, the real shift from the medial line is $<5\,mm$, and the hematoma is $<15\,mm$ thick. Most reports of successful conservative treatment concern hematomas smaller than $45\,cm^3$ (Servadei, 1997a). A shift $>5\,mm$ is significantly correlated with progression, and conservative treatment in such cases may result in failure (Chen, 1993).
- The time elapsed between trauma and CT scan is at least 6 h, or, if the first CT was obtained earlier, a repeat scan has confirmed the hematoma is still the same size. The critical time window for an evolving epidural hematoma is about 6 h from trauma, since it takes 6 to 8 h to reach its final size (Smith and Miller, 1991; Servadei and Vergoni, 1993).
- The clinical picture is stable or shows improvement. Any sign of deterioration during the initial observation period constitutes an absolute indication for surgery.

beyond the mass effect and intracranial hypertension (Gennarelli and Thibauld, 1982). Experimental studies show that the ischemia and edema typical in brain tissue around a subdural hematoma are related more to the blood and necrotoxic agents than to the mass itself (Miller et al., 1990; Chen et al., 1991; Kuroda et al., 1992). Clinical studies have brought to light a clear correlation between mortality due to acute subdural hematoma and the ratio between the thickness of the hematoma and the shift in the median line; this is called the "brain swelling factor." Survival is inversely related to this factor (Zumkeller et al., 1996). Specific criteria for surgical treatment of these patients include the following. A negative ratio between the thickness of the hematoma and the shift is an unfavorable prognostic factor, as it indicates hemispheric swelling. In such cases surgery is advisable even for lesions smaller than 25 cm^3 (Zumkeller et al., 1996). Like extradural hematomas, subdural blood may give rise to a mixed image on CT scans with high- and low-density areas, indicating the hyperacute nature of the hemorrhage, generally associated with coagulation abnormalities. Hyperacute hematomas call for immediate surgical evacuation, and correction of the coagulation disorder (Olson et al., 1989; Hoots, 1996). Posterior cranial fossa subdural hematomas implicate a high risk of abrupt neurological deterioration. Early operation is always advisable (Hecimovic et al., 1999). When a subdural hematoma is associated with other intracranial lesions, the intracranial compliance is reduced and an aggressive approach is needed.

The criteria for conservative treatment in comatose patients with acute subdural hematoma have only been discussed in the more recent literature (Servadei et al., 1997; Wong, 1995; Servadei, 1997b), as summarized in Table 18.18. Conservative treatment of subdural hematomas must always be conducted under strict medical control, with ICP monitoring, in a neurosurgical or intensive care ward with neurosurgical staff on call round the clock should urgent evacuation of the lesion become necessary.

Contusions and Lacerations

Contusions and lacerations are potentially evolving lesions causing parenchymal necrosis and hemorrhage where the CT image shows mixed low- and high-density areas. These lesions consist of areas of infarct, necrosis, edema, and hemorrhage. They may grow larger, becoming confluent, eventually looking like—and actually forming—intracerebral hematomas. There is a tendency for edema to form around the lesion, so the mass effect becomes significantly more noticeable during the acute

TABLE 18.18   Criteria for Conservative Treatment of Acute Subdural Hematoma

- Nonsurgical treatment can be considered in selected cases when the hematoma volume is <25 cm^3, the shift from the median line is <5 mm, and the hematoma is <10 mm thick. The decision to treat these cases medically or with surgery must be based on a recent or serial CT scan.
- The clinical picture is stable or shows improvement. Any sign of deterioration during the initial observation period constitutes an absolute indication for surgery.

posttraumatic phase. Intracerebral hematomas show up as uniform collections of blood with fairly sharp edges. However, it is often hard to distinguish a hemorrhagic laceration from an intracerebral hematoma, since one may so easily develop into the other. As regards the indication for surgery, a distinction must be made between single and multiple lacerations/contusions. ICP monitoring is essential in all cases.

Single Laceration/Contusion (Even in a Critical Site). For all local lesions the general criteria for surgical treatment are the same: volume $> 25\,cm^3$, shift $> 5\,mm$. For specific criteria for surgical treatment based on ICP, if ICP is less than 20 mm Hg, see Medical Treatment Criteria above; if it remains higher than 20 mm Hg despite maximal medical treatment, the lesion needs surgical debridement and possibly also internal decompression.

Multiple Foci. For specific criteria for surgical treatment based on ICP, if ICP is less than 20 mm Hg, see Medical Treatment Criteria above; if it remains higher than 20 mm Hg despite maximal medical treatment, surgical evacuation is indicated for large lesions with a marked mass effect or clinically more significant effects. The decision for surgical treatment must be taken when first-level therapy fails (mannitol, CSF drainage) but should in any event be implemented before "second-level" measures are applied—for example, barbiturate coma.

SUMMARY

Guidelines for the management of severe head injury in adults, as evolved by the Neurotraumatology Study Group of the SINch and SIAARTI are presented and discussed. Guidelines presented here are of a pragmatic nature, based on consensus and expert opinion, covering the management from accident site to intensive care unit. The importance of preventing and treating secondary insults is emphasized and the rationale on which intensive care measures are based is briefly reviewed. Aspects pertaining to specific indications for surgery and/or the possibility of conservative management of different traumatic intracranial lesions are highlighted. The importance of surgery in preventing secondary damage to the traumatized brain is emphasized.

ABBREVIATIONS

ADH	Antiolmetric hormone
BP	Blood pressure
CBF	Cerebral blood flow
CEO_2	Cerebral oxygen extraction
CPP	Cerebral perfusion pressure
CSF	Cerebrospinal fluid

CT	Computed tomography
CVP	Central venous pressure
EBIC	European Brain Injury Consortium
ECG	Electrocardiogram
EEG	Electroencephalogram
$ETCO_2$	End-expiratory carbon dioxide
GCS	Glasgow Coma Score
ICP	Intracranial pressure
ICU	Intensive care unit
MAP	Mean arterial pressure
$PaCO_2$	Arterial carbon dioxide pressure
PaO_2	Arterial oxygen pressure
SINch	Società Italiana di Neurochirurgia
SaO_2	Arterial oxygen saturation
SIAARTI	Società Italiana di Analgesia, Anestesia, Rianimazione e Terapia Intensiva
SjO_2	Jugular vein oxygen saturation
TBI	Traumatic brain injury

REFERENCES

A. R. Aitkenhead, Analgesia and sedation in intensive care, *Br. J. Anaesth.*, 63, 196–206 (1989).

P. J. D. Andrews, I. R. Piper, N. M. Dearden, and J. D. Miller, Secondary insults during intrahospital transport of head injured patients, *Lancet*, 335, 327–330 (1990).

A. P. Bricolo and M. L. Pasut, Extradural hematoma toward zero mortality. A prospective study, *Neurosurgery*, 14, 8–11 (1984).

R. Bullock, R. M. Chesnut, G. Clifton, et al., Guidelines for the management of severe head injury, *J. Neurotrauma*, 13, 643–674 (1996).

D. G. Changaris, F. McGray, J. D. Richardson, et al., Correlation of cerebral perfusion pressure and Glasgow Coma Scale to outcome, *J. Trauma*, 27, 1007–1013 (1987).

M. H. Chen, R. Bullock, D. I. Graham, et al., Ischemic neuronal damage after acute subdural hematoma in the rat: effects of pretreatment with a glutamate antagonist, *J. Neurosurg.*, 74, 944–950 (1991).

T. Y. Chen, C. W. Wong, C. N Chang, et al., The expectant treatment of asymptomatic supratentorial epidural hematomas, *Neurosurgery*, 32, 176–179 (1993).

R. Chesnut and F. Servadei, "Surgical Treatment of Post-traumatic Brain Mass Lesions", in D. Marion, Ed., *Traumatic Brain Injury*, Thieme, New York, 1999, pp. 81–101.

D. d'Avella, L. Cristofori, A. Bricolo, and F. Tomasello, Importance of MRI in the conservative management of posterior fossa acute extradural haematomas, *Acta Neurochir. (Wien)*, 142, in press (2000).

N. M. Dearden, Jugular bulb venous oxygen saturation in the management of severe head injury, *Curr. Opin. Anesthesiol.*, 4, 279–286 (1991).

N. M. Dearden, J. S. Gibson, and D. G. McDowall, Effect of high-dose dexmethasone on outcome from severe head injury, *J. Neurosurg.*, 64, 81–88 (1986).

C. Eker, B. Asgeirsson, P. O. Grande, et al., Improved outcome after severe head injury with a new therapy based on principles for brain volume regulation and preserved microcirculation, *Crit. Care Med.*, 26, 1881–1886 (1998).

H. M. Eisenberg, R. F. Frakowski, C. F. Contant, et al., High-dose barbiturate control of elevated intracranial pressure in patients with severe head injury, *J. Neurosurg.*, 69, 15–23 (1988).

T. A. Gennarelli and L. E. Thibault, Biomechanics of acute subdural hematoma, *J. Trauma*, 22, 680–686 (1982).

D. J. Gower, K. S. Lee, and J. M. McWhorter, Role of subtemporal decompression in severe closed head injury, *Neurosurgery*, 23, 417–422 (1988).

D. I. Graham, J. H. Adams, and D. Doyle, Ischaemic brain damage in fatal non missile head injury, *J. Neurol. Neurosurg. Psychiatry*, 52, 346–350 (1989).

W. K. Guerra, M. R. Gaab, H. Dietz, et al., Surgical decompression for traumatic brain swelling: indications and results, *J. Neurosurg.*, 90, 187–196 (1999).

I. Hecimovic, G. Blagus, B. Krislek, et al., Successful treatment of traumatic acute posterior fossa subdural hematoma: report of two cases, *Surg. Neurol.*, 51, 247–251 (1999).

W. K. Hoots, "Coagulation Disorders in the Head Injured Patient", in R. R. Narayan, J. E. Wilberger and J. T. Povlishock, Eds., *Neurotrauma*, McGraw-Hill, Health Profession Division, New York, 1996, pp. 673–688.

P. A. Jones, P. J. Andrews, S. Midgley, et al., Measuring the burden of secondary insults in head injured patients during intensive care, *J. Neurosurg. Anesthesiol.*, 6, 4–14 (1994).

A. M. Kaufmann and E. R. Cardoso, Aggravation of vasogenic cerebral edema by multiple dose mannitol, *J. Neurosurg.*, 77, 584–589 (1992).

Y. Kuroda, R. Bullock, Local cerebral blood flow mapping before and after removal of acute subdural hematoma in the rat, *Neurosurgery*, 30, 687–691 (1992).

R. D. Lobato, J. J. Rivas, P. A. Gomez, et al., Head-injured patients who talk and deteriorate into coma. Analysis of 211 cases studied with computerized tomography, *J. Neurosurg.*, 7. 256–261 (1991).

A. I. R. Maas, M. Dearden, G. M. Teasdale, et al., EBIC—Guidelines for management of severe head injury in adults, *Acta Neurochir.*, 139, 286–294 (1997).

A. I. R. Maas, E. W. Steyerberg, G. D. Murray, et al., Why have recent trials of neuroprotective agents in head injury failed to show convincing efficacy? A pragmatic analysis and theoretical considerations. *Neurosurgery*, 44, 1286–1298 (1999).

D. W. Marion and P. M. Carlier, Problems with initial GCS assessment caused by prehospital treatment of patients with head injuries: result of a national survey, *J. Trauma*, 36, 89–95 (1994).

D. W. Marion, L. E. Penrod, S. F. Kelsey, et al., Treatment of traumatic brain injury with moderate hypothermia, *N. Engl. J. Med.*, 336, 540–546 (1997).

L. F. Marshall, B. Toole, and S. Bowers, The National Traumatic Coma Data Bank Part 2: Patients who talk and deteriorate: Implications for treatment, *J. Neurosurg.*, 59, 285–288 (1983).

L. F. Marshall, S. B. Marshall, M. R. Klauber, et al., A new classification of head injury based on computerized tomography, *J. Neurosurg.*, 75 (Suppl. 1), 14–20 (1991).

J. D. Miller, R. Bullock, D. I. Graham, et al., Ischemic brain damage in a model of acute subdural hematoma, *Neurosurgery*, 27, 433–439 (1990).

J. P. Muizelar, A. Marmarou, J. D. Ward, et al., Adverse effects of prolonged hyperventilation in patients with severe head injury: A randomized clinical trial, *J. Neurosurg.*, 75, 731–739 (1991).

G. D. Murray, G. M. Teasdale, R. Braakman, et al., The European Brain Injury Consortium survey of head injuries, *Acta Neurochir.*, 141, 223–236 (1999).

J. D. Olson, H. H. Kaufman, J Moake, et al., The incidence and significance of hemostatic abnormalities in patients with head injuries, *Neurosurgery*, 24, 825–832 (1989).

R. S. Polin, M. E. Shaffrey, C.A. Bogaev, et al., Decompressive bifrontal craniectomy in the treatment of severe refractory posttraumatic cerebral edema, *Neurosurgery*, 41, 84–94 (1997).

C. S. Robertson, Desaturation episodes after severe head injury: influence on outcome, *Acta Neurochir.*, 59, 98–101 (1993).

B. J. Sahuquillo, C. J. Lamarca, C. J. Vilalta, et al., Acute subdural hematoma and diffuse axonal injury after severe head trauma, *J. Neurosurg.*, 68, 894–900 (1988).

F. Servadei, Prognostic factors in severely had injured adult patients with epidural haematomas, *Acta Neurochir.*, 139, 273–278 (1997a).

F. Servadei, Prognostic factors in severely head injured adult patients with acute subdural haematomas, *Acta Neurochir.*, 139, 279–285 (1997b).

F. Servadei, A. Nanni, M. T. Nasi, et al., Evolving brain lesions in the first 12 hours after head injury: analysis of 37 comatose patients, *Neurosurgery*, 37, 899–906 (1995).

F. Servadei and G. Vergoni, Extradural hematomas: surgical and nonsurgical treatment, *AJNR*, 14, 506–507 (1993).

F. Servadei, G. D. Murray, K. Penny, et al., The value of the "worst" computed tomographic scan in clinical studies of moderate and severe head injury, *Neurosurgery*, 46, 70–77 (2000).

H. K. Smith and J. D. Miller, The danger of an ultra-early computed tomographic scan in a patient with an evolving acute epidural hematoma, *Neurosurgery, 29, 258–260 (1991).*

The Study Group on Head injury of the Italian Society for Neurosurgery, Guidelines for minor head injured patients' management in adult age, *J. Neurosurg. Sci.*, 40, 11–15 (1996).

G. M. Teasdale and D. I. Graham, Craniocerebral trauma: protection and retrieval of the neuronal population after injury, *Neurosurgery*, 43, 723–738 (1998).

G. Tomei, E. Sganzerla, D. Spagnoli, et al., Posttraumatic diffuse cerebral lesions. Relationship between clinical course, CT findings and ICP, *J. Neurosurg.*, 35, 61–75 (1991).

C. W. Wong, Criteria for conservative treatment of supratentorial acute subdural haematomas, *Acta Neurochir.*, 135, 38–43 (1995).

R. A. Zimmerman and L. T. Bilaniuk, Computed tomography staging of traumatic epidural bleeding, *Radiology*, 144, 809–812 (1982).

M. Zumkeller, R. Behrmann, H. E. Heissler, H. Dietz, Computed tomographic criteria and survival rate for patients with acute subdural hematoma, *Neurosurgery*, 39, 708–713 (1996).

CHAPTER 19

HEAD INJURY CLINICAL TRIALS: UNITED STATES

J. PAUL MUIZELAAR

Department of Neurological Surgery, University of California Davis, Sacramento, California

and

LEONARD P. MILLER

San Diego, California

INTRODUCTION

There are several reasons to conduct clinical trials, including trials in head injury. For instance, one can compare two "standards of management" and determine which of the two ultimately leads to a better outcome, as was done in the trials on hyperventilation (Muizelaar et al., 1991) or hypothermia. However, in this chapter we will restrict ourselves to clinical trials designed to study effects of treatment with (new) drugs. Before embarking on treatment of head-injured patients with a new drug, some prerequisites need to be fulfilled:

1. The mechanism of the test agent must be well understood.
2. The test agent interferes with a detrimental reaction, or enhances a beneficial one, which is to be present in experimental animals and in humans.
3. The test agent leads to improved outcome—preferably clinically relevant—in experimental head injury in different animals and different types of injury.
4. The dose–response curves, time window response curves, and length of treatment must be transferable from experimental injury to human head injury.
5. The test agent is safe in human volunteers

Head Trauma: Basic, Preclinical, and Clinical Directions, Edited by Leonard P. Miller and Ronald L. Hayes, Co-edited by Jennifer K. Newcomb
ISBN 0-471-36015-5 © 2001 John Wiley & Sons, Inc.

For phase I and II studies there also need to be

6. Defined entry criteria
7. One equivocal outcome measure
8. Multiple, secondary endpoints

And, finally phase III trials also need to be

9. Randomized, preferably with prerandomization stratification
10. Placebo-controlled
11. Double-blind

Unfortunately, for various reasons, not a single clinical trial conducted so far has fulfilled all of these requirements, possibly explaining why not a single clinical trial has been able to replicate laboratory results. The present chapter will review briefly the main characteristics of the various phases of clinical development of drugs and then outline the cellular mechanisms addressed by more recent compounds that have advanced into various phases of development for head trauma.

Phase I Trial

In most cases these are dose-escalating studies. These studies are not frequently conducted in head injured patients since the majority of drugs have been tested earlier in patients with other conditions (often stroke, subarachnoid hemorrhage). However, in some instances, dose-limiting side effects in other groups of patients would not affect patients with (severe) head injuries who are comatose and on a respirator (e.g., suppression of consciousness, or respiration, or occurrence of hallucinations). The main purpose of phase I studies is to establish the safety of the maximum tolerated dose; efficacy is usually not really studied. Therefore, often patients are included who would not qualify for later studies because of low chance of success (too severely injured, outside or at the limits of expected time windows, etc.). Of course, this raises the ethical question whether one should subject patients to "experimental" treatments that have a very low chance of being beneficial for that individual although the test agents have, at that point, already shown to be tolerated in volunteers and still might have a beneficial effect.

Phase II Trials

The main purpose of phase II trials is to obtain *preliminary* efficacy data, partly to enable power calculations for later, larger trials. Often, more than one dose is tested, but now there usually is randomization and blinding. Group size is usually between 25 and 50, for a total of 100 to 150 patients. The primary outcome measure is usually clinical recovery, but some surrogate outcome measures (e.g., intracranial pressure, intracerebral hematoma development from contusions) can be used as well.

Phase III Trials

These are the large trials with over 400 patients, trying to definitely answer the question whether a drug improves outcome. Schwartz and Lellouch have proposed a distinction between explanatory trials and pragmatic trials (Schwartz and Lellouch, 1967). In the explanatory trials the effect of the drug on its specific target or a close derivative is studied: Do patients treated with oxygen radical scavengers have less oxygen radical metabolite markers in their cerebrospinal fluid? Do patients treated with tromethamine (THAM) have a lower intracranial pressure (ICP) (as a consequence of the vasoconstricting effect of THAM), and so on. However, the phase III trials are always pragmatic: Do more patients reach a good recovery when treated with the drug?

RECENT AND ONGOING MAJOR DRUG DEVELOPMENT PROGRAMS FOR HEAD TRAUMA

Enadoline (CI-977)

The pursuit of kappa opioids in head trauma clinical trials stems from a number of important preclinical observations. In particular, endogenous opioids were shown to be released following traumatic brain injury and, thus, suggested to participate in a number of the pathophysiological responses to mechanical brain injury (Lyeth and Hayes, 1992; McIntosh, 1993). In addition, beneficial effects of kappa agonists have been observed in animal models of ischemia, concussive, and peptide-induced neural injury (Tortella and DeCoster, 1994). A number of different proposals have been presented with regard to the possible mechanism of action for kappa agonist-induced neuroprotection. Enadoline, a specific and potent kappa agonist, inhibited the release of amino acids in rat hippocampus (Millan et al., 1995), potassium-evoked glutamate release from cortical slices (Lambert et al., 1991), and KCl-evoked glutamate release from cultured rat neurons (DeCoster et al., 1994). In addition, kappa agonists such as PK117302 and enadoline altered the sustained secondary rise in Ca^{2+} produced by glutamate (DeCoster et al., 1994). Moreover, the initial spike in Ca^{2+} produced by low concentrations of glutamate also appeared to be altered by these kappa agonists. Finally, kappa opioids induce diuresis that may, in part, contribute to the overall neuroprotection achieved with the systemic application of this class of compounds.

Enadoline (CI-977), an arylacetamide, is a selective kappa opioid agonist that was selected for clinical development in head trauma. Of note, this compound has also shown activity as an anticonvulsant and been examined in a number of preclinical analgesia models. CI-977 was examined in a phase IIa placebo-controlled safety and tolerability trial in a total of 50 patients from five study sites with the intent of identifying doses suitable for investigation in a phase II study. The exact results of this study were never made known. However, at higher doses the drug caused diabetes insipidus, necessitating concomitant treatment with vasopressin. Regard-

TABLE 19.1 Recent and Ongoing Major Clinical Trials for Head Trauma: United States

Drug	Sponsor	Phase	Mechanism of Action	Dosing	Patients and CTRs	Status
ACEA 1021	Cocensys/ CIBA	II	NMDA antagonist at the glycine site		120 patients	
SNX-111	Neurex/Parke Davis	I/II	Neuronal P-Ca^{2+} channel blocker	0.9 mg/kg per 24 h for 72 h	232	Trial prematurely terminated; possibly 10% increase in mortality but 5% increase in favorable outcome
Bradycor (Deltibant)	Cortech, SKB	II	BK2 receptor antagonist	3 μg/kg per min for 5 days	139p, 31 cts, GCS 3–8	No significant effect; trial terminated prematurely due to preclinical tox results; no future plans
CI-977 (Enadoline)	Parke-Davis	IIa	Kappa agonist	i.v. 0.06–18 μg/kg per h for 12 h	50 patients, 5 sites	Drug dropped from clinical development, no future plans
CP-101,606	Pfizer	II	NMDA receptor polyamine site antagonist	—	400 patients, severe head injury	Enrollment complete Aug. 2000
HU-211	Pharmos	II	Cannabinoid	i.v. 200 mg within 6 h	67 patients	Significant decrease in ICP and trend in GOS improvement. International multicenter trial of 300 patients to begin in 2000

		Phase	Mechanism	Dose	Number of patients	Result
Bay x3702	Bayer	II	5-HT1a receptor agonist/ion channel blocker			
Cerestat	Cambridge Neuroscience	II/III	NMDA antagonist		600–800 patients	No effect
THAM		III	Buffer		149	ICP control better; ameliorated danger of hyperventilation but no effect on outcome
Hypothermia	NIH	III	Multiple mechanisms affected			No effect
PEG-SOD	Sterling-Winthrop	III	Antioxidant	10,000–20,000 units per kg i.v. once	1470	Overall 4% shift to favorable outcome, $p = 0.11$. No future plans
Tirilazad	Upjohn	III	Free radical scavenger	10 mg/kg, i.v. every 6 h for 5 days	692	No benefit
Selfotel	Ciba-Geigy	III	Glutamate receptor antagonist		692	Trial terminated—excess mortality in concomitant stroke trial

less, the compound was dropped from clinical development as part of a management decision based on the difficulty and time frame of clinical development and probability for success by comparison to other clinical candidates in other indications. To the authors' knowledge, there is no intention of pursuing a follow-up compound.

Cerestat

The rationale for and merits of targeting glutamate receptors in head trauma injury has already been addressed in detail in Chapter 4. Cerestat (aptiganel) represented the first generation of EAA receptor antagonists investigated for therapeutic potential in traumatic brain injury. It is a noncompetitive NMDA (N-methyl-D-aspartate) receptor antagonist that has exhibited neuroprotection in both preclinical ischemic brain injury and head trauma models. In a controlled cortical impact injury (CCII) model applied to the left hemisphere, Cerestat was injected (2 mg/kg, i.v.) at 15 min post injury and animals were sacrificed 24 h later. In one study (Kroppenstedt et al., 1998b), Cerestat treatment reduced contusion volume, decreased hemispheric swelling and water content, lowered ICP, and improved CPP. In another similar study, Cerestat posttreatment had similar beneficial effects except that ICP was not significantly altered (Kroppenstedt et al., 1998a).

Cambridge Neuroscience in partnership with Boehringer Ingelheim commenced clinical trials of this drug in both stroke and traumatic brain injury. Over the course of these studies, safety data were accrued on up to 1000 patients. An interim analysis conducted in late 1997 indicated that continuation of these trials was unjustified. Thus, both trials were halted. A follow-up analysis of the data suggested that a subset of stroke patients may have benefited by treatment with Cerestat. Presently, no plans have been proposed for reinvestigation of this drug in either stroke or head trauma.

CP101,606

Over the past few years, a new approach to blunting excitotoxic mechanisms mediated by glutamate release has involved targeting newly uncovered glutamate receptor subtypes. In particular, recent preclinical studies in ischemic brain injury have shown that the NR2B receptor subtype is involved in neuronal cell loss. These studies were aided with the use of a specific and potent antagonist, CP101,606 [(1S,2S)-1-(4-hydroxyphenyl)-2-(4-hydroxy-4-phenylpiperidino)-1-propanol] that targets the NMDA receptor as a novel NR2B subunit antagonist. Receptor binding studies indicate that CP101,606 does not interact directly with the glutamate or glycine binding sites or with the channel pore site. Instead, inhibition of NMDA receptors results from an interaction with an allosteric modulatory site that appears closely related to that for the polyamines, since spermine and spermidine displace racemic labeled CP101,606 binding (Menniti et al., 1997). In this regard, Dingledine and co-workers (Mott et al., 1998) hypothesized that CP101,606 inhibits NMDA receptor activity by potentiating proton inhibition, a mechanism of regulation discussed in greater detail in Chapter 4 of this book. Affinity studies with

CP101,606 indicate a K_d of 10 nM at this binding site. Moreover, this compound appears to be a very selective antagonist with little activity at the alpha-1 adrenergic receptor (Chenard and Menniti, 1999).

In vivo studies revealed that CP101,606 readily crosses the blood–brain barrier and does not cause locomotor hyperactivity even at very high doses or produce vacuolization in cingulate/retrosplenial cortex (Pagnozzi et al., 1995). In efficacy studies, CP101,606 administered before ischemia to cats resulted in a significant reduction (62.9 percent) in infarct volume at 5 h post middle cerebral artery occlusion along with a decrease in dialysate lactate and cytotoxic edema as measured by diffusion coefficients (Di et al., 1997). Overall, CP101,606 reduced infarct volume caused by cerebral ischemia in two of three models. While extrapolation of these preclinical results to humans is limited due to the lack of posttrauma dosing and the extremely early time point for recording of outcome measures, the results are, nevertheless, encouraging.

CP101,606 has shown efficacy in several different rodent models of traumatic brain injury. In a lateral fluid percussion brain injury model, CP101,606-treated rats (5 mg/kg, i.p. at 15 min post injury followed by i.v. infusion for 24 h) exhibited reduced brain edema (Okiyama et al., 1998) and less deterioration in memory function and neurological score at 42 h (Okiyama et al., 1997). In a closed head injury model, CP101,606 given 15 min post injury reduced by approximately 50 percent the initial rise in intracranial pressure and completely eliminated the slower increase at the later time (Menniti et al., 1998). In a rat model of acute subdural hematoma produced by slow injection of autologous blood into the parietal subdural space, CP101,606 administration at 30 min post induction of hematoma resulted in a 29 percent and 37 percent reduction in infarct volume at 4 h (Miller et al., 1990). This effect was comparable to the neuroprotective effects observed with other NMDA antagonists studied in this same model. CP101,606, administered intravenously 30 min before a unilateral stab wound to the parietal cortex of rats inhibited c-*fos* mRNA induction in a dose-dependent manner with an ED_{50} of 4.1 mg/kg (Menniti et al., 1998). Finally, CP101,606 administered by i.v. infusion caused a dose-dependent decrease in the propagation rate of cortical spreading depression and reduced the amplitude of depolarization (Menniti et al., 1998). These results are significant in that cortical spreading depression is a detrimental process that may be involved in the cascade of events leading to CNS injury and death following head trauma. Of note, the drug is soluble at 15 mg/mL in water and, following bolus + i.v. infusion dosing, achieves steady-state bloodstream levels of around 200 ng/mL which has been established in animals as its therapeutic level. In addition, the compound has exhibited an excellent safety record which was established in phase II studies in conscious moderate head injured patients (Merchant et al., 1997; Tsuchida et al., 1997) at blood levels of the drug shown to be neuroprotective in cat studies. Moreover, the maximum tolerated mean plasma concentration of CP101,606 was 4200 ng/mL which was established in 60 healthy volunteer subjects. This concentration is approximately 20-fold higher than the putative therapeutic concentration of 200 ng/mL. Notably, the incidence of side effects, such as amnesia, confusion, dizziness, depersonalization, and somnolence, increased with increasing plasma concentrations.

CP101,606 has been examined in two small open-label studies with patients ($n = 70$) recruited from a population of mild, moderate, and severe head injury or hemorrhagic stroke (Tsuchida et al., 1997). While not powered to detect an improvement in outcome, 9 out of 11 patients presenting with severe head injury and receiving a 24 to 72 h infusion with CP101,606 had a score on the Glasgow Outcome Scale (GOS) of "good" at 6 months, with no deaths in this group, suggesting improvements in both morbidity and mortality over placebo controls. Based on this study and the supporting preclinical results, GP101,606 is now being investigated in a multi-center, double-blind, placebo-controlled study in severe head injury in approximately 400 subjects.

ACEA 1021

Another drug directed at attenuating glutamate-mediated neurotransmission in head trauma is ACEA 1021. This drug was originally developed at Cocensys Pharmaceuticals which was recently purchased by Purdue Pharmaceuticals. ACEA (7-cholo-6-methyl-5-nitro-1,4-dihydro-2,3-quinazolinedione) was shown to be a potent antagonist of NMDA receptors. In particular, ACEA is a competitive antagonist ($K_b = 7.9$ nM in oocytes, $K_b = 11$ nM in neurons) at glycine coagonist sites (see Chapter 4) and also antagonizes AMPA receptors but with a much lower potency ($K_b = 3.5$ μM in oocytes) (Ilyin et al., 1996). In vivo studies showed that this drug was neuroprotectant in a rat model of focal cerebral ischemia (Ilyin et al., 1996) and mediated a marked reduction in penumbral NMDA receptor-mediated ion channel activation after onset of an acute subdural hematoma in rat (Di and Bullock, 1996). Furthermore, ACEA administration has no effect on neuronal morphology, in contrast to MK-801 administration, which produced characteristic neuronal vacuolization and necrosis in the posterior cingulate/retrosplenial cortex (Hawkinson et al., 1997).

With regard to clinical development, ACEA, sponsored by Cocensys/Ciba, had progressed to phase II in the United States (Doppenberg et al., 1997). This trial involved a total of 120 patients. While the results of this trial have not been published, there are, to the authors' knowledge, no present plans for development of this compound in head trauma.

HU211

HU211 (dexanabinol) is a synthetic cannabinoid that has been shown also to be a noncompetitive NMDA receptor antagonist with antioxidant (Eshhar et al., 1995; Feigenbaum et al., 1989) and anti-TNF-α properties (Shohmai et al., 1997). Based on these features, this drug has been suggested as the first pluripotent cerebroprotective agent in clinical trials (Leder et al., 1999). A number of preclinical studies have profiled the neuroprotectant features of this drug (Belayer et al., 1995; Leder et al., 1999). In closed head injury models the drug exhibited protective effects (Shohami et al., 1993, 1995) and inhibited TNF-α production. In a more recent ischemic brain injury study that employed a permanent MCAO rat model, the drug was administered initially at 1 h post occlusion. HU211 administration not only resulted in a significantly decreased infarct volume but also, as with the head trauma model, lowered TNF-α levels. However, in the same study there was no apparent effect on NOS activity. To date, the drug has been evaluated in a dose escalation phase I study in normal volunteers (Brewster et al., 1997) and shown to be safe in humans in a phase II clinical trial (Biegon et al., 1997).

Hypothermia

The induction of hypothermia as a therapeutic modality in traumatic head trauma is supported by a number of successful preclinical results in both head trauma and ischemic brain injury. In particular, moderate hypothermia in the range 30 to 33°C has been shown to diminish excessive toxic neurotransmitter release and to prevent disruption of the blood–brain barrier in a rat model of fluid percussion brain injury (Jiang et al., 1991, 1992). Improved behavioral outcome and a reduction in mortality were observed in a rodent brain injury model (Clifton et al., 1992). In addition, in both global and local ischemic brain injury models, moderate hypothermia was shown to diminish neuronal loss and reduce the extent of penumbral region (Busto et al., 1989; Chopp et al., 1989). The idea of using moderate hypothermia to exert neuroprotective effects in traumatic brain injury models is not new in that the first report of its successful application occurred in 1960 (Rosomoft, 1960).

With regard to mechanism of action, recent interest has focused on the hypothermia-mediated suppression of inflammatory mediators. Cytokines such as tumor necrosis factor (TNF) or interleukin-6 (IL-6) have been shown to increase in the rat brain after fluid percussion (Taupin et al., 1993). In humans, elevated plasma and ventricular levels of IL-6 and plasma cytokine levels have been linked to the patient's clinical course of recovery (McClain et al., 1991). Additional studies have now confirmed that ventricular IL-1β was significantly lower in patients subjected to hypothermia of 32 to 33°C than in those untreated (Marion et al., 1997). More recently, human plasma IL-6 levels were shown to decrease sharply after moderate hypothermia ($n = 13$) of 4 days induced in patients admitted with a Glasgow Coma Score (GCS) of ≤ 8 versus normothermic controls ($n = 10$) (Aibiki et al., 1999). Moreover IL-6 levels were maintained at reduced levels even after rewarming. Of note, these effects on cytokine levels were observed only in patients having a better clinical course but not in those patients whose prognosis was worse.

As a treatment modality for patients, the clinical application of systemic hypothermia in patients with severe brain injury was investigated as early as 1958 (Lazorthes and Campan, 1958). Over the next 30 years, there were a number of other reports on systemic cooling in over 120 patients with severe brain injury. For the most part these investigations served as phase I studies showing that toxicity is probably low at temperatures of 30°C or greater and with durations of less than 72 h (Drake and Jory, 1962; Hendrick, 1951; Lazorthes and Campan, 1958; Sedzimar, 1959; Shapiro et al., 1974; Strachan et al., 1989). The primary toxicities observed with systemic cooling are coagulopathy, pulmonary complications, and cardiac ventricular arrhythmias. In a more recent phase II study, 46 patients with severe nonpenetrating brain injury were randomized to standard management at 37°C and to standard management with systemic hypothermia of 32 to 33°C for 48 h (Clifton et al., 1993). Mean GOS score at 3 months after injury showed an absolute increase of 16 percent in the number of patients in the Good Recovery/Moderate Disability category as compared with Severe Disability/Vegetative/Dead. In a parallel clinical trial, treatment with hypothermia for 24 h led to a beneficial effect in a stratified group of patients (Marion et al., 1997). In particular, hypothermia did not improve the outcomes of patients admitted with GCS scores of 3 or 4. However, in the patients admitted with scores of 5 to 7, hypothermia was associated with significantly improved outcomes at 3 and 6 months but not at 12 months.

Based on the results the two phase II trials, a phase III randomized, prospective multicenter placebo-controlled trial (NABISH: National Acute Brain Injury Study: Hypothermia) of moderate surface-induced hypothermia was initiated in patients with severe head injury (GCS 3 to 8). In this recently completed trial, hypothermia (33°C) was initiated within 6 h of injury and maintained for 48 h. Final enrollment was 392 patients [Hypotherma (H) = 197, normothermic (N) = 193]. The most noteworthy observation (GOS at 6 months), although not significant, was that hypothermia patients admitted with a GCS 5 to 8 and age <45 years had fewer poor outcomes ($H = 44$ percent, $N = 51$ percent) without increased complications. Also, in the hypothermia group, fewer patients experienced intracranial pressure greater than 30 mm Hg ($H = 42$ percent, $N = 61$ percent, $p = 0.0005$). Based on these overall results, the conclusion of the investigators was that hypothermia shows promise in patients with GCS 5 to 8 and <45 years old, warranting further studies.

Tirilazad Mesylate

Another pathophysiological process mediating head trauma damage, uncovered in preclinical studies, is the generation of free radicals. The topic of free radicals has been discussed in greater detail in Chapter 1. In short, free radicals, though damaging in themselves, also initiate lipid peroxidation, which is a self-propagating process that destroys cell membranes. This process is further catalyzed by the presence of ions released from micro- or macrohemorrhages into the tissue. The involvement of this process in the progression of brain damage in head trauma has been established in both in vitro and in vivo experiments. These investigations were aided with the discovery of potent inhibitors of free radical-mediated lipid peroxidation. One such compound is tirilazad mesylate, a novel 21-aminosteroid derivative with proven antioxidant potential (Hall et al., 1992). This compound was shown to be effective in various models of experimental head injury even when the head injury is combined with a secondary insult such as hypoxia (McIntosh et al., 1992). Tirilazad mesylate exhibited a good safety profile in phase II trials that led to the initiation of two large multicenter prospective trials in head injury which involved a cohort of 1120 head-injured patients (Marshall et al., 1998). Patients suffering either severe (GCS of 4 to 8) or moderate (GCS of 9 to 12) head injury received at least one dose of tirilazar mesylate. At 6 months after injury, there were no significant differences in Glasgow Outcome Scale categories of both good recovery and death between placebo and drug-treated patients. Of importance, a subgroup analysis suggested that tirilazad mesylate may be effective in reducing mortality rates in males suffering from severe head injury with accompanying traumatic subarachnoid hemorrhage. Furthermore, the authors of this trial noted a striking problem with imbalance of basic prognostic variables in spite of the large patient population studied and the institution of a block design for randomization at each center. The imbalances noted were pretreatment hypotension, pretreatment hypoxia, and the incidence of epidural hematomas.

Bradycor

Recent evidence has established a role for an acute inflammatory response associated with tissue injury. In particular, tissue injury or cell death associated with a traumatic episode stimulates an inflammatory response via activation of the contact system and the kallikrein–kinin pathway (Gallin, 1988; Kaplan and Silverberg, 1987; Kaplan et al., 1983). Recruitment of circulating neutrophils at the site of injury leads to further destructive actions mediated by oxygen radicals and hydrolases that are produced and released by these neutrophils (Weiss, 1989). Also produced at the site of injury are two highly related inflammatory mediators, kallidin and bradykinin. Both mediators act at a common B_2 receptor to augment the ongoing inflammatory response. Brakydinin, also an inflammatory mediator, is produced from plasma kallikrein-mediated cleavage of kininogen, a ubiquitous plasma protein, while kallidin is produced from kallikrein-mediated cleavage of kininogen bound to neutrophils and endothelial cell membranes (Bhoola, 1996; Figueroa et al., 1992; Henderson et al., 1992). B_2 receptor-linked mechanisms include activation of inflammatory leukocytes and stimulation of vascular endothelial cells, as well as interacting with both neuronal and nonneuronal cell populations found within brain parenchyma. The resulting actions that contribute to the overall pathophysiology of TBI include blood–brain barrier disruption, dysregulation of cerebral blood flow, edema formation, inflammatory cytokine production, and excitatory amino acid release leading to excitotoxicity (Ellis et al., 1987, 1989; Francel, 1992; Unterberg et al., 1986; Wahl et al., 1996). Based on these findings, it was suggested that interventions directed toward the bradykinin B_2 receptor might be efficacious at ameliorating the inflammatory cascade initiated by head trauma. In this regard, a recent study reported on a phase II prospective, randomized, double-blind clinical trial of Bradycor (deltibant, CP-1027), a bradykinin antagonist, conducted at 31 centers within North America in severely brain-injured patients (Marmarou et al., 1999). The results of this trial showed a positive trend in ICP, TIL, neuropsychological tests, and 3- and 6-month GOS, suggesting that a bradykinin antagonist may play a neuroprotective role in severe brain injury. However, patient enrollment was stopped prematurely at 139 patients (targeted for 160 patients) because of results of animal toxicology studies conducted during the course of this trial. Furthermore, to the authors' knowledge no future plans with regard to Bradycor or any B_2 receptor antagonist have become evident.

SNX111

SNX111 (Ziconitide, CI 1009) is a neuron-selective, voltage-gated presynaptic calcium channel blocker, which in turn leads to decreased glutamate release. A rather unique property of this compound is that in models of stroke it was still effective in reducing infarct size when given 24 h after the permanent or temporary vessel occlusion. In models of head injury it was shown to block the cerebral accumulation of calcium 48 h after injury. Extensive dose–response curves were constructed for its effect on mitochondrial dysfunction after a cortical contusion injury in the rat, finding the best effect when given as a 4 mg/kg dose 4 h post injury (rather than 15 min before injury, or 15 min, or 1 h, or 2 h post injury) with effect still being measurable when administered 10 h post injury (Verweij et al., 2000). This dose (4 mg/kg) and timing (4 h post injury) was then tested in the acceleration/deceleration rat model with severe injury paradigm (400 g from 2 m), showing improved outcome in all seven neurological and neuropsychological tests at 6 weeks (Berman et al., 93, 821–828 2000).

Although SNX had a severe side effect of causing arterial hypotension, the long time window led to great optimism for its phase II–III clinical trial, although the dose used was much lower than in the rat experiments. The trial was halted after enrollment of 232 patients when a 10 percent increase in mortality in the drug group was noted by the safety monitoring committee. However, at least half of this over-mortality could be explained by more severe injuries in the drug group, while there was also a 5 percent increase in favorable outcome. The trial was designed with prerandomization stratification in expected poor outcome and expected better outcome, but at the time of this writing the data have not been released, so that we do not know what the effect of the drug is in the different groups.

PEG-SOD (Polyethylene Glycol–Superoxide Dismutase)

Although the preclinical data with PEG-SOD were very scarce, and the drug had never been tested for its effect on outcome (neuropsychological testing) after experimental head injury, there were still convincing arguments to test it in human head injury. In a phase II trial, it was found that the highest dose used (10,000 U/kg as a one-time i.v. bolus) effected a statistically significant effect on outcome. On the basis of these data, two consecutive phase III trials, testing 10,000 U/kg and 20,000 U/kg versus placebo were conducted. In the first phase III trial, with a total of 463 patients in the three groups, the 10,000 U/kg group had a 9 percent increase in favorable outcome ($p = 0.15$), the 20,000 U/kg group a 5 percent increase ($p = 0.24$) (Young et al., 1996). In the second phase III trial 900 patients were enrolled, with both drug groups showing an approximately 3 percent shift toward better outcomes ($p \approx 0.25$). However, when all the placebo patients ($n = 485$) from the three clinical trials were compared with all the patients receiving any dose of PEG-SOD (from 2500 to 20,000 U/kg, $n = 985$), only a 4 percent shift to favorable outcomes ($p = 0.11$) was observed. It appears almost certain that with better trial design (this was one of the first large-scale clinical trials in head injury) a statistically significant and clinically sufficient effect would have been found. When the sponsoring U.S. company (Sterling Winthrop) was bought out by the French company Sanofi, the European fear of "mad cow disease" (bovine spongiform encephalopathy) dampened further interest, as the SOD was obtained from (American) cow livers.

CONCLUSION

Unfortunately, except for the European trial with the antispasm medication nimodipine in patients with major subarachnoid hemorrhage after TBI, all phase III trials in head injury have been negative (Harders et al., 1996). In our opinion, the reason for this is twofold. First, prerequisite #4 (the dose–response curves, time window response curves, and length of treatment must be transferable from experimental injury to human head injury) has usually not been met. Second, for statistical reasons it is not realistic to expect an across-the-board increase of 10% of patients reaching a good or moderately disabled outcome. What has been lacking is a good prerandomization stratification by expected outcome. This is necessary so that patients moving from the expected outcome "dead" to "vegetative" or from expected "vegetative" to "severely disabled" could still be counted as a positive effect, thus showing that the drug has a (positive) biological effect. While some drugs and treatments clearly have had a biological effect, with better trial design and patient selection an unequivocally positive trial will one day change our management of patients with (severe) head injuries.

ABBREVIATIONS

ACEA 1021	7-Chloro-6-methyl-5-nitro-1,4-dihydro-2,3-quinazolinedione
AMPA	α-Amino-3-hydroxy-5-methyl-4-isoxazole propionic acid
CCII	Controlled cortical impact injury
CI-977	Enadoline, a kappa opioid agonist
CP101,606	(1S,2S)-1-(4-Hydroxyphenyl)-2-(4-hydroxy-4-phenylpiperidino)-1-propanol (antagonist at NR2B glutamate receptor subtype)
CPP	Cerebral perfusion pressure
EEA	Excitatory amino acid
GCS	Glasgow Coma Scale
GOS	Glasgow Outcome Scale
ICP	Intracranial pressure
IL	Interleukin
MCAO	Middle cerebral artery occlusion
NMDA	N-methyl-D-aspartate

NOS	Nitric oxide synthetase
PEG-SOD	Polyethylene glycol–superoxide dismutase
PK117302	Kappa agonist
TBI	Traumatic brain injury
THAM	Tromethamine
TIL	Therapy intensity level
TNF	Tissue necrosis factor

REFERENCES

M. Aibiki, S. Maekawa, S. Ogura, Y. Kinoshita, N. Kawai, and S. Yokono, *J. Neurotrauma*, 16, 225–232 (1999).

L. Belayer, S. A. Bar, J. Adamchik, and A. Biegon, *Mol. Chem. Neuropathol.*, 25, 19–33 (1995).

R. F. Berman, B. H. Verweij, and J. P. Muizelaar, *J. Neurosurg.* 93, 821–828 (2000).

K. Bhoola, *Immunopharmacology*, 33, 247–256 (1996).

A. Biegon, N. Knoller, N. Ehrenfreund, and M. Brewster, *J. Neurotrauma*, 14, 758 (1997).

M. E. Brewster, E. Pop, R. L. Foltz, S. Reuschel, W. Griffith, S. Amselem, and A. Biegon, *Int. J. Clin. Pharmacol. Ther.*, 35, 361–365 (1997).

R. Busto, W. D. Dietrich, M. Y. T. Globus, and M. D. Ginsberg, *Stroke*, 20, 1113–1114 (1989).

B. L. Chenard and F. S. Menniti, *Curr. Pharm. Des.*, 5, 381–404 (1999).

M. Chopp, R. Knight, C. D. Tidwell, J. A. Helpern, E. Brown, and K. M. A. Welch, *J. Cereb. Blood Flow Metab.*, 9, 141–148 (1989).

G. L. Clifton, S. Allen, J. Berry, and S. M. Koch, *J. Neurotrauma*, 9, S487–S495 (1992).

G. L. Clifton, S. Allen, P. Barrodale, P. Plenger, J. Berry, S. Koch, J. Fletcher, R. L. Hayes, and S. C. Choi, *J. Neurotrauma*, 10, 263–271 (1993).

M. A. DeCoster, J. R. Conover, J. C. Hunter, and F. C. Tortella, *Neuroreport*, 5, 2305–2310 (1994).

X. Di and R. Bullock, *J. Neurosurg.*, 85, 655–661 (1996).

X. Di, R. Bullock, J. Watson, P. Fatouros, B. Chenard, F. White, and F. Corwin, *Stroke*, 28, 2244–2251 (1997).

E. M. R. Doppenberg, S. C. Choi, and R. Bullock, *Ann. N.Y. Acad. Sci.*, 825, 305–322 (1997).

C. G. Drake and T. A. Jory, *Can. Med. Assoc. J.*, 87, 887–891 (1962).

E. Ellis, M. Heizer, G. Hambrecht, et al., *Stroke*, 18, 792–795 (1987).

E. Ellis, J. Chao, and M. Heizer, *J. Neurosurg.*, 71, 437–442 (1989).

N. Eshhar, S. Striem, R. Kohen, O. Tirosh, and A. Biegon, *Eur. J. Pharmacol.*, 283, 19–29 (1995).

J. J. Feigenbaum, F. Bergmann, S. A. Richmond, and R. Mechoulam, *Proc. Natl. Acad. Sci. USA*, 86, 9584–9587 (1989).

C. D. Figueroa, L. M. Henderson, J. Kaufmann, R. A. DeLa Cadena, R. W. Colman, W. Miller-Esterl, and K. D. Bhoola, *Blood*, 79, 754–759 (1992).

P. Francel, *J. Neurotrauma*, 9, S27–S45 (1992).

J. Gallin, "Phagocytic Cells: Disorders of Function," in J. Gallin, I. Goldstein, and R. Snyderman, Eds., *Inflammation: Basic Principles and Clinical Correlates*, New York, Raven Press, 1988, pp. 493–511.

E. D. Hall, J. M. Braughler, and J. M. McCall, *J. Neurotrauma*, 9(Suppl. 1), S165–172 (1992).

A. Harders, A. Kakarieka, and R. Braakman, *J. Neurosurg.*, 85, 82–89 (1996).

J. E. Hawkinson, K. R. Haber, P. S. Sahota, H. Han Hsu, E. Weber, and M. J. Whitehouse, *Brain Res.*, 744, 227–234 (1997).

L. M. Henderson, C. D. Figueroa, W. Muller-Esterl, A. Stain, and K. D. Bhoola, *Agents Actions Suppl.* 1, 590–594 (1992).

E. B. Hendrick, *Arch. Surg.*, 79, 362–364 (1951).

V. I. Ilyin, E. R. Whittemore, M. Tran, K. Z. Shen, S. X. Cai, S. M. Kher, J. F. Keana, E. Weber, and R. M. Woodward, *Eur. J. Pharmacol.*, 310, 107–114 (1996).

J. Y. Jiang, B. G. Lyeth, G. L. Clifton, L. W. Jenkins, R. J. Hamm, and R. L. Hayes, *J. Neurosurg.*, 74, 492–496 (1991).

J. Y. Jiang, B. G. Lyeth, M. Z. Kapasi, L. W. Jenkins, and J. T. Povlishock, *Acta Neuropathol.*, 84, 495–500 (1992).

A. Kaplan and M. Silverberg, *Blood*, 70, 1–16 (1987).

A. Kaplan, J. Dunn, and M. Silverberg, *Adv. Exp. Med. Biol.*, 156, 45–61 (1983).

S. N. Kroppenstedt, G. H. Schneider, U. W. Thomale, and A. W. Unterberg, *Acta Neurochir. Suppl. (Wien)*, 71, 114–116 (1998a).

S. N. Kroppenstedt, G. H. Schneider, U. W. Thomale, and A. W. Unterberg, *J. Neurotrauma*, 15, 191–197 (1998b).

P. K. Lambert, S. Barnes, J. Hughes, G. N. Woodruff, and J. C. Hunter, *Mol. Neuropharmacol.*, 1, 77–82 (1991).

G. Lazorthes and L. Campan, *J. Neurosurg.*, 15, 162–167 (1958).

R. R. Leder, E. Shohami, O. Abramsky, and H. Ovadia, *J. Neurol.*, 162, 114–119 (1999).

B. G. Lyeth and R. L. Hayes, *J. Neurotrauma*, 9, S463–S474 (1992).

D. W. Marion, L. E. Penrod, S. F. Kelsey, W. D. Obrist, P. M. Kochanek, A. M. Palmer, S. R. Wisniewski, and S. T. DeKosky, *N. Engl. J. Med.*, 336, 540–546 (1997).

A. Marmarou, J. Nichols, J. Burgess, D. Newell, J. Troha, D. Burnham, L. Pitts, and the American Brain Injury Consortium Study Group, *J. Neurotrauma*, 16, 431–444 (1999).

L. F. Marshall, A. I. R. Maas, S. B. Marshall, A. Bricolo, M. Fearnside, F. Iannotti, M. R. Klauber, J. Lagarrigue, R. Lobato, L. Persson, J. D. Pickard, J. Piek, F. Servadei, G. N. Wellis, G. F. Morris, E. D. Means, and B. Musch, *J. Neurosurg.*, 89, 519–525 (1998).

C. McClain, D. Cohen, R. Phillips, L. Ott, and B. Young, *J. Lab. Clin. Med.*, 118, 225–231 (1991).

T. K. McIntosh, *J. Neurotrauma*, 10, 215–261 (1993).

T. K. McIntosh, M. Thomas, and D. Smith, *J. Neurotrauma*, 9, 33–46 (1992).

F. S. Menniti, B. Chenard, M. Collins, M. Ducat, I. Shalaby, and F. White, *Eur. J. Pharmacol.*, 331, 117–126 (1997).

F. S. Menniti, A. K. Shah, S. A. Williams, K. D. Wilner, W. F. White, and B. L. Chenard, *CNS Drug Rev.*, 4, 307–322 (1998).

F. S. Menniti, M. J. Pagnozzi, P. Butler, B. L. Chenard, S. S. Jaw-Tsai, and W. Frost White, *Neuropharmacology*, 39, 1147–1155 (2000).

R. E. Merchant, R. Bullock, C. A. Carmack, A. Shah, K. Wilner, and G. Ko, *J. Neurotrauma*, 14, 764 (1997).

M. T. Millan et al., *Eur. J. Pharmacol.*, 279, 75–81 (1995).

J. D. Miller, R. Bullock, D. L. Graham, M. H. Chen, and G. M. Teasdale, *Neurosurgery*, 27, 433–439 (1990).

D. D. Mott, J. J. Doherty, S. Zhang, M. S. Washburn, M. J. Fendley, P. Lyuboslavsky, S. F. Traynelis, and R. Dingledine, *Nat. Neurosci.*, 1, 659–667 (1998).

J. P. Muizelaar, A. Marmarou, J. D. Ward, H. A. Kontos, S. C. Choe, D. P. Becker, H. Gruemer, and H. F. Young, *J. Neurosurg.*, 75, 731–739 (1991).

K. Okiyama, D. H. Smith, W. F. White, and T. K. McIntosh, *Brain Res.*, 792, 291–298 (1998).

K. Okiyama, D. H. Smith, W. F. White, K. Richter, and T. K. McIntosh, *J. Neurotrauma*, 14, 211–222 (1997).

M. J. Pagnozzi, L. K. Chanbers, F. S. Menniti, B. L. Chenard, and W. F. White, *Soc. Neurosci. Abst.*, 21 (Suppl.), 1–3 (1995).

H. L. Rosomoft, *Gynecol. Obstet.* 109, 27–32 (1960).

D. Schwartz and J. Lellouch, *J. Chronic Dis.*, 20, 637–648 (1967).

C. B. Sedzimar, *J. Neurosurg.*, 16, 407–414 (1959).

H. M. Shapiro, S. R. Wyte, and J. Loeser, *J. Neurosurg.*, 40, 90–100 (1974).

E. Shohami, M. Novikov, and R. Mechonlam, *J. Neurotrauma*, 10, 109–119 (1993).

E. Shohami, M. Novikov, and R. Bass, *Brain Res.*, 674, 55–62 (1995).

E. Shohami, R. Gallily, R. Mechoulam, R. Bass, and T. Ben Hur, *J. Neuroimmunol.*, 72, 169–177 (1997).

R. D. Strachan, I. R. Whittle, and J. D. Miller, *Brain Inj.*, 3, 51–55 (1989).

V. Taupin et al., *J. Neuroimmunol.*, 42, 177–186 (1993).

F. C. Tortella and M. A. DeCoster, *Clin. Neuropharmacol.*, 17, 403–416 (1994).

E. Tsuchida, M. Rice, and R. Bullock, *J. Neurotrauma*, 14, 409–417 (1997).

A. Unterberg, C. Dautermann, A. Baethmann, and W. Muller-Esterl, *J. Neurosurg.*, 64, 269–276 (1986).

B. H. Verweij, J. P. Muizelaar, F. C. Vinas, P. L. Peterson, Y. Xiong, and C. P. Lee, *J. Neurosurg.*, 93, 829–834 (2000).

M. Wahl, E. T. Whalley, A. Unterberg, L. Schilling, A. A. Parsons, A. Baethmann, and A. R. Young, *Immunopharmacology*, 33, 257–263 (1996).

S. Weiss, *N. Engl. J. Med.*, 320, 365–376 (1989).

B. Young, J. W. Runge , K. S. Waxman, T. Harrington, J. Wilberger, J. P. Muizelaar, A. Boddy, and J. W. Kupiec, *J. Am. Med. Assoc.*, 276, 538–543 (1996).

CHAPTER 20

CLINICAL TRIALS IN HEAD INJURY: EUROPE

A.I.R. MAAS

Department of Neurosurgery, Erasmus University Medical Center, Rotterdam, The Netherlands

INTRODUCTION

Research in head injury is a dynamic field. Over the years, approaches to management have changed and new technologies have been introduced to monitoring. These have been of considerable influence on the design and conduct of clinical trials. Basic research has increased our understanding in pathophysiological mechanisms leading to secondary brain damage and has led to the development of neuroprotective agents aimed at ameliorating these mechanisms. Prior to the mid-1980s, trials were mainly initiated by investigators, but later trials on neuroprotective agents were in contrast initiated by pharmaceutical companies. The benefits and disadvantages of these changes are discussed. In response to the increasing interest in clinical evaluation of neuroprotective agents in acute brain injury, the European Brain Injury Consortium (EBIC) was founded in 1995. Besides providing significant input into design and management of clinical trials, EBIC has also concentrated on science and nontrial research. Within Europe, nine trials have been conducted on steroids, three on calcium channel blockers, one on tirilazad and four on antagonists to the glutamate/NMDA receptor. These trials are discussed in detail. Unfortunately, none of the trials has succeeded in convincingly demonstrating efficacy of agents studied in the overall population. Conversely however, neither has inefficacy been proven. Methodological aspects and specifics of the population of the head-injured patients may have been at least in part responsible for the failure to definitively prove the efficacy of agents studied. In interpreting results, such issues should be taken into consideration. The complexity of problems in clinical trial design and analysis in head injury are such that strong and sustained input and effort are required from

Head Trauma: Basic, Preclinical, and Clinical Directions, Edited by Leonard P. Miller and Ronald L. Hayes, Co-edited by Jennifer K. Newcomb
ISBN 0-471-36015-5 © 2001 John Wiley & Sons, Inc.

all experts involved in the field of neurotrauma, in order to avoid further disappointments in the future.

PROGRESS IN HEAD INJURY CARE AND ITS IMPACT ON CLINICAL TRIALS

Within Europe head injury management and research has seen some considerable achievements since the 1960s, some of which have been of major significance to initiation, design and conduct of clinical trials, also influencing characteristics of patient populations studied. Intracranial pressure (ICP) monitoring was pioneered by Guillaume and Janny (1951) and Lundberg (1960), but it was not until much later that ICP measurement was generally accepted as integral part of intensive care monitoring in severely head-injured patients. Further research on the volume–pressure relation led us to understand why some patients suddenly deteriorate (Löfgren, 1973; Miller and Pickard, 1974). ICP measurement and assessment of therapy intensity level have been proposed as possible surrogate measures of neuroprotective agents. These measures are particularly relevant to phase II trials, in order to determine whether a biological effect of the agent may be present. The therapy intensity level was first proposed by Marmarou and co-workers as a means of cross-comparing severity of injury and therapy intensity in centers participating in the Traumatic Coma Data Bank study (Maset et al., 1987).

In the 1970s, the importance of intracranial secondary insults, particularly raised ICP, was identified as one of the causes of secondary deterioration and the phrase "Patients with head injury who talk and die" was coined by Reilly et al. (1975). Systemic causes of secondary insults were further investigated in depth by Miller and co-workers and attention particularly focused on hypoxia, hypotension, hypocapnia, and hyperthermia (Andrews et al., 1990; Jones et al., 1994). Assessment of occurrence, depth, and duration of secondary insults is important when assessing comparability of placebo and treated groups in trials. Evaluation of the occurrence of secondary insults may be used as a primary endpoint in trials aimed at determining the value of different management regimes. (Robertson et al., 1999).

The 1970s also saw the introduction of the computed tomography (CT) scan to head injury management and research. From a research point of view, the CT scan affords insight in morphological changes after injury, allowing for further classification of injuries (Marshall et al., 1991) and providing prognostic information. It is interesting to note that the development of CT scanning, now considered essential to the care of neurotrauma patients, was probably indirectly sponsored by the Beatles having been initially developed by EMI, the same company that initially carried the label for the Beatles' songs. In the 1980s, guidelines for X-ray and CT scanning were introduced, showing how advantage can be taken from technical examinations.

Major improvements from the late 1970s on included the introduction of preventive measures (helmets, seat belts, airbags), improvement of intensive care monitoring and treatment, and especially also improved emergency care systems and trauma organization, including early resuscitation at the scene of the accident. The success of preventive measures has led to a decline in the incidence of severe and moderate head injury. Early resuscitation, including sedation, intubation, and ventilation, has fortunately decreased the risk of early secondary insults, but at the same time causes problems in classifying patients on the basis of clinical symptomatology. In the 1990s, treatment shifted to include cerebral perfusion pressure (CPP) management (Rosner et al., 1995), and monitoring of cerebral oxygenation was added to the intensive care setting (Robertson et al., 1989; Sheinberg et al., 1992; Gopinath et al., 1994; Kiening et al., 1996; Van Santbrink et al., 1996). In some centers microdialysis was instituted, giving some insight into metabolic derangement and disturbances at the tissue level (Persson and Hillered, 1992). Unfortunately, it has not been possible to take full advantage of possibilities provided by magnetic resonance imaging (MRI) techniques, due to practical and organizational aspects, limiting its applicability in the acute phase after head injury.

From a perspective of clinical trials, two important events occurred in the mid-1970s, namely, the introduction of the Glasgow Coma Scale (GCS) (Teasdale and Jennett, 1974) for standardized assessment of level of consciousness, and of the Glasgow Outcome Scale (GOS) (Jennett and Bond, 1975) for standardized outcome assessment.

Although it was not foreseen at that time, the GCS evolved into the main criterion for including patients in clinical trials. Severe head injury was defined as a GCS ≤ 8 and moderate head injury as GCS 9 to 12. Recently it has been proposed to include patients with a GCS of 13 in the category of moderate head injury. Appropriate classification according to the GCS is, however, complicated by the general acceptance and widespread use of early sedation, intubation, paralysis, and ventilation, causing variability in data available at the various initial time points. In a recent survey conducted by the European Brain Injury Consortium (Murray et al., 1999), the full GCS was not testable in 23 percent of patients on admission to the accident and emergency department and the motor score was not testable in 18 percent.

The GOS has become a widely accepted primary endpoint for clinical trials, seeking to demonstrate not so much a decrease in mortality but more specifically an improvement of favorable outcome. Favorable outcome is defined as the GOS categories Moderate Disability and Good Recovery. The choice to dichotomise the GOS into favorable versus unfavorable outcome was based both on clinical and social judgment. Outcome determination at six months has been chosen in the majority of trials as major endpoint and indicator of final outcome, based on clinical experience that the greatest improvement in patients occurs within six months of injury. The original description of the GOS categories is clear and concise. If definitions of the various outcome categories of the GOS are correctly interpreted and applied, interobserver variation in the use of the GOS is low (Mass et al., 1983). The use of the GOS has, however, become so widespread that such criteria may not always be followed appropriately, carrying the risk of increased observer variability. The use of standardized structural interviews, as suggested by Wilson et al. (1998), is recommended.

HISTORICAL PERSPECTIVE OF CLINICAL TRIALS

Prior to 1980 the majority of trials reported consisted of single-center studies, evaluating treatment results often in respect to historical controls. In this period various trials, focusing on efficacy of steroids, were performed. Multicenter international collaboration really started with the coma prognosis study, initiating from Glasgow by Jennett et al. (1977). In this study 700 patients were recruited in the United Kingdom (Glasgow), The Netherlands (Rotterdam and Groningen) and the United States (Los Angeles). Information obtained in this way was then used to compare treatment results between centers and countries. Gelpke et al. (1983) reported significant differences in outcome between the two Dutch centers participating and further showed that these differences could at least in part be explained by differences in referral policy and severity of patients included. Jennett et al. (1980) reported differences in management employed between countries participating and analysed whether these were related to outcome. It was shown that certain treatments were more often used in the most severely injured patients. The use of steroids or tracheostomy was not related to outcome, but patients undergoing mechanical ventilation had outcomes that were worse than expected. Whether this was a reflection of a greater degree of severity of injury in ventilated patients, or could possibly have been caused by unintended adverse effects due to overintensive hyperventilation, was not further analysed.

Such reports, resulting from standardized data collection, highlighted the need to look critically at what was being done, emphasizing the necessity to investigate comparability of series on the basis of parameter prognostic significance. The importance of this conclusion was, however, not fully recognized nor was sufficient attention paid to this aspect in subsequently conduced trials.

In the 1980s basic research increased our understanding of many different and often interrelated pathophysiological processes occurring at the biochemical level, causing secondary brain damage due to membrane dysfunction, disturbances of cellular metabolism and microvascular circulation, and ischemia. This led to the development of neuroprotective agents aimed at ameliorating these mechanisms. The number of neuroprotective drugs developed within pharmaceutical companies is not known. Some of the most promising were carried forward into clinical research. Various phase I and phase II trials have been performed, but unfortunately few of these have been reported in the medical literature. Recently a phase II trial on the use of Dexanabinol (HU-211) has been completed in Israel. The results are reported to be sufficiently promising to warrant further clinical evaluation in efficacy-directed trials. In addition, various management regimes have been described and their efficacy has been reported, again based on historical controls. An example of such a study is that reported on the Lund therapy (Asgeirsson et al., 1995). The Lund therapy aims at prevention and/or treatment of vasogenic edema by means of reducing cerebral perfusion pressure and precapillary vasoconstriction. Advocates of this approach claim good treatment results in respect to historical controls, but as yet have not shown efficacy in a prospective randomised trial. The possibility that treatment was (inadvertently) targeted to a population that may indeed have benefit remains and should be investigated. A detailed overview of these studies is outside the scope of this chapter.

The trials to be summarized will focus only on prospective treatment allocated studies. Studies performed in Europe include steroid studies, trials with the calcium antagonist nimodipine, the international tirilazad trial, conducted in Europe and Australia, and trials on antagonists of the NMDA-glutamate receptor.

INCENTIVES FOR TRIALS AND COLLABORATION WITH PHARMACEUTICAL COMPANIES

The steroid trials were primarily initiated by investigators from scientific interest, some with limited support from pharmaceutical companies. The subsequent trials on neuroprotective agents were, in contrast, initiated by pharmaceutical companies. Pressures from within these companies for rapid development and registration may have prompted some agents to be studied in patients without sufficient experimental data on efficacy and clinical data on dose relationships, including aspects of brain penetration, being available (Teasdale et al., 1999). Although investigators primarily have an academic interest, and companies a marketing interest, collaboration between companies and investigators proved beneficial to both sides. Within companies the necessary knowledge of specifics of head injury was often minimal and could be provided by investigators. The participation in trials greatly facilitated international contact and exchange of ideas and has been a significant stimulus to promoting international collaboration. This has certainly benefited head injury research in general and probably indirectly led to improved quality of care. More-over, reimbursement of personnel and material costs incurred by investigators participating in trials provided extra financial possibilities for conducting otherwise unsupported research. The increasing interest from pharmaceutical companies did, however, cause a severe inflation in financial compensation. During the European nimodipine (HIT II) trial, for instance, the average compensation to participating centers was below $1000, but reimbursement in more recent and complicated trials increased to over 10,000 US dollars per patient. Although such amounts appear extraordinarily high, they can be motivated by the cost of trial personnel, a minimum of three research nurses being required to provide a 24 hour per day cover, seven days a week. Reimbursement on a per-patient basis raises ethical questions whether such high amounts are appropriate, and whether patients and/or relatives should not also receive financial compensation, and may carry a risk of some centers including patients in trials on borderline inclusion criteria, primarily because of the high financial incentive. Costs incurred by investigating centers include overhead (personnel, organization) and per-patient costs (i.e., laboratory, CT scans). From such perspective, a fixed sum and additional reimbursement per patient may seem more appropriate. In our experience, however, pharmaceutical companies insist on compensation on a per-patient basis for reasons of company policy.

The organization and logistics of trials conducted, as well as input from investigators, varies. The nimodipine trials were organized and conducted by the

Bayer company, in close collaboration with the designated principal investigator and steering committee. Data flow and checks of case report forms (CRF) were coordinated through divisions of the company. This policy ensured frequent productive and stimulating interaction between company representatives and investigators. This approach was really only appreciated by investigators after disappointing experiences in later trials where CRF checks were performed by representatives of contract research organizations, often completely ignorant of problems in the head injury population. Frequent investigator meetings, including scientific presentations outside the scope of the trial, served to enhance medical and cultural knowledge and promote collaboration. In the HIT III nimodipine trial targeted to a population with traumatic subarachnoid hemorrhage, data entry was performed by computer and electronically transferred to the company. This approach proved extremely efficient, allowing for a fast data check and clarification, and permitted analysis of data immediately following inclusion of the last outcome data.

The international tirilazad trial, as wel as the European leg of the Selfotel trials were coordinated by the trial center in San Diego under the stimulating leadership of Larry Marshall, supported by a strong international executive committee. Experiences in these trials illustrated how important it is for the executive committee to be able to interact with pharmaceutical companies at an executive level, where decisions can be made. From the individual investigator's perspective the importance of a fast turnover and return of data clarification forms was appreciated. Both of these trials significantly promoted collaboration in head injury research between the United States, Europe, and Australia.

EBIC AND TRIALS

The selfotel trial was the last trial initiated in Europe prior to the formation of the European Brain Injury Consortium (EBIC). EBIC was founded in 1995 in response to the increasing interest in clinical evaluation of neuroprotective agents in acute brain injury (Teasdale et al., 1997). The intent of EBIC is to promote international, multicenter, interdisciplinary research aimed at improving the outcome of victims of head injury or other kinds of acute brain damage. Currently it encompasses over 150 centers from 22 countries within Europe; its work is organized by an executive committee, consisting of 10 to 12 members, acting on behalf of the consortium, developing proposals for future activities. EBIC acts as an advisory organ, working in partnership with sponsors, to ensure excellence in design, conduct, analysis, and publication of clinical trials in neuroprotection. Besides coordinating contacts between centers and pharmaceutical companies, and providing significant input into design and management of clinical trials, EBIC has also concentrated on scientific and nontrial research. Guidelines for management, aiming at a common core approach to basic management in participating centers, were formulated, based on a combination of consensus and expert opinion as well as understanding of pathophysiology, and were published in 1997 (Maas et al., 1997). A core data study was performed in 1995, including 1005 patients with severe and moderate head injury over a three-month period from 67 participating centers in 12 European countries (Murray et al., 1999). Basic demographic and clinical data from admission, aspects of treatment, and treatment complications were collected and related to six-month outcome. More detailed analysis of CT data (Servadei et al., 2000) and intensity of management (Stocchetti et al., submitted) have subsequently been reported.

Since the constitution of EBIC, all trials conducted in Europe have so far as we are aware, been discussed with EBIC. This yielded a unique perspective and overview of potentially beneficial agents. During the period up to 2000, 12 companies approached EBIC for possible further clinical evaluation of 14 agents. A total of eight trials were designed together with or coordinated through EBIC. An overview and status of these trials is given in Table 20.1.

Of the eight trials (Table 20.1), three never started and one was halted after enrollment of only two patients. The PEGSOD trial was aborted in the final stage of center recruitment when the sponsoring company, Sterling Winthrop, was taken over by Sanofi and further development of the drug was halted. The phase II trial on the bradykinin antagonist SB 238592 was halted following problems with the drug formulation, identified in preclinical studies. Following the completed phase II trial on the 5-HT-agonist Bay X 3702, in which safety was demonstrated and pharma-

TABLE 20.1   EBIC Trials

Drug	Method Under Investigation/ Type of Agent	Type of Study	Status
PEGSOD	Free radical scavenger	Phase III	Centers recruited, trial never commenced
SB 238592	Bradykinin antagonist	Phase II	Halted after enrollment of two patients
Bay X 3702	5-HT-agonist	Phase II	Completed, not published
Cerestat	Noncompetitive NMDA antagonist	Phase III	Completed, results reported, not published
Lobeluzole	Neuroprotection	Phase II	Centers recruited, trial never started
D-CPP-ene	Competitive NMDA antagonist	Phase III	Completed, Publication in preparation
Bay X 3702	5-HT-agonist	Phase II B	Centers recruited, trial never started
Nimodipine	Calcium channel blocker	Phase III/IV	Enrollment completed at August 31, 1999

cokinetic aspects further resolved, an efficacy-oriented phase IIb study was designed. Due to internal company policy decisions within the sponsoring company, however, the further preparations for initiating the trial were put on hold. The phase II study on Lobeluzole was ready to start, centers were recruited, many of which had applied to their local ethics committees, and the first investigator's meetings were held, when the decision was made within the company to stop further development, following disappointing results in just completed stroke trials. In all cases in which trials were not initiated or halted early, centers received compensation for their efforts.

Although it may be considered fair to develop plans for clinical evaluation of an agent early on in its development, the apparent relative ease with which companies halt further development, even on the very threshold of starting recruitment of patients, gives rise to concern. This is especially the case in situations in which centers have been recruited and investigators have applied to their local ethics committee. For clinicians it is difficult to understand that such developments cannot be foreseen earlier, and if so this possibility should be openly communicated to and discussed with investigators. As was also previously the experience in some other trials, company policy decisions are greatly influenced by results of studies in related fields, such as stroke.

The primary intent of phase II trials is to evaluate aspects of safety, drug dosage, and pharmacokinetics. In addition, a possible effect on monitored parameters, such as ICP and CPP may be evaluated. It is, however, inappropriate to evalute any aspect of possible efficacy on outcome in such trials, given the relatively small number of patients studied. Nevertheless, many companies wish to see some hint of efficacy in such studies before proceeding to larger phase III trials. From a scientific perspective, the decision to proceed to efficacy studies after completion of phase II trials should be based on understanding of the pathophysiological mechanism targeted, knowledge of the occurrence of such mechanisms in head injury, and results of experimental studies. It is an absolute requirement that, besides aspects of safety, the pharmacokinetics of a new drug and its availability in the target organ—the brain—should be clarified in phase II studies before proceeding to a phase III efficacy study. A more detailed report on the EBIC-conducted phase III trials is given in the following paragraph.

DETAILED OVERVIEW OF EUROPEAN EFFICACY TRIALS

European trials have concentrated on steroids, calcium channel blockers, and inhibitors of free radical damage and lipid peroxidation, as well as on antagonists of the NMDA-glutamate receptor complex. The neuroprotective agents studied are generally targeted to one specific pathophysiological mechanism, but in others, such as steroids, the mode of action is more complex and often not fully unravelled.

Corticosteroids

Corticosteroids, known to be beneficial in brain edema attributable to a tumor, have been extensively studied in many relatively small series of head injury. A chronological overview is presented in Table 20.2.

The nine reports describe eight studies; six of these can be ranked as prospective randomised clinical trials (PRCT). The study by Gobiet (1976), the first European study to describe a positive effect of steroids in human head injury, was neither blinded nor placebo controlled, as a high-dose dexamethasone group was compared to normal dose (4×4 mg) or no drug. The conclusions are therefore at best only tentative. The study reported by Zagara et al. (1987) focuses only on the effect of dexamethasone on nitrogen metabolism. No metabolic effect of treatment with steroids was found. The study described by Klöti et al. (1987) and Fanconi et al. (1988) focuses on the effect of dexamethasone on cortisol excretion after head injury. In the treated group cortisol excretion is totally suppressed but, interestingly, the authors describe in the placebo patients an increase in endogeneous cortisol up to 20 times normal values.

None of the six trials shows any convincing evidence of overall efficacy. In the study by Faupel et al. (1976) on 95 patients, a significant reduction in mortality in patients with steroids was noted. However, in this group the percentage of patients remaining unconscious or with severe neurological deficit is also considerably higher, so that overall favorable outcome is only 7 percent higher. Although announced in the literature, results of the study by Hernesniemi and Troupp (1979) have not been reported. Results have been summarized in a metaanalysis by Alderson and Roberts (1997). The study by Braakman et al. (1983) conducted in two Dutch centers showed no effect at all. This well-designed study is interesting from a scientific and methodological point of view: first, because newer statistical techniques were employed; second, because aspects of prognostic estimates were considered in the analysis. In this study a sequential statistical analysis of the one month outcome between pairs of patients from steroid and placebo groups was employed. Using a null hypothesis, 2.5 percent boundary zones were drawn, one indicating that steroids significantly improved the rate of survival and the other that they significantly lowered survival rates (95 percent probability). After the 161 patients had been studied it became clear that the upper boundary zone was impossible to reach, and the study stopped. On definitive analysis of the six-month outcome, no difference was found between the groups. In patients with an intermediate prognosis (i.e. probability of survival between 0.30 and 0.90), an 8 percent reduction in mortality was noted in the steroid-treated patients.

The study by Dearden et al. (1986) also evaluated the use of high-dose dexamethasone therapy. All patients were intensively hyperventilated and if ICP was raised were treated with mannitol and/or hypnotic infusion of barbiturates. Mortality was considerably (15 percent) higher, but not significantly in the treated group. However, in patients with raised ICP treated additionally with hypnotic infusions the mortality was significantly higher in treated patients. No increased rate of complications was noted. In the study by Gaab et al. (1994), aimed at severe and

TABLE 20.2 Recent and Ongoing Important European Clinical Trials in Head Injury

Drug	Sponsor	Dosing	Maximum Time Between Trauma and First Dose	Outcome	Number of Patients	Status
Dexamethasone	—	100 mg i.v. Days 1 to 4: 4×20 mg i.v. Days 5 to 7: 4×4 mg i.v. or i.m. Days 8, 9, 12; 12, 8, 4 mg/day	Within 6 h	Survival 1 month; GOS 6 months	161	Completed, published in 1983
Dexamethasone	—	50 mg i.v. Days 1 to 3: 100 mg/day Day 4: 50 mg Day 5: 25 mg i.v.	Not specified, approximately 70% of patients received initial drug within 8 h	GOS 6 months	130	Completed, published in 1986
Dexamethasone	—	500 mg i.v. 200 mg after 3 h 4×200 mg for 2 days	Within 3 h of injury	GOS at 10 to 14 months after injury	300	Completed, published in 1994
Triamcinolone	—	200 mg loading dose Days 1 to 4: 3×40 mg Days 5 to 8: 3×20 mg i.v.	Within 4 h of injury	GOS discharge and GOS 1 year	396	Completed, published in 1995
Nimodipine HIT I	Bayer	Initial dose 1 mg/h; increased after 2 h to 2 mg/h, continued for 7 days	Within 24 h of injury	GOS 6 months	352	Completed, published in 1991
Nimodipine HIT II	Bayer	Initial dose 1 mg/h; increased after 2 h to 2 mg/h, continued for 7 days	Within 24 h of injury and within 12 h of not obeying commands	GOS 6 months	852	Completed, published 1994

Drug	Company	Dosage	Time window	Outcome	N	Status
Nimodipine HIT III	Bayer	2 mg/h for 7 to 10 days, followed by oral treatment (360 mg daily, until day 21)	Within 12 h	GOS 6 months	123	Completed, published in 1996
Tirilazad	The Upjohn Company	10 mg/kg per day for 5 days	Within 4 h	GOS 6 months	1120	Completed, published in 1999
Eliprodil	Synthelabo	3 mg i.v. b.i.d. for 7 days followed by 10 mg orally b.i.d. for 13 days	Within 12 h	GOS 6 months	452	Completed, not published
Selfotel (CGS 19755)	Ciba-Geigy	5 mg/kg once a day for 4 days	Within 8 h of injury and within 4 hours of admission	GOS 6 months	427	Halted, problems in stroke trials
Aptiganel (Cerestat)	Cambridge Neuroscience	15 mg bolus, followed by continuous infusion of 3 mg/h for 72 h	Within 8 h of injury	1. GOS 6 months 2. disability rating scale	(47 North American and 29 European centers) 532	Halted because of low probability of showing effect. No improvement in clinical outcome at 3 or 6 months.
D-CPP-ene (CDZ EAA 494)	Sandoz	200 mg i.v. infusion twice daily for 5 days	Within 12 h of injury	GOS 6 months	924	Completed; no significant effect; publication in preparation

(continued)

TABLE 20.2 (*continued*)

Drug	Sponsor	Dosing	Maximum Time Between Trauma and First Dose	Outcome	Number of Patients	Status
Nomodipine HIT IV	Bayer	0.5 mg/h for 2 h 1 mg/h for 2 h 2 mg/h for 7 to 10 days, followed by oral treatment (360 mg daily until day 21)	Within 12 h of injury	GOS 6 months	Aimed at approximately 600 patients	Enrollment completed; analysis ongoing
Crash	Drug and placebo provided by Pharmacia Upjohn; trial supported by British Medical Research Council	2 g Methylprednisolone over 1 h; 0.4 g/h for 48 h	Within 8 h of injury	1 Death within 2 weeks 2 Death or dependence at 6 months	Aimed at enrollment of over 10,000 patients	Trial ongoing

moderate head injury, even higher doses of dexamethasone were used with a loading dose of 500 mg i.v. No significant difference on outcome or complication rate were found in the overall population. However, authors report some evidence that steroids may be effective in preventing progression of brain tissue hypodensity as evidenced on CT examination. Grumme et al. (1995), reporting on a trial conducted with triamcinolone, found a decrease of mortality by 5.5 percent and an increase in favorable outcome of 8.5 percent in the treated groups. In a subset of the population (focal lesion plus GCS ≤ 8; $n = 93$) differences were statistically significant. In this subset of the population mortality was lower in treated patients (20 percent versus 38 percent); 35 percent of treated patients had a good recovery compared to 21 percent in the placebo group. From a pathophysiological point of view this would make sense, as a focal contusion with release of substances/mediators, which in excess are brain toxic, may be likened to a tumor in which field efficacy has been proven. In both situations a cause exists for ongoing stimulation of edema.

Although perhaps ineffective in the general population of head injury, targeting steroid therapy to patients with specific focal lesions may not be inappropriate. Consequently, the "standard" of the U.S. guidelines on management of head injury (Bullock et al., 1996), stating that steroids should not be used, should be interpreted carefully according to the principles of evidence-based medicine. Such interpretation requires understanding of a pathophysiological mechanism and its consequences for therapy as well as realization of the limitations imposed by studies on the conclusions. The number of patients in studies performed on steroids in head injury is relatively small. Sample size calculations for clinical trials in head injury show that a minimum of approximately 800 patients is necessary to permit demonstration or refutation of a 10 percent difference in dichotomised outcome measures with a power of 80 percent. Since such large trials have never been conducted on steroids, some uncertainty on the use of steroids in head injury remains. In a recent metaanalysis of clinical studies on steroids in head injury, Alderson and Roberts (1997) concluded that evidence indicates a 2 percent reduction in mortality with the use of steroids. The uncertainty concerning the use of steroids in head injury has led to the initiation of the CRASH trial in the United Kingdom, which has subsequently been extended to include patients from many countries in the world. CRASH is designed as a simple pragmatic study evaluating the efficacy of steroids in the overall population of head injury. CRASH is an acronym for Corticosteroid Randomization After Significant Head Injury. Head-injured patients (judged 16 years or older) are eligible for this study if—in the absence of sedation—they have a GCS of 14 or less and treatment can be initiated within eight hours of injury. Treatment consists of a 2 g loading dose of methylprednisolone, followed by a continuous infusion of 0.4 g/h for 48 h. The study is currently ongoing. Although designed to provide the definite answer, it is questionable whether such will be the case. The design of the trial has been criticized for also including patients with mild head injury, for allowing treatment initiation up to eight hours after injury, and because outcome data obtained are not based on personal interviews.

Calcium channel blockers

Three trials on the use of the calcium channel blocker nimodipine have been performed in Europe:

HIT I (Bailey et al., 1991): A British–Finnish cooperative trial studying the effect of nimodipine in 350 patients with severe head injury.

HIT II (European Study Group of Nimodipine in Severe Head Injury, 1994): A European multicenter prospective randomised clinical trial in 872 patients.

HIT III (Harders et al., 1996): A PRCT conducted in Germany in 123 patients with head injury and evidence of traumatic subarachnoid hemorrhage on CT examination.

The primary reason for initiating the phase III trials evaluating efficacy of nimodipine in head injury was the demonstrated efficacy of this agent in patients with aneurysmal subarachnoid hemorrhage (Öhman and Heiskanen, 1988; Pickard et al., 1989), and the realization that calcium-mediated damage also occurs in head injury. Experimental studies have shown total brain tissue calcium concentration to be increased in injured areas (Fineman et al., 1993; Shapira et al., 1989) and that a sustained increase in intracellular calcium concentration initiates a series of damaging events (Siesjo et al., 1989). The calcium antagonist nimodipine has been shown to reduce brain damage in experimental models of cerebral ischemia and hemorrhage (Robinson and Teasdale, 1990). At the time of initiation of clinical trials of nimodipine in head injury, only a few experimental studies had been performed. Germano et al. (1987), in a rat model of fluid percussion injury with and without hypoxia, demonstrated improved neurological outcome and decreased lesion size after treatment with nimodipine in animals that were exposed to head injury followed by hypoxia. In a subsequent study utilizing the same model, Sanada et al. (1993) failed to show a significant benefit of nimodipine treatment when administered 10 minutes after impact.

The pharmacological effects of nimodipine are various; principally it is a selective blocker of the long lasting (L-type) voltage-sensitive channels. In neurons, approximately 30 percent of inward calcium ion current is carried by L-type channels (Fox et al., 1987). Nimodipine does not block other types of voltage-sensitive or agonist-operated calcium channels. Thus, nimodipine should be considered more as a calcium-modulating agent than as a real calcium blocker (Kakarieka, 1997). In addition, nimodipine, like other 1,4-dihydropyridines, has a vasoactive effect, causing vasodilatation of the cerebral vascular bed also. Because of additional vasodilatation of systemic vessels, a potential disadvantage of nimodipine is its hypotensive effect (Kakarieka et al., 1994).

HIT I was performed in six neurosurgical centers in Belfast, Cambridge, Helsinki, London (two centers), and Newcastle. Patients with head injury, aged 16 to 70 years, were eligible if they did not obey simple commands and could be entered within 24 h of injury. The initial dose of nimodipine was 1 mg/h, then increased after two hours to 2 mg/h if there were no adverse cardiovascular events.

The aim of the study was to detect an increase in favorable outcome from 50 percent to 65 percent. Outcome was assessed according to the GOS 6 months after injury. From 1987 to 1989, 352 patients were entered into the study. Follow-up was lost or not obtained in only two cases; thus analysis could be performed on 350 patients. In the placebo population, favorable outcome was obtained in 49 percent; this increased in the treated patients to 53 percent. Thus, a 4 percent absolute change and 8 percent relative change was obtained. Differences were not statistically significant, however. On the basis of these results, it was considered possible that a modest, but nevertheless clinically valuable, effect was achievable, and a second trial was therefore initiated.

The HIT II trial was performed between January 1, 1989 and December 31, 1991 in 21 centers located in 13 European countries. It concerned a prospective, multicenter, placebo-controlled trial in 852 patients with severe head injuries. Patients were eligible if they met the following criteria:

1. They were aged between 16 and 70 years.
2. They could not obey commands at the time of assessment for entry into the trial.
3. They had undergone computerized tomography.

Treatment was initiated within 24 h after injury and within 12 h of the patient not obeying commands. This additional inclusion criterion was selected in order to be able to include patients who initially obeyed commands, but deteriorated later. The test drug was initially given at a dose of 1 mg/h; this was increased after two hours to 2 mg/h, provided there was no adverse response, such as hypotension. The study was designed to detect an increase in favorable outcome from 50 percent to 60 percent. In the HIT II trial, nimodipine did not exhibit a statistically significant effect in the overall study population. An improvement of favorable outcome was noted from 59 percent to 61 percent and a reduction in mortality from 24 percent to 22 percent in 819 patients for whom follow-up information was available. In a secondary analysis of protocol-compliant patients, an improvement in favorable outcome from 57 percent to 61 percent and a reduction in mortality from 25 percent to 22 percent were seen. In a further subgroup of patients with traumatic subarachnoid hemorrhage, mortality and unfavorable outcome were significantly lower in the group that had received nimodipine. Fifty-one percent of the patients treated with nimodipine had an unfavorable outcome, compared to 66 percent in the placebo group. Mortality was reduced from 46 percent to 32 percent.

The findings of the HIT II trial and the analogy with spontaneous subarachnoid hemorrhage provided a logical basis for a further study, focusing on patients with CT evidence of traumatic subarachnoid hemorrhage. This was realized in the HIT III study, a prospective multicenter randomised trial of 123 patients with head injury and evidence of traumatic subarachnoid hemorrhage on the computed tomography scan. The trial was conducted in 21 German centers between January and October 1994. Patients, aged 16 to 70 years, were entered in the study within 12 h after head injury, regardless of the level of consciousness. Gunshot injuries were excluded. Treatment was initiated within 12 h after injury with 2 mg/h nimodipine for 7 to 10 days, followed by oral treatment (360 mg daily) until day 21. Outcome was assessed six months after injury, according to the GOS. In this study unfavorable outcome was lower in the nimodipine-treated group (25 percent versus 46 percent; $p = 0.02$; odds ratio 0.39; 95 percent confidence interval 0.18 to 0.86). Despite the apparently strong effect of nimodipine as demonstrated in this trial, the HIT III trial has been criticized, and doubts have been expressed about how robustly its results could be generalized. Points of concern were that 25 percent of the patients had sustained a mild head injury (GCS > 12) and that the presence of subarachnoid hemorrhage on the first CT scan could not be confirmed in 21 percent of patients when CT scans were reviewed by a committee. A pooled analysis of the combined data of the HIT I, II, and III studies has been performed by Kakarieka (1997). Analysis of 460 patients with a traumatic subarachnoid hemorrhage who were enrolled in the three nimodipine trials indicated a significant benefit from nimodipine treatment (increase in favorable outcome from 45 percent to 56 percent). The merits of such a pooled analysis, given the different patient populations and inclusion criteria for the three trials, are uncertain and it may be considered inappropriate to include in the pooled analysis results from the subgroup from which the hypothesis was generated. A retrospective analysis of patients with traumatic subarachnoid hemorrhage (tSAH), included in the HIT I trial could not support the hypothesis that nimodipine is protective in tSAH (Murray et al., 1996). A further systematic review of the relation among clinical severity, presence of tSAH and effect of nimodipine treatment would seem to be indicated. Results of the ongoing HIT IV trial, currently being conducted in the far East, Australasia, South-Africa, and some European countries are awaited before a definitive statement can be made concerning the efficacy of nimodipine in the treatment of traumatic subarachnoid hemorrhage. Enrollment of patients in this trial was completed on August 31, 1999, at which time approximately 165 patients from European centers had been included.

Free Radical Damage and Lipid Peroxidation

The process of free radical-mediated damage and its occurrence in head injury have been discussed in Chapter 1. Extensive experimental support exists for the early occurrence and pathophysiological importance of oxygen radical formation and cell membrane lipid peroxidation in traumatic brain injury (Kontos and Povlishock, 1986; Braughler and Hall, 1989; Hall and Braughler, 1989). The initiation of the chain reaction of lipid peroxidation can be blocked by inhibiting synthesis of reactive oxygen materials or by the use of antioxidant enzymes, such as superoxide dismutase or complexes of superoxide dismutase (e.g., PEGSOD). Alternatively, the propagation of lipid peroxidation may be limited by agents with so-called "membrane-stabilizing effects," such as tirilazad mesylate (Hall et al., 1994). Tirilazad mesylate has a number of actions: a radical scavenging action, and a physical chemical interaction with the cell membrane, resulting in membrane stabilization. Furthermore, it has been shown that tirilazad mesylate can protect endothelium from damage by reactive oxygen species. The compound has a high affinity for vascular endothelium and has a protective effect on the blood–brain barrier against either a traumatically induced or subarachnoid hemorrhage-induced permeability increase. Experimental studies in models of cortical impact and fluid percussion injury have demonstrated the potentially beneficial effect of tirilazad when administered early after injury (Hall et al., 1988, 1993a,b; Dimlich et al., 1990; McIntosh et al., 1992; Sanada et al., 1993). In all studies initial treatment was started within zero to 30 min of injury, which is the period during which opening of the blood–brain barrier is known to occur. The effect of tirilazad mesylate in severe and moderate head injury has been studied in two large international trials, one conducted in North America, the other in Europe and Australia. Concurrently, phase III trials in the indications stroke and subarachnoid hemorrhage have been performed.

In the European/Australian tirilazad trial the efficacy of tirilazad was studied in 1120 patients with severe and moderate heat injury (Marshall et al., 1998). Enrollment in the study began in September 1992 and was completed in November 1994. Forty neurosurgical centers in 14 European countries and Australia participated. Patients were randomized within moderate (GCS 9 to 12) or severe (GCS 4 to 8) strata aiming at the distribution of moderate to severe of 15 percent versus 85 percent. Treatment with tirilazad mesylate (10 mg/kg per day for 5 days) was initiated within 4 h of injury and continued for 5 days. In order to facilitate the start of treatment within 4 h of injury, the procedure for obtaining deferred informed consent was adopted.

The European/Australian tirilazad trial failed to show significant effect in the full population. Of the treated patients, 40 percent has made a good recovery at six months as compared with 43 percent with the placebo-treated patients. Mortality was 27 percent in the treated group and 25 percent in the placebo group. Subgroup analysis indicated a significant effect of tirilazad in reducing mortality in male patients whose CT scan showed traumatic subarachnoid hemorrhage (death: tirilazad 30 percent; placebo 41 percent; $p = 0.026$). Prior to initiating treatment there were numerical and/or statistical imbalances between the two treatment groups with regard to CT lesion type, the occurrence of pre-treatment hypoxia or hypotension, and the presence of subarachnoid hemorrhage on the pre-treatment CT scan, favoring outcome in patients treated with placebo. Similar imbalances had also been noted in the North American study conducted simultaneously. In this study the imbalances related to the Glasgow Coma Scale, the pattern of brain injury as demonstrated by the pre-treatment CT scan, and the frequency of bilaterally unreactive pupils. The tirilazad trials illustrated unexpected dosage problems, due to gender-related metabolism differences and influences of concomitant anticonvulsive medication (Fleishaker et al., 1995, 1997). Earlier multiple-dose pharmacokinetic studies demonstrated a linear relation between dosage and plasma levels over the dosage range studied, but steady state appeared to be only achieved by the fifth day of dosing (Fleishaker et al., 1993). If this is also the case in patients with traumatic brain injury, it is debatable whether the plasma concentration during the first 24 to 48 h of treatment, the period generally considered most critical in traumatic brain injury were sufficient to obtain a therapeutic effect.

Antagonists to the glutamate/NMDA receptor

Excitatory amino acids have been shown to play a major role in neuronal damage after experimental brain trauma and ischemia (Benveniste, 1991; Onodera et al., 1989; Simon et al., 1984; Zauner and Bullock, 1995). Excessive quantities of neurotransmitters, released into the extracellular fluid, may trigger a so-called excitotoxic cascade activating both glutamate *N*-methyl-D-aspartate (NMDA) and non-NMDA channels, further triggering a cascade of intracellular calcium-mediated events and disturbances of ion homeostasis resulting in a potassium shift into the extracellular space (Katayama et al., 1995; McIntosh et al., 1997). Both clinical and experimental studies have demonstrated immediate and marked increases in the extracellular concentration of excitatory amino acids following injury (Bullock et al., 1998; Faden et al., 1989; Katayama et al., 1990; Nilsson et al., 1990; Palmer et al., 1993). A detailed overview of the possible importance of glutamate excitotoxicity in trauma is provided in Chapter 1. Various glutamate antagonists, acting at different sites, have been developed, of which four were carried forward into phase III trials: Eliprodil acts at the polyamine site, Selfotel and D-CPP-ene are both competitive antagonists and Cerestat is a non-competitive antagonist, acting at the ion channel. All of these drugs have been subjected to phase III clinical trials in Europe. The Eliprodil study was performed from 1993 to 1995 in seven European centers. Inclusion criteria were patients with severe head injury as evidenced by a GCS of 4 to 8; initiation of treatment was within 12 h of injury. In total 452 patients were included in the intent to treat analysis. No significant effect was noted in the overall population, but in a subgroup of patients with CT classification 3 and 4 a significant effect was present in favor of the treated group. Unfortunately, the results have not been published. The effect of the competitive NMDA receptor antagonist Selfotel (CGS 19755) has been studied in two parallel studies, one in Canada, Western Europe, Australia and Argentine and the other in the United States and Israel (Morris et al., 1999). Patients were included with severe head injury (GCS ≤ 8) aiming at treatment initiation within 8 h of injury and within 4 h of admission. The European leg of the Selfotel trials was conducted from 1994 to 1996. The aim was to enroll 920 patients; primary endpoint was favorable outcome as determined by the GOS at six months. The study had a power of 80 percent to detect a 10 percent difference. After enrollment of 693 patients in total (427 in the international trial, 266 in the U.S./Israel trial) enrollment was stopped, because of concerns of the Safety and Monitoring Committee about an increased number of deaths and severe brain-related adverse events occurring in the drug treated groups in two contemporaneously conducted trials in stroke patients. Although analysis of the data from the head-injured patients did not show an excess of adverse events in the Selfotel treated group, further futility anlaysis indicated a low likelihood of demonstrating a major benefit on pursuing the trial to completion. Analysis of the 693 patients enrolled in both legs of the trial showed a favorable outcome in 55 percent of the Selfotel-treated group and in 58 percent of the placebo group. A further phase III trial, evaluating the efficacy of the competitive NMDA antagonist D-CPP-ene, was conducted from 1995 to 1997 in 57 European centers. Inclusion criteria consisted of patients not obeying commands with at least one reactive pupil. Initiation of treatment was within 12 h of injury. In this study 924 patients were enrolled. Preliminary analysis of the results has been presented at various international meetings. The definitive publication of results is however still awaited. No efficacy in the overall population could be demonstrated. In the treated group a higher incidence of seizures was noted.

A phase III trial of the effect of aptiganel (Cerestat), a noncompetitive NMDA antagonist was initiated in patients with severe head injury in 1996. This study aimed at an enrollment of 700 patients with an 80 percent power to detect a 12 percent increase in favorable outcome. The study was halted in September 1997, on the basis of review of the results from the planned interim analysis on the first 340 patients. The distribution of the GOS at three months after injury showed a difference of only 1.1 percent in favor of Cerestat. The decision to terminate this trial was also made against the background of concern about effects of the agent in patients with stroke. In total 532 patients were enrolled; on final analysis of the six months outcome the percentage of patients with favorable outcome in the treated group was 59 percent versus 58.5 percent in the placebo group.

CONCLUSIONS AND LESSONS FOR THE FUTURE

As has been the experience in trials conducted in other continents, results of phase III trials on neuroprotective agents in severe and moderate head injury have been disappointing, and none of the trials performed so far has succeeded in meeting the predetermined hypothesis of increasing the absolute percentage of patients with favorable outcome by at least 10 percentage points. A common misconception is that consequently these agents are ineffective. Efficacy may not have been proven at this predetermined level, but conversely neither has inefficiency been proven. In fact, many trials demonstrate some increase, albeit nonsignificant, in treated patients and in others a beneficial effect was noted in subgroups. In the current era of evidence-based medicine, the limitations imposed by the patient population itself, as well as by the clinical trial design and analysis, should be taken into consideration. Decisions for initiating phase III trials in head injury have been strongly influenced by preclinical and clinical experience in related disorders, such as subarachnoid hemorrhage and ischemia. However, questions can be raised concerning the validity and robustness of preclinical and clinical data from phase II trials, relating to the field of head injury (Bullock, 1999; Maas et al., 2000). Important aspects are that the agent under investigation has been shown to inhibit relevant pathophysiological processes in models, that the process is known to occur in patients, and that the agent can be administered safely, in a regimen that is appropriate therapeutically in terms of dosage, brain penetration, and time scale. The tirilazad trial illustrated unexpected dosage problems, due to gender-related metabolism differences and influences of concomitant anticonvulsive medication. Aspects of brain penetration of this drug had not been fully investigated on initiation of trials. Recent studies have shown tirilazad to be concentrated primarily in the microvascular bed and it has been postulated that the main effect may be a protective effect on the endothelium. Excitatory amino acid neurotoxicity, specifically due to glutamate excess, although probably an important pathophysiological mechanism in some patients with head injury, does certainly not occur in all patients. Microdialysis studies have shown this mechanism to be more relevant in patients with focal contusions, acute subdural hematomas, or secondary ischemic events (Bullock et al., 1998), but less likely to occur in patients without structural brain lesions on CT scan, or without ischemic episodes. Such patients may constitute up to 40 percent of the overall head injury population. Attempting to demonstrate efficacy in the overall population, based on a possible effect on the targeted mechanism, which probably only occurs in just over half of the patients, may be considered extremely difficult. Moreover, brain penetration for competitive glutamate/NMDA receptor antagonist is poor and concentrations achieved are considerably lower than concentrations reported in dialysis from the extracellular fluid in patients with glutamate release (Zauner et al., 1996). As these agents are competitive, it is debatable whether the local concentrations obtained are sufficient to provide a neuroprotective effect.

The heterogeneity of the population of head-injured patients studied poses particular problems. In both tirilazad trials imbalances were noted between placebo and treatment groups concerning important prognostic variables. Imbalances can be reduced by stratifying patients according to baseline risk variables at the moment of randomization. Alternatively, imbalances can be corrected for at the time of analysis by adjusting for baseline characteristics using multivariable statistical techniques. Such adjustment should be prospectively specified in the protocol and permits individualizing treatment effect in contrast to the current procedures of pulled outcome analysis. Stratification can only be performed for a limited number of variables and preferably a combination of prognostic variables should be taken into account, identifying patients with a certain risk profile.

Not only does the heterogeneity of the population of head-injured patients cause problems concerning risk of imbalances, but the degree to which the prognostic effect determines outcome may have consequences for the calculation of sample sizes. Series of severe head injuries include by definition some patients with an a priori poor chance of survival, as well as those with a high chance of favorable outcome. Patients at low risk for unfavorable outcome are unlikely to benefit from a new therapy and conversely in patients with a high risk for unfavorable outcome it may be very difficult to show any efficacy. Jennett et al. stated in 1980 that prediction of outcome soon after injury would make it possible to recognize these patients, and attention could then be focused on those whose outcome was in doubt and therefore liable to be influenced. In this way the efficacy of a particular therapeutic technique would likely be detected much more rapidly, because its benefit would not be submerged or obscured by its use in many patients whose outcome was already determined. Jennett further states that probably a quarter of the patients will do well with conventional intensive management and another quarter are obviously destined to die, because the brain damage is so severe is inconceivable. In the megadose steroid study reported by Braakman et al. (1983), the number of patients with a less than 10 percent chance for survival or death was approximately 25 percent. In this study, furthermore, the treatment effect was analysed in relation to an estimated probability of survival in individual patients. Although results were nonsignificant, an 8 percent reduction in mortality rate in the steroid treated patients was noted, if the initial probability of survival was between 0.30 and 0.90. On review of these data it may be considered appropriate to target clinical trials to patients with an intermediate prognosis. In a study involving statistic modelling of potential head injury trials, Machado et al., (1999) demonstrated that targeting trials to patients with an intermediate prognosis would allow a reduction in sample size by 30 percent with no reduction in statistical power.

Utilizing the dichotomised GOS as primary endpoint in phase III trials of neuroprotective agents poses particular problems. In unselected populations of severe head injury the outcome distribution is typically U-shaped: a substantial proportion of patients die (25 percent to 40 percent) and another substantial proportion recover largely to their previous lifestyle (30 percent to 45 percent). An extensive analysis of problems incurred as a result of utilizing the dichotomized GOS has been presented by Maas et al. (1999). It was demonstrated that even a substantial change in outcome distribution need not necessarily be reflected in the dichotomised GOS. Theoretically, an improvement of favorable outcome can be obtained by upgrading a patient over one, two, or three of the categories of the full GOS. Taking the outcome distribution from the HIT II nimodipine trial as an example, it was shown that upgrading 50 percent of patients by one category, or by 25 percent over two or three categories would not meet trial requirements of improving favorable outcome by 10 percent. Yet, such a shift would represent a powerful biological effect and substantial reduction of mortality.

It has been argued that the Glasgow Outcome Scale is insensitive, especially in patients with more favorable outcomes, and that this insensitivity may be one of the reasons for inability to detect a significant benefit in head injury trials. For this reason a modification to the GOS was proposed by Jennett and colleagues in 1981, designed to numerically widen the scale to eight points. Problems of a higher interrater variability in the use of the extended Glasgow Outcome Scale may be overcome by using structured interviews as proposed by Wilson et al. (1998). Various other outcome measures as possible endpoints in clinical trials have been discussed by Bullock, (1999).

Following the disappointing results of phase III trials conducted, dark clouds have subsequently covered the European field of neuroprotection in traumatic brain injury, and interest from pharmaceutical companies on embarking on new trials has significantly decreased. However, it may not all be doom and gloom. Metaanalysis conducted over data from 10 phase III trials on neuroprotective agents in head injury showed an overall odds ratio of 0.90 (0.70 to 1.06), which may be considered supportive of the concept that some efficacy of neuroprotective agents in head injury is present (Maas et al., 1999). Moreover, in two trials efficacy in subgroups of the overall population has been demonstrated. This was the case in the European nimodipine HIT II trial as well as in the triamcinolone trial. Unfortunately subgroups

TABLE 20.3 Coricosteroid Studies

Author	Drug and Dosage	No. of Patients	Type of Study	Outcome	Result
Gobiet (1976)	Dexamethasone 12×8 mg versus no drug or 4×4 mg	93	Open study	Mortality	Mortality lower, significantly fewer ICP increases over 50 mm Hg
Faupel et al., (1976)	Dexamethasone Low dose: 12 mg loading, 4×4 mg 8 days High dose: 100 mg i.v., 100 mg i.m. after 6 h, 4×4 mg 8 days	95	PRCT	Mortality/ disability at discharge	Significant reduction of mortality, no difference in unfavorable outcome
Hernesniemi and Troupp (1979)	Betamethasone 100 mg i.v. on admission 80 mg/day i.v. for 7 days	169	Double-blind prospective	Mortality plus disability 6 or 12 months	No difference in mortality or disability
Braakman et al. (1983)	Dexamethasone 100 mg i.v. Day 1 to 4: 4×20 mg i.v. Days 5 to 7: 4×4 mg i.v.	161	PRCT[a]	Survival 1 month GOS 6 months[b]	No effect on mortality or GOS 6 months
Dearden et al. (1986)	Dexamethasone 50 mg i.v. bolus Days 1 to 3: 100 mg i.v. Day 4: 50 mg Day 5: 25 mg continuous infusion	130	PRCT	GOS 6 months	No significant difference; 15% higher mortality in treated patients

Reference	Treatment	No.	Trial type	Outcome measure	Results
Zagara et al. (1987)	0.36 mg/kg per 24 h Dexamethasone i.v. for 9 days	24	Phase II trial investigating effect on nitrogen metabolism	GOS 3 months	No significant difference in mortality; no difference in GOS 3 months
Klöti et al. (1987) Fanconi et al. (1988)	Dexamethason 1 mg/kg per day, days 1 to 3	24	Phase II trial studying effect of dexamethasone on cortisol excretion; prospective randomised trial	GOS 6 months	Suppressioin of cortisol excretion in patients treated with dexamethasone; in placebo patients, elevation of endogenous cortisol excretion to 20 times normal values
Gaab et al. (1994)	Dexamethason 500 mg i.v. $\leq$ 3 h 200 mg after 3 h, 4×200 mg for 2 days	300	PRCT	GOS 12 months	No difference in outcome or complications
Grumme et al. (1995)	Triamcinolone 200 mg loading dose within 4 h Days 1 to 4: 4 × 40 mg Days 5 to 8: 3×20 mg	396	PRCT	GOS discharge and 1 year	Decrease of mortality by 5.5%; increase in favorable outcome 8.5%; in subgroup of patients with GCS $\leq$ 8 and focal lesions, significant difference in favor of treatment

[a]PRCT, prospective randomised clinical trial.
[b]GOS, Glasgow Outcome Scale.

455

were not specified in advance and consequently no definite conclusion can be drawn. Further evidence for the possible efficacy of nimodipine in traumatic subarachnoid hemorrhage was provided by a study by the HIT III trial.

A major advantage of trials on neuroprotective agents in head injury has been the facilitation of contact and collaboration between neurotraumatological centers. The support of pharmaceutical companies in this regard is well recognized by investigators and highly appreciated. The complexity of problems occurring in clinical trial design and analysis in head injury is such that strong and sustained input and effort are required from all experts involved in the field of neurotrauma in order to avoid further disappointments in the future.

ABBREVIATIONS

CPP	Cerebral perfusion pressure
CRASH	Corticosteroid Randomization After Significant Head Injury
CRF	Case Report Form
CT	Computed Tomography
EBIC	European Brain Injury Consortium
GCS	Glasgow Coma Scale
GOS	Glasgow Outcome Scale
HIT	Head Injury Trial (nimodipine trials)
ICP	Intracranial pressure
MRI	Magnetic Resonance Image
NMDA	N-methyl-D-aspartate
PEGSOD	Polyethylene glycol—superoxide dismutase
PRCT	Prospective randomized clinical trial
TSAH	Traumatic subarachnoid hemorrhage

REFERENCES

P. Alderson and I. Roberts, *Br. Med. J.*, 314, 1855–1859 (1997).

P. J. D. Andrews, I. R. Piper, N. M. Dearden, and J. D. Miller, *Lancet*, 327–330 (1990).

B. Asgeirsson, P.-O. Grände, and C.-H. Nordström, *Acta Anaesthesiol. Scand.*, 39, 112–114 (1995).

I. Bailey, A. Bell, J. Gray, R. Gullan, O. Heiskanan, P. V. Marks, H. Marsh, D. A. Mendelow, G. Murray, and J. Ohman, *Acta Neurochir. (Wien)*, 110, 97–105 (1991).

H. Benveniste, *Cerebrovasc. Brain Metab. Rev.*, 3, 213–245 (1991).

R. Braakman, H. J. A. Schouten, M. Blaauw-van Dishoeck, and J. M. Minderhoud, *J. Neurosurg.*, 58, 326–330 (1983).

J. M. Braughler and E. D. Hall, *Free Radic. Biol. Med.*, 6, 289–301 (1989).

R. Bullock, *Neurosurgery*, 45, 207–220 (1999).

R. Bullock, R. M. Chesnut, G. Clifton, J. Ghajar, D. W. Marion, R. K. Narayan, D. W. Newell, L. H. Pitts, M. J. Rosner, and J. E. Wilberger, *J. Neurotrauma*, 13, 643–734 (1996).

R. Bullock, A. Zauner, J. J. Woodward, J. Myseros, S. C. Choi, S. C. Kaura, J. D. Ward, A. Marmarou, and H. F. Young, *J. Neurosurg.*, 89, 507–518 (1998).

N. M. Dearden, J. S. Gibson, D. G. McDowall, R. M.Gibson, and M. M. Cameron, *J. Neurosurg.*, 64, 81–88 (1986).

R. V. W. Dimlich, P. A. Tornheim, R. M.Kindel, E. D. Hall, J. M. Braughler, and J. M. McCall, in D. A. Long, Ed., *Advances in Neurology*, Vol. 52, Raven Press, New York, 1990, pp. 365–375.

European Study Group of Nimodipine in Severe Head Injury, *J. Neurosurg.*, 80, 797–804 (1994).

A. I. Faden, P. Demediuk, S. S. Panter, and R. Vink, *Science*, 244, 798–800 (1989).

S. Fanconi, J. Klöti, M. Meuli, H. Zaugg, and M. Zachmann, *Intensive Care Med.*, 14, 163–166 (1988).

G. Faupel, H. J. Reulen, D. Müller, and K. Schürmann, in H. M. Pappius, and W. Feindle, Eds., *Dynamics of Brain Edema*, Springer-Verlag, Berlin, 1976, pp. 337–343.

I. Fineman, D. A. Hovda, M. Smith, A. Yoshino, and D. P. Becker, *Brain Res.*, 624, 94–102 (1993).

J. C. Fleishaker, G. R. Peters, K. S. Cathcart, and R. C. Steenwyk, *J. Clin. Pharmacol.*, 33, 182–190 (1993).

J. C. Fleishaker, L. K. Hulst-Pearson, and G. R. Petrs, *Am. J. Ther.* 2, 553–560 (1995).

J. C. Fleishaker, R. N. Straw, and C. J. Cross, *J. Pharm. Sci.*, 86, 434–437 (1997).

A. P. Fox, M. C. Nowycky, and R. W. Tsien, *J. Physiol. (Lond.)* 394, 149–172 (1987).

M. R. Gaab, H. A. Trost, A. Alcantara, A. Karimi-Nejad, D. Moskopp, R. Schultheiss, W. J. Bock, J. Piek, H. Klinge, F. Scheil, P. Osterwald, M. Samii, A. Brawanski, J. Meixensberger, K. Schürmann, R. Schubert, H. Arnold, U. Kehler, K. Deisenroth, G. Benker, J. C. Vester, and H. Dietz, *Zentralbl. Neurochir.*, 55, 135–143 (1994).

G. J. Gelpke, R. Braakman, D. F. Habbema, and J. Hilden, *J. Neurosurg.*, 59, 745–750 (1983).

B. Germano, L. Pitts, and N. Islinge, *Abstract, International Symposium on Calcium Antagonists*, New York (1987).

W. Gobiet, W. J. Bock, J. Liesegang, and W. Grote. J. W. F. Beks, D. A. Bosch, and M. Brock, Eds., *Intracranial Pressure III*, Springer-Verlag, Berlin, 1976, pp. 231–235.

S. P. Gopinath, C. S. Robertson, C. F. Contant, C. Hayes, Z. Feldman, R. K. Narayan, and R. G. Grossman, *J. Neurol. Neursurg. Psychiatry*, 57, 717–723 (1994).

T. Grumme, A. Baethmann, D. Kolodziejczyk, J. Krimmer, M. Fischer, B. v. Eisenhart Rothe, R. Pelka, H. Bennefeld, E. Pöllauer, H. Koston, F. Leheta, S. Necek, G. Neeser, W. Sachsenheimer, J. Sommerauer, and F. Verhoeven, *Res. Exp. Med.*, 195, 217–229 (1995).

J. Guillaume and P. Janny, *Rev. Neurol.*, 84, 31–142 (1951).

E. D. Hall and J. M. Braughler, *Free Radic. Biol. Med.*, 6, 303–313 (1989).

E. D. Hall, P. A. Yonkers, and J. M. McCall, *J. Neurosurg.*, 68, 456–461 (1988).

E. D. Hall, S. L. Smith, P. K. Andrus, and J. R. Zhang, *J. Neurotrauma*, 10 (Suppl. 1), 87 (1993a).

E. D. Hall, P. K. Andrus, and P. A. Yonkers, *J. Neurochem.*, 60, 588–594 (1993b).

E. D. Hall, J. M. McCall, and E. D. Means, *Adv. Pharmacol.*, 28, 221–268 (1994).

A. Harders, A. Kakarieka, R. Braakman, and the German tSAH Study Group, *J. Neurosurg.*, 85, 82–89 (1996).

J. Hernesniemi and H.Troupp, *Acta Neurochir.*, Suppl. 28, 499 (1979).

B. Jennett and M. Bond, *Lancet*, 480–484 (1975).

B. Jennett, G. Teasdale, S. Galbraith, J. Pickard, H. Grant, R. Braakman, C. Avezaat, A. Maas, J. Minderhoud, C. J. Vecht, J. Heiden, R. Small, W. Caton, and T. Kurze, *J. Neurol. Neurosurg. Psychiatry*, 40, 291–298 (1977).

B. Jennett, G. Teasdale, J. Fry, R. Braakman, J. Minderhoud, J. Heiden, and T. Kurze, *J. Neurol. Neurosurg. Psychiatry*, 43, 289–295 (1980).

B. Jennett, J. Snoek, M. R. Bond, and N. Brooks, *J. Neurol. Neurosurg. Psychiatry*, 44, 285–293 (1981).

P. A. Jones, P. J. Andrews, S. Midgley, S. I. Anderson, I. R. Piper, J. L. Tocher, A. M. Housley, J. A. Corrie, L. Slattery, and N. M. Dearden, *J. Neurosurgery. Anesthisiol.*, 6, 4–14 (1994).

A. Kakarieka, *Traumatic Subarachnoid Hemorrhage*, Springer-Verlag, Berlin, 1997.

A. Kakarieka, E. H. Schakel, and J. Fritze, *J. Neural. Transm.* (Suppl.) 43, 13–21 (1994).

Y. Katayama, D. P. Becker, T. Tamura, and D. A. Hovda, *J. Neurosurg.* 73, 889–900 (1990).

Y. Katayama, T. Maeda, M. Koshinaga, T. Kawamata, and T. Tsubokowa, *Brain Pathol.*, 5, 427–435 (1995).

K. L. Kiening, A. W. Unterberg, T. F. Bardt, G. H. Schneider, and W. R. Lanksch, *J. Neurosurg.*, 85, 751–757 (1996).

J. Klöti, S. Fanconi, M. Zachmann, and H. Zaugg, *Child's Nerv. Syst.*, 3, 103–105 (1987).

H. A. Kontos and J. Povlishock, *CNS Trauma*, 2, 257–263 (1986).

J. Löfgren, "Pressure–Volume Relationships of the Cerebrospinal Fluid System," Thesis, University of Göteborg, 1973.

N. Lundberg, *Acta Psyciatr. Neurol. Scand.*, 36 (Suppl.), 149 (1960).

A. I. R. Maas, R. Braakman, H. J. A. Schouten, J. M. Minderhoud, and A. H. van Zomeren, *J. Neurosurg.* 58, 321–325 (1983).

A. I. R. Maas, M. Dearden, G. M. Teasdale, R. Braakman, F. Cohadon, F. Iannotti, A. Karimi, F. Lapierre, G. Murray, J. Ohman, L. Persson, F. Servadei, N. Stocchetti, and A. Unterberg on behalf of the European Brain Injury Consortium, *Acta Neurochir.*, 139, 286–294 (1997).

A. I. R. Maas, E. W. Steyerberg, G. D. Murray, et al., *Neurosurgery*, 44, 1286–1298 (1999).

A. I. R. Maas, "Assessment of Agents for the Treatment of Head Injury: Problems and Pitfalls in Trial Design", *CNS Drugs*, 13(2), 139–154 (2000).

S. G. Machado, G. D. Murray, and G. M. Teasdale on behalf of the European Brain Injury Consortium, *J. Neurotrauma*, 16 (12) 1131–1138 (1999).

L. F. Marshall, S. Bowers Marshall, M. R. Klauber, M. Van Berkum Clark, H. M. Eisenberg, J. A. Jane, T. G. Luerssen, A. Mamarou, and M. A. Foulkes, *J. Neurosurg.*, 75 (Suppl.), S14–S20 (1991).

L. F. Marshall, A. I. R. Maas, S. Bowers Marshall, A. Bricolo, M. Fearnside, F. Iannotti, M. L. Klauber, J. Lagarrigue, R. Lobato, L. Persson, J. D. Pickard, J. Piek, F. Servadei, G. N. Wellis, G. F. Morris, E. D. Means, and B. Musch, *J. Neurosurg.*, 89, 519–525 (1998).

A. L. Maset, A. Marmarou, J. D. Ward, S. Choi, H. A. Lutz, D. Brooks, R. J. Moulton, A. DeSalles, J. Muizelaar, and H. Turner, *J. Neurosurg.*, 67, 832–840 (1987).

T. K. McIntosh, M. Thomas, and D. Smith, *J. Neurotrauma*, 9, 33–46 (1992).

T. K. McIntosh, K. E. Saatman, and R. Raghupathi, *Neuroscientist* 3, 169–175 (1997).

J. D. Miller and J. D. Pickard, *Injury*, 5, 65–268 (1974).

G. F. Morris, R. Bullock, S. Bowers Marshall, A. Marmarou, A. I. R. Maas, the Selfotel Investigators, and L. F. Marshall, *J. Neurosurg.*, 91, 737–743 (1999).

G. D. Murray, G. M. Teasdale, and H. Schmitz, *Acta Neurochir. (Wien)*, 138, 1163–1167 (1996).

G. D. Murray, G. M. Teasdale, R. Braakman, F. Cohadon, M. Dearden, F. Iannotti, A. Karimi, F. Lapierre, A. Maas, J. Ohman, L. Persson, F. Servadei, N. Stocchetti, T. Trojanowski, and A. Unterberg, on behalf of the European Brain Injury Consortium, *Acta Neurochir. (Wien)*, 141, 223–236 (1999).

P. Nilsson, L. Hillered, U. Ponten, and U. Ungerstedt, *J. Cereb. Blood Flow Metab.*, 10, 631–637 (1990).

J. Öhman and O. Heiskanen O, *J. Neurosurg.*, 69, 683–686 (1988).

H. Onodera, T. Araki, and K. Kogure, *J. Cereb. Blood Flow Metab.*, 9, 623–628 (1989).

A. M. Palmer, D. W. Marion, M. L. Botscheller, P. E. Swedlow, S. D. Sturren, and S. T. De Kosky, *J. Neurochem.*, 61, 2015–2024 (1993).

L. Persson, and L. Hillered, *J. Neurosurg.*, 76, 72–80 (1992).

J. D. Pickard, G. D. Murray, R. Illingsworth, M. D. Shaw, G. M. Teasdale, P. M. Foy, P. R. Humphrey, D. A. Lang, R. Nelson, and P. Richards, *J. Neurol. Neurosurg. Psychiatry*, 52, 140 (1989).

P. L. Reilly, D. I. Graham, J. H. Adams, and B. Jennett, *Lancet*, 2, 375–377 (1975).

C. S. Robertson, R. K. Narayan, Z. L. Gokaslan, R. Pahwa, R. G. Crossmann, P. Caram, and E. Allen, *J. Neurosurg.*, 70, 222–230 (1989).

C. S. Robertson, A. B. Valadka, H. J. Hannay, C. F. Contant, S. P. Gopinath, M. Cormio, M. Uzura, and R. G. Grossmann, *Crit. Care Med.*, 27, 2086–2095 (1999).

M. J. Robinson and G. M. Teasdale, *Cerebrovasc. Brain Metab. Rev.*, 2, 205–226 (1990).

M. J. Rosner, S. D. Rosner, and A. H. Johnson, *J. Neurosurg.*, 83, 949–962 (1995).

T. Sanada, T. Nakamura, M. C. Nishimura, K. Isayama, and L. H. Pitss, *J. Neurotrauma*, 10, 65–71 (1993).

H. van Santbrink, A. I. R. Maas, and C. J. J. Avezaat, *Neurosurgery*, 38, 21–31 (1996).

F. Servadei, G. Murray, K. Penny, et al., *Neurosurgery*, 46, 70–77 (2000).

Y. Shapira, G. Yadid, S. Cotev, and E. Shohami, *Neurol. Res.*, 11, 169–172 (1989).

M. Sheinberg, J. M. Kanter, C. S. Robertson, C. F. Contant, R. K. Narayan, and R. G. Grossmann, *J. Neurosurg.*, 76, 212–217 (1992).

B. K. Siesjo and F. Bengtsson, *J. Cereb. Blood Flow Metab.*, 9, 127–140 (1989).

R. P. Simon, J. H. Swan, T. Griffiths, and B. S. Meldrum, *Science*, 226, 850–852 (1984).

N. Stocchetti, K. Penny, M. Dearden, R. Braakman, F. Cohadon, F. Iannotti, F. Lapierre, A. Karimi, A. I. R. Maas, G. D. Murray, J. Öhman, L. Persson, F. Servadei, G. M. Teasdale, T. Trojanowski, and A. Unterberg, on behalf of the European Brain Injury Consortium, *Intensive Care Med.*, submitted, (2001).

G. Teasdale and B. Jennett, *Lancet*, 81–84 (1974).

G. M. Teasdale, R. Braakman, F. Cohadon, M. Dearden, F. Iannotti, A. Karimi, F. Lapierre, A. Maas, G. Murray, J. Öhman, L. Persson, F. Servadei, N. Stocchetti, T. Trojanowski, and A. Unterberg. The European Brain Injury Consortium, *Acta Neurochir. (Wien)*, 139, 797–803 (1997).

G. M. Teasdale, A. Maas, F. Iannotti, J. Öhman, and A. Unterberg, *Acta Neurochir. Suppl.*, 73, 111–116 (1999).

J. L. T. Wilson, L. E. L. Pettigrew, and G. M. Teasdale, *J. Neurotrauma*, 15, 573–585 (1998).

G. Zagara, P. Scaravilli, C. Carmen Belluci, and M. Seveso, *J. Neurosurg. Sci.*, 31, 207–212 (1987).

A. Zauner and R. Bullock, *J. Neurotrauma*, 12, 547–554 (1995).

A. Zauner, R. Bullock, A. J. Kuta, J. Woodward, and H. F. Young, *Acta Neurochir. Suppl. (Wien)*, 67, 40–44 (1996).

CHAPTER 21

CLINICAL TRIALS IN HEAD INJURY: ASIA

SADAHIRO MAEJIMA, M.D., Ph.D. and YOICHI KATAYAMA, M.D., Ph.D.
Department of Neurological Surgery, Nihon University School of Medicine, Japan

INTRODUCTION

At present, two kinds of therapeutic drugs for head trauma (for disturbance of consciousness associated with head trauma) are available on the market in Japan: CDP-choline (cytidine diphosphate choline, Nicholin®) and protirelin tartrate [L-pyroglutamyl-1-histidyl-L-prolinamide-L-tartrate monohydrate, TRH (thyrotropin-releasing hormone) analogue, Hirtonin®]. Of these, CDP-choline is presently marketed in Europe and is undergoing clinical trials (phase III) in the United States. Another TRH analogue, NS-3 (montirelin hydrate), is currently submitted to the Ministry of Health and Welfare for approval.

In Japan, the clinical trials for three drugs were aborted in phase II: JTP-2942 (TRH analogue), aptiganel (aptaguanal hydrochloride, NMDA antagonist) and lazaroids (21-aminosteroid tirilazad mesylate; lipid peroxidase inhibitor, radical scavenger). In the United States, the clinical trial for lazaroids was aborted in phase III.

Currently, two drugs are in phase II in Japan for head trauma. These are BAY-X-3702 (5-HT1A receptor antagonist) and TAK-218 (5-aminocoumarans, inhibitor of lipid peroxidation and dopamine release). BAY-X-3702 is also in phase II in Western countries, and TAK-218 is in phase I in the United States. While eliprodil (NMDA antagonist) is undergoing clinical trials (phase III) in Western countries, no clinical trial is being planned in Japan (Table 21.1).

Head Trauma: Basic, Preclinical, and Clinical Directions, Edited by Leonard P. Miller and Ronald L. Hayes, Co-edited by Jennifer K. Newcomb
ISBN 0-471-36015-5   © 2001 John Wiley & Sons, Inc.

TABLE 21.1   Development of Therapeutic Medicines for Head Trauma in Various Countries

Compound (Company)	Mechanism	Development Status		
		Japan	United States	Europe
CDP-Choline (Takeda)		Marketed	Phase III	Marketed (France)
Protirelin tartrate (Takeda)	TRH analogue	Marketed		
NS-3 (Nippon Shin'yaku)	TRH analogue	Approval		
JTP-2942 (Japan Tobacco)	TRH analogue	Aborted (phase II)		
Lazaroids (Upjohn)	Inhibitor of lipd peroxidation	Aborted (phase II)	Aborted (phase III)	
Aptiganel (Boehringer Ingelheim)	NMDA antagonist	Aborted	Phase II	Phase III (U.K.)
BAY-X-3702 (Bayer)	5-HT1A agonist	Phase II	Phase II	Phase II
TAK-218 (Takeda)	Inhibitors of lipid peroxidation and dopamine release	Phase II	Phase I	
Eliprodil (Synthelabo)	NMDA antagonist ifenprodil analogue		Phase III	Phase III

DRUGS AVAILABLE IN THE MARKET IN JAPAN

CDP-Choline (Nicholin®)

History of Development. CDP-choline was developed on the basis of biochemical and pharmacological studies on disorders of phospholipid metabolism and consciousness, brain function, and pathology associated with brain trauma. It was approved in 1966 as a therapeutic drug for disturbance of consciousness associated with head trauma and brain surgery. Its efficacy was confirmed in combined treatment with cholinolytic agent against Parkinson's disease in 1976, in promoting the recovery of upper limb function in patients with postapoplectic hemiplegia in 1977, and in improving disturbance of consciousness in the acute phase of cerebral infarction in 1987. As a subsequent review failed to reconfirm the drug's usefulness in Parkinson's disease, the relevant efficacy and effectiveness were deleted on March 7, 1997.

Pharmacological Action. CDP-Choline administration leads to the repair of membranes of cerebral nerves by promoting the respiration of mitochondria within neurons and the biosynthesis of lecithin. It was thought, therefore, that the drug is effective for attenuating disturbances of consciousness and hemiplegia on the basis of improvement of brain metabolism (rabbits, rats, and dogs) (Takamiya, 1966; Koike et al., 1970; Aizawa et al., 1971; Watanabe et al., 1971; Kono, 1972; Nagai et al., 1985; Kakihana et al., 1985), improvement of circulation in the brain (dogs) (Miyazaki et al., 1968; Suzuki et al., 1969), stimulation of the ascending reticular activation system of the brain stem (rats and monkeys) (Sato et al., 1974; Fukuda et al., 1985; Saji et al., 1975; Yoshimoto et al., 1976), and reactivation of residual functions of the pyramidal and extra-pyramidal tracts in rabbits, cats, and rats (Kakihana et al, 1985; Fukuda et al., 1985; Yasuhara et al., 1974).

Preclinical Results. The administration of CDP-choline at 60 mg/kg or greater to mice with disturbance of consciousness induced by experimental head trauma caused significant improvement in comparison to a control group. The model of consciousness disturbance involves dropping a Bakelite rod of diameter 10 mm weighing 20 g from a height of 30 cm onto an immobilized male mouse head (Manaka et al., 1978).

Clinical Results. The drug improves consciousness and EEG of patients suffering from disturbance of consciousness in association with head trauma and brain surgery. In particular, improving effects have been reported in patients without evident brain stem symptoms (Yokoyama et al., 1968; Ishii et al., 1964).

In a small clinical trial involving 46 head trauma patients with serious disturbance of consciousness, the improvement of consciousness was examined through a double-blind study with CDP-choline administered to 22 patients, and placebo to 24. It was reported that the level of consciousness was restored faster and the percentage of recovery was significantly higher ($p = 0.04$) in the CDP-choline group compared to placebo control (Espagno et al., 1979).

For 390 patients with acute-phase disturbance of consciousness within 2 weeks after the onset of cerebral apoplexy (cerebral infarction 272, cerebral hemorrhage 115, others 3, with the consciousness level poorer than III-1 of the Japan Coma Scale), the improvement of consciousness was examined in a double-blind study for CDP-choline 1000 mg/day administered intravenously every day for two weeks. In the cases of cerebral infarction, the improvement of consciousness level was significantly higher ($p < 0.05$) in test groups than in placebo group, while no significant difference was recognized in case of cerebral hemorrhage (Tazaki et al., 1986).

Side effects were recognized in 15 out of 1304 cases (1.15 percent) suffering disturbance of consciousness associated with head trauma or brain surgery and administered CDP-choline by injection. They included headache (1 case, 0.08 percent), salivation (1 case, 0.08 percent), anxiety and psychoneurotic symptom (1 case, 0.08 percent), vomiting and alimentary canal symptom (1 case, 0.08 percent), head fever (1 case, 0.08 percent), facial fever (1 case, 0.08 percent), hypotension and circulatory system symptom (6 cases, 0.46 percent).

Pharmacokinetic Profile. CDP-Choline was injected into the caudal vein of mice of dd strain (weight about 20 g), and the radioactivity in various organs was measured at 1, 3, 6, and 16 h later. The distribution over 1 to 6 hours was 30 percent in liver, 10 percent in kidney and 3 percent in pancreas (Ijichi et al., 1972).

[^{3}H]CDP-Choline was admininstered into the portal vein of mice, and 30 min later the liver was excised for measurement of the radioactivity derived from cytidine. It was found that about 16 percent of administered drug was taken up into the metabolic system of the liver within 30 min, and distributed broadly in the cytidine-derived nucleotide pool.

[^{3}H]CDP-Choline was administered into the cervical artery of rats, and 5 min later the liver was excised for measurement of the radioactivity derived from choline. It was found that choline parts were taken into lecithin or decomposed into phosphorylcholine, chloline, and betaine to be incorporated quickly into the liver metabolic system (Yonekawa et al., 1970).

[^{3}H]CDP-Choline was administered into the vein of mice, and the radioactivity in urine was measured. Of [^{3}H]CDP-choline-derived radioactivity recovered from various organs (12 percent recovered), the excretion in urine accounted for ~ 20 percent in 6 h, and ~ 55 percent in 16 h (Yonekawa et al., 1970).

[^{3}H]CDP-Choline 10 mg/kg was administered intravenously to rats of a brain trauma group ($n = 2$) and a control group ($n = 3$). The brain was excised for measurement of the radioactivity 10, 30, 60 min, and 3, 5, and 24 h after administration. The distribution decreased up to 30 min after administration, and subsequently, a peak was attained 3 h later in the damaged side and the intact side for the brain trauma group, but 60 h later for the control group. It was found that at these peaks the intake of CDP-choline decreased in the order damaged side, intact side of the brain trauma group, and control group (Hashizume et al., 1970).

Protirelin Tartrate (Hirtonin®)

History of Development. Protirelin tartrate injection was developed on the basis of biochemical and pharmacological studies on the central nervous system activation and pathology of thyrotropin-releasing hormone (TRH). It was approved in 1978 as a therapeutic drug for prolonged disturbance of consciousness associated with head trauma and subarachnoid hemorrhage.

Pharmacological Action. Protirelin tartrate acts upon the midbrain limbic system (nucleous accumbens) to prompt release of dopamine and upon the hypothalamus and the reticular formation of the brain stem. Consequently, the spontaneous movement is augmented (rats) (Miyamoto et al., 1977, 1979; Plotnikoff et al., 1972), emergence is accelerated (mice, cats) (Manaka et al., 1977; Doi et al., 1978), and EEG is activated (cats) (Saji et al., 1977; Fukuda et al., 1979), attenuating prolonged disturbance of consciousness.

Preclinical Results. Protirelin tartrate injection was administered to male rats of SD strain intraperitoneally or into bilateral mid-brain limbic nuclei, and the spontaneous movement was measured. The control group was administered physiological saline. The augmentation of spontaneous movements, such as ambulation, rearing, grooming and preening was dependent on dose, showing a peak around 20 to 30 min after the administration, followed by gradual decay. The total amount of spontaneous movement in 60 min was nearly equal for a group of administered protirelin tartrate at 20 mg/kg into the peritoneal cavity and a group administered 10 μg into the midbrain limbic nuclei bilaterally. A significant augmentation of spontaneous movement was recognized ($p < 0.01$) in groups administered 5 mg/kg or more protirelin tartrate in comparison to control (Miyamoto et al., 1977, 1979).

A model of disturbance of consciousness was developed with a male mouse of dd strain onto whose vertex a Bakelite rod of 10 mm diameter and 20 g weight was dropped from 30 cm. Time from onset of coma by drop impact to the emergence of righting reflex and that of spontaneous movement was measured. Protirelin tartrate was administered into the caudal vein 10 min before giving impact at doses 5, 2.5, 1.25, 0.63, 0.32, 0.16, 0.08, and 0.04 mg/kg. For the control group, physiological saline was administered. When protirelin tartrate was administered at doses 0.16 mg/kg or higher, the time required for emergence of righting reflex and spontaneous movement was significantly shortened ($p < 0.01$) (Manaka et al., 1977).

Adult cats weighing 2.5–3.3 kg were anesthetized with ether and immobilized with *d*-tubocurarine chloride (1 mg/kg), and EEG from neocortex (suprasylvian gyrus) and hippocampus was recorded through bipolar leads. Within 4 to 6 s after the intravenous administration of protirelin tartrate 0.1 mg/kg or more, EEG of the neocortex exhibited increased low-amplitude, fast waves, and that of hippocampus had increased q-wave (hippocampal arousal wave), demonstrating EEG activation and arousal effects of this drug. The efferent sympathetic discharge showed a monophasic increase, and after a short delay, the contraction of nicitating membrane, rise of blood pressure, and increase of amplitude of efferent discharge in phlenic nerve were recognized (Saji et al., 1977).

Clinical Results. To examine the usefulness of protirelin tartrate injection for delayed disturbance of consciousness, a nationwide comparative trial based on double-blind test (group-to-group comparison) was carried out involving 110 institutions for eight months from December 1997 to August 1998.

Five hundred and fourteen patients suffered from disturbance of consciousness for three weeks or longer with the level of consciousness stabilized at II-1 or better of Japan Coma Scale for one week or longer. As a test drug, protirelin tartrate injection (as protirelin tartrate) 2 or 0.5 mg or an inert placebo (physiological saline) was administered intravenously either by injectin or by drip infusion once a day for 10 days. The consciousness level and clinical symptom were assessed at six times: −7 day before administration; the day before administration; days 3, 7, and 11 (the day after the last administration); and day 18 (7th day after the end) of administration). The overall effects were evaluated on the 11 in terms of overall improvement (in seven steps: markedly, improved, slightly improved, unchanged, slightly aggravated, aggravated, and markedly aggravated), overall safety (degree of side effects in four steps: none, slight, moderate, and marked), and overall usefulness (in seven steps: very useful, fairly useful, slightly useful, not useful, slightly unfavorable, and markedly unfavorable).

Diseases of the subjects were broken down as follows: head trauma 112 cases (Hirtonin® injection 2 mg 36 cases, 0.5 mg 36 cases, and control 40 cases); cerebral infarction 41 cases (Hirtonin® injection 2 mg 15 cases, 0.5 mg 11 cases, and control 15 cases); cerebral hemorrhage 74 cases (Hirtonin® injection 2 mg 25 cases, 0.5 mg 24 cases, and control 25 cases); subarachnoid hemorrhage 137 cases (Hirtonin® injection 2 mg 42 cases, 0.5 mg 51 cases, and control 44 cases); brain tumor 41 cases (Hirtonin® injection 2 mg 16 cases, 0.5 mg 9 cases, and control 16 cases); and others 16 cases.

In head trauma cases, the overall improvement with Hirtonin® at 2 mg was 50 percent and was 27.5 percent in the control, indicating a trend of improvement ($p < 0.10$), while the overall usefulness with Hirtonin® at 2 mg was 50 percent, and was 22.5 percent in the control, indicating a significant improvement ($p < 0.05$).

In subarachnoid hemorrhage cases, for those with disturbance of consciousness lasting for three weeks or longer and consciousness level locked for three weeks or shorter, the overall improvement with Hirtonin® at 2 mg was 65.2 percent, and was 33.3 percent in the control, indicating a trend of improvement ($p < 0.10$), while the overall usefulness with Hirtonin® at 2 mg was 52.2 percent, and was 19.0 percent in the control, indicating a significant improvement ($p < 0.05$).

Side effects were examined in 514 cases, and it was found that the side effects occurred in 8/173 (4.6 percent) in the Hirtonin® injection 2 mg group, in 13/171 (7.6 percent) in the Hirtonin® injection 0.5 mg group, and in 8/170 (4.7 percent) in the control group. No significant difference was recognized among the three groups. Side effects were recognized in 194 of 4217 cases (4.60 percent): psychoneurotic 16 (0.38 percent), liver and bile system 83 (1.97 percent), digestive system 25 (0.59 percent). The subjective complaints included nausea, fever, and eruption, while the objective symptoms involved rises in S-GOT, S-GPT and AL-P (Sano et al., 1979).

Pharmacokinetic Profile. Protirelin tartrate labelled with tritium was administered intravenously to male rats of SD strain, the radioactivity in the blood disappeared quickly with a half-life about 8 min. The serum contained 34.8 percent of free [³H]TRH 30 min after intravenous administration, and the relative contents of free [³H]TRH in the tissue radioactivity were 6.6 percent, 4.0 percent, and 3.0 percent for the hypophysis, liver, and kidney, respectively. The urinary excretion rates were 33.4 percent in 4 h and 40.8 percent in 24 h after intravenous administration. Urine taken 4 h after the administration contained [³H]TRH corresponding to about a half of the administered radioactivity, indicating rapid excretion through the kidney. In 96 h after intravenous administration, [³H]TRH was excreted 45.9 percent in urine, 5.1 percent in feces, 4.8 percent in exhalation, with 28.4 percent retained in the body. Similar pharmacokinetics was observed with subcutaneous administration (Uda et al., 1976).

DRUGS SUBMITTED FOR APPROVAL

Montirelin Hydrate (NS-3)

This drug $(-)$-N-{[(3R,6R)-6-methyl-5-oxo-3-thiomorpholinyl]-carbonyl}-L-histi-dyl-L-prolinamide tetrahydrate], developed by Nippon Shin'yaku, is an analog of thyrotropin-releasing hormone (L-pyroglutamyl-L-histidyl-L-prolinamide, TRH). It was developed on the basis of biochemical and pharmacological studies on its central nervous activation and pathology.

History of Development. TRHs activate the central nervous system, and one of them, protirelin tartrate has been widely used for improving the disturbance of consciousness in clinical applications (Sano et al., 1979). It is hypothesized that TRH improves disturbance of consciousness by activating the dopamine-based nerves in nucleus accumbens, of the midbrain limbic system and acetylcholine (ACh)-based nerves in the hypothalamus and brain stem reticular system (Manaka et al., 1988). However, TRH is readily metabolized within the body (Jacklson et al., 1979; Nagai et al., 1980) and the activation of the central nervous system is too. Grunenthal A.G. of Germany developed montirelin hydrate (NS-3), a derivative of TRH with higher resistance to metabolism and longer duration of action (Bauer, 1979; Flohe et al., 1983).

Montirelin hydrate has pharmacological effects of activating cerebral acetylcholinergic neurons (Itoh et al., 1994a), noradrenergic neurons (Itoh et al., 1994b), and dopaminergic neurons (Itoh et al., 1996). It has been confirmed with various models for disturbance of consciousness that montirelin hydrate is 10 to 100 times more effective than TRH at activating the CNS (Ogasawara et al., 1993; Ukai et al., 1996a; Mushiroi et al, 1996), 5 to 10 times as long in duration (Ithoh et al., 1994a,b), and about 25 times as high in permeability (Itoh et al., 1995). In addition, the drug is known to increase local cerebral blood flow (Adachi et al., 1990) and improve the cerebral utilization of glucose under anesthetization with pentobarbital (Ukai et al., 1996b). Montirelin hydrate has completed phase I (Nakajima et al., 1996; Miyake et al., 1996), phase II (Takakura et al., 1996a,b), and phase III studies (Takahura et al., 1996c); Montirelin hydrate is currently submitted to the Ministry of Health and Welfare for approval.

Preclinical Results. Montirelin hydrate and TRH were administered intravenously to evaluate their EEG activating effects in adult cat models with damaged midbrain reticular system and posterior hypothalamus and with transient brain ischemia. In cats with damaged midbrain reticular system, both montirelin hydrate and TRH extended the duration of EEG activation in a dose-dependent manner; the minimum effective dose was 0.001 mg/kg for montirelin hydrate and 0.03 mg/kg for TRH. In cats with posterior hypothalamus damage, both montirelin hydrate and TRH extended the duration of EEG activation in a dose-dependent manner; the minimum effective dose was 0.003 mg/kg for montirelin hydrate and 0.1 mg/kg for TRH. With models of transient brain ischemia, latent time from starting reperfusion to emergence of cortical EEG and hippocampal rhythm was studied. The administration of montirelin hydrate at a dose higher than 0.03 mg/kg significantly reduced the latent time for emergence of cortical EEG ($p < 0.05$) and at 0.3 mg/kg that for emergence of hippocampal rhythm ($p < 0.05$). On the other hand, the administration of 10 mg/kg TRH did not affect the latent time for EEG emergence (Ukai et al., 1996a). In mouse models of coma induced by head impact and pentobarbital anesthesia, the antagonistic action of montirelin hydrate was studied in terms of recovery time of righting reflex. It was found that the administration of montirelin hydrate at a dose of 0.3 mg/kg reduced the recovery time of righting reflex significantly ($p < 0.05$) with intensity of action about 10 to 30 times as high as that of TRH (Mushiroi et al., 1996).

Clinical Results

Phase III Studies with Montirelin Hydrate (NS-3). A multi-institutional double-blind comparative study was carried out for the purpose of determining the effect of montirelin hydrate (NS-3) to patients suffering from disturbance of consciousness with protirelin tartrate (Hirtonin®) as a placebo. Patients with disturbance of consciousness caused by head trauma and subarachnoid hemorrhage were selected. The level of consciousness before starting administration was limited from I-2 (2) to III-1 (100) on the Japan Coma Scale (JCS), the fixation of conscious level was longer than a week and shorter than three months, and the duration of disturbance of consciousness longer than a week and shorter than six months. Montirelin hydrate (NS-3) 0.5 mg or protirelin tartrate 2 mg was dissolved in 10 to 20 ml physiological saline and slowly administered intravenously once a day for 14 days continuously. The efficacy was assessed on the basis of improvement of consciousness disturbance (JCS, GCS); improvement of clinical symptoms related to disturbance of consciousness (in four steps); general improvement of consciousness disturbance (combined evaluation of improvement of consciousness disturbance with improvement of clinical symptoms related to disturbance of consciousness); assessment of motor paralysis (in six steps); general improvement of different symptoms (in six steps; involving subjective complaints, psychic symptoms, neurological findings, and daily activity); and finally with overall improvement (in six steps), general safety (in five steps), and usefulness (in six steps). The data were analyzed by χ^2-test and Wilcoxon's rank-sum test. The vital signs before and after the administration were analyzed by Dunnett's multiple comparison with ±5 percent level of significance and ±15 percent deviation of background. For the analysis of major evaluation items (overall improvement, general safety, and usefulness), the protocol-compatible (PC) analysis was used, and for the overall evaluation, the intent-to-treat (ITT) analysis was applied to cases including those excluded from the PC analysis. The percentage improvement of conscious level on the 7th day of administration (day 7), the day following the final administration (day 15), and two weeks after the time administration (day 28) was 18.0 percent, 35.6 percent, and 44.5 percent, respectively, for the montirelin hydrate group, and 13.7 percent, 24.0 percent, and 40.4 percent, respectively, for the protirelin tartrate group. The improvement on the day before the end of administration tended to be higher in the montirelin hydrage group than in the protirelin tartrate group ($p = 0.066$, by χ^2-test). The percentage improvement of clinical symptoms related to consciousness disturbance on days 7, 15, and 28 was 18.9 percent, 45.8 percent, and 53.6 percent, respectively, for the montirelin hydrate group, and 16.1 percent, 38.4 percent, and 54.4 percent, respectively, for the protirelin tartrate group, presenting no significant difference between the two groups. The percentage overall improvement of consciousness disturbance on days 7, 15, and 28 was 23.0 percent, 51.7 percent, and 57.3 percent, respectively, for the montirelin hydrate group, and 15.3 percent, 37.6 percent, and 54.4 percent, respectively, for the protirelin tartrate group. On the day next to the end of administration, the percentage improvement in the montirelin hydrate group was significantly higher than in the protirelin tartrate group ($p = 0.037$, by χ^2-test). The percentage improvement of neurological findings on days 7, 15, and 28 was 6.1 percent, 17.7 percent, and 25.4 percent, respectively, for the montirelin hydrate group, and 3.2 percent, 7.5 percent, and 16.5 percent, respectively, for the protirelin tartrate group. The improvement of neurological findings on the day next to the end of administration tended to be higher in the montirelin hydrate group than in the protirelin tartrate group ($p = 0.072$, by χ^2-test). The percentage improvement of daily life behavior on days 7, 15, and 28 was 6.4 percent, 28.6 percent, and 37.1 percent, respectively, for the montirelin hydrate group, and 7.0 percent, 25.2 percent, and 37.7 percent, respectively, for the protirelin tartrate group, presenting no significant differences between the two groups. The percentage occurrence of side effects was 17.7 percent (23 out of 130 cases) in the montirelin hydrate group, and 10.7 percent (14 out of 131 cases), presenting no significant difference between the two groups. Major side effects included hepatic function disorder, vomiting, nausea, and fever, all of which were transient. The total number of subjects was 276, with the 137 in montirelin hydrate group and 139 in the protirelin tartrate group. No difference was recognized between the backgrounds of the two groups. The percentage overall improvement on days 7, 15, and 28, the percentage "general safety," and the percentage "usefulness" were evaluated based on PC analysis (Table 21.2) and ITT analysis (Table 21.3) (Takakura et al., 1996c).

DRUGS IN PHASE II

JTP-2942 (TRH Analogue)

JTP-2942   (Na-[(1S,2R)-2-methyl-4-oxocyclopentylcarbonyl]-L-histidyl-L-prolin-amide monohydrate; CAS131404-34-7) is a thyrotropin-releasing hormone (L-pyroglutamyl-L-histidyl-L-prolinamide, TRH) analogue that was developed by the Institute of Japan Tobacco. The development was carried out on the basis of biochemical and pharmacological studies on its central nervous system activation and pathology.

History of Development. In 1969, Boler et al. reported that TRH not only induces the anterior lobe of hypophysis to release thyrotropin and prolactin, but also

TABLE 21.2   PC Analysis of Percentage of Overall Improved, "General Safety," and Usefulness" with Montirelin Hydrate (NS-3)

Overall Percentage Improvement

Day	Drug	% Improvement	χ^2-test	Wilcoxon Rank-Sum Test
7	Montirelin hydrate	27/121 (22.3%)	$p = 0.158$ N.S.	$p = 0.791$ N.S.
	Protirelin tartrate	18/124 (14.5%)		
15	Montirelin hydrate protirelin tartrate	61/117 (52.1%) 46/125 (36.8%)	$p = 0.023*$	$p = 0.040*$
28	Montirelin hydrate	63/110 (57.3%)	$p = 0.666$ N.S.	$p = 0.040$ N.S.
	Protirelin tartrate	61/114(53.5%)		

General Safety

Drug	% Safety	χ^2-Test	Wilcoxon Rank-Sum Test
Montirelin hydrate	108/130 (83.1%)	$p = 0.140$ N.S.	$p = 0.079**$
Protirelin tartrate	118/131 (90.1%)		

Usefulness

Drug	% Usefulness	χ^2-Test	Wilcoxon Rank-Sum Test
Montirelin hydrate	58/122 (47.5%)	$p = 0.097**$	$p = 0.291$ N.S.
Protirelin tartrate	45/124 (36.3%)		

Evaluation based on protocol-compatible (PC) analysis.
N.S. no significance; $*p = 0.05$; $**p < 0.01$.

is widely distributed in the amygdala, medulla, cortex, septum, and hippocampus (Boler et al., 1969; Brownstein et al., 1974; Morley, 1979; Yarbrough, 1979; Emson et al., 1981; Parker et al., 1983). In 1984, Pilotte et al. found that TRH receptors exist at a number of sites in the amygdala, hippocampus, hypothalamus, and other central nervous system areas (Pillote et al., 1984). These findings suggested that TRH might also play an important role as a neurotransmitter and/or modulator of other neurotransmitters such as acetylcholine (ACh) or dopamine (Horita et al., 1986). Subsequently, a number of studies indicated that TRH and its analogues accelerate ACh turnover by augmenting the extracellular ACh level and improve memory and learning capability and antagonism of pentobarbital-induced anesthesia (Yarbrough, 1979; Breese et al., 1975; Schmidt, 1977; Brunello et al., 1981; Narumi et al., 1983; Yamamoto et al., 1987; Horita et al., 1989; Giovannini et al., 1991; Okada et al.,

Table 21.3   ITT Analysis of Percentage of Overall Improvement, "General Safety," and Usefulness" with Montirelin Hydrate (NS-3)

Overall Percentage Improvement

Day	Drug	% Improvement	χ^2-test	Wilcoxon Rank-Sum Test
7	Montirelin hydrate	29/133 (21.8%)	$p = 0.177$ N.S.	$p = 0.958$ N.S.
	Protirelin tartrate	20/136 (14.7%)		
15	Montirelin hydrate	68/133 (51.1%)	$p = 0.019*$	$p = 0.048*$
	Protirelin tartrate	50/138 (36.2%)		
28	Montirelin hydrate	77/131 (58.8%)	$p = 0.497$ N.S.	$p = 0.312$ N.S.
	Protirelin tartrate	70/130(53.8%)		

General Safety

Drug	% Safety	χ^2-Test	Wilcoxon Rank-Sum Test
Montirelin hydrate	114/136 (83.8%)	$p = 0.202$ N.S.	$p = 0.119$ N.S.
Protirelin tartrate	123/137 (89.8%)		

Usefulness

Drug	% Usefulness	χ^2-Test	Wilcoxon Rank-Sum Test
Montirelin hydrate	65/134 (48.5%)	$p = 0.045**$	$p = 0.097$ N.S.
Protirelin tartrate	49/137 (35.8%)		

Evaluation based on intent-to-treat (ITT) analysis.
N.S. no significance; $*p = 0.05$.

1991; Yamamura et al., 1991). Clinically, it was reported that TRH is effective for curing damage of the spinal cord, head trauma, and Alzheimer's disease (Griffiths, 1986, 1987; Faden et al., 1992). The clinical trial of this drug was discontinued in phase II because of the unexpected side effects such as severe drug allergy.

Preclinical Results. JTP-2942 at 0.3 mg/kg or TRH at 3 mg/kg was administered intraperitoneally to male rats of SD strain, and levels of acetylcholine (ACh) in the frontal lobe and hippocampus and extracellular choline level were determined by microdialysis. With JTP-2942, the release of ACh in the frontal lobe and hippocampus increased to 300 percent, while TRH increased the release in the frontal lobe alone to 200 percent. Both drugs decreased the extracellular choline level in both frontal lobe and hippocampus. JTP-2942 (0.001 to 1 mM) has more potent effects, about 1000 times as high as TRH (1 and 10 mM), on the release of ACh and extracellular choline levels in frontal lobe and hippocampus (Toide et al., 1993).

The effects of JTP-2942 and TRH on the central nervous system were examined with mice of ICR strain and rats of SD strain. When JTP-2942 or TRH was administered subcutaneously to compare their effects on hypothermia induced by reserpine, the effect of JTP-2942 was about 80 times as high as that of TRH. When JTP-2942 or TRH was administered intravenously to compare their effects on the flexor reflex in spinal rats, the effect of JTP-2942 was about 16 times as high as that of TRH. When JTP-2942 or TRH was administered orally to compare their effects on the motor suppression caused by chlorpromazine, JTP-2942 exerted an antagonistic action while TRH did not. When JTP-2942 or TRH was administered intraperitoneally to compare their effects on the anesthesia induced by pentobarbital and the disturbance of consciousness model induced by brain concussion, the effect of JTP-2942 was about 30 and 3 times, respectively, as high as that of TRH. On the other hand, when JTP-2942 or TRH was administered into the abdominal aorta to compare their effects on the release of thyroid-stimulating hormone (TSH), the effect of JTP-2942 was about 1/3 as high as that of TRH (Matsushita et al., 1993).

The mechanism of JTP-2942 antagonization of reserpine-induced hypothermia was studied. It was conjectured that JTP-2942 exerts its effects mainly through the adrenal gland and autonomic nervous system, but rarely through the hypothalamus–hypophysis–thyroid system like TRH (Matsushita et al., 1995a). JTP-2942 or TRH was administered intravenously to examine their effects on anesthesia induced by pentobarbital. Both drugs reduced emergence time in a dose-dependent manner. The minimum effective dose was 0.03 mg/kg for JTP-2942 and 1 mg/kg for TRH. The effect of JTP-2942 is about 30 times as high as that of TRH owing to accelerated turnover of ACh (Matsushita et al., 1995b).

Aptaguanal Hydrochloride (Aptiganel)

This drug (N-1-naphthyl-N'-3-ethylphenyl-N'-methylguanidine) developed by Cambridge Neuroscience, is an NMDA antagonist. It was developed on the basis of biochemical and pharmacological studies on its central nervous system activation and pathology. In other countries, the development of this drug is cerebral apoplexy was aborted on consideration of risk–benefit ratio. After examination of data from the phase III study, its efficacy for cerebral apoplexy was confirmed, and the development was resumed. At present, its use for attenuating neuropathology associated with head trauma is being studied. In Japan, the development of aptiganel was carried out for the indication of cerebral apoplexy and head trauma, but the clinical trial was discontinued in phase II.

History of Development. Aptiganel is a selective and non-competitive NMDA receptor-blocking agent, developed for improving brain function. The drug prevents neurons from perishing after damage to the head or spinal cord, by blocking NMDA receptors and attenuating Ca^{2+} entry via ligand-gated ion channels.

Preclinical Studies. The nerve-protecting effect of this drug was evaluated by diffusion-weighted MRI using the middle cerebral artery occlusion models produced in male rats of SD strain. When aptiganel was administered 15 min after occlusion, the infarct volume was reduced by 66 percent in comparison to that in control animals (Minematsu et al., 1993a). In a similar model of middle cerebral artery occlusion using male rats of SD strain, bolus injection of aptiganel 1.13 mg/kg 15 min after occlusion was followed by intravenous drip infusion of 0.785 mg/per h for 165 min, to evaluate the nerve-protecting effect by diffusion and perfusion MRI. It was found that the administration of aptiganel reduced the occlusion volume to about 1/5 of the control, securing more effective circulation (Minematsu et al., 1993b).

A controlled cortical impact injury (impact depth 2 mm, impact velocity 7 mm/s) was given to left side temporoparietal lobe of male rat of SD strain. Aptiganel (2 mg/kg) was administered 15 min after the injury, and the nerve-protecting effect of aptiganel was assessed on the basis of volume of brain contusion 24 h after the injury. In the test group, the volume of brain contusion was reduced by 13.6 percent ($p < 0.05$) in comparison to the control, hemispheric swelling by 31.5 percent, and percent water content (control, 82.78 ± 0.12 percent; aptiganel HCl, 82.30 ± 0.18 percent; $p < 0.05$). In addition the intracranial pressure was decreased and the cerebral perfusion pressure was significantly increased ($p < 0.05$) (Kroppenstedt et al., 1998a,b).

Tirilazad Mesylate (Lazaroid)

This drug was developed by Pharmacia and Upjohn. Tirilazad mesylate is an aminosteroid of the lazaroid series with an amino group at position 21: {21-[4-(2,6-di-1-pyrrolidynyl-4-pyrimidinyl)-1-piperazinyl]-16α-methylpregna-1,4,9(11)-triene-3,20-dione monomethanesulfonate}. It was developed on the basis of biochemical and pharmacological studies on its central nervous system protection and pathology. In 1997, the development of tirilazad for head trauma and ischemic brain injury was discontinued because of safety problems observed in the course of clinical trial (phase III). In Japan, the clinical trial (phase II) of indication for subarachnoid hemorrhage and head trauma was aborted because of unaccountable mortality from brain edema and augmentation of intracranial pressure.

History of Development. Tirilazad mesylate is an aminosteroid compound with a tissue-protecting action in ischemic brain damage through the inhibition of iron-dependent lipid peroxidation and scavenging of free radicals. It has been also confirmed that the drug protects endothelial function from damage by reactive oxygen species. The usefulness of this drug as a therapeutic agent for spinal cord injury has been demonstrated, and its protective effect for ischemic brain injury caused by cerebral vasospasm and anti-flammatory effect has been reported. It is also under development as a therapeutic agent against atherosclerosis and graft-rejection reaction.

Preclinical Results. Antiperoxidative action of tirilazad mesylate was evaluated using excised aorta ring of rabbit based on endotheline-dependent relaxation. It was found that this drug protects vascular endothelium from injury due to peroxidation by active oxygen (Rosemary et al., 1995).

With a spinal cord compression model (180 g, 5 min at L3, under sodium pentobarbital anesthesia) using an adult cat, the effect of tirilazad mesylate was assessed through pial blood flow (laser Doppler flowmetry). Tirilazad mesylate, which is a nonglucocorticoid 21-aminosteroid lipid peroxidation inhibitor, had no inhibitory action on Ca^{2+}-dependent phospholipase A_2. The drug suppressed the pial hyperperfusion of injured spinal cord in the acute phase of spinal cord injury at 1 and 4 h without inhibiting eicosanoids production (Edwards et al., 1995).

The anti-inflammatory effect of tirilazad mesylate was assessed on the basis of survival rate and degree of hepatic injury using a rat model of endotoxic shock and acute liver failure (induced by 20-min perfusion of ischemic liver and administration of *Salmonella enteritidis* endotoxin 0.5 mg/kg). The drug improved hepatic injury by 60 percent 4 h after perfusion, and survival rate from 18 percent to 55 percent. On the basis of pathophysiological studies, it was hypothesized that the drug reduces the early tissue injury directly through inhibition of lipid peroxidation and/or membrane stabilization and inhibits later neurotrophil-induced injury (Peitan et al., 1994).

A blinded, randomized placebo-controlled study was carried out using a baboon model of middle cerebral artery occlusion (balloon occlusion for 3 h). In the test group with tirilazad mesylate (3 mg/kg) administered 15 min before starting the perfusion, the occlusion volume was reduced by 40 percent in comparison to control, and neurological score and remission were improved (Mori et al., 1995).

Clinical Results. A randomized, double-blind study was carried out with 245 patients with subarachnoid hemorrhage (SAH) caused by ruptured cerebral arterial flow in 12 Canadian institutions. Within 72 h after the onset, tirilazad mesylate was intravenously administered at three doses (0.6, 2, and 6 mg/kg day) for 10 days. In the group administered 2 mg/kg tirilazad mesylate, the symptomatic vasospasm was reduced from 41 percent to 21 percent ($p < 0.05$) in comparison with the control, and the favorable outcome (good recovery or moderate disability on the GOS) was increased from 70 percent to 90 percent ($p < 0.05$). No serious side effect was observed (Clarke et al., 1995). In Europe and Australia, phase II/III studies (randomized studies) were carried out with 1015 patients with subarachnoid hemorrhage (SAH) caused by ruptured cerebral arterial flow. Within 48 h after onset, tirilazad mesylate was intravenously administered at three doses (0.6, 2, and 6 mg/kg per day) for 10 days. The symptomatic vasospasm occurred in 25.7 percent of the control group, while in the test group (with doses of 0.6, 2, and 6 mg/kg per day) it occurred in 22.7 percent, 26.5 percent, and 18.4 percent, respectively. There was no significant difference between the control and the high-dose groups ($p = 0.047$). The mortality rate was significantly lower ($p < 0.01$) in the test group (11.2 percent) than in the control group (19.8 percent). In the highest-dose group, the improvement was seen only in male patients. The major side effect was phlebitis (Dorsch et al., 1995).

5-HT1A Receptor Agonist (BAY X3702)

This drug, developed by Bayer, is a 5-HT1A receptor agonst: $(-)$-(R)-2-{4-[(3,4-dihydro-2H-1-benzopyran-2-yl)methyl]aminobutyl}-1,2-bennzisothiazol-3-(2H)-one 1,1-dioxide monohydrochloride. It was developed on the basis of biochemical and pharmacological studies of its central nervous system protection and pathology.

History of Development. BAY X3702 is a selective 5-HT1A receptor agonist and developed as a brain function-protecting agent. The drug suppresses glutamate-induced depolarization, which increases at the time of brain ischemia and trauma by inducing hyperpolarization through the control of potassium (K^+) current. Additionally, the activation of 5-HT1A receptors localized at glutamatergic terminals inhibits release of glutamate. On the basis of these facts, the drug is hypothesized to suppress the delayed neural cell death following brain ischemia and head trauma.

In Japan, the drug is in phase II for brain ischemia and head trauma.

Preclinical Results. The brain-protecting effects of this drug were evaluated with a computer-assisted image analysis system on the basis of infarct volume on the 7th day after the onset of ischemia using one-side middle cerebral artery occlusion (permanent electrocoagulation) model of Long-Evans rats. The drug was administered by multiple i.v. bolus injection (0.0003 to 0.1 mg/kg) and 4-h continuous i.v. infusion (0.0003 to 0.3 mg/kg per h). In case of multiple i.v. bolus injection, a dose-dependent brain-protecting effect was recognized at doses of 0.001 to 0.01 mg/kg, and the infarct volume was reduced by up to 73 percent. In case of 4-h continuous i.v. infusion, a dose-dependent brain-protecting effect was recognized at doses of 0.001 to 0.01 mg/kg per h, and the infarction focus volume was reduced by 59 percent to 65 percent (Jean De Vry et al., 1997).

Cultured hippocampal neurons were exposed to 0.5 mM L-glutamate for 1 h, and 18 h later the brain-protecting effect of BAY X3702 was assessed on the basis of trypan blue staining and cell morphology. The drug prevented neural death at doses of 0.001 to 1 μM, and the effect of 0.1 μM BAY X3702 was comparable to that of 1 μM WAY 100635 (Semkova et al., 1998).

In a rat transient middle cerebral artery occlusion model (modified intraluminal filament occlusion technique), perfusion was resumed 1 h after the onset of ischemia, while BAY X3702 was administered at a dose of 0.001 mg/kg per h through continuous i.v. infusion for 4 h. Two days later, the brain-protecting effect of the drug was assessed on the basis of occlusion volume. In the test groups, the occlusion volume was reduced by 81 percent in the cerebral cortex, 67 percent in the caudate/putamen, and nearly 100 percent in the hippocampus (Jean De Vry et al., 1997).

In a rat acute subdural hematoma model (produced by unilateral autohematic injection into subdural space on somatosensory cortex), the brain-protecting effect of the drug was assessed on the basis of infarction volume of crebral cortex on the 7th day after injury using conventional histological study and computer-assisted image analysis system. In case of multiple i.v. bolus injection (given immediately and 2 h and 4 h after injury), infarct volume was reduced by up to 60 percent to 64 percent at doses 0.01 and 0.1 mg/kg. In case of continuous i.v. infusion (0.00003 to 1 mg/kg per h) for 4 h starting immediately after injury, infarct volume was reduced by up to 76 percent at a dose 0.001 mg/kg per h. When the continuous i.v. infusion (0.01 mg/kg per h) was started 3 or 5 h after injury, infarct volume was reduced by 74 percent or 54 percent, respectively. If it was administered 5 h or longer after injury, no therapeutic effect was recognized (Jean De Vry et al., 1997).

5-Aminocoumarans (TAK-218)

TAK-218, developed by Takeda Chemical Industries, Ltd, is one of 2,3-dihydro-5-benzofuranamines: (S)-2,3-dihydro-2,4,6,7-tetramethyl-2-[(4-phenyl-1-piperidinyl)-methyl]-5-benzofuranamine dihydrochloride. It was developed on the basis of biochemical and pharmacological studies on its central nervous system protection and pathology.

History of Development. TAK-218 is one of the 5-aminocoumarans and was developed as a brain function-protecting agent for brain ischemia and head trauma. In the event of brain ischemia, excitatory amino acids such as glutamate, and also dopamine are released in extraordinary amounts, produced free radical affect mitrochondrial functions and expand tissue damage. TAK-218 is hypothesized to suppress secondary brain damage following brain ischemia and head trauma through dual inhibition of lipid peroxidation and dopamine release.

Preclinical Results. In a male rat transient global ischemia model (four-vessel occlusion model), 3 mg/kg of TAK-218 or its *R*-isomer was administered intraperitoneally immediately and 2 h and 24 h after starting perfusion. The brain-protecting effects of the drug were assessed on the basis of survival rate 1, 3, 5, 7, 10, and 14 days after starting perfusion. TAK-218 and its *R*-isomer improved the survival rate significantly better than the control ($p < 0.05$). TAK-218 improved the mortality at days 1 to 7 after starting perfusion significantly better than its *R*-isomer ($p < 0.05$) (Ohkawa et al., 1997).

In a male Wistar rat penetration-induced brain injury model (injury produced by inserting a gloss rod of 1.5 mm diameter from the cortex to the striatum through a burr hole using a stereotactic technique), TAK-218 or its *R*-isomer was administered intraperitoneally immediately and 2 h after injury at doses 0.03, 0.1, 0.3, and 1 mg/kg to assess its brain-protecting effects. The assessment was based on the degree of damage in the nigrostriatal system through apomorphine-induced circling at 1, 3, 7, and 14 days after trauma. TAK-218 reduced the functional disturbance in dose-dependent manner significantly better than the control ($p < 0.01$). The effective minimum dose was 0.1 mg/kg, while the *R*-isomer reduced the functional disturbance only at a dose of 1 mg/kg on day 14 after injury ($p < 0.01$) (Ohkawa et al., 1997).

CONCLUSION

Basic studies on the central nervous system disorder caused by the head trauma have been significantly advanced, and the mechanism of secondary brain damage associated with the trauma is becoming understood. On the basis of these studies, protection of the brain from irreversible damage has been clinically studied. In Japan, clinical studies with NMDA antagonists, lazaroids and inhibitors of lipid peroxidation, have been carried out, but no clinical application has yet been achieved because of side effects and other problems.

At present 5-HT1A agonist (BAY X-6702) and dual inhibitors of lipid peroxidation and dopamine release (TAK-218) are in the course of clinical development (phase II), but no clinical report is available, and their efficacy and side effects are undefined. For TRH analogues (NS-3), the clinical trial (phase III) was finished in 1996, and the application has been submitted. The efficacy of NS-3 has been demonstrated through a double-blind comparative test with TRH analogue (protirelin tartrate) which has been used widely in clinical applications. The drug needs to be used in the clinical field at an earlier stage for proper evaluation.

Currently, only two agents for improving the central nervous system (improving disturbance of consciousness) are being marketed: CDP-choline (Nicholin®) and protirelin tartrate (Hirtonin®), while none of the central nervous system protecting agents is available in the market. Accelerated development of these drugs is desirable in these underdeveloped fields.

ABBREVIATIONS

ACh	Acetylcholine
CDP	Cytidine diphosphate
EEG	Electroencephalogram
Hirtonin	Protirelin tartrate
ITT	Intent to treat
JCS	Japan Coma Scale
NMDA	N-methyl-D-aspartate
NS-3	Montirelin hydrate
PC	Protocol-compatible
SAH	Subarachnoid hemorrhage
TRH	Thyrotropin-releasing hormone
TSH	Thyroid-stimulating hormone
S-GOT	Serum glutamic oxaloacetic transaminase
S-GPT	Serum glutamic pyruvic transaminase
AL-P	Alkaline phosphatase
MRI	Magnetic resonance imaging

REFERENCES

T. Adachi, H. Horita, and K. Ohno *Jiritsu Shinkei*, 27, 442–448 (1990) [In Japanese].

T. Aizawa, K. Mori, and K. Komi, *Nihon Iji Shinpo*, 2450, 43–46 (1971) [In Japanese].

K. Bauer, *Hoppe-Seyler's Z. Physiol. Chem.*, 360, 1126 (1979).

J. F. Boler, M. Enzmann, K. Folkers, C. Bowers, and A. V. Schalley, *Biochem. Biophys. Res. Commun.*, 37, 705 (1969).

G. R. Breese, J. M. Cott, B. R. Cooper, A. J. Prange, M. A. Lipton, and N. P. Plotnikoff, *J. Pharmacol. Exp. Ther.*, 193, 11 (1975).

M. J. Brownstein, M. Palkovits, J. M. Saavedra, R. M. Bassiri, and R. D. Utiger, *Science*, 185, 267 (1974).

N. Brunello and D. L. Cheney, *J. Pharmacol. Exp. Ther.*, 219, 489 (1981).

E. Clarke Haley Jr., N. F. Kassell, W. M. Alves, B. K. A. Weir, and C. A. Hansen, *J. Neurosurg.* 82, 786–790 (1995).

T. Doi, Y. Saji, and Y. Nagawa, *Yakuri To Chiryo*, 6, 3229–3237 (1978) [In Japanese].

N. W. C. Dorsh, E. D. Means, and N. F. Kassel, *J. Cereb. Blood Flow Metab. (Suppl.)* 15, 1 (1995).

D. H. Edwards, et al., *J. Neurotrauma*, 12, 245–256 (1995).

P. C. Emson, G. W. Bennett, and M. N. Rossor, *Neuropeptides*, 2, 115 (1981).

A. I. Faden and S. Salzman, *Trends Pharmacol. Sci.*, 13, 29 (1992).

L. Flohe, K. Bauer, and E. Friderichs, "Biological Effect of Degradation-stabilized TRH Analogues," in E. C. Griffiths and G. W. Bennett, Eds. *Thyrotropin-Releasing Hormone*, Raven Press, New York, 1983, pp. 327–340.

N. Fukuda, Y. Saji, and Y. Nagawa, *Folia Pharmacol. Japon*, 75, 321–331 (1979) [In Japanese].

N. Fukuda, K. Ikeda, and Y. Saji, *Yakuri To Chiryo*, 13, 5021–5029 (1985) [In Japanese].

M. G. Giovannini, F. Casamenti, A. Nistri, F. Paoli, and G. Pepeu, *Br. J. Pharmacol.*, 102, 363 (1991).

E. C. Griffiths, *Nature*, 322, 212 (1986).

E. C. Griffiths, *Clin. Sci.*, 73, 449 (1987).

K. Hashizume, K. Arai, T. Tsuchida, H. Masuzawa, H. Kamano, and M. Nagai, *Saigailgaku*, 13, 1022–1037 (1970) [In Japanese].

A. Horita, M. A. Carino, and H. Lai, *Annu. Rev. Pharmacol. Toxicol.*, 26, 311 (1986).

A. Horita, M. A. Carino, J. Zabawska, and H. Lai, *Peptides*, 10, 121 (1989).

H. Ijichi, A. Kizu, Y. Hino, and H. Kiyamura, *Yakubutsu Ryoho*, 5, 67–74 (1972) [In Japanese].

S. Ishii, *No To Shinkei*, 16, 281 (1964) [In Japanese].

Y. Itoh, Ogasawara, T., T. Mushiroi, A. Yamazaki, and Y. Ukai, *J. Pharmacol. Exp. Ther.*, 271, 884–890 (1994a).

Y. Itoh, T. Ogasawara, A. Yamazaki, Y. Ukai, A. Miura, and K. Kimura, *J. Pharmacol. Exp. Ther.*, 268, 255–261, (1994b).

Y. Itoh, T. Sugimoto, Y. Ukai, A. Morino, and K. Kimura, *J. Pharm. Pharmacol.*, 47, 833–836 (1995).

Y. Itoh, A. Yamazaki, Y. Ukai, Y. Yoshikuni, and K. Kimura, *Pharmacol. Toxicol.*, 78, 421–428 (1996).

I. M. D. Jackson, P. D. Papapertrou, and S. Reichlin, *Endocrinology*, 104, 1292–1298 (1979).

Jean De Vry, D. Hartmut, G. Thomas, H. Hang-Georg, H. Ervin, J. Reinhard, M. Thomas, M. Frank, O. Wolfgang, S. Dietrich, S. L. Rudolf, and S. Thomas, *Drugs of the Future*, 22, 341–349 (1977).

J. Espango, M. Tremoulet, M. Gigaud, and Ch. Espagno, *La Vio Medicale*, 3, 195–196 (1979).

M. Kakihana, J. Kato, S. Narumi, and A. Nagoaka, *Yakuri To Chiryo*, 13, 5043–5054 (1985) [In Japanese].

Y. Koike, S. Izawa, S. T. Murai, and T. Subokawa, *Shin'yaku To Rinsho*, 19, 1815–1819 (1970) [In Japanese].

S. Kono, *Okayama Igakukai Zasshi*, 84, 289–305 (1972) [In Japanese].

S. N. Kroppenstedt, G. H. Schneider, U. W. Thomale, and A. W. Unterberg, *J. Neurotrauma*, 15, 191–197 (1998a).

S. N. Kroppenstedt, G. H. Schneider, U. W. Thomale, and A. W. Unterberg, *Acta Neurochir. Suppl. (Wien)*, 71, 114–116 (1998).

S. Manaka, *Igaku No Ayumi*, 104, 253 (1978) [In Japanese].

S. Manaka, *Igaku No Ayumi*, 146, 482–486 (1988) [In Japanese].

S. Manaka and K. Sano, *Igaku No Ayumi*, 102, 867–869 (1977) [In Japanese].

M. Matsushita, F. Yonemori, N. Furukawa, A. Ohta, K. Toide, I. Uchida, and K. Iwata, *Arzneim.-Forsch./Drug Res.*, 43, 813–817 (1993).

M. Matsushita, F. Yonemori, A. Ohata, and K. Iwata, *Arzneim.-Forsch./Drug Res.*, 45, 708–711 (1995a).

M. Matsushita, F. Yonemori, A. Hamada, K. Toide, and K. Iwata, *Eur. J. Pharmacol.* 276, 177–182 (1995b).

K. Minematsu, M. Fisher, L. Li, M. A. Davis, A. G. Knapp, R. E. Cotter, R. N. McBurney, and C. H. Stoak, *Neurology*, 43, 397–403 (1993a).

K. Minematsu, M. Fisher, L. Li, and C. H. Stoak, *Stroke*, 24, 2074–2081 (1993b).

M. Miyamoto and Y. Nagawa, *Eur. J. Pharmacol.*, 44, 143–152 (1977).

M. Miyamoto, S. Narumi, and Y. Nagai, *Jpn. J. Pharmacol.*, 29, 335–347 (1979).

Y. Mikaye and H. Sasaki, *Rinsho Iyaku*, 12, 1013–1029 (1996) [In Japanese].

M. Miyazaki, *Gendai No Rinsho*, 2, 61–64 (1968) [In Japanese].

E. Mori, et al., *Cerebrovasc. Dis.*, 5, 342–349 (1995).

J. E. Morley, *Life Sci.* 25, 1539 (1979).

T. Mushiroi, T. Shibahara, Y. Tamura, *Nihon Yakurigaku Zasshi*, 107, 273–284 (1996) [In Japanese].

Y. Nagai, S. Narumi, and Y. Nagawa, *J. Neurochem.*, 35, 963–971 (1980).

Y. Nagai and A. Nagaoka, *Yakuri To Chiryo*, 13, 5037–5041 (1985) [In Japanese].

S. Narumi, Y. Nagai, M. Miyamoto, and Y. Nagawa, *Life Sci.*, 32, 1637 (1983).

T. Ogasawara, Y. Ukai, and M. Tamura, *Biomed. Res.*, 14, 317–328 (1993).

S. Ohkawa, K. Fukatsuk, S. Miki, T. Hashimoto, J. Sakamoto, T. Doi, Y., Nagai, and T. Aono, *J. Med. Chem.*, 40, 559–573 (1997).

M. Okada, *J. Neurochem.* 56, 1544 (1991).

C. R. Parker, Jr. and J. C. Porter, *J. Neurochem.*, 41, 1614 (1983).

L. Peitan, S. L. Vonderfecht, G. M. McGuire, M. A. Fisher, A. Farhood, and H. Jaeschke, *Exp. Ther.*, 27, 438–445 (1994).

N. S. Pilotte, N. A. Sharif, and D. R. Burt, *Brain Res.*, 293, 372 (1984).

N. P. Plotnikoff, A. J. Prange, Jr., G. R. Breese, M. S. Anderson, and I. C. Wilson, *Science*, 178, 417–418 (1972).

M. K. Rosemary, P. L. Munns, K. L. Leach, and W. R. Mathews, *Methods Fund. Exp. Clin. Pharmacol.*, 17, 279–292 (1995).

Y. Saji, Y. Nagawa, K. Mizuno, and H. Hibino, *Kiso To Rinsho*, 9, 262–272 (1975) [In Japanese].

Y. Saji, T. Mikoda, and Y. Nagawa, *J. Takeda Res. Lab.*, 36, 39–45 (1977) [In Japanese].

K. Sano, K. Kitamura, K. Takeuchi, M. Tsuru, H. Kanaya, J. Suzuki, K. Ueki, N. Nakamura, T. Kuwabara, N. Kageyama, S. Yamamoto, H. Handa, H. Mogami, N. Nishimoto, T. Uozumi, S. Kuramoto, Y. Matsukado, S. Manaka, M. Kagawa, M. Ogashiwa, R. Ishii, A. Kuwayama, Y. Yagyu, and N. Tachibana, *Adv. Neurol. Sci.*, 23, 184–210 (1979).

H. Sato, K. Kimura, Y. Handa, H. Saito, and H. Ito, *Rinsho To Kenkyu*, 51, 2256–2260 (1974) [In Japanese].

D. E. Schmidt, *Commun. Psychopharmacol.*, 1, 469 (1977).

I. Semkova, P. Wolz, and J. Krieglstein, *Eur. J. Pharmacol.*, 359, 251–260 (1998).

K. Suzuki, K. Yasuda, Y. Kumagaya, T. Takeya, and T. Yoshida, *Yakbutsu Ryoho*, 2, 948–952 (1969) [In Japanese].

K. Takakura, I. Saito, M. Ogashiwa, and S. Manaka, *Rinsho Iyaku*, 12, 1031–1049 (1996a) [In Japanese].

K. Takakura, I. Saito, T. Yoshimoto, M. Ogashiwa, S. Manaka, H. Kikuchi, T. Hayakawa, K. Matsumoto, M. Fukui, T. Asakura, and T. Nakashima, *Rinsho Iyaku*, 12, 1051–1078 (1996b) [In Japanese].

K. Takakura, I. Saito, T. Yoshimoto, T. Kirino, M. Ogashiwa, S. Manaka, YH. Kikucyi, T. Hayakawa, K. Matsumoto, M. Fukui, T. Asakura, and T. Nakashima, *Rinsho Iyaku*, 12, 1079–1111, (1996c) [In Japanese].

Y. Takamiya, *Kurume Kgakukai Zasshi*, 29, 985–1005 (1996) [In Japanese].

Y. Tazaki, E. Ohtomo, T. Kutsuzawa, M. Kameyama, T. Omae, and M. Fujishima, *Igaku No Ayumi*, 136, 791–817 (1986) [In Japanese].

K. Toide, M. Shinoda, M. Takase, K. Iwata, and H. Yoshida, *Eur. J. Pharmacol.*, 233, 21–28 (1993).

F. Uda, A. Fujino, T. Manzai, N. Motyizuki, T. Tokiwa, and M. Nakazawa, *Yakuri To Chiryo*, 4, 515–544 (1976) [In Japanese].

Y. Ukai, T. Ogasawara, Y. Yoshikuni, and K. Kimura, *Folia Pharmacol. Japan*, 107, 273–284 (1996a) [In Japanese].

Y. Ukai, M. Watanabe, and Y. Hirata, *Oyo Yakuri*, 51, 147–153 (1996b) [In Japanese].

M. Watanabe, S. Kono, K. Mitsunobu, T. Suzuki, and S. Otsuki, *No To Shinkei*, 23, 721–725 (1971) [In Japanese].

M. Yamamoto, and KM. Shimizu, *Arch. Pharmacol.*, 336, 561 (1987).

M. Yamamura, K. Kinoshita, H. Nakagawa, and R. Ishida, *Jap. J. Pharmacol.*, 55, 69 (1991).

G. G. Yarbrough, *Prog. Neurobiol.*, 12, 291 (1979).

M. Yasuhara, and H. Naito, *Curr. Ther. Res.*, 16, 346–374 (1974).

I. Yokoyama, N. Matuoka, T. Kamitsuka, Y. Miura, Z. Miyakawa, and K. Otsuka, *Shinryo*, 21, 1894–1900 (1968) [In Japanese].

Y. Yonekawa and K. Seta, *No To Shinkei*, 22, 871–875 (1970) [In Japanese].

T. Yoshimoto and Z. Suzuki, *Yakuri To Chinryo*, 4, 823–829 (1976) [In Japanese].

APPENDIX

WEB SITE NAME	ADDRESS
American Brain Injury Consortium	www.abic.vcu.edu
American Assoc Neurol Surgeons	www.neurosurgery.org/aans/
American Assoc Adv Science	www.aaas.org
American Society For Neurochemistry	www.ASNeurochem.org
Antibody Resource Page	www.antibodyresource.com/findantibody.html
Biotech Clinical Trial (Recombinant Capital)	http://recap.com/mainweb.nsf/HTML/clinical+frame?OpenDocument
Brain Information Technology	http://www.brainit.gla.ac.uk/brainit
Brain Injury Association (USA)	www.biausa.org
ClinicalTrials.gov (service of NIH)	www.clinicaltrials.gov
Clinical Trials in Head Injury	http://www.ninds.nih.gov/news_and_events/headinjurywkshp.htm

Food & Drug Administration	www.fda.gov
Internet Grateful Med	http://igm.nlm.nih.gov
JCBFM	http://www.jcbfin.com/
Journal of Neurosurgery	http://www.neurosurgery.org/ aans/journals/jns/index.html
Journal of Neurotrauma	http://www.liebertpub.com/ neu/default1.asp
MedMatrix	www.medmatrix.org
MedScape	www.medscapc.com
National Center for Biotech Information (USA)	www.ncbi.nlm.nih.gov/
National Institutes of Health (USA)	www.nih.gov
National Institute of Neurological Disorders and Stroke (USA)	www.ninds.nih.gov
National Neurotrauma Society	www.edc.gsph.pitt.edu/ neurotrauma
Neurosurgery Online	http://www.neurosurgery-online.com
NINDS Traumatic Brain Injury Info Page	www.ninds.nih.gov/ health_and_medical/disorders/ tbi_doc.htm
National Library of Medicine (USA)	www.nlm.nih.gov
Neurosciences on the Internet	www.Neuroguide.com
Society for Neuroscience	www.sfn.org
The Whole Brain Atlas	www.med.harvard.edu/AANLIB
Trauma image bank (has some neurotrauma pix)	http://www.trauma.org/ imagebank/imagebank.html
Trauma org	www.trauma.org
University of Florida Brain Institute	www.ufbi.ufl.edu
Univ of Penn Head Injury Center	http://bioeng.seas.upenn.edu/ tbilab
University of Pitt Safar Center for Resuscitation Research	www.safar.pitt.edu

AUTHOR	EMAIL ADDRESS
Sharon Brown, Ph.D.	sbrown@bcm.tmc.edu
Dominico d'Avella, M.D.	davellan@unime.it
C. Edward Dixon, Ph.D.	edixon@neuronet.pitt.edu
Alan Faden, M.D.	fadena@giccs.georgetown.edu
Seth P. Finklestein, M.D.	finklestein@helix.mgh.harvard.edu
Ronald L. Hayes, Ph.D.	mcelroy@ufbi.ufl.edu
David A. Hovda, Ph.D.	dhovda@mednet.ucla.edu
Dr. Katayma, M.D., Ph.D.	ykataym@med.nihon-u.ac.jp
Anthony E. Kline, Ph.D.	akline@neuronet.pitt.edu
Patrick Kochanek, M.D.	kochanek@smtp.anes.upm.edu
C. P. Lee, Ph.D.	cplee@med.wayne.edu
Philipp M. Lenzlinger, M.D.	lenzling@mail.med.upenn.edu
Harvey S. Levin. Ph.D.	hlevin@bcm.tmc.edu
Bruce Lyeth, Ph.D.	bglyeth@ucdavis.edu
A. I. R. Maas, M.D.	maas@neur.azr.nl
Sadahiro Maejima, M.D.	smaejima@med.nihon-u.ac.jp
Tony Marmarou, Ph.D.	Marmarou@abic.vcu.edu
Lawrence F. Marshall, M.D.	lfmarshall@ucsd.edu
Tracy K. McIntosh, Ph.D.	mcintosh@seas.upenn.edu
Leonard P. Miller, Ph.D.	miller4atc@aol.com
J. Paul Muizelaar, M.D.	j.paul.muizelaar@ucdmc.ucdavis.edu
Jennifer K. Newcomb, Ph.D.	jnfernandez1@yahoo.com
Brian R. Pike, Ph.D.	pike@ufbi.ufl.edu
John T. Povlishock, Ph.D.	jpovlishock@hsc.vcu.edu
Ramesh Raghupathi, Ph.D.	rramesh@mail.med.upenn.edu
Meredith Temple, Ph.D.	templem@ninds.nih.gov
David Thurman, M.D.	dxt9@cdc.gov
Marike Zwienenberg, M.D.	mzwien@aol.com

INDEX